A Quarter Century
of Community Psychology

Readings from the *American Journal
of Community Psychology*

A Quarter Century of Community Psychology

Readings from the *American Journal of Community Psychology*

Edited by

Tracey A. Revenson, Senior Editor
*The Graduate Center of the City
    University of New York
New York, New York*

Anthony R. D'Augelli
*Pennsylvania State University
University Park, Pennsylvania*

Sabine E. French
*University of California
Riverside, California*

Diane L. Hughes
*New York University
New York, New York*

David Livert
*The Graduate Center of the City
    University of New York
New York, New York*

Edward Seidman
*New York University
New York, New York*

Marybeth Shinn
*New York University
New York, New York*

Hirokazu Yoshikawa
*New York University
New York, New York*

Kluwer Academic / Plenum Publishers
New York   Boston   Dordrecht   London   Moscow

Library of Congress Cataloging-in-Publication Data

A quarter century of community psychology: readings from the American journal of
community psychology/edited by Tracey A. Revenson ... [et al.].
    p.   cm.
   Includes bibliographical references and index.
   ISBN 0-306-46729-1—ISBN 0-306-46730-5 (pbk.)
     1. Community psychology. I. Revenson, Tracey A. II. American journal of community
psychology.

RA790.55 .Q37 2002
362.2′2—dc21

                            2002022224

ISBN 0-306-46729-1 (hardbound)
    0-306-46730-5 (paperback)

© 2002 Kluwer Academic/Plenum Publishers, New York
233 Spring Street, New York, New York 10013

http://www.wkap.nl

10 9 8 7 6 5 4 3 2 1

To our mentors, who took us
under their wing and empowered us

Contributors

Luleen S. Anderson, Private Practice, 330 Military Cutoff Road, Arbor Court, Wilmington, North Carolina 28405

Chester Bennett (deceased)

Craig Blakely, Department of Health Policy and Management, Texas A&M University School of Rural Public Health, College Station, Texas 77843

Ana Marie Cauce, Department of Psychology, University of Washington, Seattle, Washington 98195

David M. Chavis, Association for the Study and Development of Community, 312 South Frederick Avenue, Gaithersburg, Maryland 20877

Cary Cherniss, Graduate Studies in Applied and Professional Psychology, Rutgers University, Piscataway, New Jersey 08854

Florence Collins, San Rafael City Schools, San Rafael High School, San Rafael, California 94901

Joan Cone, West Contra Costa Unified School District, El Cerrito High School, El Cerrito, California 94530

Saul Cooper, 1050 Wall Street, Ann Arbor, Michigan 48105

Emory L. Cowen, (deceased)

Anthony R. D'Augelli, Department of Human Development and Family Studies, The Pennsylvania State University, University Park, Pennsylvania 16802

William S. Davidson II, Department of Psychology, Michigan State University, East Lansing, Michigan 48823

Laura Dean, Columbia University School of Public Health, New York, New York 10032

Darlene DeFour, Department of Psychology, Hunter College, City University of New York, New York, New York 10021

Barbara Snell Dohrenwend (deceased)

James G. Emshoff, Department of Psychology, Georgia State University, Atlanta, Georgia 30303

Robert D. Felner, Department of Education and the National Center on Public Education and Social Policy, University of Rhode Island, Kingston, Rhode Island 02881

Jennifer Fisher, Mayo Clinic, Rochester, Minnesota 55905

Sabine E. French, Department of Psychology, University of California, Riverside, California 92521

Ruth J. Friedman, Department of Psychology, Arizona State University, Tempe, Arizona 85287

Marc Garcia (deceased)

Melanie A. Ginter, P. O. Box 215, 100 United Drive, North Haven, Connecticut 06473

Nancy Gonzalez, Department of Psychology, Arizona State University, Tempe, Arizona 85287

Rand Gottschalk, Aon Consulting, Human Resources Consulting Group, Chicago, Illinois 60606

William Hall (deceased)

Leonard Hassol (deceased)

Barton J. Hirsch, School of Education, Northwestern University, Evanston, Illinois 60208

Carollee Howes, Department of Education, UCLA Graduate School of Education & Information Studies, Los Angeles, California 90095-1521

Diane L. Hughes, Department of Psychology, New York University, New York, New York 10003

Donald C. Klein, Graduate College of the Union Institute, Columbia, Maryland 21044

David Livert, Department of Psychology, The Graduate Center of the City University of New York, New York, New York 10016

Julie Lustig, Division of Adolescent Psychology, University of California, San Francisco, California 94109

Art Martin (deceased)

John Martin (deceased)

Craig A. Mason, Department of Psychology, University of Miami, Coral Gables, Florida 33124

Kenneth Maton, Department of Psychology, University of Maryland/ Baltimore County, Baltimore, Maryland 21250

Jeffrey P. Mayer, Department of Community Health, Saint Louis University, St. Louis, Missouri 63104

Michelle Melhorn, 6359 Kensington Avenue, Richmond, California 94805

Deborah Phillips, Department of Psychology, Georgetown University, Washington, DC 20057-1001

Richard H. Price, Institute for Social Research, University of Michigan, Ann Arbor, 48106

Judith Primavera, Department of Psychology, Fairfield University, Fairfield, Connecticut 06430

Julian Rappaport, Department of Psychology, University of Illinois, Urbana, Illinois 61820

Tracey A. Revenson, Doctoral Program in Psychology, The Graduate Center of the City University of New York, New York, New York 10016–4309

Stephanie Riger, Women's Studies Program, University of Illinois, Chicago, Illinois 60607

David B. Roitman, Organization Consultant, P.O. Box 1147, Wilton, New Hampshire 03086

Gershen Rosenblum, 346 Setucket Road, Dennis, Massachusetts 02638–2517

Irwin N. Sandler, Department of Psychology, Arizona State Universtiy, Tempe, Arizona 85287

Neal Schmitt, Department of Psychology, Michigan State University, East Lansing, Michigan 48823

Yaacov Schul, Institute for Social Research, University of Michigan, Ann Arbor, Michigan 48106

Edward Seidman, Department of Psychology, New York University, New York, New York 10003

Marybeth Shinn, Department of Psychology, New York University, New York, New York 10003

Karen Simontacchi, West Contra Costa Unified School District, El Cerrito High School, El Cerrito, California 94530

Charles Soulé, Pediatric Psychiatry, New York Presbyterian Hospital, New York, New York 10032

Jenn-Yun Tein, Department of Pychology, Arizona State University, Tempe, Arizona 85287

Abraham Wandersman, Department of Psychology, University of South Carolina, Columbia, South Carolina 29208

Edison J. Trickett, Department of Psychology, University of Illinois at Chicago, Chicago, Illinois 60607

Rhona S. Weinstein, Department of Psychology, University of California, Berkeley, California 94720

Stephen G. West, Department of Psychology, Arizona State University, Tempe, Arizona 85287

Susan Westover, 4455 East Camelback Road, Suite 160E, Phoenix, Arizona 85018

Marcy Whitebook, Center for the Study of Child Care Employment, University of California, Berkeley, California 94720–5555

Sharlene Wolchik, Department of Psychology, Arizona State University, Tempe, Arizona 85287

Amiram D. Vinokur, Institute for Social Research, University of Michigan, Ann Arbor, Michigan 48106

Hirokazu Yoshikawa, Department of Psychology, New York University, New York, New York 10003

Preface

Looking back over the past quarter century or so, it becomes apparent that Community Psychology has developed a rich tradition of theory, empirical research, action, and innovative methods. Within the field of psychology, community psychology challenges traditional ways of thinking. It considers not only the person but also whole ecological systems, recognizing that the linkages between persons and systems may be as important as either factor alone. It examines both top-down and bottom-up change; it recognizes the need for cultural diversity; and it recognizes the need for both research and praxis—actually, their interaction, which is termed "action research" or "action science."

Many of the important writings have been published in the *American Journal of Community Psychology (AJCP)*.[1] As such, the intellectual history of the field is embedded in this journal. In 1996, The Publications Committee of the Society for Community Research and Action (SCRA, Division 27 of the American Psychological Association), in cooperation with Plenum Publishing Corporation, published a call for an editor or editorial team to "develop a volume which will use the most impactful papers from the [*AJCP*] to portray the rich tradition of ... action research ... " (Call for Nominations, 1996, p. 17). The editors of the volume you are holding answered that call and were subsequently asked to bring the project to fruition.

As the concepts and tenets of Community Psychology are embedded in a social-historical perspective, we feel it is important to identify the factors that converged to prompt such a volume at the time. First, Community Psychology had become a legitimate area of inquiry with its own paradigms, values, and assumptions; it was no longer in the throes of an adolescent identity crisis. Second, the *AJCP* had become a rich resource of current thinking in the area, publishing theoretical advances, original research, and critical reflections on the field by those in the field. Third, and most important, Community Psychology was beginning to experience its "radiating effects" (Kelly, 1971) on other areas of psychology, other social and behavioral sciences, policy, and the helping professions.

In a letter to the first author at the time the book was announced, Richard Price, a Past President and Distinguished Contribution Recipient from the Division, wrote, "This is an enormously ambitious project. ... [I]t's pretty hard for me to think of articles that would stand out above the rest. Instead, let me suggest some characteristics of articles that might recommend them to you for the book: (1) articles that powerfully articulate the values and ideals of the field; (2) articles that set an exemplary standard for empirical community research; (3) articles that describe "turning points" in the history of the field; and (4) articles about the future of community psychology." We took Rick's advice to heart, as no single approach would be sufficient to represent the field of Community Psychology. A traditional approach might have been to organize the readings in terms of content, selecting the important theoretical, methodological, empirical and action research papers under each heading. Or, one could simply select the most frequently cited papers exemplifying theory, research, and action. Instead, we wanted to present a picture of the field that provided an implicit illustration of the growth of a field, of progress and change, and of the setbacks along the way. To place the reprinted articles in context, we have written four "capstone" essays specifically for this volume. Each essay follows a single theme and can be read as a reflection of the field over the past three decades and, hopefully, a blueprint for where it is going. The capstone essays raise critical issues, scrutinize the evolution of an area over time, and propose ideas for future work. They portray the ongoing struggles or dialectics within the field, and focus on enduring themes over the past quarter century. They address questions that are only partially answered and present new challenges to the field that go beyond its original focus on mental health. But, most important, these essays capture not only what makes community psychology unique but also its demons: the problems, frames, and dilemmas that community psychology continues to struggle with but has not resolved: How do you conceptualize communities? How does diversity become incorporated into theory? Into practice? Where do you induce change (persons, settings, policies)?

The capstone essays make this volume of readings unique. Most collections are usually concept-oriented in their organization, dealing with the contemporary meaning of the concept and failing to understand the evolution and change of the concept over time. Take the theme of diversity as an example. There has been attention to the need for including diverse populations in Community Psychology research and action from its inception; however, the definition of diversity and its influence on research methodologies has changed over time—from implying that one should include underserved populations in research studies and action programs to examining our assumptions underlying the research questions and variables. Similarly, diversity has broadened its range from a singular focus on gender and ethnicity to include sexual orientation, levels of competence, and cultural origin. The selected readings are presented chronologically in order to provide the reader with a sense of the progression of ideas and research. This ordering provides clues as to what the social concerns were at the time the articles were written. We wanted to include articles that both reflected the enduring values of the field and that sparked the field to move forward. In fact, most of the articles cross-cut several themes. For example an article on mutual-help groups would be salient to themes of prevention, stress, support, and empowerment.

For scholars in social science and social work, health care professionals, and policymakers, this volume may be their introduction to both community psychology and the *AJCP*. We hope it whets your appetite for more. For many "younger" community psychologists and students this volume fills a gap on their shelves before their subscription to *AJCP* started.[2] And, although senior community psychologists are likely to have dusty volumes of *AJCP* on their shelves, this book will invite them to return to past writings with a contemporary gaze.

ACKNOWLEDGMENTS

Our thanks go first of all to Irwin Sandler and Christopher Keys, who guided the Society for Community Research and Action (SCRA or Division 27 of the American Psychological Association) as it embarked on this project. As Publications Chair and President of SCRA at the time, they coordinated the process of framing the project and selecting an editorial team. We hope that "the gang from New York City" has fulfilled your expectations. We also thank Jodi Kellar and Jenni Hoffman for their untiring help with "cataloguing" the hundreds of articles in the *American Journal of Community Psychology* during the two-year selection process.

Eliot Werner, our Executive Editor at Plenum, shepherded this book through the publication process. Eliot is no stranger to community psychology, having nurtured the *American Journal of Community Psychology* for nearly 20 years and produced the *Handbook of Community Psychology*. We are glad that he had the insight to realize that the time had come for a collection of classic articles and grateful for his flexibility as the book split into two volumes, this one and *Ecological Research to Promote Social Change: Methodological Advances from Community Psychology* (2002). We will miss him and wish him luck with the next stage of his career.

We also want to pay tribute to the four editors of *AJCP* during the quarter century we reviewed: Charles Spielberger (1973–1976), John C. Glidewell (1977–1988), Julian Rappaport (1989–1992), and Edison J. Trickett (1993–1997). Although editors may be captives of the material submitted to their journals (J. Rappaport, personal communication, January

13, 1994), they can influence the field at the margins by improving what gets submitted and encouraging diversity in submissions. These four men did just that; they worked hard to generate exciting submissions and keep the journal on the cutting edge. But such tasks are not carried out in isolation— so hats off the all the Associate Editors, Editorial Board members, Student Board members, and ad hoc reviewers who labored (often anonymously) in the fields of the *AJCP*.

TRACEY A. REVENSON
ANTHONY R. D'AUGELLI
SABINE E. FRENCH
DIANE L. HUGHES
DAVID LIVERT
EDWARD SEIDMAN
MARYBETH SHINN
HIROKAZU YOSHIKAWA

NOTES

1. Although community psychologists read and publish in a wide variety of venues, the call read: "For over two decades, [*AJCP*] has been the major publication outlet of the emerging field of community psychology" (1996, p. 17).
2. Fewer than 200 people held individual subscriptions to *AJCP* before the journal became a benefit of membership of the Society for Community Research and Action in 1988.

REFERENCES

Call for Nominations (1996, Spring). *The Community Psychologist, 29*(1), 17.

French, S. E. & D'Augelli, A. R. (2002). Diversity in community psychology. In T. A. Revenson, A. R. D'Augelli, S. E. French, D. L. Hughes, D. Livert, E. Seidman, M. Shinn, & H. Yoshikawa (Eds), *A quarter century of community psychology: Readings from the* American Journal of Community Psychology (pp. 65–77). New York: Kluwer Academic/Plenum Publishers.

Kelly, J. G. (1971). The quest for valid preventive interventions. In G. Rosenblum (Ed.), *Issues in community psychology and preventive mental* health (pp. 109–139). New York: Behavioral Publications.

Livert, D. & Hughes, D. L. (2002). The ecological paradigm: Persons in settings. In T. A. Revenson, A. R. D'Augelli, S. E. French, D. L. Hughes, D. Livert, E. Seidman, M. Shinn, & H. Yoshikawa (Eds.), *A quarter century of community psychology: Readings from the* American Journal of Community Psychology (pp. 51–63). New York: Kluwer Academic/Plenum Publishers.

Revenson, T. A. & Seidman, E. (2002). Looking backward and moving forward. In T. A. Revenson, A. R. D'Augelli, S. E. French, D. L. Hughes, D. Livert, E. Seidman, M. Shinn, & H. Yoshikawa (Eds.), *A quarter century of community psychology: Readings from the* American Journal of Community Psychology (pp. 3–31). New York: Kluwer Academic/Plenum Publishers.

Yoshikawa, H. & Shinn, M. (2002). Facilitating change: Where and how should community psychology intervene? In T. A. Revenson, A. R. D'Augelli, S. E. French, D. L. Hughes, D. Livert, E. Seidman, M. Shinn, & H. Yoshikawa (Eds.). *A quarter century of community psychology: Readings from the* American Journal of Community Psychology (pp. 33–49). New York: Kluwer Academic/Plenum Publishers.

A Note to Instructors

Many faculty members want to use original research and writings in their teaching but feel frustrated by the enormous amount of work to make the syllabi readings easily accessible to students. We suspect that many of us (or rather our students) spend a good deal of time and money making copies of the articles that are reprinted in this volume. One of the reasons for producing this book of readings was to facilitate this process. The volume can be used as a primary text or as a supplemental reader for advanced undergraduate, master's-level, or doctoral-level Community Psychology courses.

An instructor could build a course around this volume in an historical fashion, bringing in the social history of American psychology or American politics to frame the articles. Alternately, she or he could use the capstone essays to define units, assigning those articles cited in the capstone essays and reprinted in the book. Or, an instructor could integrate the capstone essays and reprinted readings into a more traditional, topical syllabus. Finally, the volume can stand by itself as an introduction to community psychology for students in social work, public policy, community health, applied developmental psychology, applied social psychology, and clinical psychology.

To aid instructors in organizing a course, the chart in Appendix A organizes the 19 *American Journal of Community Psychology* articles reprinted in this volume by construct, topic, population, and setting. Appendices B–D provide additional suggestions for important articles in the field. Appendix B provides a listing and reference information for the Awards for Distinguished Contributions to Theory and Research in Community Psychology from the Society for Community Research and Action. Appendix C provides similar information for the Awards for Distinguished Practice in Community Psychology. Appendix D lists all Special Issues and Special Sections of the *American Journal of Community Psychology*—Special Issues and Special Sections cluster a number of articles devoted to a specific topic.

Contents

xix

APPENDICES

I

Capstone Essays

1

Looking Backward and Moving Forward: Reflections on a Quarter Century of Community Psychology

Tracey A. Revenson and Edward Seidman

If all of us in this room lived for a thousand years and did research every day, we would still not know enough. The question now as it always has been is not "do we know enough?" but "are we willing to help society solve its human problems with what we do know?"

FAIRWEATHER, 1986, p. 135

The turn of the century and the approach toward middle age mark a good time to take stock of accomplishments and achievements, to do a little soulsearching, and to make midcourse adjustments. Thirty-five years ago, "a pioneering band of [clinical] psychologists met at Swampscott, Massachusetts ... named themselves for the first time as community psychologists, and ... talked out the basic principles of the field" (Brody, 1986, p. 139). The times they were a-changin', and the emergence of this new field was part and parcel of the sociopolitical context of the 1960's, in particular

Tracey A. Revenson • Doctoral Program in Psychology, The Graduate Center of the City of New York, New York, New York 10016-4309 **Edward Seidman** • Department of Psychology, New York University, New York, New York 10003.

A Quarter Century of Community Psychology: Readings from the American Journal of Community Psychology, edited by Tracey A. Revenson *et al.* Kluwer Academic/Plenum Publishers, New York, 2002.

the Community Mental Health Movement, the War on Poverty, and the Great Society (Bloom, 1978; Cowen, Gardner, & Zax, 1967; Merritt, Greene, Jopp, & Kelly, 1999; Yoshikawa & Shinn, Chapter 2, this volume).

In looking back over the past 35 years and ahead to the next 35, we kept returning to a comment made by Richard Price in a letter dated January 27, 1997, to the senior editor. Rick suggested that as important as it was to examine the values and ideals of the field, we should think about the turning points in the history of the field. A turning point is a point at which a decisive change takes place; at which something changes direction. This led us to think: What made community psychology so exciting, so different, so "outside the envelope," so dangerous for us—not only at the time it emerged, but at the time each of us was introduced to it? Why had we chosen this field or left other areas of psychology (or other careers) to pursue it? What were the ideas that were so powerful, so convincing, so on the mark, that they galvanized people to disrupt the traditions of American (clinical and experimental) psychology and work in a new paradigm?

Such an approach is obviously personal and skips over many important contributions to the field. As we were writing this essay, we continually struggled with our chosen metaphor of turning points. Were these really turning points in the field? Were they the *only* turning points? By using this metaphor, were we missing many other important developments that occurred and moved the field forward in an evolutionary if not revolutionary manner? (Unequivocally, yes.) Thankfully, the three other capstone essays in this volume do an excellent job of demonstrating how specific themes and phenomena of interest in Community Psychology have endured and/or transmogrified over the past quarter century (French & D'Augelli, Chapter 4, this volume; Livert & Hughes, Chapter 3, this volume; Yoshikawa & Shinn, Chapter 2, this volume).

Reading twenty-five volumes of a single journal is a sobering experience. Once you make your way through, one fact comes into focus: The field (as reflected through the eyes of its premier journal) is as stable as it is changeable, and as with most developmental processes, the changes are neither linear, lockstep, nor universal. Many of the central phenomena of interest, such as prevention, have existed from the beginning. Some have lasted, and some have waxed and waned. The turning points we have chosen retrospectively may not have been turning points at the time, but created fresh ideas or social innovations whose power would become evident only with a historical review. So with the opening bars of *Thus Spake Zarathustra* playing on the computer's CD, we offer up our version of the critical moments when community psychology changed course.

TURNING POINT 1: THE EMERGENCE OF A FIELD

The Boston Conference on the Education of Psychologists for Community Mental Health held from May 4–8, 1965 was a turning point in the most simple fashion. Known forever as the Swampscott Conference because of its location, it has come to be seen as the founding event for the field of community psychology. Newbrough wrote in the first volume of the *American Journal of Community Psychology* (AJCP), " 'Community' is a word that found its way into psychology formally through the Swampscott Conference" (1973, p. 201).

At Swampscott, several significant chords were struck. Most important were new ideas as to who should provide psychological services, what should be provided, to whom, and to what ends (Bennett *et al.*, 1966). There was a growing recognition that many mental health services were inaccessible to—if not inappropriate for—a wide variety of people and problems (Cowen *et al.*, 1967). Moreover, difficulties were (and still are) overrepresented among those marginalized people or those in the lowest socioeconomic strata of society; these difficulties included classic mental health problems, such as delinquency or chronic mental illness, as well as a variety of debilitating problems-in-living, such as poverty-related despair, substandard educational experiences, unemployment, and stress induced by undesirable living conditions. The conference conveners stated unequivocally, "the time had come to expand psychology's area of inquiry and action" (Bennett *et al.*, 1966, p. 4).

The domain of Community Psychology was defined by the Swampscott conferees as "behavior *in* its social context" (Bennett *et al.*, 1966, p. 1, italics added) and "the study of general psychological processes that *link* social systems with individual behavior in complex interaction" (Bennett *et al.*, 1966, p. 7, italics added). This conceptualization of community psychology accomplished two things. First, it shifted the gaze from the amelioration of mental illness to the prevention of mental illness *and* the promotion of mental health. Second, it moved from a reactive position of delivering services to individuals already designated as ill to designing preventive interventions developed in collaboration with community leaders and "responsible laymen" (Bennett *et al.*, 1966, p. 1). This new field of community psychology would be "related to, yet independent of, community mental health" (Kelly, 1990, p. 769). There was a commitment to prevention (vs. treatment), the generation and dissemination of new knowledge, and the application of that knowledge "in the community."

A number of roles were deemed central to the activities of a community psychologist: "Community psychologists were characterized as change agents, social systems analysts, consultants in community affairs, and students generally of the whole man [sic] in relation to all his [sic] environments (Bennett et al., 1966, p. 26). The responsibility of community psychologists to be social activists was not resolved fully at that time. (Nor is it now.) Education and training were to be grounded in a broad interdisciplinary orientation, i.e., community psychologists should be generalists who have the ability to use information from many different perspectives and different disciplines. As we continue to struggle with the issues of prevention and the facilitation of social change, these same themes reemerge. Many of the chords that were struck at Swampscott continue to reverberate.

Looking back (and perhaps at the time as well), it is apparent that the conference ideas were not fully articulated. The values, conceptions, and strategies of research and action in the community did not simply erupt at Swampscott. Rather, the "swamp" was a rich primordial soup from which innovative and radical notions (at least for American psychology at the time) bubbled up. The outlines for this new field had appeared, but were to be filled in over the next decades.

In the late 1960s and early-to mid-1970s, card-carrying community psychologists (and others not as excited to wear this new badge) developed a wide variety of innovative action programs (e.g., Goldenberg, 1971; Reppucci, 1973). One breakthrough innovation was the relocation of a group of chronic mental patients into the community where they could live and work and call upon mental health professionals when they—and not the professionals—perceived the need (Fairweather, Sanders, Maynard, & Cressler, 1969; Fairweather, Sanders, & Tornatzky, 1974). Although Fairweather's Lodge was an example of tertiary prevention, it possessed two other features that were pivotal for community psychology: first, it involved the creation of a setting in which residents could experience different kinds of role relationships with each another and with mental health professionals, and second, it defined the social experiment as a method to evaluate social innovations.

Innovative treatment programs were common during the first decade of community psychology. Many focused on redefining the role and training of "helpers," for example, using college students to work on a one-to-one level with chronic mental patients (Rappaport, Chinsky, & Cowen, 1971) or teaching neighbors to provide support and understanding to friends in distress (Ehrlich, D'Augelli, & Conter, 1981). Many focused on strengths instead of deficits, e.g., in Fairweather's lodges, psychiatric patients were viewed as capable of governing themselves; using paraprofessionals built on community strengths. Despite the fact that the Swampscott participants had "intentionally acknowledged that community psychology was more than and separate from community mental health" (Kelly, 1987, p. 517), these innovative programs often remained housed within national and local systems of mental health services that emphasized the remediation of individual deficits.

There was a loud call for earlier, more preventive interventions. Cowen exhorted the field to move toward primary prevention efforts (1977, 1980, 1982, 1985), but for some time, early detection/secondary prevention programs remained the norm. Prevention programs varied in the populations they targeted, including economically disadvantaged preschool children, school-aged children with academic or behavioral difficulties, adolescents in legal jeopardy, college students in distress, the mentally ill, and elderly people living alone (Cowen *et al.*, 1967; Denner & Price, 1973; Seidman & Rappaport, 1974). These programs were innovative in that they employed volunteers and paraprofessionals to intervene with individuals showing early manifestations of mental dysfunction and problem behaviors. Issues of AJCP from 1973–1978 contain many descriptions and evaluations of such programs, including crisis counseling programs, telephone hotlines within community mental health centers, and programs within elementary school classrooms.

Community psychologists found themselves increasingly in the role of consultants to agencies and grassroots organizations (Cherniss, 1976, Chapter 6, this volume; Dworkin & Dworkin, 1975). In this role, they performed needs assessments, worked with professional and lay helpers to improve their skills, recommended services, and developed programs in schools, prisons, and mental health agencies (Kelly, 1979; Murrell, 1973).

Provocative concepts, ideas, methods, and the beginnings of new paradigms also catalyzed the early development of the field. Many of these notions, once again, emerged from the "swamp" and reflected the political and cultural climate of the times (Kelly, 1990). *Blaming the Victim* (Ryan, 1971) not only was a book that captured the hearts and minds of community psychologists, but also was a salient concept that has endured the test of time. Similarly, over the course of the decade (and the following ones), Seymour Sarason (1971, 1974, 1975, 1976, 1978) provided numerous critical analyses and penetrating insights into the problem of change, the psychological sense of community, and the creation of settings. His work influenced community psychologists, and many others, particularly in the field of education, and continues to do so to this day. Ira Iscoe (1974) directed our attention to the "competent community." Rudolph Moos (1973) wrote a seminal article describing different ways of conceptualizing human environments, and developed numerous scales for assessing the social climates of different kinds of settings. Individually and collectively, these and other ideas forced us to look towards settings and communities for solutions. No longer could we be content to limit our focus to individuals and their families.

During the same era, community psychologists and fellow travelers were further developing conceptual frameworks to link individuals and communities, providing the groundwork for theories of interlocking contexts (e.g., Bronfenbrenner, 1977). Robert Reiff (1968, 1975) introduced the sociological construct of "levels of analysis" that would continue to frame our work conceptually and methodologically for the next two decades (e.g., Shinn & Rapkin, 2000). Even more importantly, Reiff argued that relationships *within* and *between* levels should serve as loci for assessment and intervention. James Kelly (1971b) gave us a framework for understanding and studying the radiating effects of interventions, which he and other scholars would develop further in the next two decades (Kelly, 1986, 1990; Kelly, Ryan, Altman, & Stelzber, 2000). Using a "levels of analysis" schema embedded in a systems theory framework, Stanley Murrell (1973) gave Community Psychology its first full textbook at a time when the field was in its infancy.[1]

Although we argue that the innovative programs and provocative concepts of the early years of Community Psychology originated in the Swampscott meetings, they were clearly reflective of a larger set of social, political, and policy changes taking place at the time as part of the "Great Society"—the Civil Rights Movement, the Women's Liberation Movement, the Community Mental Health Act, the War on Poverty, Head Start and Follow-Through. Within the context of these sociopolitical events, the elements for a discipline of community psychology to move forward were fully in place (Kelly, 1990).

TURNING POINT 2: THE WORD IS OUT

The publication of two vital books on Community Psychology in the same year (1977) crystallized the conceptual frameworks, values, and assumptions of the newly developing field. Julian Rappaport's *Community Psychology: Values, Research, and Action* and Kenneth Heller and John Monahan's *Psychology & Community Change* demonstrated that Community Psychology possessed a substantive body of knowledge and a theory (or set of theories). These volumes presented the basic tenets, values, methods, and approaches of the field, backed up by exemplary empirical community research. The volumes legitimized the field and gave it a public face.

Rappaport's book, to many, served as a touchstone, locating the field within existing American psychology, yet clearly distinct from it. Its contributions are manifold: explication of the values of the field (and at that time, even suggesting that psychological science *had* values was an advanced idea); reframing social problems in terms of second-order vs. first-order change; advancing the first comprehensive theory of social change, involving multiple levels of analysis, multiple stakeholders, power relationships, resources, and unintended costs; and lodging this within an ecological paradigm and a strengths-based perspective. Rappaport was not the first to bring all these ideas to the table; for example, the strengths-based perspective finds its roots in the work of Marie Jahoda (1958) and George Albee (1982a), and the idea of second- vs. first-order change was first explicated by Watzlawick, Weakland, and Fisch (1974). But *Community Psychology: Values, Research, and Action* was the first time these ideas were woven together into a unified paradigm of social change. The fact that portions of Rappaport's original volume remain on many current-day community psychology syllabi reflects the essential nature of the ideas as well as the volume's continuing contributions to the field.

Heller and Monahan's book, published the same year, also provided detailed knowledge about the elements necessary for social change to happen. It linked these elements with the percolating ideas in public health, community organizing, law, and public policy, as well as clinical psychology and community mental health. As a result, *Psychology & Community Change* was highly accessible to researchers and interventionists from many disciplines that wanted to be the change agents that were the subject of debate at the Swampscott Conference. The book also influenced the direction the field would take in its second decade, by introducing the importance of social strains (stress), formal and informal social networks, and community infrastructures to the idea of effective social interventions.

With these two volumes, Community Psychology "took off." More so than earlier mental health work, research and interventions were lodged within an ecological paradigm: People were viewed as integral parts of a social system or overlapping systems, with the understanding that change in one brings about change in the other(s). Many studies explicitly or implicitly adopted a person–environment fit perspective (French, Rodgers, & Cobb, 1974), in which the person wasn't always seen as the defective "component."

The new interest in personal and social stress led to an explosion of empirical research on the protective factors that could buffer individuals from the deleterious effects of stressful life events (Moos, 1984). Accordingly, the issues of the AJCP published in the late 1970s and the 1980s are filled with articles on stress, formal and informal support systems, mutual help, social skills training, and enhancing competence among both individuals and communities (Glidewell, 1988). Barbara Snell Dohrenwend's theory of social stress (1978, Chapter 7, this volume; Dohrenwend & Dohrenwend, 1981), guided much of this work. (Interestingly, it included an intervention component that is often overlooked by contemporary readers.)

The twin topics of social networks and social support received the lion's share of attention (and journal pages). Manuel Barrera (1986) elucidated an elegant framework for this growing research area while others contributed to stress-buffering theory (e.g., Wilcox, 1981), the ecology of support (Hirsch & Rapkin, 1986), and measurement development (e.g., Procidano & Heller, 1983; Vaux, Riedel, & Stewart, 1987). Others examined the impact of social support and mental health through the mechanism of self-help or mutual-help groups (e.g., Borkman, 1991; Maton, 1989, Chapter 12, this volume), or the connection of support to existing network structures, which were sometimes limited by culture (DeFour & Hirsch, 1990, Chapter 15, this volume). Mutual help was viewed not only as a coping resource (e.g., Gottlieb, 1988; Levine, 1988), but also as a social movement in its own right (Rappaport et al., 1985).

The work of George Albee (1982b), Emory Cowen (1982, 1985), Steven Danish and Anthony D'Augelli (1980); Maurice Elias (e.g., Elias et al., 1986), Myrna Shure and George Spivack (e.g., Spivack & Shure, 1985), Irwin Sandler (e.g., Sandler, 2001; Wolchik et al., 1993, Chapter 20, this volume), and Roger Weissberg (e.g., Weissberg, Caplan, & Harwood, 1991) brought the notions of building competence and social coping skills into school- and community-based prevention programs, and disseminated their knowledge to the community at large. Was this enough? In many ways, the interventions that many community psychologists were pursuing involved social changes with a lower case "s." Facilitating social support in families, schools, and small groups was more the norm than grappling with income inequity or poverty. Although these "small wins" (Weick, 1984) can be very effective, why weren't the grander goals articulated in Rappaport's book pursued more vigorously? Were there more developmental tasks for the adolescent discipline of community psychology to master first? Or was this restraint a reflection of the larger sociopolitical zeitgeist? After all, in the 1980s and 1990s there was a strong national reaction against the activism and grand social change goals of the 1960s and 1970s.

TURNING POINT 3: EMPOWERING OTHERS

The publication of Julian Rappaport's article, *In Praise of Paradox: A Social Policy of Empowerment Over Prevention* (1981, Chapter 8, this volume) brought the field yet another magnetizing construct that precisely reflected the discipline's underlying values and fueled larger-scale second-order change interventions. "By empowerment I mean that our aim should be to enhance the possibilities for people to control their own lives" (Rappaport, 1981, p. 15). This reaches back to the original ideas of the Swampscott Conference: Community psychologists realized that the solutions to many of society's problems lay in the developing of existing community resources rather than blaming society's victims (Ryan, 1971) and that interventions should be developed in collaboration with community leaders and "responsible laymen" [*sic*] (Bennett *et al.*, 1966, p. 1).

Rappaport's ideas on empowerment drew heavily from a monograph (Berger & Neuhaus, 1977) that focused on settings or key mediating structures such as family, neighborhood, church, and voluntary organizations as the vehicles for empowerment. Rappaport stated,

> We need to recognize that many settings which are successful in the creation of opportunities, niches, and resources for empowerment will not concern themselves with mental health in our rather narrow disciplinary sense. ... We need to learn from [*the people in the settings*] what the range of solutions is really like and then to encourage social policies that enable more people to develop their own solutions (1981, pp. 19–20).

These words shattered two basic assumptions: first, the central tenet of American psychology that people should trust in the knowledge and power of the professional, and second, community psychology's singular emphasis on mental health outcomes. Even community psychologists had become shackled by these assumptions, because of both their Western mindset and training as clinical psychologists (Sarason, 1981). Coming from a different mold, empowerment theory suggested that the delivery of services, mental health and otherwise, need no longer be our *raison d'être*. In collaboration with people in settings we could help discover and define new solutions, and in the process, people would create their own opportunities to empower themselves.[2]

It is difficult to locate an article in AJCP since 1981 that doesn't explicitly or explicitly refer to empowerment processes, but this ubiquity has diluted the concept. Empowerment has been variously called a theory, a value, a paradigm, a process, a mechanism, a phenomenon of interest, a technology, a guiding metaphor, and a sacred concept (Bond, Hill, Mulvey, & Terenzio, 2000c; Perkins & Zimmerman, 1995; Rappaport, 1987; Swift & Levin, 1987; Trickett, Watts, & Birman, 1993). It is a noun, a verb, and an adjective. Zimmerman and Perkins (1995) distinguish between empowering processes and outcomes (see also Zimmerman [2000] for the distinction between empower*ing* and empower*ed* people and communities). The construct of empowerment fluidly linked and incorporated many existing concepts within community psychology: natural helping systems, a strengths-based perspective, proactive helping, and second-order change. It also defined community psychologists' role relationships with people, policies, programs, and professionals (Rappaport, 1987).

The concept of empowerment also joined easily with Community Psychology's renewed interest in settings and environments. At about the same time, Richard Price (1980) wrote a small but pivotal chapter about risky situations that redirected our attention from persons to settings. Edward Seidman (1988, Chapter 11, this volume) underscored the importance of settings as a critical unit of analysis and locus of intervention (see also O'Donnell, Tharp, & Wilson, 1993). Marybeth Shinn (1987) echoed this sentiment, exhorting community psychologists to expand their domains beyond mental hospitals and halfway houses to schools, neighborhoods, religious institutions, and organizations (see also Keys & Frank, 1987). Kenneth Maton (1989, Chapter 12, this volume; Maton & Salem, 1995), among others, took Shinn's words to heart, exploring the setting-level characteristics of churches, self-help groups, and senior centers, such as facilitation of meaningful role and social support provision, that led to greater well-being on the individual level.

Abraham Wandersman, David Chavis, and their colleagues pioneered the study of neighborhoods as essential to social intervention and change (e.g., Chavis & Wandersman, 1990, Chapter 14, this volume; McMillan & Chavis, 1986; McMillan, Florin, Stevenson, Kerman, & Mitchell, 1995; Rich, Edelstein, Hallman, & Wandersman, 1995). They focused not only on neighborhoods as the core unit of analysis of person–environment fit, but also on community coalitions to develop and implement social change efforts, and illustrated how social change proceeds. Their long-term program of action research with neighborhood organizations demonstrates that citizen participation in neighborhood organizations improves both "objective" features of the community, such as safety, housing, and crime, as well as the more subjective psychological sense of community or belongingness (Wandersman & Florin, 1990). This work also linked the notions of prevention and empowerment: Efforts to prevent social problems included efforts to empower local neighborhood, school, and church organizations.

Schools have long been a place where psychologists have intervened, as described earlier. However, the focus on settings led community psychologists to develop innovative programs that would more directly alter the social ecology of schools and relationships among students and teachers, invoking both first- and second-order change (e.g., Felner, Ginter, & Primavera 1982, Chapter 9, this volume; Gruber & Trickett, 1987; Weinstein et al., 1991, Chapter 16, this volume). An early and influential example was Felner, Ginter, and Primavera's (1982) high school intervention to restructure the role relationships of students to each other, to teachers, and to the setting itself (i.e., what happens in "homeroom"). Rhoda Weinstein and her colleagues (1991) also worked to change structural features of school, and the relations among different groups within it, to maximize the communication of positive expectancies and minimize school failure. They targeted not only standard features of the high school environment (e.g., curriculum, grouping, student leadership opportunities), but also restructured relations between teachers and students, between parents and teachers, and between the classroom and the school administration. Moreover, programs were developed collaboratively with teachers and administrators. Interventions such as these can create empowering organizations (Zimmerman, 2000) that emphasize the linkages among different constituent groups, but these efforts may not always minimize the inequalities and redistribute power (Gruber & Trickett, 1987).

At the core of both these interventions was what Sarason (1971) termed behavioral regularities, later reconceptualized as social regularities (Seidman, 1988, Chapter 11, this volume). Social regularities are the patterns of social transactions, relations, connections, or linkages between people or between people and settings. Seidman (1988), among others, has argued that these linkages between persons and settings need to become the focal point of intervention.

The concept and imagery of empowerment stimulated collaboration between scientists and citizens (Rappaport et al., 1985; Serrano-García, 1984; Wandersman & Florin, 1990).[3] Kelly reminded us of our responsibility: "The prefix 'community,' coming before the word psychology, carries cogent and clear expectations for the conduct of research. If our research unwittingly exploits those with whom we work, we become, in fact, a pollutant, as we limit their personal and cultural development" (Kelly, 1980, cited in Altman, 1986, p. 577). Chavis, Stuckey, and Wandersman (1983) pointed out the interdependence between scientists and citizens, and the need to build coalitions between the two groups. Perhaps most importantly, the imagery of empowerment gave voice to a variety of groups whose voices had previously been silent or silenced—among them, people who had been discriminated against, people in poverty, people with physical or mental disabilities, feminists, and gay and lesbian communities (Serrano-García & Bond, 1994).

We have depicted the many beneficial aspects of the introduction of empowerment to community psychology, a construct that continues to be central to the field. However, our own analysis of the empowerment construct is not unequivocally positive. Despite the focus on the more proximal mediating structures that would foster empowering person–environment transactions within larger more impersonal settings, too many community psychologists have fallen back on person-centered language or methods to assess empowerment or its effects:

> Despite the vast proliferation of programs and policies claiming to be based on the concept of empowerment, the connections between policy or program content and empowerment theory and research are often tenuous at best, especially at the legislative and administrative policy level (Perkins, 1995, p. 788).

Riger's (1993, Chapter 19, this volume) penetrating analysis of empowerment concluded that the assumptions and values implicit in its definition and operationalization are limiting. The first assumption is that of individualism, with its potential to lead to competition and conflict among those who are empowered. The second assumption is the preference for masculine concepts such as mastery, power, and control (versus more feminine concerns of communion and cooperation) to undergird the construct. Moreover, most methods of assessing empowerment are reduced to measures that involve outcomes among individuals or aggregates of individuals. "While our rhetoric continues to emphasize the role of empowering values and social organizations and environments, studies of community process are scarce" (Heller, 1989, p. 1). Perkins (1995) offers several important recommendations to move us closer to this goal, for example: using collective conceptions of empowerment instead of individualistic ones; becoming familiar with policy processes, particularly on the local level; and remaining collaborative throughout the entire effort, from program planning to evaluation to information dissemination for policy change (see also Wolff, 1987).

Again, the sociopolitical context may help us understand how the original considerations of empowerment have evolved. The 1980s was the decade of Reaganomics, and getting government out of the business of trying to solve social problems, counting instead on those thousand (individual) points of light. Human and social problems were to be left to the voluntary organizations, churches, the tax write-offs of large corporations, and the good will of others.[4] It is an interesting historical note that the monograph that first brought the concept of empowerment to Community Psychology's attention ("To Empower People") was published by the American Enterprise Institute, a conservative think tank. Placing the onus of responsibility on mediating structures (e.g., churches and voluntary organizations)—as opposed to larger government structures and policies, and federal, state, and local budgets—was an effective way of keeping the solution to social problems out of the government's bailiwick. It also led community psychologists to begin thinking more seriously about influencing social policy (e.g., Jason, 1998; Phillips, Howes, & Whitebook, 1992, Chapter 18, this volume; Zigler, 1990).

TURNING POINT 3–3/4: LINKING HUMAN DIVERSITY WITH/WITHIN COMMUNITY PSYCHOLOGY'S TRADITIONS

As this book goes to press, we believe that we are witnessing a turning point that has needled the field since its inception—a change in the way diversity is defined, researched, and discussed; making it not an idea to be incorporated into current work, but an idea that shapes the work and transforms the theories. Community psychology has always had a long-standing commitment to diversity (French & D'Augelli, Chapter 4, this volume) and to "serving the underserved" (Snowden, 1982). Community psychologists have always been willing to engage in difficult dialogues related to gender, race, and sexual orientation. Defining values of the field always have included a cultural pluralism that both respects and fosters differences among people (e.g., Iscoe, 1987).

Despite this long-standing commitment to diversity, its expression within our research and practice has been less than successful, "still hazy after all these years" to use Trickett's musical metaphor (Trickett, Watts, & Birman, 1993). Twenty years after the Swampscott Conference, Snowden commented that a major task facing community psychology was "to improve its sensitivity and effectiveness in working on the problems of minority communities ... "(1987, pp. 581) as well as to be more appealing to ethnic minority psychologists. Only very recently has Community Psychology moved closer to—in Serrano-García and Bond's (1994) elegant phrase—empowering the silent ranks.

In its first two decades, Community Psychology paid less attention to women and ethnic minority groups in both research and practice than would have been expected, given the confluence of the national zeitgeist of the Civil Rights Movement and the Women's Liberation Movement with the guiding values of the field. A similar phenomenon occurred in its next decade, as the Gay Rights Movement gained momentum and prominence. The lack of research about and interventions with women, people of color, gay and lesbian people, and individuals who are differently abled has been documented in many reviews of what we publish in our journals, particularly during the early years of the field (Bernal & Enchautegui-de-Jésus, 1994; Garnets & D'Augelli, 1994; Loo, Fong, & Imawasa, 1988; Lounsbury, Cook, Leader, & Meares, 1985; Lounsbury, Leader, Meares, & Cook, 1980; Martin et al., 1999; Novaco & Monahan, 1980; Speer et al., 1992). The singular conclusion of these articles: Some progress has been made, but more needed to be done.

Studies in the early years of the field did not even disclose the gender or ethnicity of participants. Later studies would add the demographic descriptors, but continued to frame studies or the definition of social problems in terms of between-group differences, with an implicit white–male–heterosexual norm. Many studies (unknowingly) adopted a "deficit model": the nonmainstream group was depicted as less competent than the mainstream groups, or social problems were framed in terms of a high-risk demographic population, e.g., teen pregnancy was studied only with lower-income, African–American girls. Bernal and Enchautegui-de-Jésus (1994) provide a cogent illustration of this phenomenon with respect to Latino/Latina populations. Cause for "population-based" social problems was socially constructed as a result of the debilitating aspects of oppression. This moved the locus of causality from inside to outside the person/group, but did little to reframe the social problem in terms of social structural factors.

Unlike other areas within American psychology, community psychology did not view nonmainstream groups as inherently inferior (as a result of biology or personality, etc.), but still used "compassionate stereotypes," whereby concern and advocacy for a group is based on their problems, infirmities, and helplessness. Despite the attribution to oppression or social forces, interventions were still focusing on "helping" the target group—sometimes helping them to be(come) more empowered, but sometimes helping them to be(come) more mainstream. The pull toward a deficit model—despite the tenets of empowerment and competence-building—may have been a remnant of psychology's traditional individual differences approach, and/or it may have stemmed from our overriding value to help "those in need " —which often turned out to be people of color, and/or people in poverty. It was time for a change.

That change came in a new approach to human diversity delineated by Edison Trickett, Meg Bond, Irma Serrano-García, and Roderick Watts, among others. Trickett and his colleagues (Trickett, Watts, & Birman, 1993, 1994; Trickett, 1994, 1996) proposed an overarching framework that placed diversity *within* community psychology's guiding principles/theories/exemplars: empowerment, prevention, behavior in context, and a strengths-based perspective. The core of this framework is an ecological perspective, emphasizing the interdependence of people and their environments (Livert & Hughes, Chapter 3, this volume). In order to understand a particular ecology, one must be familiar with and value the cultural context, i.e., "how social values, reflected in social structures and policies, differentially affect the experience of different groups ... how power and other social resources [are distributed]" (Trickett *et al.*, 1993, p. 273), and how ascribed statuses such as race, class, and gender, affect these processes. Woven within this framework are notions of valuing the strengths of diverse groups, empowering diverse people within diverse settings, and changing the settings themselves (Trickett, 1996).

If one adopts this framework, then the dominant perspective must change from an androcentric, heterosexist, European-American worldview to a more social-constructionist perspective that encompasses a wide(r) variety of people. This new worldview, in turn, influences the entire research process, from problem definition to methodology to interpretation (Hughes & Seidman, 2002; Watts, 1993) while restructuring the relationships among those involved in the research process (Bond, Hill, Mulvey, & Terenzio, 2000a, 2000b; Miller & Banyard, 1998; Roosa & Gonzales, 2000). Meg Bond (1999) elaborates on this, emphasizing the importance of active collaboration among diverse groups and recognizing the diversity *within* groups. To this end, Trickett's ecological human diversity paradigm and the research that grows from it are not just about understanding or incorporating multiple perspectives into our work, but about social justice.

Current research in community psychology suggests that this framework already has had an influence. There has been a greater visibility of feminist approaches and research on different groups of women (e.g., Bond *et al.*, 2000a, 2000b; Campbell, 1998; Swift, Bond, & Serrano-García, 2000), culturally-anchored approaches (e.g., Hughes & DuMont, 1993; Maton, Hrabowski, & Grelf, 1998; Seidman, Hughes, & Williams, 1993) and gay/lesbian concerns (e.g., Garnets & D'Augelli, 1994; Martin, Dean, Garcia, & Hall, 1989, Chapter 13, this volume; Waldo, Hesson-McInnis, & D'Augelli, 1998) in both science and action. We have thought hard about the contexts of poor families and families of color and how parenting, peer, and community influences interact (Gonzales, Cauce, Friedman, & Mason, 1996, Chapter 24, this volume; Maton, Hrabowski, & Greif, 1998; Seidman, 1991; Seidman *et al.*, 1999; Wilson, 1997). We have asked the people we are studying how to understand their lives (e.g., Dumka, Gonzales, Wood, & Formoso, 1998; Hughes & DuMont, 1993; Riger, 2001; Watts, 1993) and brought this information together with existing constructs (e.g., Gibbs & Fuery, 1994). Moreover, many of these studies have opened up the canon of methodologies, using more qualitative and context-dependent approaches when called for (Bond *et al.*, 2000b; Miller & Banyard, 1998), and allowing us to acknowledge "multiple realities" (Bond, 1999, p. 341).

A central premise of Community Psychology always has been the importance of developing theory, research, and action which examine the interdependence of people and context, and locates individuals, social settings, and communities in a sociocultural context (Bond, 1999; Trickett, 1996). Only in the past few years, however, has context moved from a rich heuristic concept to a essential component of the research enterprise, bringing forward the notion of the unequal distribution of power and privilege that was elucidated in the early years of the field (e.g., Watts, Griffith, & Abdul-Adil, 1999). Because a decisive change has not yet taken place, we decided not to label this as a full turning point. As Harry Potter had to have faith that he would be able to cross through to the invisible Platform 9-3/4 to catch the Hogwart's Express (Rowling, 1998)—actually, faith that a magical opening existed at all between Gates 9 and 10—we have faith that looking back several years from now, the melding of human diversity and context will open up new vistas in theory, research, and action.

BACK TO THE FUTURE ... AGAIN

To not be the victims of history we must build upon it, not repeat it.
FAIRWEATHER, 1986, p. 133

What has Community Psychology accomplished in its first quarter century? What role has Community Psychology played in the larger field of psychology? What should we expect of the field at the dawn of the 21st century?

Without resting on our laurels, it is obvious that Community Psychology has made substantive contributions to the well-being of diverse individuals and has influenced American Psychology in significant but sometimes nonacknowledged ways. Before we had much to give away, Kelly (1971a) talked about "giving away the by-line," i.e., developing "people and communities without seeking visibility and public applause for his [sic] service" (pp. 902–903). In an American Psychological Association symposium reflecting on the 20th anniversary of Swampscott, Snowden (1987) referred to the "peculiar successes" of the field—instances where we can see tangible achievements (for example, in bringing mental health services to the poor and to minorities) and where community psychology should claim credit (if not full credit).

In the past 30 years, Community Psychology has given a lot away, through two different routes: collaboration with grassroots stakeholders (e.g., Chavis & Wandersman, 1990, Chapter 14, this volume; Saegert & Winkel, 1996; Serrano-García, 1984, 1994) and research that informs policy (e.g., Jason, 1998; Shinn, 1992, Chapter 17, this volume, 1997; Phillips, Howes, & Whitebook, 1992, Chapter 18, this volume). Heeding the calls of Rappaport (1981, 1987) and Shinn (1987), community psychology has applied its knowledge base in multiple settings and addressed many issues beyond mental health, including health care (e.g., Jason, 1998; Petersen, 1998; Revenson & Schiaffino, 2000), religious institutions (e.g., Maton, 1989, Chapter 12, this volume; Pargament & Maton, 2000), legal institutions (e.g., Melton, 2000; Reppucci, 1999), and the welfare system (e.g., Knitzer, 2000; Knitzer, Yoshikawa, Cauthen, & Aber, 2000).

The ranks of community psychologists are small, leading some to say that its influence is dwindling. We may have given a lot away, but our basket is hardly empty. Community psychology has made unique contributions to social change over the past quarter century that other disciplines have not, and these contributions will continue to be valuable in this century. Community psychology integrates concerns with schools, families, and ecological processes in ways that developmental psychology has only come to recently. Community psychology weaves psychological, organizational, and setting-level processes in a way that is unfamiliar but crucial to public policy analysis. Community psychology brings knowledge of how human diversity is played out in a cultural context to the development of programs and policies in a way that cultural psychology has not. Community psychology links micro- and macro-social processes together with health behavior in a way that public health does not. And in a true transactional fashion, other disciplines bring us important approaches and methods that have only begun to enrich Community Psychology, but have not been fully integrated into the field, such as the methods of applied anthropology.

Community psychologists were (and remain) at the frontier of the design of preventive interventions (Durlak & Wells, 1997; Kellam, Koretz, & Mościcki, 1999a, 1999b; Koretz, 1991; Sandler, 2001). A wide array of well-documented early detection and intervention (secondary prevention) programs, developed, in large measure, by community psychologists, have been incorporated into the mainstream of clinical, counseling, and school psychology (see *Fourteen Ounces of Prevention*, Price, Cowen, Lorion, & Ramos-McKay, 1988). Community psychologists also have been major players in the development of population-centered primary prevention programs, many under the aegis of the Preventive Intervention Research Centers sponsored by the National Institutes of Mental Health (Koretz, 1991). (Three of the four original centers were lead by community psychologists: George Spivak & Myrna Shure, Richard Price, and Irwin Sandler.) These and other developments over the last decade recently culminated in the creation of an interdisciplinary Society for Prevention Research and a journal, *Prevention Science*.

Moreover, community psychologists were pioneers in developing many of the methodological innovations for preventive intervention research. At Swampscott, "the conferees recognized that community psychologists would need to be strong researchers, armed with strong methods for dealing with anecdotal data, multivariate interactions, and the assessment of change at various points in time" (Elias, 1987, p. 542). More complex ecological models demanded more complex research designs and statistics, and community psychologists met this challenge (e.g., Linney, 2000; Seidman, 1993; Shinn & Rapkin, 2000). A number of the innovations in research design, ecological assessment, and culturally anchored methods published in the *American Journal of Community Psychology* are gathered together in a companion volume, *Ecological Research to Promote Social Change: Methodological Advances from Community Psychology* (Revenson *et al.*, 2002).

As discussed earlier, community psychology was one of the first areas within psychology to grapple with issues of human diversity, bringing them into theory, research, and action. Many of the themes discussed at the recent National Multicultural Conference and Summit sponsored by the American

Psychological Association (Sue, Bingham, Porché-Burke, & Vasquez, 1999) are reiterations of concerns and solutions posed by community psychologists over the past three decades. In this way, Community Psychology stands as the "conscience" of organized American psychology, speaking up for and empowering disenfranchised groups before other practitioners and researchers did. In part because of the strides in this area, community psychology continues to affirm and sanction multiple and alternative approaches to inquiry (Kelly, Ryan, Altman, & Stelzner, 2000; Miller & Banyard, 1998; Riger, 1993, Chapter 19, this volume; Shinn, 1997; Trickett, 1996, Chapter 23, this volume).

Concepts that emerged from within community psychology not only have influenced other areas of psychology and social science, but have also been "discovered" by these fields. For example, community psychology's long-term emphasis on building resources and competencies, and looking for strengths and not just weaknesses presaged the American Psychological Association's current zeitgeist of "positive psychology" (Sheldon & King, 2001). The topic of social support, the most written about topic in the *AJCP* in the 1980s (Speer *et al.*, 1992) is now a central area of interest within health psychology, medical sociology, and public health. Developmental psychology has recently realized the importance of neighborhood influences on child and adolescent development. Our longstanding commitment to action science has increasingly been adopted by the emerging sub-disciplines of applied developmental and applied social psychology. Clinical psychology has made great strides in providing context- and culturally-specific mental health services to ethnic minority populations (Snowden, Martinez, & Morris, 2000).

While we are feeling proud, it is important to remind ourselves that our work is not done. Tensions still exist between local collaborations/community-driven research and the accumulation of knowledge (Blakely *et al.*, 1987, Chapter 10, this volume). How do we figure out the key ingredients inside the black box of social interventions? How do we work with the local community to figure out how to adapt interventions that work elsewhere so that they will work here? Or does each locally driven collaborative action research project have to start from scratch, as though we had never done anything similar somewhere else? Understanding process is a partial solution—to the extent that we know how things work, we are better able to pull out key ingredients for replication or to modify approaches to achieve the same processes in new contexts, and thus, are better able to discard unneeded baggage that may not fit the new context. But as Trickett (1996, Chapter 23, this volume) and others have warned us, that process must be understood within and respectful of the cultural context of the community. Despite the knowledge we have accumulated, we know relatively little about how social structure and community structure affect people's lives and how these structures are amenable to change (Heller, 1989).

For a while now, Community Psychology has advocated moving away from secondary prevention and person-centered interventions toward systems-level and sociopolitical preventive interventions, in order for the interventions to have staying power (e.g., Linney, 1990; Seidman, 1988, Chapter 11, this volume; Watts, *et al.*, 1999). In the future we need to look more closely at the relations between assessment and intervention *across* systems. Seidman (1991) points out that adolescents may experience problems (and get services) in multiple domains—school failure, delinquency and status offenses, early pregnancy, substance use/abuse, and later in life, welfare—but that these may be the same adolescents, having multiple risk factors and existing within overlapping service domains. This also has been documented with people with mental illness, who get bounced from homeless shelters to jails to mental hospitals to substance abuse treatment programs, without anybody taking a real look at the process (Shinn, 1992, Chapter 17, this volume, 1997). An early article by Tausig (1987) detailed these "cracks" in the service system, but this has not been a central focus of community psychology to date. It also might be useful to understand how these individuals bounce from system to system, and work on coordinated, community-based approaches. Further, Community Psychology might benefit from reaching into new arenas or renewing their involvement in old ones, such as continued racial tensions and conflicts, nuclear disarmament, abortion rights, the diminishing safety net for America's poor, welfare reform, increases in immigration to the United States, and grassroots movements arising from the globalization of trade.

Community Psychology provides an intellectual and social space for scientists, practitioners, and citizens to work together and to integrate many areas of scholarship to find common ground for analyzing social systems and social change. Slightly over a decade ago, Price wrote:

> The fundamental question is whether (or even if) a better understanding of social and community life actually can bring about improved social conditions. A second question is how does one go about translating social insights derived from research and scholarship into improved conditions for families, organizations, and communities (1989, p. 151).

These always will remain fundamental questions for the field. In the 21st century, however, we reask them with the knowledge we have gained over the past thirty-five years: solutions for one group may mean fewer resources for another, and many current interventions often leave the underlying context unchanged.

We give Seymour Sarason the last words:

> The last sentence of most dissertations is that "further research is indicated".... At the top of my agenda [for community psychology] are these

questions: How do we justify our field? What overarching vision do we have in common? Further soul searching is needed (2000, p. 929).

While social problems and communities continually change, these questions always will be with us, for it is the struggle to find answers and reframe questions that defines what community psychologists do.

NOTES

1. Zax and Specter published a text in 1974 titled *An Introduction to Community Psychology* (John Wiley & Sons), but the volume dealt almost exclusively with community mental health concepts and programs.
2. We acknowledge that Fairweather was empowering people with psychiatric problems through self-governing communities (as were some of his contemporaries) long before Rappaport brought the word into community psychology. The concept of mediating structures, however, was new to the field.
3. Applied community psychologists have been the leaders in developing tools with which to work with community organizations and create effective community coalitions. A good resource is the Community Toolbox, found at http://ctb.ukans.edu.
4. The political forces behind these innovations did not come to a halt with the end of the Kennedy and Johnson administrations. President Nixon approved a series of negative income tax experiments that reinforced being employed without removing welfare benefits. However, a near-sighted evaluation halted the experiments rather quickly, citing an individual-level "disincentive motivation" to work while receiving benefits. Later evaluations found that there were long-term effects on employment and quality of life, particularly for women who had used the additional income for schooling, resulting in better-paying employment several years down the line. The negative tax experiments are an exemplary illustration of experimental social innovations.

REFERENCES

Note: An asterisk preceding an entry denotes an award address to a recipient of the Award for Distinguished Contribution to Community Psychology and Commmunity Mental Health.

Albee, G. W. (1982a). Preventing psychopathology and promoting human potential. *American Psychologist, 37,* 1043–1050.
*Albee, G. W. (1982b). The politics of nature and nurture. *American Journal of Community Psychology, 10,* 4–36.
Altman, D. G. (1986). On defining a role for community psychology: The contributions of James G. Kelly. *American Journal of Community Psychology, 14,* 573–579.
Barrera, M. (1986). Distinctions between social support concepts, measures, and models. *American Journal of Community Psychology, 14,* 413–446.
Bennett, C. C., Anderson, L. S., Cooper, S. Hassol, L., Klein, D. C., & Rosenblum, G. (1966). *Community psychology: A report of the Boston Conference on the Education of Psychologists for Community Mental Health.* Boston, MA: Boston University, and Quincy, MA: South Shore Mental Health Center.
Berger, P. L. & Neuhaus, R. J. (1977). *To empower people: The role of mediating structures in public policy.* Washington, DC: American Enterprise Institute for Public Policy Research.

Bernal, G. & Enchautegui-de-Jésus, N. (1994). Latinos and Latinas in community psychology: A review of the literature. *American Journal of Community Psychology*, 22, 531–558.

Blakely, C. H., Mayer, J. P., Gottschalk, R. G., Schmitt, N., Davidson, W. S., Roitman, D. B., & Emshoff, J. G. (1987). The fidelity-adaptation debate: Implications for the implementation of public sector programs. *American Journal of Community Psychology*, 15, 253–268.

*Bloom, B. L. (1978). Community psychology: Midstream and middream. *American Journal of Community Psychology*, 6, 205–217.

Bond, M. A. (1999). Gender, race, and class in organizational contexts. *American Journal of Community Psychology*, 27, 327–355.

Bond, M. A., Hill, J., Mulvey, A., & Terenzio, M. (Eds.). (2000a). Feminism and community psychology: I [Special issue]. *American Journal of Community Psychology*, 28(5).

Bond, M. A., Hill, J., Mulvey, A., & Terenzio, M. (Eds.). (2000b). Feminism and community psychology: II [Special issue]. *American Journal of Community Psychology*, 28(6).

Bond, M. A., Hill, J., Mulvey, A., & Terenzio, M. (2000c). Weaving feminism and community psychology: An introduction to the special issue. *American Journal of Community Psychology*, 28, 585–597.

Borkman, T. J. (Ed.). (1991). Self-help groups [Special issue]. *American Journal of Community Psychology*, 19(5).

Brody, J. G. (1986). Community psychology in the eighties: A celebration of survival. *American Journal of Community Psychology*, 14, 139–146.

Bronfenbrenner, U. (1977). Toward an experimental ecology of human development. *American Psychologist*, 32, 513–531.

Campbell, R. (1998). The community response to rape: Victims' experiences with the legal, medical, and mental health systems. *American Journal of Community Psychology*, 26, 355–379.

Chavis, D., Stuckey, P. E., & Wandersman, A. (1983). Returning basic research to the community: A relationship between scientist and citizen. *American Psychologist*, 38, 424–434.

Chavis, D. M. & Wandersman, A. (1990). Sense of community in the urban environment: A catalyst for participation and community development. *American Journal of Community Psychology*, 18, 55–81.

Cherniss, C. (1976). Preentry issues in consultation. *American Journal of Community Psychology*, 4, 13–24.

Cowen, E. L. (1977). Baby-steps toward primary prevention. *American Journal of Community Psychology*, 5, 1–22.

*Cowen, E. L. (1980). The wooing of primary prevention. *American Journal of Community Psychology*, 8, 258–284.

Cowen, E. L. (Ed.). (1982). Research in primary prevention in mental health [Special issue]. *American Journal of Community Psychology*, 10(3).

Cowen, E. L. (1985). Person-centered approaches to primary prevention in mental health: Situation-focused and competence-enhancement. *American Journal of Community Psychology*, 13, 31–48.

Cowen, E. L., Gardner, E. A., & Zax, M. (Eds.) (1967). *Emergent approaches to mental health problems*. New York: Appleton-Century-Crofts.

Danish, S. J. & D'Augelli, A. R. (1980). Promoting competence and enhancing development through life development intervention. In L. A. Bond & J. C. Rosen (Eds.), *Primary prevention of psychopathology*, vol. 4 (pp. 105–129). Hanover, NH: University Press of New England.

DeFour, D. C. & Hirsch, B. J. (1990). The adaptation of black graduate students: A social network approach. *American Journal of Community Psychology*, 18, 487–503.

Denner, B. & Price, R. H. (1973). *Community mental health: Social action and community reaction.* New York: Holt, Rinehart and Winston.

Dohrenwend, B. S. (1978). Social stress and community psychology. *American Journal of Community Psychology, 6,* 1–14.

*Dohrenwend, B. S. & Dohrenwend, B. P. (1981). Socioenvironmental factors, stress, and psychopathology. *American Journal of Community Psychology, 9,* 129–164.

Dumka, L. E., Gonzales, N. A.,Wood, J. L., & Formoso, D. (1998). Using qualitative methods to develop conceptually relevant measures and preventive interventions: An illustration. *American Journal of Community Psychology, 26,* 605–638.

Durlak, J. & Wells, A. M. (1997). Primary prevention mental health programs for children and adolescents: A meta-analytic review. *American Journal of Community Psychology, 25,* 115–152.

Dworkin, A. L. & Dworkin, E. P. (1975). A conceptual overview of selected consultation models. *American Journal of Community Psychology, 3,* 151–160.

Ehrlich, R. P., D'Augelli, A. R., & Conter, K. R. (1981). Evaluation of a community-based system for training natural helpers. I: Effects on verbal helping skills. *American Journal of Community Psychology, 9,* 321–337.

Elias, M. J. (1987). Establishing enduring prevention programs: Advancing the legacy of Swampscott. *American Journal of Community Psychology, 15,* 539–554.

Elias, M. J., Gara, M., Ubriaco, M., Rothbaum, P. A., Clabby, J. F., & Schuyler, T. (1986). Impact of a preventive social problem solving intervention on children's coping with middle-school stressors. *American Journal of Community Psychology, 14,* 259–276.

*Fairweather, G. W. (1986). The need for uniqueness. *American Journal of Community Psychology, 14,* 128–137.

Fairweather, G. W., Sanders, D. H., Maynard, H., & Cressler, D. L. (1969). *Community life for the mentally ill: An alternative to institutional care.* Chicago: Aldine.

Fairweather, G. W., Sanders, D. H., & Tornatzky, L. G. (1974). *Creating change in mental health organizations.* New York: Pergamon.

Felner, R. D., Ginter, M., & Primavera, J. (1982). Primary prevention during school transitions: Social support and environmental structure. *American Journal of Community Psychology, 10,* 277–290.

French, J. R. P., Jr., Rodgers, W., & Cobb, S. (1974). Adjustment as person-environment fit. In G. V. Coelho, D. A. Hamburg, & J. E. Adams (Eds.), *Coping and adaptation* (pp. 316–333). New York: Basic Books.

French, S. E. & D'Augelli, A. R. (2002). Diversity in community psychology. In T. A. Revenson, A. R. D'Augelli, S. E. French, D. L. Hughes, D. Livert, E. Seidman, M. Shinn, & H. Yoshikawa (Eds.). *A quarter century of community psychology: Readings from the* American Journal of Community Psychology (pp. 65–77). New York: Kluwer Academic/Plenum Publishers.

Garnets, L. D & D'Augelli, A. R. (1994). Empowering lesbian and gay communities: A call for collaboration with community psychology. *American Journal of Community Psychology, 22,* 447–470.

Gibbs, J. T. & Fuery, D. (1994). Mental health and well-being of Black women: Toward strategies of empowerment. *American Journal of Community Psychology, 22,* 559–582.

Glidewell, J. C. (1988). Reflections on thirteen years of editing AJCP. *American Journal of Community Psychology, 16,* 759–770.

Goldenberg, I. I. (1971). *Build me a mountain.* Cambridge, MA: The MIT Press.

Gonzales, N. A., Cauce, A., Friedman, R. J., & Mason, C. A. (1996). Family, peer, and neighborhood influences on academic achievement among African American adolescents: One-year prospective effects. *American Journal of Community Psychology, 24,* 365–387.

Gottlieb, B. H. (Ed.). (1988). *Marshalling social support: Formats, processes, and effects.* Newbury Park, CA: Sage.

Gruber, J. & Trickett, E. J. (1987). Can we empower others? The paradox of empowerment in the governing of an alternative public school. *American Journal of Community Psychology, 15,* 353–371.

Heller, K. (1989). The return to community. *American Journal of Community Psychology, 17,* 1–15.

Heller, K. & Monahan, J. (1977). *Psychology and community change.* Homewood IL: The Dorsey Press.

Hirsch, B. J. & Rapkin, B. D. (1986). Social networks and adult social identities: Profiles and correlates of support and rejection. *American Journal of Community Psychology, 14,* 395–412.

Hughes, D. L. & DuMont, K. (1993). Using focus groups to facilitate culturally anchored research. *American Journal of Community Psychology, 21,* 775–806. Reprinted in T. A. Revenson, A. R. D'Augelli, S. E. French, D. L. Hughes, D. Livert, E. Seidman, M. Shinn, & H. Yoshikawa (Eds.). (2002). *Ecological research to promote social change: Methodological advances from community psychology* (pp. 257–289). New York: Kluwer Academic/Plenum Publishers.

Hughes, D. L. & Seidman, E. (2002). In pursuit of a culturally anchored methodology. In T. A. Revenson, A. R. D'Augelli, S. E. French, D. L. Hughes, D. Livert, E. Seidman, M. Shinn, & H. Yoshikawa (Eds.). *Ecological research to promote social change: Methodological advances from community psychology* (pp. 243–255). New York: Kluwer Academic/Plenum Publishers.

Iscoe, I. (1974). Community psychology and the competent community. *American Psychologist, 29,* 607–613.

Iscoe, I. (1987). From Boston to Austin and points beyond: The tenacity of community psychology. *American Journal of Community Psychology, 15,* 587–590.

Jahoda, M. (1958). *Current concepts of positive mental health.* New York: Basic Books.

*Jason, L. A. (1998). Tobacco, drug, and HIV prevention media interventions. *American Journal of Community Psychology, 26,* 151–188.

Karetz, D. S. (1991). Preventive Intervention Research Centers [Special issue]. *American Journal of Community Psychology, 19*(4).

Kellam, S. G., Koretz, D., & Mościcki, E. K. (Eds.). (1999a). Prevention Science, Part I [Special issue]. *American Journal of Community Psychology, 27*(4).

Kellam, S. G., Koretz, D., & Mościcki, E. K. (Eds.). (1999b). Prevention Science, Part II [Special issue]. *American Journal of Community Psychology, 27*(5).

Kelly, J. G. (1971a). Qualities for the community psychologist. *American Psychologist, 26,* 897–903.

Kelly, J. G. (1971b). The quest for valid preventive interventions. In G. Rosenblum (Ed.), *Issues in community psychology and preventive mental health* (pp. 109–139). New York: Behavioral Publications.

*Kelly, J. G. (1979). Tain't what you do, it's the way that you do it. *American Journal of Community Psychology, 7,* 244–261.

Kelly, J. G. (1986). Context and process: An ecological view of the interdependence of practice and research. *American Journal of Community Psychology, 14,* 581–590.

Kelly, J. G. (1987). Some reflections on the Swampscott conference. *American Journal of Community Psychology, 15,* 515–518.

Kelly, J. G. (1990). Changing contexts and the field of community psychology. *American Journal of Community Psychology, 18,* 769–792.

Kelly, J. G., Ryan, A. M., Altman, B. E., & Stelzner, S. S. (2000). Understanding and changing social systems: An ecological view. In J. Rappaport & E. Seidman (Eds.), *Handbook of community psychology* (pp. 133–159). New York: Kluwer Academic/Plenum Publishers.

Keys, C. B. & Frank, S. (Eds.). (1987). Organizational perspectives in community psychology [Special issue]. *American Journal of Community Psychology*, *15*(3).

Knitzer, J. (2000). Helping troubled children and families: A paradigm of public responsibility. In J. Rappaport & E. Seidman (Eds.), *Handbook of community psychology* (pp. 541–563). New York: Kluwer Academic/Plenum Publishers.

Knitzer, J., Yoshikawa, H., Cauthen, N., & Aber, J. L. (2000). Welfare reform, family support, and child development: Perspectives from policy analysis and developmental psychopathology. *Development and Psychopathology*, *12*, 619–632.

Koretz, D. S. (Ed.) (1991). Preventive intervention research centers [Special issue]. *American Journal of Community Psychology*, *19* (4).

*Levine, M. (1988). An analysis of mutual assistance. *American Journal of Community Psychology*, *16*, 167–188.

Linney, J. A. (1990). Community psychology into the 1990s: Capitalizing opportunity and promoting innovation. *American Journal of Community Psychology*, *18*, 1–18.

Linney, J. A. (2000). Assessing ecological constructs and community context. In J. Rappaport & E. Seidman (Eds.) *Handbook of community psychology* (pp. 647–667). New York: Kluwer Academic/Plenum Publishers.

Livert, D. & Hughes, D. L. (2002). The ecological paradigm: Persons in settings. In T. A. Revenson, A. R. D'Augelli, S. E. French, D. L. Hughes, D. Livert, E. Seidman, M. Shinn, & H. Yoshikawa (Eds.). *A quarter century of community psychology: Readings from the American Journal of Community Psychology* (pp. 51–63). New York: Kluwer Academic/Plenum Publishers.

Loo, C., Fong, K. T., & Iwamasa, G. (1988). Ethnicity and cultural diversity: An analysis of work published in community psychology journals. *Journal of Community Psychology*, *16*, 332–349.

Lounsbury, J. W., Cook, M. P., Leader, D. S., & Meares, E. P. (1985). In E. C. Susskind & D. C. Klein (Eds.). *Community resarch: Methods, paradigms, and applications* (pp. 39–106). New York: Praeger.

Lounsbury, J. W., Leader, D. S., Meares, E. P., & Cook, M. P. (1980). An analytic review of research in community psychology. *American Journal of Community Psychology*, *8*, 415–441.

Martin, J. L., Dean, L., Garcia, M., & Hall, W. (1989). The impact of AIDS on a gay community: Changes in sexual behavior, substance use, and mental health. *American Journal of Community Psychology*, *17*, 269–293.

Martin, P., Lounsbury, D., Nguyen, H., Randall, K., Legaspi, A., Thomas, O., Siebold, W., Lewis, K., & Davidson, W. (1999, June). An analytic review of the *American Journal of Community Psychology* (1993–1998): A preliminary report. Paper presented at the Biennial Conference of the Society for Community Research and Action, New Haven, CT.

Maton, K. I. (1989). Community settings as buffers of life stress? Highly supportive churches, mutual help groups, and senior centers. *American Journal of Community Psychology*, *17*, 203–232.

Maton, K. I. & Salem, D. A. (1995). Organizational characteristics of empowering community settings: A multiple case study approach. *American Journal of Community Psychology*, *23*, 631–656.

Maton, K. I., Hrabowsi, F. A. III, & Grelf, G. L. (1988). Preparing the way: A qualitative study of high achieving African-American males and the role of the family. *American Journal of Community Psychology*, *26*, 639–668.

McMillan, B. & Chavis, D. (1986). Sense of community: A definition and theory. *Journal of Community Psychology*, *14*, 6–23.

McMillan, B., Florin, P., Stevenson, J., Kerman, B., & Mitchell, R. E. (1995). Empowerment praxis in community coalitions. *American Journal of Community Psychology*, *23*, 699–728.

Melton, G. (2000). Community change, community stasis, and the law. In J. Rappaport & E. Seidman (Eds.), *Handbook of community psychology* (pp. 523–539). New York: Kluwer Academic/Plenum Publishers.

Merritt, D. M., Greene, G. J., Jopp, D. A., & Kelly, J. G. (1999). A history of Division 27 (Society for Community Research and Action). In D. A. Dewsbury (Ed.), *Unification through division: Histories of the divisions of the American Psychological Association*, Vol. III (pp. 73–99). Washington, DC: American Psychological Association.

Miller, K. E. & Banyard, V. L. (1998). Qualitative research in community psychology [Special issue]. *American Journal of Community Psychology*, 26(4).

Moos, R. H. (1973). Conceptualizations of human environments. *American Psychologist, 28*, 652–665.

*Moos, R. H. (1984). Context and coping: Toward a unifying conceptual framework. *American Journal of Community Psychology, 12*, 5–36.

Murrell, S. A. (1973). *Community psychology and social systems*. New York: Behavioral Publications.

Newbrough, J. R. (1973). Community psychology: A new holism. *American Journal of Community Psychology, 1*, 201–211.

Novaco, R. & Monahan, J. (1980). Research in community psychology: An analysis of work published in the first six years of the *American Journal of Community Psychology*. *American Journal of Community Psychology, 8*, 131–146.

O'Donnell, C. R., Tharp, R. C., & Wilson, K. (1993). Activity settings as the unit of analysis: A theoretical basis for community intervention and development. *American Journal of Community Psychology, 21*, 501–520.

Pargament, K. I. & Maton, K. I. (2000). Religion in community life. In J. Rappaport & E. Seidman (Eds.). *Handbook of community psychology* (pp. 495–522). New York: Kluwer Academic/Plenum Publishers.

Perkins, D. D. (1995). Speaking truth to power: Empowerment ideology as social intervention and policy. *American Journal of Community Psychology, 23*, 765–794.

Perkins, D. D. & Zimmerman, M. A. (1995). Empowerment theory, research, and application. *American Journal of Community Psychology, 23*, 569–580.

Peterson, J. L. (Ed.). (1998). HIV/AIDS prevention through community psychology [Special issue]. *American Journal of Community Psychology*, 26(1).

Phillips, D. A., Howes, C., & Whitebook, M. (1992). The social policy context of child care: Effects on quality. *American Journal of Community Psychology, 20*, 25–51.

Price, R. H. (1980). Risky situations. In D. Magnusson (Ed.), *Toward a psychology of situations: An interactional perspective* (pp. 103–112). Hillsdale, NJ: Erlbaum.

*Price, R. H. (1989). Bearing witness. *American Journal of Community Psychology, 17*, 151–167.

Price, R. H., Cowen, E. L., Lorion, R. P., & Ramos-McKay, J. (Eds.) (1988). *Fourteen ounces of prevention: A casebook for practitioners*. Washington, DC: American Psychological Association.

Procidano, M. E. & Heller, K. (1983). Measures of perceived social support from friends and from family: Three validation studies. *American Journal of Community Psychology, 11*, 1–24.

Rappaport, J. (1977). *Community psychology: Values, research, and action*. New York: Holt, Rinehart and Winston.

Rappaport, J. (1981). In praise of paradox: A social policy of empowerment over prevention. *American Journal of Community Psychology, 9*, 10–25.

*Rappaport, J. (1987). Terms of empowerment/exemplars of prevention: Toward a theory for community psychology. *American Journal of Community Psychology, 15*, 121–145.

Rappaport, J., Chinsky, J. M., & Cowen, E. L. (1971). *Innovations in helping chronic patients: College students in a mental institution*. New York: Academic Press.

Rappaport, J., Seidman, E., Toro, P., McFadden, L. S., Reischl, T. M., Roberts, L. J., Salem, D. A., Stein, C. H., & Zimmerman, M. A. (1985). Collaborative research with a mutual help organization. *Social Policy, 15*, 12–24.

Reiff, R. (1968). Social intervention and the problem of psychological analysis. *American Psychologist, 23*, 524–531.

*Reiff, R. (1975). Of cabbages and kings. *American Journal of Community Psychology, 3*, 187–196.

Reppucci, N. D. (1973). The social psychology of institutional change: General principles for intervention. *American Journal of Community Psychology, 1*, 330–341.

*Reppucci, N. D. (1999). Adolescent development and juvenile justice. *American Journal of Community Psychology, 27*, 307–326.

Revenson, T. A., D'Augelli, A. R., French, S. E., Hughes, D. L., Livert, D., Seidman, E., Shinn, M., & Yoshikawa, H. (Eds.). (2002). *Ecological research to promote social change: Methodological advances from community psychology.* New York: Kluwer Academic/Plenum Publishers.

Revenson, T. A. & Schiaffino, K. M. (2000). Community-based health interventions. In J. Rappaport & E. Seidman (Eds.), *Handbook of community psychology* (pp. 471–493). New York: Kluwer Academic/Plenum Publishers.

Rich, R. C., Edelstein, M., Hallman, W. K., & Wandersman, A. H. (1995). Citizen participation and empowerment: The case of local environmental hazards. *American Journal of Community Psychology, 23*, 657–676.

Riger, S. (1993). What's wrong with empowerment. *American Journal of Community Psychology, 21*, 279–292.

*Riger, S. (2001). Transforming community psychology. *American Journal of Community Psychology, 29*, 69–81.

Roosa, M. W. & Gonzales, N. A. (Eds.). (2000). Minority issues in prevention [Special issue]. *American Journal of Community Psychology, 28*(2).

Rowling, J. K. (1998). Harry Potter and the sorcerer's stone. New York: Scholastic Books.

Ryan, W. (1971). *Blaming the victim.* New York: Random House.

Saegert, S. & Winkel, G. (1996). Paths to community empowerment: Organizing at home. *American Journal of Community Psychology, 24*, 517–550.

*Sandler, I. (2001). Quality and ecology of adversity as common mechanisms of risk and resilience. *American Journal of Community Psychology, 29*, 19–61.

Sarason, S. B. (1971). *The culture of the school and the problem of change.* Boston: Allyn & Bacon.

Sarason, S. B. (1974). *The psychological sense of community: Prospects for a community psychology.* San Francisco: Jossey Bass.

*Sarason, S. B. (1976). Community psychology and the anarchist insight. *American Journal of Community Psychology, 4*, 246–261.

Sarason, S. B. (1976). Community psychology, networks, and Mr. Everyman. *American Psychologist, 31*, 317–328.

Sarason, S. B. (1978). The nature of problem-solving in social action. *American Psychologist, 33*, 370–380.

Sarason, S. B. (1981). An asocial psychology and a misdirected clinical psychology. *American Psychologist, 36*, 827–836.

Sarason, S. B. (2000). Barometers of community change: Personal reflections. In J. Rappaport & E. Seidman (Eds.), *Handbook of community psychology* (pp. 919–929). New York: Kluwer Academic/Plenum Publishers.

Seidman, E. (1988). Back to the future, community psychology: Unfolding a theory of social intervention. *American Journal of Community Psychology, 16*, 3–24.

*Seidman, E. (1991). Growing up the hard way: Pathways of urban adolescents. *American Journal of Community Psychology, 19*, 173–205.
Seidman E. (Ed.). (1993). Methodological issues in prevention research [Special issue]. *American Journal of Community Psychology, 21*(5).
Seidman, E. & Rappaport, J. (1974). The educational pyramid: A paradigm for research, training, and manpower utilization community psychology. *American Journal of Community Psychology, 2*, 119–130.
Seidman, E., Hughes, D., & Williams, N. (Eds.). (1993). Cultural phenomena and the research enterprise. *Toward a culturally anchored methodology* [Special issue]. *American Journal of Community Psychology, 21*(6).
Seidman, E., Chesir-Teran, D., Friedman, J. L., Yoshikawa, H., Allen, L., Roberts, A., & Aber, J. L. (1999). The risk and protective functions of perceived family and peer microsystems among urban adolescents in poverty. *American Journal of Community Psychology, 27*, 211–238.
Serrano-García, I. (1984). The illusion of empowerment: Community development within a colonial context. *Prevention in Human Services, 3*(2/3), 173–200.
Serrano-García, I. (1994). The ethics of the powerful and the power of ethics. *American Journal of Community Psychology, 22*, 1–20.
Serrano-García, I. & Bond, M. A. (Eds.). (1994). Empowering the silent ranks [Special issue]. *American Journal of Community Psychology, 22*(4).
Sheldon, K. M. & King, L. (2001). Positive psychology. [Special section] *American Psychologist, 56*(3), 216–263.
Shinn, M. (1987). Expanding community psychology's domain. *American Journal of Community Psychology, 15*, 555–574.
Shinn, M. (1992). Homelessness: What is a psychologist to do? *American Journal of Community Psychology, 20*, 1–24.
*Shinn, M. (1997). Family homelessness: State or trait? *American Journal of Community Psychology, 25*, 755–769.
Shinn, M. & Rapkin, B. D. (2000). Cross-level research without cross-ups in community psychology. In J. Rappaport & E. Seidman (Eds.), *Handbook of community psychology* (pp. 669–695). New York: Kluwer Academic/Plenum Publishers.
Snowden, L. R. (Ed.). (1982). *Reaching the underserved: Mental health needs of neglected populations.* Beverly Hills, CA: Sage.
Snowden, L. R. (1987). The peculiar successes of community psychology: Service delivery to ethnic minorities and the poor. *American Journal of Community Psychology, 15*, 575–586.
Snowden, L. R., Martinez, M., & Morris, A. (2000). Community psychology and ethnic minority populations. In J. Rappaport & E. Seidman (Eds.), *Handbook of community psychology* (pp. 833–855). New York: Kluwer Academic/Plenum Publishers.
Speer, P., Dey, A., Griggs, P., Gibson, C., Lubin, B., & Hughey, J. (1992). In search of community: An analysis of community psychology research from 1984–1988. *American Journal of Community Psychology, 20*, 195–210.
*Spivack, G. & Shure, M. B. (1985). ICPS and beyond: Centripetal and centrifugal forces. *American Journal of Community Psychology, 13*, 226–244.
Sue, D. W., Bingham, R. P., Porché-Burke, L., & Vasquez, M. (1999). The diversification of psychology: A multicultural revolution. *American Psychologist, 54*, 1061–1069.
Swift, C. A., Bond, M. A., & Serrano-García, I. (2000). Women's empowerment: A review of community psychology's first twenty-five years. In J. Rappaport & E. Seidman (Eds.). *Handbook of community psychology* (pp. 857–895). New York: Kluwer Academic/Plenum Publishers.

Swift, C. & Levin, G. (1987). Empowerment: An emerging mental health technology. *Journal of Primary Prevention*, 8, 71–94.

Tausig, M. (1987). Detecting "cracks" in mental health service systems: Application of network analytic techniques. *American Journal of Community Psychology*, 15, 337–351. Reprinted in T. A. Revenson, A. R. D'Augelli, S. E. French, D. L. Hughes, D. Livert, E. Seidman, M. Shinn, & H. Yoshikawa (Eds.). (2002). *Ecological research to promote social change: Methodological advances from community psychology* (pp. 171–186). New York: Kluwer Academic/Plenum Publishers.

Trickett, E. J. (1994). Human diversity and community psychology: Where ecology and empowerment meet. *American Journal of Community Psychology*, 22, 583–592.

*Trickett, E. J. (1996). A future for community psychology: The contexts of diversity and the diversity of contexts. *American Journal of Community Psychology*, 24, 209–234.

Trickett, E. J., Watts, R., & Birman, D. (1993). Human diversity and community psychology: Still hazy after all these years. *Journal of Community Psychology*, 21, 264–279.

Trickett, E. J., Watts, R., & Birman, D. (1994). In E. J. Trickett, R. J. Watts, & D. Birman (Eds.). *Human diversity: Perspectives on people in context* (pp. 7–26). San Francisco: Jossey-Bass.

Vaux, A., Riedel, S., & Stewart, D. (1987). Modes of social support: The social support behaviors (SS-B) scale. *American Journal of Community Psychology*, 15, 209–237.

Waldo, C. R., Hesson-McInnis, M. S., & D'Augelli, A. R. (1998). Antecedents and consequences of victimization of lesbian, gay, and bisexual young people: A structural model comparing rural university and urban samples. *American Journal of Community Psychology*, 26, 307–334.

Wandersman, A. & Florin, P. (1990). Citizen participation, voluntary organizations, and community development: Insights for empowerment through research. [Special section] *American Journal of Community Psychology*, 18(1), pp. 41–177.

Watts, R. J. (1993). Community action through manhood development: A look at concepts and concerns from the frontline. *American Journal of Community Psychology*, 21, 333–360.

Watts, R. J., Griffith, D. M., & Abdul-Adil, J. (1999). Sociopolitical development as an antidote for oppression–Theory and action. *American Journal of Community Psychology*, 27, 255–271.

Watzlawick, P., Weakland, J. H., & Fisch, R. (1974). *Change: Principles of problem formation and problem resolution*. New York: Norton.

Weick, K. E. (1984). Small wins: Redefining the scale of social problems. *American Psychologist*, 39, 40–49.

Weinstein, R. S., Soulé, C. R., Collins, F., Cone, J., Mehlhorn, M., & Simontacchi, K. (1991). Expectations and high school change: Teacher–researcher collaboration to prevent school failure. *American Journal of Community Psychology*, 19, 333–364.

Weissberg, R. P., Caplan, M. Z., & Harwood, R. L. (1991). Promoting competence enhancing environments: A systems-based perspective on primary prevention. *Journal of Consulting and Clinical Psychology*, 59, 830–841.

Wilcox, B. (1981). Social support, life stress, and psychological adjustment: A test of the buffering hypothesis. *American Journal of Community Psychology*, 9, 371–386.

Wilson, M. N. (Ed.). (1997). Women of color: Social challenges of dual minority status and competing community contexts [Special issue]. *American Journal of Community Psychology*, 25(5).

Wolchik, S. A., West, S. G., Westover, S., Sandler, I. N., Martin, A., Lustig, J., Tein, J.-Y., & Fisher, J. (1993). The children of divorce parenting intervention: Outcome evaluation of an empirically based program. *American Journal of Community Psychology*, 21, 293–331.

Wolff, T. (1987). Community psychology and empowerment: An activist's insights. *American Journal of Community Psychology*, *15*, 151–166.

Yoshikawa, H. & Shinn, M. (2002). Facilitating change: Where and how should community psychology intervene? In T. A. Revenson, A. R. D'Augelli, S. E. French, D. L. Hughes, D. Livert, E. Seidman, M. Shinn, & H. Yoshikawa (Eds.). *A quarter century of community psychology: Readings from the* American Journal of Community Psychology (pp. 33–49). New York: Kluwer Academic/Plenum Publishers.

*Zigler, E. (1990). Shaping child care policies and programs in America. *American Journal of Community Psychology*, *18*, 183–216.

Zimmerman, M. A. (2000). Empowerment theory: Psychological, organizational, and community levels of analysis. In J. Rappaport & E. Seidman (Eds.), *Handbook of community psychology* (pp. 43–63). New York: Kluwer Academic/Plenum Publishers.

Zimmerman, M. A. & Perkins, D. D. (Eds.). (1995). Empowerment theory, research, and application [Special issue]. *American Journal of Community Psychology*, *23*(5).

2

Facilitating Change: Where and How Should Community Psychology Intervene?

Hirokazu Yoshikawa and Marybeth Shinn

The main focus on prevention has led to a necessary concern with the interaction between social system structures and functions and the mental health of populations ... It was pointed out that community psychology would frequently be involved with facilitating change rather than with preventing anything.

BENNETT *et al.*, 1966, pp. 6–7

Struggles over where and how to facilitate social change have remained central to the field of Community Psychology since its birth at Swampscott, Massachusetts in the spring of 1965. Difficult issues within the field, ranging from debates over empowerment versus prevention, to the challenges of culturally relevant intervention and the facilitation of community-wide change, all can be linked back to the two central questions of *where* and *how*. Community psychologists' answers to these questions over the past 25 years reveal much about the values, assumptions, and practices of the field.

Hirokazu Yoshikawa and **Marybeth Shinn** • Department of Psychology, New York University, New York, New York 10003.

A Quarter Century of Community Psychology: Readings from the American Journal of Community Psychology, edited by Tracey A. Revenson *et al.* Kluwer Academic/Plenum Publishers, New York, 2002.

WHERE SHOULD COMMUNITY
PSYCHOLOGISTS INTERVENE?

The question of where community psychologists should intervene hinges on the more general question of where the change process takes place, in terms of settings or ecological levels of analysis. Clinical psychologists typically conceptualize change as occurring within the individual or the family system. Community psychology emerged because of dissatisfaction with an apparent gap between services and change conceptualized at the individual or family level, and the need for change to address institutional problems central to American society at the time, such as poverty and racism. Concerns about the disparity between the ideals versus the reality of social change were initially voiced by those working within the mental health system. In response to the report of the Joint Commission on Mental Health and Illness (1961), legislation mandating the establishment of community mental health centers was passed, and principles were developed to guide their implementation (Smith & Hobbs, 1966). These included community control and governance of mental health centers, and the importance of prevention, to be accomplished through strengthening of the criminal justice system and the schools. The change in focus from clinical issues affecting individuals to factors affecting entire settings or communities is reflected in the Swampscott conference report (Bennett *et al.*, 1966, Chapter 5, this volume).

Expanding from individual to setting-wide or population-based change was thus a central concern of community psychology at its inception, and remains a guiding principle to this day. Some of the most innovative early inventions created alternative settings, which emphasized fundamental changes in the structure of professional–client role relationships traditionally associated with service systems such as mental health or juvenile justice. Such changes contrasted with traditional, individual-based modes of service delivery. For example, Fairweather's lodge system created an alternative to traditional outpatient care for formerly hospitalized patients (Fairweather, Sanders, & Tornatzky, 1974). Lodges, located in the community, differed from standard residential "halfway houses" by radically equalizing traditional professional–client power relationships. Residents of the lodge managed all of their own daily needs; supervision was provided as needed, but eventually was phased out as group autonomy increased. Rates of rehospitalization were dramatically lower and rates of employment much higher in the lodge group compared to a control group receiving usual outpatient services (Fairweather, Sanders, & Tornatzky, 1974).

The lodge program demonstrated several strengths of community psychology in its early years. First, as an intervention, its locus of change was the setting or population level, rather than the individual. Second, the focus of change was on relationships among groups of people, or social regularities, as defined by the setting (Seidman, 1988, Chapter 11, this volume). This shift in focus brought about the possibility of change at multiple ecological levels, with effects on both the setting (e.g., the democratization of roles) and individuals (mental health and employment outcomes). Third, the lodge intervention created an alternative setting where none had previously existed.

Community psychology also began to initiate setting- and population-based interventions in social systems in areas other than mental health. Schools were a major setting for community psychology efforts. These efforts included consultation (Sarason, Levine, Goldenberg, Cherlin, & Bennett, 1966), school-based mental health programs, with education and training for parents as well as staff (Glidewell, Gildea, & Kaufman, 1973; Kantor, Gildea, & Glidewell, 1969), and the use of paraprofessionals to provide services to children deemed at risk (Cowen, Hightower, Pedro-Carroll, Work, & Wyman, 1996). Moreover, many of the early interventions focused on changing role relationships within schools for the benefit of staff and students (Felner, Ginter, & Primavera 1982, Chapter 9, this volume; Sarason, 1971; Weinstein et al., 1991, Chapter 16, this volume). The STEP program (Felner, Ginter, & Primavera 1982, Chapter 9, this volume), for instance, expanded the roles of homeroom teachers to include those of general academic advisor and primary link to home. At the same time, the STEP program created an alternative setting within large high schools by establishing "mini-schools" within a larger school: Students in particular homerooms stayed together as a social unit through all of their primary subjects. In this way, social regularities were changed not only between teacher and student, but also between students and peers, and among academic units.

Community psychologists also developed early interventions in proximal settings other than schools (Livert & Hughes, Chapter 3, this volume). Goldenberg (1971), for example, created a residential program for delinquent youth, which, like Fairweather's lodge, utilized a radically democratic, horizontal organizational structure rather than a hierarchical one, including nonprofessional helpers in collaboration with more traditional mental health professionals. Presently, successful interventions to improve physical and mental health outcomes have been developed in settings as varied as mutual help groups (Rappaport et al., 1985), gay bars (Miller, Klotz, & Eckholdt, 1998), and homes (Olds & Korfmacher, 1997).

Perhaps most important, as communities themselves became a subject of study (Chavis & Wandersman, 1990, Chapter 14, this volume; Heller, 1989; Martin, Dean, Garcia, & Hall, 1989, Chapter 13, this volume; Sarason,

1974), efforts to facilitate change at the community level were undertaken (Chavis, 1995; Hawkins, Catalano, and Associates, 1994; Serrano-García, 1984). The shift to community posed a challenge in that communities were not just another setting in which to intervene, but represented a more distal ecological level of intervention. Community coalition-building, for example, implied working with multiple stakeholders and settings within a community, and could be conceptualized as a mesosystem intervention, focusing on relationships among microsystems such as families, community agencies, or schools (Bronfenbrenner, 1979). Moreover, a community coalition could become a locus of change in itself, rather than simply a partner in installing a predetermined intervention (Chavis, 1995; D'Augelli & Hart, 1987). Outcomes could include not just individual-level goals such as reductions in aggressive behavior or drug use, but also community-level outcomes such as increases in aggregate sense of community or neighborhood-level resources.

Creating population-based interventions has proven quite difficult, in part because of the complexity of social and political forces, and in part because traditional evaluation designs such as randomized controlled trials were often less practical at the setting or systems level. Efforts to evaluate or intervene in systems of care have aimed to integrate fragmented service systems (Bickman et al., 1995; Tausig, 1987). Other efforts focused on reforming individual systems such as juvenile justice. Rappaport, Seidman, and Davidson (1979), for example, created a successful early diversion program to replace traditional court adjudication for juvenile delinquents with paraprofessional support and advocacy.

Interventions at the public policy level have been scant, despite the importance of considering psychological outcomes of social policies. Community psychologists have made contributions in some policy-relevant areas. Research such as Phillips, Howes, and Whitebook's work (1992, Chapter 18, this volume) on documenting effects of state-level child care legislation on quality of care in childcare centers enriches both the fields of public policy analysis and community psychology by illuminating connections between macro-level influences and psychological outcomes. Other examples of policy work in community psychology include work on homelessness (Shinn, 1992, Chapter 17, this volume) tobacco control legislation (Jason, 1991, 1998), and welfare policy (Yoshikawa & Hsueh, 2001; Yoshikawa, Rosman, & Hsueh, 2001).

The choice of an ecological level or setting in which to intervene still leaves open the question of *where* change should occur. Despite their label, setting-level interventions often focus on change at the individual level. A program aimed at a relatively distal ecological level (such as policy) can still be individual-focused (e.g., campaigns to sway politicians on a particular issue; Jason & Rose, 1984). Rappaport (1977), drawing on work of Watzlawick, Weakland, & Fisch (1974), has noted that mismatches may occur between the goals of an intervention and its actual effects, if they are targeted at different levels (for example, individual-level treatment programs with community-level goals). More forcefully, Albee (1982) has argued that prevention programs focused on individual-level change will never have an impact on population-level incidence of problems. Seidman (1987) also suggested that setting- or systems-level interventions must first focus on proximal outcomes at those levels, and should expect changes at the individual level to follow only as distal outcomes of setting-level change. Despite these calls for setting- or systems-level intervention, only recently have interventions been conceptualized as facilitating change at multiple, nested ecological levels. As a result, methodologies have been developed to untangle change at such levels (Bryk & Raudenbush, 1992; Perkins & Taylor, 1996), and have begun to be applied to the analysis of population-based interventions (e.g., Pentz, 1994).

The work of community psychology has expanded in these ways beyond its historical roots in community mental health. The *where* of community psychology as a field of action now incorporates a wide range of settings and ecological levels that may influence the well-being of populations. We now turn to the question of *how*.

HOW SHOULD COMMUNITY PSYCHOLOGISTS INTERVENE?

The question of *how* in intervention in community psychology, as much as *where*, has historical roots in the societal forces of the 1960s. The importance of community participation in institutions and social programs, the empowerment of disenfranchised groups, and the emphasis on democratic rather than hierarchical power structures all represent values central to Community Psychology. These values reflect, in large part, fundamental tenets of the civil rights movement and the War on Poverty.

Community psychology has made its greatest contributions in answering the question of how to intervene by its persistent examination of the values that guide interventions. The transition from assuming individual-level change as the goal of an intervention to making concrete attempts to address setting-level or population-based change has already been discussed. Other turning points in the field include transitions from prevention of mental illness to promotion of well-being, and from "top-down" interventions to "bottom-up" or grassroots efforts propelled by those who will be affected by the changes.

QUESTIONING THE OUTCOME: FROM ILLNESS PREVENTION TO HEALTH PROMOTION

Community psychology's emphasis on prevention grew out of interests in expanding outcomes from physical diseases, traditionally targeted in public health efforts, to mental illness (see Jahoda, 1958, and Caplan, 1969, for early discussions). Emerging out of the community mental health movement and using the language of public health, environmental models, focusing on contextual factors such as poverty, replaced biological models of disease prevention in the 1960s (Bloom, 1965). Despite the national excitement about community mental health at that time and the advocacy of well-known community psychologists (Albee, 1982; Cowen et al., 1975; Cowen, 1980), relatively little research in the years immediately following the Swampscott report focused on primary prevention (that is, prevention efforts initiated before early signs of problem or illness development). Instead, much of the work characterized as prevention involved early detection and intervention for existing mental health problems, and innovative alternatives to institutionalization, such as Fairweather's lodge program.

Although prevention has been cited as a goal of federal mental health policy since the 1960s (Kennedy, 1963; President's Commission on Mental Health, 1978), it is only in more recent years that the field has fully established its own institutions and federal funding streams. The setting of national research agendas to further the work of prevention (Institute of Medicine, 1994; National Institute of Mental Health, 1993) is one reflection of the institutional respect which prevention has earned. The accumulated research documenting the successes of prevention programs has contributed to the growing prominence of the field (Cowen, 1994, Chapter 21, this volume; Durlak & Wells, 1997; Price, Cowen, Lorion, & Ramos-McKay, 1988).

The scope of prevention programs to date encompasses many ecological levels, from small-group interventions focused on interpersonal cognitive factors (e.g., Shure, 1979) to interventions encompassing multiple settings in people's lives (e.g., prevention programs for children with separate classroom- and family-focused components; Wolchik et al., 1993/Chapter 20, this volume) to the development of community coalitions (Chavis, 1995; Kegeles, Hays, & Coates, 1996). Methodological advances address the increasingly complex questions of how preventive interventions achieve their effects, and for whom they work best. Mediational models explore whether prevention programs attain their intended results through effects on hypothesized intervening variables (Van Ryn & Vinokur, 1992), while moderational models identify subgroups for whom programs are more or less effective (Vinokur, Price, & Schul, 1995, Chapter 22, this volume; Wolchik et al., 1993/Chapter 20, this volume).

The preventive intervention research cycle (Institute of Medicine, 1994; National Institute of Mental Health, 1993), currently the dominant conceptual model of the field, has as its goal the prevention of mental illness. The steps outlined in the cycle consist of:

1. identifying risk and protective factors associated with the incidence of mental disorders;
2. modifying them in small-scale randomized intervention trials (reducing risk factors, strengthening protective factors);
3. revising the interventions based on quantitative evaluation of outcomes; and
4. expanding to larger-scale replications.

The framework has been used, under varying labels, as the conceptual basis of several large-scale prevention programs (Vinokur, Price, & Schul, 1995, Chapter 22, this volume; Wolchik et al., 1993, Chapter 20, this volume; Conduct Problems Prevention Research Group, 1993). The preventive intervention research cycle has been valuable in drawing together generative and evaluative phases of prevention research into one coherent, empirically-based model, and in emphasizing developmental specificity in choosing risk and protective factors to modify. Although previous work had explored the value of risk and protective factors as a basis for intervention (Price, 1987) and issues of replication and dissemination (Blakely et al., 1987, Chapter 10, this volume), these efforts had not been integrated into a comprehensive model until now.

Cowen and others have challenged the preventive intervention research for its emphasis on disorder-based models of prevention (Cowen, 1994, Chapter 21, this volume; Shore, 1998). Cowen has advocated the enhancement of competencies and psychological wellness as a complementary goal to preventing illnesses. Implications of this challenge include considering competence-enhancing processes as intervention strategies, rather than simply the reduction of risk factors. For example, a growing group of programs for school-age children aim to enhance competence, rather than prevent pathology (Elias, Gara, Schuyler, Branden-Muller, & Sayette, 1991; Weissberg, Caplan, & Harwood, 1991). A recent meta-analysis of effects of prevention programs for children and adolescents concluded that many prevention programs have enhanced positive outcomes, and that effect sizes for positive outcomes were comparable to those for problem outcomes (Durlak & Wells, 1997).

QUESTIONING WHO SHOULD GUIDE SOCIAL CHANGE: EMPOWERMENT

In the early years of the community mental health movement, community psychologists employed paraprofessionals and nonprofessionals as change agents. Even when role relationships were redefined as part of the intervention, however, most prevention programs were developed by psychologists. These programs were designed to solve problems as defined by psychologists, sometimes drawing on a community needs assessment or other forms of community input. In a seminal paper, Rappaport (1981, Chapter 8, this volume) questioned this traditional approach in favor of one in which those affected take control and guide change. He proposed *empowerment* as an alternative paradigm to prevention, defining empowerment as the process by which persons, organizations, and communities gain mastery over their affairs. Rappaport contrasted a "needs" perspective inherent in many prevention programs with a "rights" perspective characteristic of empowerment. The needs perspective might also be characterized as the "risk" perspective upon which the preventive intervention research cycle rests; it implied a top-down approach to intervention in which target populations were viewed as "dependent persons to be helped, socialized, trained, given skills, and have their illnesses prevented" (Rappaport, 1981, p. 11, Chapter 8, this volume, page 131). In contrast, the rights perspective viewed people as having a range of rights and competencies within settings that can enable them to gain mastery over their affairs.

Rappaport's 1981 article was a turning point in the field of community psychology because it raised the provocative question of not where or how to intervene, but *whether* to intervene, if interventionists did not understand how settings influence people's control over their lives. Rappaport's model of empowerment reasserted the values upon which community psychology was founded, specifically, the valuing of democratic, participatory models of decision-making over hierarchical ones. Empowerment has since been operationalized in a variety of ways in research, including perceptions of personal control and critical understanding of one's sociopolitical environment (Zimmerman, 1990), citizen participation in community life (Rappaport, 1987; Rich, Edelstein, Hallman, & Wandersman, 1995), and positive organizational climate (McMillan, Florin, Stevenson, Kerman, & Mitchell, 1995).

Community psychologists have elaborated the relationship between empowerment and intervention since the publication of Rappaport's article. Rappaport himself (1987) modified the seeming incompatibility between prevention and empowerment perspectives, distinguishing between empowerment as the basis for theory development in the area of intervention, and prevention as the actual strategy for intervention. Others had, in the interim, put forward ways in which preventive interventions might be consistent with empowerment: specifically, those that emphasize collaborating with target populations, allocating resources for competency-building, and augmenting cultural sensitivity (Felner, Jason, Moritsugu, & Farber, 1983).

Riger's critique of empowerment, based in part on feminist theory and research, pointed out some assumptions regarding power that may limit empowerment theory (Riger, 1993, Chapter 19, this volume). She argued that empowerment perpetuates an individualist perspective, critiquing Rappaport's emphasis on mastery as potentially creating competition and conflict among empowered groups. Riger called for greater integration of notions of empowerment with those of communion and connectedness. Implications for empowerment-based interventions from Riger's analysis included attention to larger contexts, which may subvert attempts to equalize power. Serrano-García (1984) described a coalition-building intervention, based on empowerment theory, to address needs perceived by residents of a community in Puerto Rico. The intervention was based explicitly on values of cultural relativity and diversity. Following an initial needs assessment, community psychologists worked with residents to form two task forces, which worked towards the twin goals of disseminating information to the community and meeting social and recreational needs. Although the intervention was successful in meeting some of the interventionists' goals and increasing citizen participation in community affairs, Serrano-García concluded that the project was not completely successful. The interventionists could not deal with the central question of Puerto Rico's political status, or succeed to a greater degree in consciousness raising, because their affiliation with a public university required a nonpartisan stance. In fact, the success of the project vis-à-vis the goals that it did achieve may have been possible because it did not "choose to deal with problems which directly confront governmental institutions" (Serrano-García, 1984, p. 198). This observation reflected concerns of other community psychologists (Elias, 1987; Gruber & Trickett, 1987) that interventions, whether prevention- or empowerment-based, pay adequate attention to larger contexts that may constrain their effects.

FUTURE DIRECTIONS IN INTERVENTION AND SOCIAL CHANGE

Community psychology has made considerable progress in its first quarter century toward understanding where and how to facilitate change. Many of its ideas about prevention have worked their way into the mainstream, as witnessed by the Institute of Medicine's 1994 report. The early successes of the field have laid the groundwork for increasingly sophisticated approaches in three areas which continue to challenge interventionists, and where community psychologists may be expected to take the lead in the future: Understanding how culture and context influence social interventions, expanding the scope and targets of intervention, and developing methods for understanding contextual change.

We are only beginning to understand the ways in which culture and context may enhance or constrain the effectiveness of interventions, and hence, how to tailor strategies for diverse populations. Such work must be based on studies of the ways that contexts shape naturally occurring processes that might be targets of intervention. Important recent studies have shown, for example, that: optimal levels of maternal restrictiveness depend on levels of neighborhood risk (Gonzales, Cauce, Friedman, & Mason, 1996, Chapter 24, this volume); optimal sources of social support vary by social context and the race of the recipient (Maton, Teti, Corns, & Vieira-Baker, 1996); and the nature of children's friendships depends on the ecological context of their care (Rizzo & Corsaro, 1995). Researchers have described how a collaborative research effort played out in a particular school setting (Weinstein *et al.*, 1991, Chapter, 16, this volume) or how an intervention to reduce the risk for AIDS infection based on diffusion of information among male prostitutes worked differently in different "hustler" bars and with different racial groups (Miller, Klotz, & Eckholdt, 1998). Others have provided more general guidance about modifying strategies for prevention research in diverse communities (Morrissey *et al.*, 1997). Community psychologists are rising to the challenge of understanding how contexts shape intervention, but additional knowledge is needed on how interventions are affected by characteristics of their host settings (Elias, 1987).

We must also increase our understanding of how to conduct intervention research that reflects the worldviews of diverse populations. Issues of cultural, gender, or sexual diversity have rarely been integrated explicitly into the conceptualization or content of interventions (French & D'Augelli, Chapter 4, this volume). Trickett (1996, Chapter 23, this volume), Hughes and Seidman (2002), Marin (1993), and Watts (1992), among others, have challenged us to do so.

Some examples of culturally anchored intervention research currently exist and raise challenges to more traditional methods. Watts (1993), for example, utilized qualitative methods in a descriptive study of black manhood development programs, which have as their goal the empowerment of black male youth. He found that activists in these programs valued aspects of their work which would not be considered as outcomes in mainstream social science evaluation research; in particular, emphases on spirituality and giving back to black communities. Other noteworthy interventions that were developed from the perspective of diverse communities include efforts to promote tobacco control policies in Northwest Indian tribes (Lichtenstein, Lopez, Glasgow, Gilbert-McRae, & Hall, 1996), an HIV prevention intervention for black adolescents (Jemmott, Jemmott, & Fong, 1998), and an intervention which successfully decoupled the link between negative stereotyping and academic underachievement for black college freshmen

(Steele, 1997). Culturally anchored interventions have not been limited to those serving racial or ethnic minority populations. Successful HIV prevention interventions have been created, for example, by and for young gay men in community settings (Kegeles, Hays, & Coates, 1996; Miller, Klotz, & Eckholdt, 1998).

The scope and targets of intervention efforts should be expanded. Although community psychologists have long focused intervention strategies on adults (e.g., Fairweather, Sanders, & Tornatzky, 1974; Serrano-García, 1984), prevention programs are too often confined to children and adolescents. The Michigan JOBS intervention, which focused on improving coping after job loss (Vinokur, Price, & Schul, 1995, Chapter 4, this volume), and the interventions for gay men just mentioned are excellent but too-rare examples of prevention directed at adults. Prevention efforts too often remain directed at individual change, despite community theory about the importance of contextual influences on behavior. Recent work on community-wide prevention and empowerment models (Hawkins, Catalano, and Associates, 1994), and efforts to build community coalitions and communities' capacity to mobilize their own resources (Chavis, 1995) are exciting counterexamples on which to build. Finally, we need to expand efforts to change social policy to promote well-being. Jason's work (1991, 1998) demonstrates that not all social policy is set by elected representatives. He has shown, for example, the importance of working with law enforcement officials to enforce rules prohibiting the sale of cigarettes to minors (leading to new legislation that permitted easier enforcement), and working with media outlets to broadcast a variety of prevention and health promotion messages.

Methods must keep pace with theory, and the methods for assessing effects and processes of experimental interventions are becoming increasingly sophisticated (West, Aiken, & Todd, 1993). We now have methods to conceptualize and measure change at multiple levels (e.g., Bryk & Raudenbusch, 1992; Pentz, 1994). However, we need better tools to examine the effects of interventions or efforts at empowerment in settings and communities, where the number of sites is often small, and where designs involving random assignment can be problematic. In-depth, longitudinal, qualitative studies (e.g., Gruber & Trickett, 1987; Serrano-García, 1984), ethnographic methods that better incorporate the voices of research participants (Burawoy et al., 1991; Burton, Allison, & Obeidallah, 1995), quasi-experimental longitudinal designs that manipulate the timing of interventions in a small number of communities or settings (Biglan et al., 1996; Miller, Klotz, & Eckholdt, 1998), and methods that focus as much on community processes as on outcomes (Goodman, Wandersman, Chinman, Imm, & Morrissey, 1996), may be well-suited to such efforts. Techniques to measure changes in empowerment have been developed (Zimmerman, 1990), but not often applied to intervention strategies.

The issues identified by participants in the Swampscott Conference in 1965 remain central to community psychology today. Facilitating change, fostering empowerment, promoting competence, and preventing dysfunction are still challenges, although we have many more examples to guide our efforts. In the past quarter century, community psychology has expanded the social sciences' understanding of social system structures and functions, and placed a new emphasis on the diversity of populations. It has expanded the focus of intervention from individuals to social systems, and developed innovative methods for assessing contextual change. In the next quarter century, community psychology should seek even more innovative ways to do justice to the contexts and complexity of human experience in the service of social change.

REFERENCES

Albee, G. W. (1982). Preventing psychopathology and promoting human potential. *American Psychologist, 37,* 1043–1050.

Bennett, C. C., Anderson, L. S., Cooper, S., Hassol, L., Klein, D. C., & Rosenblum, G. (1966). *Community psychology: A report of the Boston Conference on the Education of Psychologists for Community Mental Health.* Boston, MA: Boston University and Quincy, MA: South Shore Mental Health Center.

Bickman, L., Guthrie, P. R., Foster, E. M., Lambert, E. W., Summerfelt, W. T., Breda, C. S., & Heflinger, C. A. (1995). *Evaluating managed mental health services: The Fort Bragg experiment.* New York: Plenum Press.

Biglan, A., Ary, D., Koehn, V., Levings, D., Smith, S., Wright, Z., James, L., & Henderson, J. (1996). Mobilizing positive reinforcement in communities to reduce youth access to tobacco. *American Journal of Community Psychology, 24,* 625–638.

Blakely, C. H., Mayer, J. P., Gottschalk, R. G., Schmitt, N., Davidson, W. S., Roitman, D. B., & Emshoff, J. G. (1987). The fidelity-adaptation debate: Implications for the implementation of public sector programs. *American Journal of Community Psychology, 15,* 253–268.

Bloom, B. L. (1965). The "medical model," miasma theory, and community mental health. *Community Mental Health Journal, 1,* 333–338.

Bronfenbrenner, U. (1979). *The ecology of human development.* Cambridge, MA: Harvard University Press.

Bryk, A. & Raudenbush, S. W. (1992). *Hierarchical linear models: Applications and data analysis methods.* Newbury Park, CA: Sage.

Burawoy, M., Burton, A., Ferguson, A. A., Fox, K. J., Gamson, J., Gartrell, N., Hurst, L., Kurzman, C., Salzinger, L., Schiffman, J., & Ui, S. (1991). *Ethnography unbound: Power and resistance in the modern metropolis.* Berkeley, CA: University of California Press.

Burton, L. M., Allison, K. W., & Obeidallah, D. (1995). Social context and adolescence: Perspectives on development among inner-city African–American teens. In L. J. Crocker & A. C. Crouter (Eds.), *Pathways through adolescence: Individual development in relation to social contexts* (pp. 119–138). Hillsdale, NJ: Lawrence Erlbaum Associates.

Caplan, R. B. (1969). *Psychiatry and the community in nineteenth century America: The recurring concern with the environment in the prevention and treatment of mental disorder*. New York: Basic Books.

Chavis, D. M. (1995). Building community capacity to prevent violence through coalitions and partnerships. *Journal of Health Care for the Poor and Underserved, 6*, 234–245.

Chavis, D. M. & Wandersman, A. (1990). Sense of community in the urban environment: A catalyst for participation and community development. *American Journal of Community Psychology, 18*, 55–81.

Conduct Problems Prevention Research Group (1993). A developmental and clinical model for the prevention of conduct disorder: The FAST Track Program. *Development and Psychopathology, 4*, 509–527.

Cowen, E. L. (1980). The wooing of primary prevention. *American Journal of Community Psychology, 8*, 258–284.

Cowen, E. L. (1994). The enhancement of psychological wellness: Challenges and opportunities. *American Journal of Community Psychology, 22*, 149–179.

Cowen, E. L., Hightower, A. D., Pedro-Carroll, J. L., Work, W. C., & Wyman, P. A. (1996). *School-based prevention for at-risk children: The Primary Mental Health Project*. Washington, DC: American Psychological Association.

Cowen, E. L., Trost, M. A., Lorion, R. P., Dorr, D., Izzo, L. D., & Isaacson, R. V. (1975). *New ways in school mental health: Early detection and prevention of school maladaptation*. New York: Human Sciences Press.

D'Augelli, A. R. & Hart, M. M. (1987). Gay women, men, and families in rural settings: Toward the development of helping communities. *American Journal of Community Psychology, 15*, 79–93.

Durlak, J. A. & Wells, A. M. (1997). Primary prevention mental health programs for children and adolescents: A meta-analytic review. *American Journal of Community Psychology, 25*, 115–152.

Elias, M. J. (1987). Establishing enduring prevention programs: Advancing the legacy of Swampscott. *American Journal of Community Psychology, 15*, 539–553.

Elias, M. J., Gara, M. A., Schuyler, T. F., Branden-Muller, L. R., & Sayette, M. A. (1991). The promotion of social competence: Longitudinal study of a school-based program. *American Journal of Orthopsychiatry, 61*, 409–417.

Fairweather, G. W., Sanders, D. H., & Tornatzky, L. G. (1974). *Creating change in mental health organizations*. New York: Pergamon Press.

Felner, R. D., Ginter, M., & Primavera, J. (1982). Primary prevention during school transitions: Social support and environmental structure. *American Journal of Community Psychology, 10*, 277–290.

Felner, R. D., Jason, L. A., Moritsugu, J. N., & Farber, S. S. (1983). Preventive psychology: Evolution and current status. In R. D. Felner, L. A. Jason, J. N., Moritsugu, & S. S. Farber (Eds.), *Preventive psychology: Theory, research and practice* (pp. 3–10). New York: Pergamon Press.

French, S. E. & D'Augelli, A. R. (2002). Diversity in community psychology. In T. A. Revenson, A. R. D'Augelli, S. E. French, D. L. Hughes, D. Livert, E. Seidman, M. Shinn, & H. Yoshikawa (Eds.), *A quarter century of community psychology: Readings from the* American Journal of Community Psychology (pp. 65–77). New York: Kluwer Academic/Plenum Publishers.

Glidewell, J. C., Gildea, M. C. L., & Kaufman, M. K. (1973). The preventive and therapeutic effects of two school mental health programs. *American Journal of Community Psychology, 1*, 295–329.

Goldenberg, I. I. (1971). *Build me a mountain*. Cambridge, MA: The MIT Press.

Gonzales, N. A., Cauce, A. M., Friedman, R. J., & Mason, C. A. (1996). Family, peer, and neigh-borhood influences on academic achievement among African–American adolescents: One-year prospective effects. *American Journal of Community Psychology, 24*, 365–387.

Goodman, R. M., Wandersman, A., Chinman, M., Imm, P., & Morrissey, E. (1996). An ecologi-cal assessment of community-based interventions for prevention and health promotion: Approaches to measuring community coalitions. *American Journal of Community Psychology, 24*, 33–61.

Gruber, J. & Trickett, E. J. (1987). Can we empower others? The paradox of empowerment in the governing of an alternative public school. *American Journal of Community Psychology, 15*, 353–371.

Hawkins, J. D., Catalano, R., and Associates (1994). *Communities that care: Action for drug abuse prevention*. San Francisco, CA: Jossey Bass.

Heller, K. (1989). The return to community. *American Journal of Community Psychology, 17*, 1–15.

Hughes, D. & Seidman, E. (2002). In pursuit of a culturally anchored methodology. In T. A. Revenson, A. R. D'Augelli, S. E. French, D. L. Hughes, D. Livert, E. Seidman, M. Shinn, & H. Yoshikawa (Eds.). *Ecological research to promote social change: Methodological advances from community psychology* (pp. 243–255). New York: Kluwer Academic/Plenum Publishers.

Institute of Medicine (1994). *Reducing risks for mental disorders: Frontiers for preventive inter-vention research*. Washington, DC: National Academy Press.

Jahoda, M. (1958). *Current concepts of positive mental health*. New York: Basic Books.

Jason, L. A. (1991). Participating in social change: A fundamental value for our discipline. *American Journal of Community Psychology, 19*, 1–16.

Jason, L. A. (1998). Tobacco, drug, and HIV prevention media interventions. *American Journal of Community Psychology, 26*, 151–188.

Jason, L. A. & Rose, T. (1984). Influencing the passage of child passenger restraint legislation. *American Journal of Community Psychology, 12*, 485–495.

Jemmott, J. B., Jemmott, L. S., & Fong, G. T. (1998). Abstinence and safer sex HIV risk-reduction interventions for African American adolescents. *Journal of the American Medical Association, 279*, 1529–1536.

Joint Commission on Mental Health and Illness (1961). *Action for mental health*. New York: John Wiley.

Kantor, M. B., Gildea, M. C. L., & Glidewell, J. C. (1969). Preventive and therapeutic effects of maternal attitude change in the school setting. *American Journal of Public Health, 59*, 490–502.

Kegeles, S. M., Hays, R. B., & Coates, T. J. (1996). The Mpowerment Project: A community-level HIV prevention intervention for young gay men. *American Journal of Public Health, 86*, 1129–1136.

Kennedy, J. F. (1963, February 5). Message from the President of the United States relative to mental illness and mental retardation. Washington, DC: The White House.

Lichtenstein, E., Lopez, K., Glasgow, R. E., Gilbert-McRae, S., & Hall, R. (1996). Effectiveness of a consultation intervention to promote tobacco control policies in Northwest Indian tribes. *American Journal of Community Psychology, 24*, 639–655.

Livert, D. & Hughes, D. (2002). The ecological paradigm: Persons in settings. In T. A. Revenson, A. R. D'Augelli, S. E. French, D. L. Hughes, D. Livert, E. Seidman, M. Shinn, & H. Yoshikawa (Eds.), *A quarter century of community psychology: Readings from the American Journal of Community Psychology* (pp. 51–63). New York: Kluwer Academic/Plenum Publishers.

Marin, G. (1993). Defining culturally appropriate community interventions: Hispanics as a case study. *Journal of Community Psychology, 21*, 149–161.

Martin, J. L., Dean, L., Garcia, M., & Hall, W. (1989). The impact of AIDS on a gay community: Changes in sexual behavior, substance use, and mental health. *American Journal of Community Psychology, 17,* 269–293.

Maton, K. I., Teti, D. M., Corns, K. M., & Vieira-Baker, C. C. (1996). Cultural specificity of support sources, correlates, and contexts: Three studies of African–American and Caucasian youth. *American Journal of Community Psychology, 24,* 551–587.

McMillan, B., Florin, P., Stevenson, J., Kerman, B., & Mitchell, R. E. (1995). Empowerment praxis in community coalitions. *American Journal of Community Psychology, 23,* 699–728.

Miller, R. L., Klotz, D., & Eckholdt, H. M. (1998). HIV prevention with male prostitutes and patrons of hustler bars: Replication of an HIV preventive intervention. *American Journal of Community Psychology, 26,* 97–132.

Morrissey, E., Wandersman, A., Seybolt, D., Nation, M., Crusto, C., & Davino, K. (1997). Toward a framework for bridging the gap between science and practice in prevention. *Evaluation and Program Planning, 20,* 367–377.

National Institute of Mental Health (1993). *The prevention of mental disorders: A national research agenda.* Rockville, MD: Author.

Olds, D. L. & Korfmacher, J. (Eds.). (1997). Prenatal and early childhood home visitation I: Evolution of a program of research [Special issue]. *Journal of Community Psychology, 25* (1).

Pentz, M. A. (1994). Adaptive evaluation strategies for estimating effects of community-based drug abuse prevention programs. [Monograph] *Journal of Community Psychology, CSAP Special Issue, 22,* 26–51.

Perkins, D. D. & Taylor, R. B. (1996). Ecological assessments of community disorder: Their relationship to fear of crime and theoretical implications. *American Journal of Community Psychology, 24,* 63–108. Reprinted in T. A. Revenson, A. R. D'Augelli, S. E. French, D. L. Hughes, D. Livert, E. Seidman, M. Shinn, & H. Yoshikawa (Eds.) (2002). *Ecological research to promote social change: Methodological advances from community psychology* (pp. 127–170). New York: Kluwer Academic/Plenum Publishers.

Phillips, D. A., Howes, C., & Whitebook, M. (1992). The social policy context of child care: Effects on quality. *American Journal of Community Psychology, 20,* 25–51.

President's Commission on Mental Health (1978). *Report of recommendations.* Washington, DC: US Government Printing Office.

Price, R. H. (1987). Linking intervention research and risk factor research. In J. A. Steinberg & M. M. Silverman (Eds.), *Preventing mental disorders: A research perspective* (pp. 48–56). US Department of Health and Human Services Document No. ADM 87-1492.

Price, R. H., Cowen, E. L., Lorion, R. P., & Ramos-McKay, J. (Eds.) (1988). *Fourteen ounces of prevention: A casebook for practitioners.* Washington, DC: American Psychological Association.

Rappaport, J. (1977). *Community psychology: Values, research, and action.* New York: Holt, Rinehart and Winston.

Rappaport, J. (1981). In praise of paradox: A social policy of empowerment over prevention. *American Journal of Community Psychology, 9,* 1–25.

Rappaport, J. (1987). Terms of empowerment/exemplars of prevention: Toward a theory for community psychology. *American Journal of Community Psychology, 15,* 121–145.

Rappaport, J., Seidman, E., & Davidson, W. S. (1979). Demonstration research and manifest versus true adoption: The natural history of a research project to divert adolescents from the legal system. In R. F. Muñoz, L. R. Snowden, & J. G. Kelly (Eds.), *Social and psychological research in community settings* (pp. 101–131). San Francisco: Jossey Bass.

Rappaport, J., Seidman, E., Toro, P., McFadden, L. S., Reischl, T. M., Roberts, L. J., Salem, D. A., Stein, C. H., & Zimmerman, M. A. (1985). Collaborative research with a mutual help organization. *Social Policy, 15,* 12–24.

Rich, R. C., Edelstein, M., Hallman, W. K., & Wandersman, A. H. (1995). Citizen participation and empowerment: The case of local environmental hazards. *American Journal of Community Psychology, 23*, 657–676.

Riger, S. (1993). What's wrong with empowerment. *American Journal of Community Psychology, 21*, 279–292.

Rizzo, T. A. & Corsaro, W. A. (1995). Social support processes in early childhood friendship: A comparative study of ecological congruences in enacted support. *American Journal of Community Psychology, 23*, 389–417. Reprinted in T. A. Revenson, A. R. D'Augelli, S. E. French, D. L. Hughes, D. Livert, E. Seidman, M. Shinn, & H. Yoshikawa (Eds.). (2002). *Ecological research to promote social change: Methodological advances from community psychology* (pp. 187–216). New York: Kluwer Academic/Plenum Publishers.

Sarason, S. B. (1971). *The culture of the school and the problem of change.* Boston: Allyn & Bacon.

Sarason, S. B. (1974). *The psychological sense of community: Prospects for a community psychology.* San Francisco: Jossey Bass.

Sarason, S. B., Levine, M., Goldenberg, I. I., Cherlin, D. L., & Bennett, E. M. (1966). *Psychology in community settings: Clinical, educational, vocational, social aspects.* New York: John Wiley.

Seidman, E. (1987). Toward a framework for primary prevention research. In J. A. Steinberg & M. M. Silverman (Eds.), *Preventing mental disorders: A research perspective* (pp. 2–19) (DHHS Publication No. ADM 87-1492). Washington, DC: US Department of Health and Human Services.

Seidman, E. (1988). Back to the future, community psychology: Unfolding a theory of social intervention. *American Journal of Community Psychology, 16*, 3–24.

Serrano-García, I. (1984). The illusion of empowerment: Community development within a colonial context. *Prevention in Human Services, 3*(2/3), 173–200.

Shinn, M. (1992). Homelessness: What is a psychologist to do? *American Journal of Community Psychology, 20*, 1–24.

Shore, M. F. (1998). The making, unmaking, and remaking of primary prevention. *Journal of Mental Health, 7*, 471–477.

Shure, M. B. (1979). Training children to solve interpersonal problems: A preventive mental health program. In R. E. Muñoz, L. R. Snowden, & J. G. Kelly (Eds.), *Social and psychological research in community settings* (pp. 30–68). San Francisco: Jossey Bass.

Smith, M. B. & Hobbs, N. (1966). The community and the community mental health center. *American Psychologist, 15*, 113–118.

Steele, C. M. (1997). A threat in the air: How stereotypes shape intellectual identity and performance. *American Psychologist, 52*, 613–629.

Tausig, M. (1987). Detecting "cracks" in mental health service systems: Application of network analytic techniques. *American Journal of Community Psychology, 15*, 337–351. Reprinted in T. A. Revenson, A. R. D'Augelli, S. E. French, D. L. Hughes, D. Livert, E. Seidman, M. Shinn, & H. Yoshikawa (Eds.). (2000). *Ecological research to promote social change: Methodological advances from community psychology* (pp. 171–186). New York: Kluwer Academic/Plenum Publishers.

Trickett, E. J. (1996). A future for community psychology: The contexts of diversity and the diversity of contexts. *American Journal of Community Psychology, 24*, 209–234.

Van Ryn, M. & Vinokur, A. D. (1992). How did it work? An examination of the mechanisms through which an intervention for the unemployed promoted job-search behavior. *American Journal of Community Psychology, 20*, 577–597.

Vinokur, A. D., Price, R. H., & Schul, Y. (1995). Impact of the JOBS intervention on unemployed workers varying in risk for depression. *American Journal of Community Psychology, 23*, 39–74.

Watts, R. J. (1992). Elements of a psychology of human diversity. *Journal of Community Psychology, 20,* 116–131.

Watts, R. J. (1993). Community action through manhood development: A look at concepts and concerns from the frontline. *American Journal of Community Psychology, 21,* 333–359.

Watzlawick, P., Weakland, J. H., & Fisch, R. (1974). *Change: Principles of problem formation and problem resolution.* New York: W. W. Norton.

Weinstein, R. S., Soule, C. R., Collins, F., Cone, J., Mehlhorn, M., & Simontacchi, K. (1991). Expectations and high school change: Teacher-researcher collaboration to prevent school failure. *American Journal of Community Psychology, 19,* 333–363.

Weissberg, R. P., Caplan, M. Z., & Harwood, R. L. (1991). Promoting competence enhancing environments: A systems-based perspective on primary prevention. *Journal of Consulting and Clinical Psychology, 59,* 830–841.

West, S. G., Aiken, L. S., & Todd, M. (1993). Probing the effects of individual components in multiple component prevention programs. *American Journal of Community Psychology, 21,* 571–605. Reprinted in T. A. Revenson, A. R. D'Augelli, S. E. French, D. L. Hughes, D. Livert, E. Seidman, M. Shinn, & H. Yoshikawa (Eds.). (2002). *Ecological research to promote social change: Methodological advances from community psychology* (pp. 9–42). New York: Kluwer Academic/Plenum Publishers.

Wolchik, S. A., West, S. G., Westover, S., Sandler, I. N., Martin, A., Lustig, J., Tein, J.-Y., & Fisher, J. (1993). The children of divorce parenting intervention: Outcome evaluation of an empirically based program. *American Journal of Community Psychology, 21,* 293–331.

Yoshikawa, H. & Hsueh, J. (2001). Child development and public policy: Toward a dynamic systems perspective. *Child Development, 72,* 1887–1903.

Yoshikawa, H., Rosman, E. A., & Hsueh, J. (2001). Variation in teenage mothers' experiences of child care and other components of welfare reform: Selection processes and developmental consequences. *Child Development, 72,* 299–317.

Zimmerman, M. (1990). Taking aim on empowerment research: On the distinction between psychological and individual conceptions. *American Journal of Community Psychology, 18,* 169–177.

3

The Ecological Paradigm:
Persons in Settings

David Livert and Diane L. Hughes

Community psychology in this view is devoted to the study of general psychological processes that link social systems with individual behavior in complex interaction ... The community psychologist should have the knowledge and skill to assess and modify the reciprocal relationships between individuals and the social systems with which they interact.

BENNETT *et al.*, 1966, p. 7

A central theme of community psychology is the idea that people live in a variety of social settings that influence their well-being. Any explanation of individual behavior without reference to these influential contexts is incomplete and may lead to misdirected efforts at social change. The term "Community Psychology" itself implies a junction of setting ("Community") and individual ("Psychology") processes. At the time it was founded, the concept of studying "persons within settings" was advanced as one that was central to the field. Inquiry and action should address social system structures as a means to attaining the goal of prevention of mental health disorders (Bennett *et al.*, 1966, Chapter 5, this volume).

David Livert • Doctoral Program in Psychology, The Graduate Center of the City University of New York, New York, New York 10016-4309   **Diane L. Hughes** • Department of Psychology, New York University, New York, New York 10003.

A Quarter Century of Community Psychology: *Readings from the* American Journal of Community Psychology, edited by Tracey A. Revenson *et al.* Kluwer Academic/Plenum Publishers, New York, 2002.

Because the focus on "persons within settings" is in opposition to psychology's dominant traditions of individual-centered inquiry, Community Psychology has drawn upon two distinct social science intellectual traditions: the study of individual psychology and the study of community/societal processes (Keys & Frank, 1987a). American psychology has gone through periods of greater emphasis on the "situation" or setting; during the late 1960s many areas of psychology raised questions about person–culture–environment interactions that were similar to those posed at the Swampscott Conference (e.g., Gergen, 1973). In contrast, Community Psychology has maintained its focus on "persons in settings" as a core facet. Over the years, however, Community Psychology has expanded its conceptualization of settings, the relationship of settings to the individuals and groups who inhabit them, and the ways to study them.

A central tenet of Community Psychology is that proximal and distal environments can exert considerable influence on individual behavior, thus providing both opportunities and constraints for psychological well-being. Understanding and potentially changing behavior requires analysis of the psychological and nonpsychological characteristics of settings that create boundary conditions for the individual. Although most psychological approaches conceptualize behavior as a function of the person *and* the setting, environmental variables generally are in the background (Moos, 1973) and only unidimensional causality is examined. Community Psychology moves the settings and ecologies of human behavior into the foreground and examines the dynamic reciprocal relationships between persons and settings (Bronfenbrenner, 1977; Seidman, 1988, Chapter 11, this volume).

Community Psychologists study settings that vary considerably in size and form. Perhaps the simplest, and most common, way to define a setting is as a distinctive, physically and temporally bounded environment such as a classroom or church. Settings may also be a combination of physical milieux and the behavior within them, such as in Barker's concept of behavior settings (Schoggen, 1989). Homerooms (Felner, Ginter, & Primavera, 1982, Chapter 9, this volume), community coalitions (Chavis & Wandersman, 1990, Chapter 14, this volume), religious congregations (Maton, 1989, Chapter 12, this volume; Pargament, Silverman, Johnson, Echemendia, & Snyder, 1983), and neighborhoods (Coulton, Korbin, & Su, 1996; Perkins & Taylor, 1996) have been studied as examples of behavior settings. Settings also include the proximate social systems or networks in which the individual is embedded, such as family, workplace, or mutual-help groups; these settings may be associated with varying physical locations or may have none at all. For example, nongeographic relational communities that develop through the Internet may furnish a meaningful and influential setting, which endows members with a sense of community. Finally, societal practices or governmental policies represent broader settings or macrosystems (Bronfenbrenner, 1977) that can influence behavior in immediate environments such as the classroom (Phillips, Howes, & Whitebook, 1992, Chapter 18, this volume).

CONCEPTUAL APPROACHES TO SETTINGS

An examination of ways in which community psychologists have studied persons in settings over the past 30 years reveals considerable diversity in the definition of setting (as noted above), the phenomena of interest, and the relationship between the two. A dominant paradigm or theory has not emerged: the study of persons in settings has been as diverse as the types of settings in which we live. What emerge instead are several overlapping conceptual approaches.

Behavior Settings

Barker's pioneering study of behavior settings actually predates the founding of the field. According to behavior setting theory, settings vary in terms of "molar behaviors" or units of observed, goal-directed, person–environment interactions specific to that setting (Schoggen, 1989). Because they are temporal in nature, multiple behavior settings may be found in the same physical location: the behavior setting "school car wash" occurs in the same physical space as "school bus loading," but at different times. In addition to studying specific behavior settings, Community Psychologists have examined the commonalities within behavior settings. For example, Luke, Rappaport, and Seidman (1991) used a cluster analysis of behavioral interactions within mutual assistance groups to identify four subtypes of this behavior setting; patterns of member participation and psychological well-being varied significantly among the subtypes.

Structural Characteristics

Settings such as organizations and workplaces also vary in their structural characteristics, which include communication patterns, power distributions, and rules. Structural characteristics of settings of interest to community psychologists include staffing ratios or per-student expenditures (Moos, 1973). For example, Kelly's examination of the effects of student turnover rates on teacher perceptions of student behavior demonstrates the influence of a structural characteristic on individual interaction (1979).

Research on the construct of "manning" (later called "personing") or "staffing" also underscores the importance of structural characteristics for individual well-being, in part because these constructs represent one form of person–environment fit (French, Rodgers, & Cobb, 1974). Each setting possesses a certain number of behavioral "programs," carried out by the occupants of the setting. Understaffed settings contain a less than optimal number of occupants to carry out the programs, thus providing positive challenges in the form of multiple responsibilities and tasks, whereas over-staffed settings lead to less challenge, responsibility, and press to participate (Oxley & Barrera, 1984; Perkins, 1982). Thus, through the mechanism of fit (or misfit), settings influence mental health.

Aggregate Personal and Behavior Characteristics

Determination of person–environment fit may alternatively involve the "compositional qualities" of a setting. Compositional qualities involve the aggregate or average characteristics of setting inhabitants, such as age, ethnicity, household income, or achievement test scores—variables that hold important consequences for behavior and well-being. An overlooked study of statistical minorities (Kaufman, Gregory, & Stephan, 1990) demonstrates the power of such compositional qualities. Student adjustment was compared across elementary school classrooms which were either predominately Anglo, Hispanic, or a balance of the two; students in the statistical minority were more aggressive or withdrawn (depending on ethnic predominance) than students in the majority.

Social Climate

In contrast to the aggregate characteristics of a setting, social climate approaches explore the influence of aggregate perceptions of a setting. The concept of *social climate* received considerable research attention from community psychologists in the late 1970s and through the 1980s. An aggregation of individual phenomenological experiences of an environment, a social climate is characterized by dimensions such as the quality of relationships, opportunities for personal growth, and goal clarity within the setting (Trickett & Moos, 1974; Wright & Cowen, 1982). Social climate has been studied within families, residences, schools, spiritual communities, community organizations, and psychiatric treatment facilities. Dimensions of climate often are correlated with well-being. For example, in a study by Trickett and Moos (1974), student satisfaction and emotional adjustment in a particular class were positively related to aspects of the social climate in that class, such as teacher–student relationship, teacher effectiveness, and rule clarity. These environmental features, however, were not related to students' overall satisfaction with their school, illustrating the localized nature of social climate influences. Studying religious communities, Pargament and his colleagues (1983) found that the social climate of a congregation was related to aspects of member satisfaction: for example, individuals in congregations with high autonomy reported greater life satisfaction than those in congregations with less autonomy. Climate also varied systematically across affiliation; Catholic congregations were found to be higher in activity dimensions while predominately white Protestant churches were lower in flexibility dimensions.

RELATIONS BETWEEN PEOPLE AND SETTINGS

An integral part of Community Psychology's approach to studying persons in context is to understand the relationships, or transactions, that emerge among individuals in settings. Such relations are features that cannot be discerned from the study of individuals or settings in isolation. Sarason's (1971) landmark concept of *behavioral regularities* within a setting refers to the patterns of individual behavior or transactions between individuals. Sarason also stresses the importance of *programmatic regularities*—the formal and informal practices in settings—that result in behavioral regularities. For example, programmatic regularities in school curricula may lead teachers to rely primary upon lecture-oriented teaching styles that discourage student-initiated questions and deeper comprehension. Both Sarason (1977) and Wicker (1987) advise that community psychologists should endeavor to identify behavioral regularities as a means of understanding settings and the behaviors within them; such regularities are typically overlooked and unquestioned by those populating the setting. Seidman's definition of *social regularities* (1988, Chapter 11, this volume) expands the construct to include the relations or connections among people in that setting *that are sustained and repeated over time* (cf. Barker's notion of standing patterns of behavior).

Just as individuals are located in settings, settings themselves are nested in broader social systems. In our view, Bronfenbrenner (1977) provided the most influential articulation of a nested systems framework. *Microsystems* consist of role relations and interpersonal structures in an immediate setting containing the focal individual, such as family, work, or school. Throughout one's day and one's lifespan, individuals engage in a series of settings and associated microsystems. Microsystems are themselves part of a relational system, termed the *mesosystem*. An adult's mesosystem might consist of home, family, work, or religious and volunteer organizations. Formal and informal social structures that do not contain the focal person but which affect microsystems are called *exosystems*. For example, a parent's stress at work may lead to subsequent undesirable interactions with his or her children at home.

Bronfenbrenner's framework has been used by community psychologists in theory development (e.g., Seidman, 1988, Chapter 11, this volume), inquiry (e.g., Phillips, Howes, & Whitebook, 1992, Chapter 18, this volume) and intervention (e.g., Felner, Ginter, & Primavera, 1982, Chapter 9, this volume). Similar frameworks can be found in Berger and Neuhaus' discussion of the potential mediating structures linking individual and society (1981), and Wicker's expansion of Barker's behavior setting theory (1987), a revision that addresses the geographic, historical, and organizational context of behavior settings.

Network analysis also has been used to understand the social structural influences on settings and individual behavior. For example, DeFour and Hirsch (1990, Chapter 15, this volume) found that African–American graduate students whose social networks were more dense (i.e., interconnected) were more satisfied with their graduate experience. Contact with black faculty members outside of the university setting was also associated with adjustment, illustrating a social regularity maintained across settings (the mesosystem level). Network analyses need not use individuals as the unit of analysis. Tausig (1987) examined the mesosystem level network of mental health service agencies in a single community. Identification of the links between agencies (or lack thereof) could then be used to improve service delivery at the system level.

Phillips and her colleagues (1992, Chapter 18, this volume) exemplify how distal influences such as state regulatory environments affect microlevel settings. More desirable teacher–student interaction styles in day care settings were found in states with more stringent regulatory environments; better quality interactions were also more likely to be found in nonprofit centers. Studies of the relationship between regional economic variation and mental health care utilization similarly straddle system levels (e.g., Banziger, Smith, & Foos, 1982; Cahill, 1983; Frank, 1981).

AN EMPIRICAL EXAMPLE OF
"PERSONS-IN-SETTINGS": NEIGHBORHOODS

Over the past 25 years, community psychologists have generated a substantial and diverse body of empirical research and interventions that embody ecological approaches to understanding and changing selected phenomena of interest. In particular, a great deal of research has examined how an individual's proximate neighborhood influences psychological outcomes, the behavioral regularities within that setting, and as a consequence, behavior in other settings. Neighborhood influences have been studied in terms of adolescent academic achievement (Brooks-Gunn, Duncan, Klebanov, & Sealand, 1993; Gonzales, Cauce, Friedman, & Mason, 1996, Chapter 24, this volume), adolescent drug use and other problem behaviors (Allison et al., 1999), and fear of crime (Perkins & Taylor, 1996; Riger, LeBailly, & Gordon, 1981).

Community psychologists have also examined how citizen participation may be linked to neighborhood context. One of the field's distinctive concepts, a psychological sense of community, originally was developed by Sarason (1974) and operationalized by community psychologists such as McMillan and Chavis (1986), Davidson and Cotter (1993), and Plas and Lewis (1996). A sense of community arises from the relationship between an individual and others within a territorial or relational community. It has been shown to influence individual participation in neighborhood organizations and fear of crime; reciprocally, participation in one's neighborhood environment may increase one's sense of community and feelings of empowerment (Chavis & Wandersman, 1990, Chapter 14, this volume; Perkins, Florin, Rich, Wandersman, & Chavis, 1990; Saegert & Winkel, 1996; Taylor, Gottfredson, & Brower, 1985).

MODELS OF INFLUENCE

As community researchers have intensified efforts to elucidate the relationship between individuals and settings, they have conceptualized these linkages in a variety of ways. Approaches in which environmental characteristics directly influence phenomena of interest within that setting could be termed *main effects* models. These models are probably the most widely tested in studies found in the *American Journal of Community Psychology* (*AJCP*) (Gonzales, Cauce, Friedman, & Mason, 1996, Chapter 24, this volume). For example, social climate studies, such as that of Wright and Cowen (1982), describe linkages between the classroom environment and student-level outcomes. Rizzo and Corsaro's ethnographic study of friendship (1995) is another exemplar of main effects: different classroom tasks and emotional requirements prompted friendships that differed in form and function.

Distal environments may also alter individual-level outcomes or social regularities through their influence on more proximate settings. Such *mediational* approaches can explicate the links between the individual and greater macrosocial influences. Simmons, Johnson, Beaman, Conger, & Whitbeck (1996) found that the effects of community impoverishment on adolescent adjustment and deviant behavior were mediated by parenting and peer behavior. Sampson, Raudenbush, and Earls (1997) provide a sophisticated demonstration of how perceptions of collective efficacy can mediate the relationship between poverty and crime in Chicago neighborhoods.

Environmental/ecological studies also examine *moderatoral models* or interaction effects, in which the influence of individual characteristics is conditioned by setting, underscoring the importance of "fit" between individual and environment. One of community psychology's unique contributions has been inquiry that describes how the elements of sociocultural diversity interact with settings (Trickett, 1996, Chapter 23, this volume). For example, immigrants' experience of assimilation may be influenced strongly by the community in which it takes place: Russian immigrants who settle in Washington, DC may assimilate more quickly than those in New York City who have moved into more homogeneous immigrant communities.

Settings may also moderate individual-level psychological processes. Maton (1989, Chapter 12, this volume) examined the process of coping with stress across three types of behavior settings: religious congregations, self-help groups, and senior citizen centers. In church congregations and self-help groups, the impact of stressful events on coping reactions was moderated by the social climate of the setting, whereas in senior citizens centers, stress was related to coping in the same way across different perceptions of social climate. Likewise, Gonzales and colleagues (1996, Chapter 24, this volume) found that the influence of parenting styles and peer interactions on children's academic achievement was moderated by characteristics of the neighborhood. In low-risk neighborhoods greater maternal control was associated with lower grade point averages (GPAs), however peer support did not influence achievement. In contrast, in high-risk neighborhoods, neither maternal control nor peer support was predictive of higher GPAs.

If explanations for individual behavior and psychological well-being are incomplete without an understanding of settings, then attempts to improve well-being are incomplete without changes in setting-level phenomena. A distinct contribution of Community Psychology has been the demonstration of effective interventions based at the school, neighborhood, or community level, instead of traditionally individual-centered interventions for the same problems (Kelly, 1990). Yoshikawa and Shinn (Chapter 2, this volume) review how community psychologists have formulated and implemented interventions that utilize ecological approaches to improve well-being.

TAKING ACCOUNT AND LOOKING AHEAD

The past 25 years have witnessed greater emphasis on environmental factors in community psychology, as well as in social psychology, psychiatry, psychobiology, and medicine (Moos, 1996). However, psychologists generally continue to devote most of their efforts to the understanding of individual-based phenomena, leaving context in the background (Shinn, 1996). Even within community psychology, many argue that the contextual or ecological orientation has achieved, at best, "partial paradigm acceptance" (Trickett, 1996, Chapter 23, this volume).

Although community psychologists have examined contextual influences in an increasing variety of settings outside of the laboratory and mental health center, many of the major environments remain understudied (Shinn, 1987). Moos (1996) urged more study of settings' influences over time, to understand what kinds of settings have enduring influences on people, and how settings jointly influence behavior. A special issue of *AJCP* on organizational settings (Keys & Frank, 1987b) foretold Moos's call for more community research on settings themselves as phenomena of interest, particularly investigations of their dynamic and configural properties. Settings can be studied as phenomena with developmental stages (Bartunek & Betters-Reed, 1987; Moos, 1996); similarly, Kelly (1990), among others, has emphasized the need for longitudinal approaches to understanding contexts. Including a temporal dimension will provide insight regarding how settings influence ongoing regularities and individual development over time.

Although studies of persons and settings have also generally utilized single methodical approaches, the methodologies for studying persons-in-settings is becoming more diverse and sophisticated. A recent special issue of *AJCP* devoted entirely to ecological assessment detailed a variety of strategies used by community psychologists to assess setting features, and to link features at different levels of analysis to individual phenomena (Shinn, 1996). For example, self-reports, observations, and media reports can provide complementary measures of crime and disorder within the same neighborhood (Perkins & Taylor, 1996). In addition, community psychologists are beginning to use qualitative methodologies that can be particularly effective avenues for understanding individuals' experience of settings, and how influences may vary across cultures (Hughes & DuMont, 1993, Plas & Lewis, 1996). At the same time, recent statistical advances will help researchers understand different levels of ecological influence (Bronfenbrenner, 1977). Techniques such as multi-level modeling (Bryk & Raudenbush, 1992) offer community psychologists more powerful ways to analyze individual, setting, and macrosocial data.

By expanding ecological approaches and developing original conceptual paradigms, community psychologists have delineated a broad range of
theoretical frameworks for inquiry and action. Concurrently, an expanding
toolbox of ecological methods has emerged for inquiry within these frameworks. "Grand" or macro theories are not likely to unify these diverse
approaches to understanding the interplay of persons and settings. Taking
settings seriously may be antithetical to the development of general theories
that apply to all settings. Rather, future studies will probably continue to
occupy the theoretical "middle range" with a focus on specific settings or
types of settings. Regardless of what theories emerge, Community
Psychology appears to be committed to continuing its study of the multifac-
eted relationships between persons and settings through the next 25 years.

REFERENCES

Allison, K. W., Crawford, I., Leone, P. E., Trickett, E., Perez-Febles, A., Burton, L. M., &
    LeBlanc, R. (1999). Adolescent substance use: Preliminary examinations of school and
    neighborhood context. *American Journal of Community Psychology, 27*, 111–141.
Banziger, G., Smith, R. K., & Foos, D. (1982). Economic indicators of mental health service
    utilization in Rural Appalachia. *American Journal of Community Psychology, 10*,
    669–686.
Bartunek, J. M. & Betters-Reed, B. L. (1987). The stages of organizational creation. *American
    Journal of Community Psychology, 15*, 287–304.
Bennett, C. C., Anderson, L. S., Cooper, S., Hassol, L., Klein, D. C., & Rosenblum, G. (1966).
    *Community psychology: A report of the Boston Conference on the education of psycholo-
    gists for community mental health.* Boston: Boston University Press.
Berger, P. L. & Neuhaus, R. J. (1981). *To empower people.* Washington, DC: American
    Enterprise Institute for Public Policy Research.
Bronfenbrenner, U. (1977). Toward an experimental ecology of human development.
    American Psychologist, 32, 513–531.
Brooks-Gunn, J., Duncan, G. J., Klebanov, P. K., & Sealand, N. (1993). Do neighborhoods influ-
    ence child and adolescent development? *American Journal of Sociology, 99*, 353–395.
Bryk, A. S. & Raudenbush, S. W. (1992). *Hierarchical linear models: Applications and data
    analysis methods.* Newbury Park, CA: Sage.
Cahill, J. (1983). Structural characteristics of the macroeconomy and mental health:
    Implications for primary research. *American Journal of Community Psychology, 11*,
    553–571.
Chavis, D. M. & Wandersman, A. (1990). Sense of community in the urban environment: A cat-
    alyst for participation and community development. *American Journal of Community
    Psychology, 18*, 55–81.
Coulton, C. J., Korbin, J. E., & Su, M. (1996). Measuring neighborhood context for young chil-
    dren in an urban area. *American Journal of Community Psychology, 24*, 5–32. Reprinted
    in T. A. Revenson, A. R. D'Augelli, S. E. French, D. L. Hughes, D. Livert, E. Seidman, M.
    Shinn, & H. Yoshikawa (Eds.), *Ecological research to promote social change:
    Methodological advances from community psychology* (pp. 99–126). New York: Kluwer
    Academic/Plenum Publishers.

Davidson, W. B. & Cotter, P. R. (1993). Psychological sense of community and support for public school taxes. *American Journal of Community Psychology, 21*, 59–66.

DeFour, D. C. & Hirsch, B. J. (1990). The adaptation of black graduate students: A social network approach. *American Journal of Community Psychology, 18*, 487–503.

Felner, R. D., Ginter, M., & Primavera, J. (1982). Primary prevention during school transitions: Social support and environmental structure. *American Journal of Community Psychology, 10*, 277–290.

Frank, J. A. (1981). Economic change and mental health in an uncontaminated setting. *American Journal of Community Psychology, 9*, 395–410.

French, J. P., Rodgers, W., & Cobb, S. (1974). Adjustment as person-environment fit. In: G. V. Coelho, D. A. Hamberg, & J. E. Adams (Eds.), *Coping and adjustment* (pp. 316–333). New York: Basic Books.

Gergen, K. J. (1973). Social psychology as history. *Journal of Personality and Social Psychology, 26*, 309–320.

Gonzales, N. A., Cauce, A. M., Friedman, R. J., & Mason, C. A. (1996). Family, peer, and neighborhood influences on academic achievement among African–American adolescents: One-year prospective effects. *American Journal of Community Psychology, 24*, 365–387.

Hughes, D. & DuMont, K. (1993). Using focus groups to facilitate culturally-anchored research. *American Journal of Community Psychology, 21*, 775–806. Reprinted in T. A. Revenson, A. R. D'Augelli, S. E. French, D. L. Hughes, D. Livert, E. Seidman, M. Shinn, & H. Yoshikawa (Eds.), *Ecological research to promote social change: Methodological advances from community psychology* (pp. 243–255). New York: Kluwer Academic/Plenum Publishers.

Kaufman, K. Gregory, W. L., & Stephan, W. G. (1990). Maladjustment in statistical minorities within ethnically unbalanced classrooms. *American Journal of Community Psychology, 18*, 757–765.

Kelly, J. G. (Ed.) (1979). *Adolescent boys in high schools: A psychological study of coping and adaptation*. Hillside, NJ: Lawrence Erlbaum Associates.

Kelly, J. G. (1990). Changing contexts and the field of community psychology. *American Journal of Community Psychology, 18*, 769–792.

Keys, C. B. & Frank, S. (1987a). Community psychology and the study of organizations: A reciprocal relationship. *American Journal of Community Psychology, 15*, 239–252.

Keys, C. B. & Frank, S. (1987b). Organizational perspectives in community psychology. [Special issue]. *American Journal of Community Psychology, 15*(3).

Luke, D. A., Rappaport, J., & Seidman, E. (1991). Setting phenotypes in a mutual help organization: Expanding behavior setting theory. *American Journal of Community Psychology, 19*, 147–167. Reprinted in T. A. Revenson, A. R. D'Augelli, S. E. French, D. L. Hughes, D. Livert, E. Seidman, M. Shinn, & H. Yoshikawa (Eds.), *Ecological research to promote social change: Methodological advances from community psychology* (pp. 217–238). New York: Kluwer Academic/Plenum Publishers.

Maton, K. I. (1989). Community settings as buffers of life stress? Highly supportive churches, mutual help groups, and senior centers. *American Journal of Community Psychology, 17*, 203–232.

McMillan, D. W. & Chavis, D. M. (1986). Sense of community: A definition and theory. *Journal of Community Psychology, 14*, 6–23.

Moos, R. H. (1973). Conceptualizations of human environments. *American Psychologist, 28*, 652–665.

Moos, R. H. (1996). Understanding environments: The key to improving social processes and program outcomes. *American Journal of Community Psychology, 24*, 193–201.

Oxley, D. & Barrera, M. (1984). Undermanning theory and the workplace: Implications of setting size for job satisfaction and social support. *Environment and Behavior, 16*, 211–234.

Pargament, K. I., Silverman, W., Johnson, S., Echemendia, R., & Snyder, S. (1983). The psychosocial climate of religious congregations. *American Journal of Community Psychology, 11*, 351–381.

Perkins, D. D. & Taylor, R. B. (1996). Ecological assessments of community disorder: Their relationship to fear of crime and theoretical implications. *American Journal of Community Psychology, 24*, 63–108. Reprinted in T. A. Revenson, A. R. D'Augelli, S. E. French, D. L. Hughes, D. Livert, E. Seidman, M. Shinn, & H. Yoshikawa (Eds.), *Ecological research to promote social change: Methodological advances from community psychology* (pp. 127–170). New York: Kluwer Academic/Plenum Publishers.

Perkins, D. D., Florin, P., Rich, R. C., Wandersman, A., & Chavis, D. M. (1990). Participation and the social and physical environment of residential blocks: Crime and community context. *American Journal of Community Psychology, 18*, 83–115.

Perkins, D. V. (1982). Individual differences and task structure in the performance of a behavior setting: An experimental evaluation of Barker's Manning Theory. *American Journal of Community Psychology, 10*, 617–634.

Phillips, D. A., Howes, C., & Whitebook, M. (1992). The social policy context of child care: Effects on quality. *American Journal of Community Psychology, 20*, 25–52.

Plas, J. M. & Lewis, S. E. (1996). Environmental factors and sense of community in a planned town. *American Journal of Community Psychology, 24*, 109–143.

Riger, S., LeBailly, R. K., & Gordon, M. T. (1981). Community ties and urbanites' fear of crime: An ecological investigation. *American Journal of Community Psychology, 9*, 653–666.

Rizzo, T. A. & Corsaro, W. A. (1995). Social support processes in early childhood friendship: A comparative study of ecological congruences in enacted support. *American Journal of Community Psychology, 23*, 389–417. Reprinted in T. A. Revenson, A. R. D'Augelli, S. E. French, D. L. Hughes, D. Livert, E. Seidman, M. Shinn, & H. Yoshikawa (Eds.), *Ecological research to promote social change: Methodological advances from community psychology* (pp. 187–216). New York: Kluwer Academic/Plenum Publishers.

Saegert, S. & Winkel, G. (1996). Paths to community empowerment: Organizing at home. *American Journal of Community Psychology, 24*, 517–550.

Sampson, R. J., Raudenbush, S. W., & Earls, F. (1997). Neighborhoods and violent crime: A multilevel study of collective efficacy. *Science, 277*, 918–924.

Sarason, S. B. (1971). *The culture of the school and the problem of change.* Boston: Allyn & Bacon.

Sarason, S. B. (1974). *The psychological sense of community: Prospects for a community psychology.* San Francisco, CA: Jossey-Bass.

Sarason, S. B. (1977). A "cultural" limitation of system approaches to educational reform. *American Journal of Community Psychology, 5*, 277–288.

Schoggen, P. (1989). *Behavior settings: A revision and extension of Roger G. Barker's ecological psychology.* Stanford, CA: Stanford University Press.

Seidman, E. (1988). Back to the future, community psychology: Unfolding a theory of social intervention. *American Journal of Community Psychology, 16*, 3–24.

Shinn, M. (1987). Expanding Community Psychology's domain. *American Journal of Community Psychology, 15*, 555–574.

Shinn, M. (1996). Ecological assessment: Introduction to the special issue. *American Journal of Community Psychology, 24*, 1–4.

Simmons, R. L., Johnson, C., Beaman, J., Conger, R. D., & Whitbeck, L. B. (1996). Parents and peer groups as mediators of the effect of community structure on adolescent problem behavior. *American Journal of Community Psychology, 24*, 145–172.

Tausig, M. (1987). Detecting "cracks" in mental health service systems: Application of network analytic techniques. *American Journal of Community Psychology*, *15*, 337–351. Reprinted in T. A. Revenson, A. R. D'Augelli, S. E. French, D. L. Hughes, D. Livert, E. Seidman, M. Shinn, & H. Yoshikawa (Eds.), *Ecological research to promote social change: Methodological advances from community psychology* (pp. 171–186). New York: Kluwer Academic/Plenum Publishers.

Taylor, R. B., Gottfredson, S. D., & Brower, S. (1985). Attachment to place: Discriminant validity, and impacts of disorder and diversity. *American Journal of Community Psychology*, *13*, 525–542.

Trickett, E. J. (1996). A future for community psychology: The contexts of diversity and the diversity of contexts. *American Journal of Community Psychology*, *24*, 209–234.

Trickett, E. J. & Moos, R. H. (1974). Personal correlates of contrasting environments: Student satisfactions in high school classrooms. *American Journal of Community Psychology*, *2*, 1–12.

Wicker, A. W. (1987). *Behavior settings reconsidered: Temporal stages, resources, internal dynamics, context.* In D. Stokols & I. Altman (Eds.) *Handbook of Environmental Psychology* (pp. 613–653), New York: John Wiley.

Wright, S. & Cowen, E. L. (1982). Student perception of school environment and its relationship to mood, achievement, popularity, and adjustment. *American Journal of Community Psychology*, *10*, 687–704.

Yoshikawa, H. & Shinn, M. (2002). Facilitating change: Where and how should community psychology intervene? In T. A. Revenson, A. R. D'Augelli, S. E. French, D. L. Hughes, D. Livert, E. Seidman, M. Shinn, & H. Yoshikawa (Eds.), *A quarter century of community psychology: Readings from the* American Journal of Community Psychology (pp. 33–49). New York: Kluwer Academic/Plenum Publishers.

4

Diversity in Community Psychology

Sabine E. French and Anthony R. D'Augelli

The community psychologist should have the knowledge and skills to assess and modify the reciprocal relationships between individuals and the social systems with which they interact.

BENNETT *et al.*, 1966, p. 7

What does diversity mean for community psychology? What has it meant in the past, what should it mean in the future? Community psychology has always held as an ideal a focus on the rich variability of individual behaviors in diverse community and cultural contexts; however, a focus on diversity in community psychology research often has fallen short of this ideal. Beyond its meaning as an analysis of individual differences or sociodemographic classifiers, diversity in community psychology has taken on a more complex contemporary meaning. We begin this discussion with an examination of how the definition of diversity has evolved, and how it has been represented in community psychology research.

    The attention to diversity in community psychology reflects the convictions of the field's originators that conceptual approaches and empirical research on mental health problems that ignored the social context would inevitably "blame the victim" (Ryan, 1971, 1994) by locating the causal mechanisms for problems in individual deficits or predispositions. Such

Sabine E. French • Department of Psychology, University of California, Riverside, California 92521   **Anthony R. D'Augelli** • Department of Human Development and Family Studies, The Pennsylvania State University, University Park, Pennsylvania 16802.

A Quarter Century of Community Psychology: *Readings from the* American Journal of Community Psychology, edited by Tracey A. Revenson *et al*. Kluwer Academic/Plenum Publishers, New York, 2002.

analyses were not only inadequate as explanations, but also had the potential to perpetuate problems by displacing a focus from social structural factors of power and privilege. As a paradigm, community psychology would transcend traditional individual psychology, whose epistemology might result in research that informed approaches to changing individuals, but was inadequate for research that would inform change at the community level. Moreover, some argued that traditional psychology was woefully inadequate to the task of empowering individuals, families, and communities. Without a community perspective, groups that were historically marginalized in society would remain so; a rigorous analysis of social and community life could immensely help such groups.

With such goals in mind, a consistent theme in the field's history has been diversity. Diversity has become a common, yet imprecisely used term that has been reconceptualized continually over the last 25 years (Trickett, Watts, & Birman, 1993). Most frequently, discussions of diversity have centered on increasing the representation of racial and ethnic groups in programs or studies. At first, diversity was explored by paying attention to the diverse social contexts of people's lives. Later, it would become a framework by which distinct groups in society could be understood, and their problems remedied or prevented. Most recently, diversity has become a framework for understanding cultural and subcultural variability, broadly defined—a conceptual model for understanding and researching people in their cultural contexts as well as a strategy for designing and evaluating ecologically valid social and community interventions. These more inclusive views will continue to influence the way that community psychologists do their work (Trickett, 1996, Chapter 23, this volume).

THE DIVERSITY OF SOCIAL CONTEXTS

An appreciation of how individual behavior is elicited, shaped, and reinforced by differing social contexts was the first approach community psychologists took to embodying diversity in their work. Both proximal and distal social circumstances affect behavior in community settings. Over 20 years ago, leaders in the field were making impassioned pleas for the field to focus on connections between people and settings. Rieff (1975) urged the field to understand "the relationship between history and biography, between the individual's becoming and history as it is emerging" (p. 189). A year later, Sarason (1976) wrote "community psychologists ... are people who would like to change the world," (p. 258) but warned that a naïve interest in change would likely backfire. Social settings have idiosyncratic histories that must be understood, and early work in community psychology involved attempts to chart the nature of the diverse social settings of people's lives (Moos, 1976).

Defining settings of interest and their parameters was, and continues to be, an enormous challenge (Livert & Hughes, Chapter 3, this volume). Should the community psychologist focus on the neighborhood, the school, the entire community, or on social policies? Clearly, no one approach could address the issue, and community psychologists developed the concept of multiple levels of analysis, to allow for the study of different social contexts and, under the best of conditions, the simultaneous study of interlocking social settings. Dohrenwend's (1978, Chapter 7, this volume) classic paper on the linkages between social stressors and mental health outcomes exemplifies the conceptual breakthroughs that community psychology could produce. Such a complex model of community stress generates many different approaches to change, and Dohrenwend's list of interventions ranging from crisis intervention to political action for disadvantaged groups shows the generativity of a conceptual model that has diversity at its core.

The durability of Dohrenwend's model can be seen a decade later in Martin, Dean, Garcia, and Hall's (1989, Chapter 13, this volume) work about how the AIDS epidemic, a community stressor, dramatically changed the sexual behavior of gay men in one particular context within one particular time period. Other investigators would focus on different levels of social impact. Phillips, Howes, and Whitebook's (1992, Chapter 18, this volume) analysis charts the impact of legislation (child care regulations) on individuals (children) in diverse settings (child care facilities). Using a more proximal influence model, Maton's (1989, Chapter 12, this volume) research not only focuses on community groups that influence people's adaptation, but also distinguishes among three kinds of settings (churches, mutual help groups for bereaved parents, and senior citizen centers), and shows how the settings work in different ways to buffer people from common life stressors. A number of other community psychologists have also shown how different settings operate in different ways to buffer people from common life stressors. For instance, the work of Felner and colleagues (1982, Chapter 9, this volume), DeFour and Hirsch (1990, Chapter 15, this volume), and Weinstein and colleagues (1991, Chapter 16, this volume) demonstrates how the social structures of different school settings affect students' (and teachers') lives. Their research emphasizes how the broad category of social structure must be carefully deconstructed to more precisely capture the impact of distinctive environments on adaptation and change.

As early as 1974, community psychologists were exploring how differences in school environments affected students (Trickett & Moos, 1974). By 1996, Gonzales, Cauce, Friedman and Mason's work (1996, Chapter 24, this volume) showed what over 20 years could accomplish in studying the diversity of settings. By showing how academic achievement among African–American adolescents is influenced by a complex array of family, peer, and neighborhood factors, Gonzales and her colleagues revealed how community psychologists' understanding of the diverse contexts of people's lives has grown richer and more complex. Recently, an entire issue of the journal was devoted to prevention research in rural communities (Muehrer, 1997). The core question—how very different settings influence people—remains simple, but its articulation has become increasingly sophisticated, as have the research methodologies used to explore the question (Bryk & Raudenbush, 1992; Coulton, Korbin, & Su, 1996; Luke, Rappaport, & Seidman, 1991; Perkins & Taylor, 1996; Rizzo & Corsaro, 1995; Shinn & Rapkin, 2000; Tausig, 1987).

DIVERSITY AS A TOOL FOR UNDERSTANDING DISADVANTAGE

In another approach to the issue of diversity, community psychology has provided conceptual and methodological tools through which the lives of people in communities who had historically been disenfranchised could be understood. Working to improve the lives of the poor, especially those from marginalized ethnic and racial groups in inner cities, was the first challenge the field confronted, and it remains an important focus today. An excellent example is Shinn's important work on homeless families (1997, Chapter 17, this volume). Shinn shatters the stereotype that homelessness results from mental dysfunction, showing that the availability of housing—a contextual or social structural factor—plays a crucial role.

The destructive power of cultural stereotypes that purport to explain the difficult lives of people living outside the mainstream can be reduced by a careful review of how social contextual factors contribute to families' problems. Initially, community mental health workers were ahead of researchers in confronting issues of diversity. By moving from psychiatric hospitals and other institutional settings into the community to provide services to underserved populations, they directly confronted the diversity of people's social contexts. This experience inevitably created skepticism about the appropriateness of the mental health services that professionals provided. To what extent was individual psychotherapy, even if provided in a storefront clinic, the solution to the complex life challenges faced by people in their everyday lives? Not only was it impossible to train enough professionals to provide such help, but there was the unavoidable question of its effectiveness. At minimum, this scrutiny led to the use of local nonprofessionals, whether called "indigenous paraprofessionals" or "community helpers," to serve helping functions, based on the premise that resistance to change could be mitigated by a familiar change agent who could translate general principles of help-giving into locally relevant language and custom.

An early example of this is a community mental health program for American Indians living on reservations, a group that had been seriously underserved (Kahn *et al.*, 1975). A more recent example of how community psychologists work to meet the needs of disadvantaged people in their own settings can be seen in an HIV-prevention intervention that uses the social networks of intravenous drug users as agents of change (Latkin, Mandell, Vlahov, Oziemkowska, & Celentano, 1996). Another example is the collaboration by community psychologists at the University of Illinois, Urbana-Champaign with a mutual help organization for people with mental illness (Zimmerman *et al.*, 1991). The rich array of self-help and mutual help organizations now in place in most communities reflects the recognition that different community intervention approaches are needed to deal with different life experiences. Community psychologists have often taken the lead in these projects to provide empirical data that address the issue of such programs' effectiveness.

RESEARCHING AND AFFIRMING CULTURAL DIVERSITY

Despite the values of the field, it would take time for diversity to make its way into research conducted by community psychologists. In the first decade of the *American Journal of Community Psychology* (*AJCP*), it was not uncommon for study participants' racial and ethnic backgrounds to be omitted from sample descriptions. Such oversights led to homogenization of communities and an overgeneralization of research findings to "the community." As diversity was increasingly acknowledged in the empirical enterprise of community psychology, researchers made greater efforts to include nonwhite participants and identify them as such.

Progress has been slow. One of the first empirical analyses of how community psychology had fared in its commitment to diversity was published by Loo, Fong, and Iwamasa (1988). Summarizing 20 years of published work in community psychology journals, they found that only 11% of the articles related to ethnic minority communities. Few studies had lived up to the field's "original goals of furthering cultural diversity and devoting greater research and service to ethnic minority populations" (p. 341). Those studies that did accomplish these goals were of several types: studies of single ethnic minority groups; comparisons of particular ethnic minority groups with white samples; studies of international populations; or comparisons between ethnic minority groups. Among the small number of articles published on single ethnic minority groups, half were on African Americans, 30% were on Hispanic or Puerto Rican people, 12% were on Asian Americans, and only 4% studied Native Americans. Bernal and Enchautegui-de-Jesus (1994) reviewed the status of Latinos and Latinas in the community psychology literature from 1973 through 1992, and concluded that about 4% of all published papers focused on this population or had samples with a minimum of 15% Latino/a participants. Serious concerns have also been raised about the field's treatment of women and gender (Mulvey, 1988; Swift, Bond, & Serrano-García, 2000) and lesbian and gay populations (Garnets & D'Augelli, 1994). A study of empowerment of people with physical disabilities (Fawcett et al., 1994) is one of the few in community psychology that has focused on that population.

Community psychology first approached incorporating diverse populations into its research with studies in which data on ethnic minority groups were compared to findings on European Americans, who served as a normative comparison group. In this approach, diversity is essentially a demographic construct. In addition, the issues studied evolved from a majority worldview, i.e., with topics and research questions framed on and tested with European–American samples being extended to other populations. Community psychology's next step was intensive studies of "underrepresented groups," most notably, analyses of individual ethnic/racial minority groups or of women. Some projects compared two or more minority groups to one another, and did not use European Americans as a normative comparison group. This shift was partly a result of the growing numbers of psychologists from underrepresented groups asserting their interests, and advocating for the study of particular groups. Nonetheless, the topics studied were not culturally anchored (Hughes & Seidman, 2002; Hughes, Seidman, & Williams, 1993), and were often replications of earlier studies.

More recently, community psychologists have studied diversity by researching issues salient to particular groups—women; racial/ethnic minority groups; and lesbian, gay, and bisexual populations. Research in this vein has tended to highlight the challenges faced by the particular group involved, with the general goal of bringing these problems to the attention of policymakers, funding sources, and social scientists. These studies of single groups often have a problem or deficit focus. Without an understanding of the social contextual factors that contribute to the problems shown by a particular group, such studies inadvertently reinforce the view that the group has deficits. Hughes and Dodge's (1997) study of how workplace discrimination and bias affect the lives of African–American women is an excellent example of how community psychologists can study particular groups in ways that avoid blaming the victims by systematically attending to differences in settings and contextual stressors.

Community psychology has thus evolved into a psychological discipline that makes important contributions to careful studies of differences between groups and within groups. An excellent example of the field's ability to carefully compare across settings and people is Rizzo and Corsaro's (1995) ethnography of preschool children's friendships. Rizzo and Corsaro observed three different groups of children, two European–American and one African–American, in their different preschool settings. The European–American children were from families of middle- to upper-level socioeconomic status and the African–American children were predominantly working class, so that socioeconomic status, a powerful diversity factor, also was taken into account. Each group was described individually, with observations tied to the goals of each school and the nature of each community. The researchers' understanding of children's communities greatly aided their understanding of what they observed. For instance, they noted that teachers of the African–American children often did not intervene in disputes. Without an appreciation of the community, the researchers might conclude that the teachers were not demonstrating appropriate care for their students. But, taking both ecological features and cultural diversity into account, Rizzo and Corsaro concluded that the teachers' actions were intended to promote independence, enabling the youngsters to learn how to take care of themselves in their particular community. Moreover, the goal of this study was not to compare and contrast the friendships of white students with that of African–American students, but instead, to examine common threads of friendship and support in the context of the demands and constraints of different preschools. The researchers did not hold the friendships of the African–American preschoolers up to those of the white preschoolers as a standard for comparison. This study was informative about differences, yet did not reduce the richness among contexts and people in these contexts to a simple set of group comparisons.

Within-group differences are also important to study. Martin, Dean, Garcia, and Hall's (1989, Chapter 13, this volume) work documented the stress experienced by the gay community during early years of the HIV epidemic, and Gonzales and her colleagues (1996, Chapter 24, this volume) carefully considered the neighborhoods of the African–American students they studied. Both research teams went to great lengths to include diversity within their "homogenous" samples, despite the fact that both populations— gay men and African–American youths—are often difficult to recruit for participation in psychological research. Martin and his colleagues contacted numerous gay organizations, recruited at a gay pride festival, and had study participants recruit friends so as to obtain an ethnically and socioeconomically diverse group of gay men. In order to sample socioeconomically diverse African–American youths, Gonzales and her colleagues recruited in public places such as an African–American cultural fair in addition to recruiting at schools. These diverse recruitment practices demonstrate the importance of flexibility and creativity when studying people in their natural settings.

Researching diversity in community psychology involves conducting research in distinctive ways (Hughes & Seidman, 2002; Hughes, Seidman, & Williams, 1993; Sasao & Sue, 1993; Vega, 1992). One approach is to ensure that measurement tools used on mainstream populations are relevant to other groups (e.g., Knight, Verdin, Ocampo, & Roosa, 1994; see also Hughes & Seidman, 2002). Another focus is to determine if community characteristics influence problem behaviors, as Mitchell and Beals (1997) found in a study of American Indian adolescents from different community settings. But incorporating diversity into community research ultimately involves modifications in all phases of the research, from problem formulation to the interpretation of the results (Hughes & Seidman, 2002; Hughes, Seidman, & Williams, 1993). Indeed, perhaps the most important challenge is the definition of the phenomenon of interest. The development of the research problem must take diversity into account, as the framing of the problem generally structures the nature of the findings. Sasao and Sue (1993) argue that such "metamethodological" issues have been given inadequate attention in past research on diversity, and this must change if community psychology is to consistently produce research informed by a culturally anchored perspective.

To attain this goal, community psychologists must first give careful attention to the articulation of the "cultural category" under study (Vega, 1992). This can be accomplished in part by including the group being studied in all phases of the development of a research project, especially in the beginning, when the problem is formulated. An excellent example of this is Hughes and Dumont's (1993) examination of racial stressors at work and their effects on the racial socialization of children. This study used focus groups to uncover the types and perceptions of workplace racial stressors that are salient to the lives of African–American workers. Rather than impose an expected set of stressors, these researchers allowed the participants to discuss relevant experiences with each other in a group setting. These group discussions allowed the participants to agree or disagree with each other, and permitted the clarification of all topics. Further, the groups were then able to explore the relationship between their experiences and the ways in which they prepared their children to deal with future encounters with racism. Although the researchers entered the setting with specific questions in mind, they allowed the participants to define the constructs so that the researchers could be confident that they were culturally relevant.

FUTURE DIRECTIONS FOR COMMUNITY PSYCHOLOGY IN ITS COMMITMENT TO DIVERSITY

The power of community psychology to contribute to our understanding of human diversity has long been recognized by the field's leaders. Trickett's (1996, Chapter 23, this volume) paper is in this tradition, providing both a strong restatement of the field's commitment to diversity and a framework for the future. The sweeping breadth of Trickett's critique—suggesting the incorporation of a contextual philosophy of science and a set of methodological guidelines—shows that community psychology, even decades after its birth, must continually review its own contributions to social analysis and social change. In such critiques, it is crucial to determine to what extent the field demonstrates its promise to understand, in Trickett's words: "the contexts of diversity and the diversity of contexts." Against these demanding expectations, community psychology will always fall short. Social and cultural change is rapid in post-industrial, technologically-driven societies; thus, the contexts in which the research questions are being asked are in flux, and an understanding of a particular social problem must always be incomplete. Community psychology is nonetheless ideally suited to the dynamic study of change in community settings.

Community psychology will continue to study the unique problems and lives of different groups in their distinctive social and cultural settings, taking into account both the differential impacts of diverse settings, and differences among and within groups living in specific settings. Community psychology must examine the challenges faced by groups facing special stressors imposed by social circumstances or social policies. An understanding of the challenges faced by specific groups must also include an appreciation of the history, traditions, and current cultural practices of the group, and of its patterns and social regularities (Seidman, 1988, Chapter 11, this volume). Not all research on historically marginalized groups inevitably leads to social interventions to remedy their inequitable positions, but rigorously conducted research clearly has an impact. Paradoxically, research focusing on the problems faced by marginalized groups might inadvertently reinforce negative stereotypes, if such research is not balanced by an examination of the strengths of these groups. Fortunately, the field has evolved beyond a conceptual model that simply identifies a problem in adaptation, coping, or social support in one particular demographic group or community, and then substitutes another group or community for comparative study.

Community psychology is rapidly becoming the psychological study of cultural diversities in different social contexts, with increasingly precise distinctions within groups being made. For instance, community psychology research increasingly differentiates among different ethnic groups such as Latinos (Puerto Rican, Colombian, Mexican, etc.), Blacks (African–American, Caribbean–American, etc.) or Asians (Chinese, Korean, Japanese, etc.) as well as European–American groups who retain a strong ethnic identity (Italian–American, Irish–American, etc.). A recent paper, for instance, documents the distinctive experiences of African–American women who also are college athletes (Sellers, Kuperminc, & Damas, 1997). Even sexual orientation groups will be studied with greater differentiation. For example, Miller, Klotz, and Eckholdt (1998) described an intervention conducted at a particular kind of gay social setting in New York City. As Trickett suggests, when we aggregate people—whether by age, gender, racial or ethnic background, sexual orientation, or disability status—we erase their different histories and experiences, and make a careful and meaningful study of their lives impossible. The work of community psychology must reflect, amid its complexity, the cultural diversity of the people whose lives we study.

A psychology that homogenizes people by placing them in broad social categories is not the kind that the forefathers of community psychology envisioned. Nor is it one that our more diverse set of current leaders would endorse (Serrano-García & Bond, 1994). Community psychology has made tremendous progress in its focus on diversity since the Swampscott Conference. Yet much more must be done, so that the field accurately reflects the diversity of our current cultural landscape. The challenge of redefining diversity will always be a central task for community psychologists. Our responses to the challenge, if based on our progress to date, will become increasingly thoughtful and sophisticated; our responses also will become increasingly diverse. Both conceptual and methodological tools have advanced to meet the challenge. The "problem of diversity" will never be resolved. We will never feel completely satisfied with our efforts to understand differences between people in communities, since the way that the field conceptualizes diversity will continue to change. Nonetheless, community psychology—its core assumptions, analytic frameworks, and methodologies as reflected in 25 years of work—remains psychology's most powerful approach to "the study of general psychological processes that link social systems with individual behavior in complex interaction" (Bennett et al., 1966, p. 7, Chapter 5, this volume).

REFERENCES

Bennett, C. C., Anderson, L. S., Cooper, S., Hassol, L., Klein, D. C., & Rosenblum, G. (1966). *Community psychology: A report of the Boston Conference on the education of psychologists for community mental health.* Boston: Boston University Press.

Bernal, G. & Enchautegui-de-Jesus, N. (1994). Latinos and Latinas in community psychology: A review of the literature. *American Journal of Community Psychology*, *22*, 531–557.

Bryk, A. S. & Raudenbush, S. W. (1992). *Hierarchical linear models: Applications and data analysis methods.* Newbury Park, CA: Sage.

Coulton, C. J., Korbin, J. E., & Su, M. (1996). Measuring neighborhood context for young children in an urban area. *American Journal of Community Psychology*, *24*, 5–32. Reprinted in T. A. Revenson, A. R. D'Augelli, S. E. French, D. L. Hughes, D. Livert, E. Seidman, M. Shinn, & H. Yoshikawa (Eds.). (2002). *Ecological research to promote social change: Methodological advances from community psychology* (pp. 99–126). New York: Kluwer Academic/Plenum Publishers.

DeFour, D. C. & Hirsch, B. J. (1990). The adaptation of Black graduate students: A social network approach. *American Journal of Community Psychology*, *18*, 487–503.

Dohrenwend, B. S. (1978). Social stress and community psychology. *American Journal of Community Psychology*, *6*, 1–14.

Fawcett, S. R., White, G. W., Balcazar, F. E., Suarez-Balcazar, Y., Mathews, R. M., Paine-Andrew, A., Seekins, T., & Smith, J. F. (1994). A contextual-behavioral model of empowerment: Case studies involving people with physical disabilities. *American Journal of Community Psychology*, *22*, 471–496.

Felner, R. D., Ginter, M., & Primavera, J. (1982). Primary prevention during school transitions: Social support and environmental structure. *American Journal of Community Psychology*, *10*, 277–290.

Garnets, L. D. & D'Augelli, A. R. (1994). Empowering lesbian and gay communities: A call for collaboration with community psychology. *American Journal of Community Psychology*, *22*, 447–470.

Gonzales, N. A., Cauce, A., Friedman, R. J., & Mason, C. A. (1996). Family, peer, and neighborhood influences on academic achievement among African American adolescents: One-year prospective effects. *American Journal of Community Psychology*, *24*, 365–387.

Hughes, D. & Dodge, M. A. (1997). African American women in the workplace: Relationships between job conditions, racial bias at work, and perceived job quality. *American Journal of Community Psychology*, *25*, 581–599.

Hughes, D. L. & Dumont, K. (1993). Using focus groups to facilitate culturally anchored research. *American Journal of Community Psychology*, *21*, 775–806. Reprinted in T. A. Revenson, A. R. D'Augelli, S. E. French, D. L. Hughes, D. Livert, E. Seidman, M. Shinn, & H. Yoshikawa (Eds.). (2002). *Ecological research to promote social change: Methodological advances from community psychology* (pp. 257–289). New York: Kluwer Academic/Plenum Publishers.

Hughes, D. L. & Seidman, E. (2002). In pursuit of a culturally anchored methodology. Reprinted in T. A. Revenson, A. R. D'Augelli, S. E. French, D. L. Hughes, D. Livert, E. Seidman, M. Shinn, & H. Yoshikawa (Eds.), *Ecological research to promote social change: Methodological advances from community psychology* (pp. 243–255). New York: Kluwer Academic/Plenum Publishers.

Hughes, D., Seidman, E., & Williams, N. (1993). Cultural phenomena and the research enterprise: Toward a culturally anchored methodology. *American Journal of Community Psychology*, *21*, 687–703.

Kahn, M. W., Williams, C., Galvez, E., Lejero, L., Conrad, R., & Goldstein, G. (1975). The Papago Psychology Service: A community mental health program on an American Indian reservation. *American Journal of Community Psychology*, *3*, 81–98.

Knight, G. P., Virdin, L. M., Ocampo, K. A., & Roosa, M. (1994). An examination of cross-ethnic equivalence of measures of negative life events and mental health among Hispanic and Anglo-American children. *American Journal of Community Psychology*, *22*, 767–783.

Latkin, C. A., Mandell, W., Vlahov, D., Oziemkowska, M., & Celentano, D. D. (1996). The long-term outcome of a personal network-oriented HIV prevention intervention for injection drug users: The SAFE study. *American Journal of Community Psychology, 24,* 341–364.

Livert, D. & Hughes, D. L. (2002). The ecological paradigm: Persons in settings. In T. A. Revenson, A. R. D'Augelli, S. E. French, D. L. Hughes, D. Livert, E. Seidman, M. Shinn, & H. Yoshikawa (Eds.). *A quarter century of community psychology: Readings from the American Journal of Community Psychology* (pp. 51–63). New York: Kluwer Academic/Plenum Publishers.

Loo, C., Fong, K. T., & Iwamasa, G. (1988). Ethnicity and cultural diversity: An analysis of work published in community psychology journals, 1965–1985. *Journal of Community Psychology, 16,* 332–349.

Luke, D. A., Rappaport, J., & Seidman, E. (1991). Setting phenotypes in a mutual help organization: Expanding behavior setting theory. *American Journal of Community Psychology, 19,* 147–167. Reprinted in T. A. Revenson, A. R. D'Augelli, S. E. French, D. L. Hughes, D. Livert, E. Seidman, M. Shinn, & H. Yoshikawa (Eds.). (2002). *Ecological research to promote social change: Methodological advances from community psychology* (pp. 217–238). New York: Kluwer Academic/Plenum Publishers.

Martin, J. L., Dean, L., Garcia, M., & Hall, W. (1989). The impact of AIDS on a gay community: Changes in sexual behavior, substance use, and mental health. *American Journal of Community Psychology, 17,* 269–293.

Maton, K. I. (1989). Community settings as buffers of life stress? Highly supportive churches, mutual help groups, and senior centers. *American Journal of Community Psychology, 17,* 203–232.

Miller, R. L., Klotz, D., & Eckholdt, H. M. (1998). HIV prevention with male prostitutes and patrons of hustler bars: Replication of an HIV preventive intervention. *American Journal of Community Psychology, 25,* 97–131.

Mitchell, C. M. & Beals, J. (1997). The structure of problem and positive behavior among American Indian adolescents: Gender and community differences. *American Journal of Community Psychology, 25,* 257–288. Reprinted in T. A. Revenson, A. R. D'Augelli, S. E. French, D. L. Hughes, D. Livert, E. Seidman, M. Shinn, & H. Yoshikawa (Eds.). (2002). *Ecological research to promote social change: Methodological advances from community psychology* (pp. 291–321). New York: Kluwer Academic/Plenum Publishers.

Moos, R. H. (1976). Evaluating and changing community settings. *American Journal of Community Psychology, 4,* 313–326.

Muehrer, P. (1997). Introduction to the special issue: Mental health prevention science in rural communities and contexts. *American Journal of Community Psychology, 25,* 421–424.

Mulvey, A. (1988). Community psychology and feminism: Tensions and commonalities. *Journal of Community Psychology, 16,* 70–83.

Perkins, D. D. & Taylor, R. B. (1996). Ecological assessments of community disorder: Their relationship to fear of crime and theoretical implications. *American Journal of Community Psychology, 24,* 63–108. Reprinted in T. A. Revenson, A. R. D'Augelli, S. E. French, D. L. Hughes, D. Livert, E. Seidman, M. Shinn, & H. Yoshikawa (Eds.). (2002). *Ecological research to promote social change: Methodological advances from community psychology* (pp. 127–170). New York: Kluwer Academic/Plenum Publishers.

Phillips, D. A., Howes, C., & Whitebook, M. (1992). The social policy context of child care: Effects on quality. *American Journal of Community Psychology, 20,* 25–51.

Rieff, R. (1975). Of cabbages and kings. *American Journal of Community Psychology, 3,* 187–196.

Rizzo, T. A. & Corsaro, W. A. (1995). Social support processes in early childhood friendship: A comparative study of ecological congruences in enacted support. *American Journal of*

Community Psychology, *23*, 389–417. Reprinted in T. A. Revenson, A. R. D'Augelli, S. E. French, D. L. Hughes, D. Livert, E. Seidman, M. Shinn, & H. Yoshikawa (Eds.). (2002). *Ecological research to promote social change: Methodological advances from community psychology* (pp. 187–216). New York: Kluwer Academic/Plenum Publishers.

Ryan, W. (1971). *Blaming the victim*. New York: Random House.

Ryan, W. (1994). Many cooks, brave men, apples and oranges: How people think about equality. *American Journal of Community Psychology*, *22*, 25–35.

Sarason, S. (1976). Community psychology and the anarchist insight. *American Journal of Community Psychologist*, *4*, 246–259.

Sasao, T. & Sue, S. (1993). Toward a culturally anchored ecological framework of research in ethnic-cultural communities. *American Journal of Community Psychology*, *21*, 705–727.

Seidman, E. (1988). Back to the future, community psychology: Unfolding a theory of social intervention. *American Journal of Community Psychology*, *16*, 3–24.

Sellers, R. M., Kuperminc, G. P., & Damas, A. (1997). The college life experiences of African American women athletes. *American Journal of Community Psychology*, *27*, 699–720.

Serrano-García, I. & Bond, M. A. (1994). Empowering the silent ranks: Introduction. *American Journal of Community Psychology*, *22*, 433–445.

Shinn, M. (1992). Homelessness: What's a psychologist to do? *American Journal of Community Psychology*, *20*, 1–24.

Shinn, M. (1997). Family homelessness: State or trait? *American Journal of Community Psychology*, *25*, 755–769.

Shinn, M. & Rapkin, B. (2000). Cross-level analysis without cross-ups in community psychology. In J. Rappaport & E. Seidman (Eds.), *Handbook of community psychology* (pp. 669–695). New York: Kluwer Academic/Plenum Publishers.

Swift, C., Bond, M., & Serrano-García, I. (2000). Women's empowerment: A review of community psychology's first twenty-five years. In J. Rappaport & E. Seidman (Eds.), *Handbook of community psychology* (pp. 857–895). New York: Kluwer Academic/Plenum Publishers.

Tausig, M. (1987). Detecting "cracks" in mental health services: Application of network analytic techniques. *American Journal of Community Psychology*, *15*, 337–351. Reprinted in T. A. Revenson, A. R. D'Augelli, S. E. French, D. L. Hughes, D. Livert, E. Seidman, M. Shinn, & H. Yoshikawa (Eds.). (2002). *Ecological research to promote social change: Methodological advances from community psychology* (pp. 171–186). New York: Kluwer Academic/Plenum Publishers.

Trickett, E. J. (1996). A future for community psychology: The contexts of diversity and the diversity of contexts. *American Journal of Community Psychology*, *24*, 209–234.

Trickett, E. J. & Moos, R. H. (1974). Personal correlates of contrasting environments: Student satisfactions in high school classrooms. *American Journal of Community Psychology*, *2*, 1–12.

Trickett, E. J., Watts, R., & Birman, D. (1993). Human diversity and community psychology: Still hazy after all these years. *Journal of Community Psychology*, *21*, 264–279.

Vega, W. A. (1992). Theoretical and pragmatic implications of cultural diversity for community research. *American Journal of Community Psychology*, *20*, 375–391.

Weinstein, R. S., Soulé, C. R., Collins, F., Cone, J., Mehlhorn, M., & Simontacchi, K. (1991). Expectations and high school change: Teacher–researcher collaboration to prevent school failure. *American Journal of Community Psychology*, *19*, 333–363.

Zimmerman, M., Reischl, T. M., Seidman, E., Rappaport, J., Toro, P. A., & Salem, D. A. (1991). Expansion strategies of a mutual help organization. *American Journal of Community Psychology*, *19*, 251–278.

II
The Origin

5

Psychology and the Community

Chester C. Bennett, Luleen Anderson, Saul Cooper, Leonard Hassol, Donald C. Klein, and Gershen Rosenblum

Intense, candid, and task-oriented small group discussion at the beginning of the Conference led to a strongly expressed recognition that the participants were occupied not only with an interest in the community mental health movement, but more importantly, with a general sense that the time had come to expand psychology's area of inquiry and action. Participants referred to psychologists' participation in such diverse areas of national life as the Peace Corps, the anti-poverty effort, a broad movement into the field of education, and the development of the consultation function in an array of settings, as evidence of the fact that both knowledge about, and competence in, social change activities have developed in psychology over the past several decades. A deep stirring and metamorphosis was seen as being in process. The Conference participants, while holding diverse views on how to define and interpret these changes, decided to expand the Conference mandate and move toward the conception of a new field, tentatively labeled "Community Psychology."

It was acknowledged that this decision would imply some major realignments within the training and practice structures of the profession. Some participants voiced a degree of personal surprise at their own willingness to move in this direction after only three days of conference exploration, and the point was made that a good deal of fermentation of this idea must have been in the background of everyone's thinking for some time. As detailed

SOURCE: Community Psychology: A Report of the Boston Conference on the Education of Psychologists for Community Mental Health, Chapter II, pp. 4–8.

A Quarter Century of Community Psychology: Readings from the American Journal of Community Psychology, edited by Tracey A. Revenson *et al.* Kluwer Academic/Plenum Publishers, New York, 2002.

discussion proceeded, a number of factors emerged as contributing to this sense of readiness to test new conceptions.

Psychologists have been involved for some time in a range of social change functions which include activities in the mental health-mental illness area but are not limited to it. Conference members described current activities, such as helping school administrators to restructure the communication patterns within their school systems so as to ease the transition to junior high school for elementary school children; advising the administrators of cooperative housing projects on the design and evaluation of the governmental and social structures which tenants in such projects evolve; advising governors of states and legislative committees on a wide range of public policy decisions; and in some instances taking the initiative toward starting new public programs. This involvement of psychologists in a broadened range of social action was seen as developing rapidly.

Many psychologists have moved into these areas from a primary training in, and identification with, mental health. They remain active in mental health but see this approach as having decreasing strategic leverage and validity for helping to answer some of the growing problems of our complex society. The point was emphasized that if psychology wants to make an impact on large social processes (and a majority of this sample of psychologists accepted that goal), it will have to step out of its immersion in strictly clinical-medical settings.

Acceptance of the goal of participation in a larger range of social processes did not, however, preclude a sharp division within the Conference as to how this is to be accomplished and how much policy responsibility psychologists should assume. One group, coming most recently from an ardent involvement in anti-poverty programs, felt that the traditional reluctance of psychologists to step out of the advisory role into the decision-making role usually results in a distortion, or at least watering down, of their views. They further felt that psychologists have shown a capacity to develop projects and programs that break open traditional conceptual constraints and that are susceptible to evaluation. It was asserted that psychologists, by virtue of their training and interests, are in a strong position to make the kinds of policy decisions which allow meaningful evaluation to proceed. This group also advocated a far more active role for psychologists in initiating and advancing legislation, and in influencing administrative decisions and the execution of public policy.

Running counter to this position was another strongly held view that society has not given psychology a mandate to tackle most social ills, that the knowledge and competence claimed in the area of social change is yet to be demonstrated, and that if psychologists want to take on public policy decision-making, they should stand for public office. While agreement was reached on the need for wider activity under the roof of community psychology, the extent of psychological activism was left open for further demonstration and discussion.

Another strong influence upon the thinking of the conference members was the emergence of the Federal Community Mental Health Centers program about which considerable ambivalence was freely voiced. It was felt that the Federal program may serve to legitimize certain emerging practices, such as consultation, which promise a wider possibility of impact. To that extent, an opportunity exists for developing and testing creative approaches. It was felt that psychology may have a good chance to work with and to influence the Federal program so that concepts and methods independent of the medical model can emerge. On the other hand, the conference members were agreed that the Federal Community Mental Health Centers program represents only a consolidation of past advances in technique within a fairly narrow medical view of behavior disorder, that the present order of priorities embodied in the regulations for this program will not allow for any important preventive gains, and that therefore the program will have difficulty in becoming a major focus for the kind of social change functions connoted by the term "Community Psychology."

Participants were at pains to point out that movement in the direction of community psychology is dictated by intrinsic professional judgment and feelings of competence and not in reaction to extrinsic factors such as the Federal program or availability of other funds. In fact, an explicit warning was voiced concerning the seductive and distorting influence which funds earmarked for predetermined purposes can have on the direction of scientific development in this new area. Finally, but perhaps most important, the point was made that an excessive immersion in mental health-illness concerns imposes half realized but very effective limitations on the range of issues which psychological science will attempt to meet and, therefore, narrows the potential contribution which psychology can expect to make to scientific knowledge and to human betterment.

As the conference discussions proceeded the groups moved toward a conception of community psychology as the major field, with community mental health as one area of interest in this field. It was recognized that certain clinically trained psychologists now active in the community mental health area, and some recruits from social and other areas of psychology, are the current closest approximations of community psychologists. Most of these individuals did not receive formal training in either community mental health or anything resembling community psychology. Presumably then, much of the training in clinical psychology has major relevance for this new area. However, awareness was also voiced of the fact that the self-selection of psychologists now active in community mental health programs may have resulted in a group atypical of psychology in general, a group whose involvement and skill in this area may have developed subsequent to, and independently of, their clinical training.

Intense efforts to come up with a working definition of the field of community psychology led to the not unexpected finding that a rigorous definition was presently beyond our grasp. Descriptively, however, a number of elements of a definition were proposed, tested, and reworked. The product of these labors is presented here in two sections: a brief, very general field description, and an attempt to describe the role of that newly discovered form of life, the community psychologist.

Existing community mental health programs provided the takeoff points for attempts to define community psychology. The conceptual and programmatic dimensions of community mental health were seen as stemming, in large measure, from a public health prevention framework. This has led to such innovations as changing the location of services in time and place, instituting new patterns of service, and experimenting with a range of manpower innovations, including the planned utilization of strategically or naturally situated helping resources. The main focus on prevention has led to a necessary concern with the interaction between social system structures and functions and the mental health of populations. Attempts at intervention in social systems, with a preventive emphasis, become a logical extension of community mental health services.

One group of conference members was therefore willing to see this framework expanded beyond the concern with mental health and mental illness. Community psychology in this view is devoted to the study of general psychological processes that link social systems with individual behavior in complex interaction. Conceptual and experimental clarifications of such linkages were seen as providing the basis for action programs directed toward improving individual, group, and social system functioning. Included in the area of investigation would be studies of planned change, social system analysis, psychological ecology, social action evaluation, normal human development within various social settings, conflict resolution, mental health and illness in the broad sense, intergroup relations, community organization and dynamics, etc. Some of the members who advanced this view felt that this mere listing of interest areas could be interpreted as suggesting a touch of megalomania. That impression, it was felt, usually vanishes under actual contact with the thicket of theoretical, methodical and human relations problems that confront any attempt to make the slightest dent in any one of these problem areas.

Other participants felt that it was far too early to attempt a structuring of community psychology in terms of any currently available model. Discomfort was voiced with the purely analogical concurrence between the public health prevention model and the much broader range of social change functions included within community psychology. It was pointed out that community psychology would frequently be involved with facilitating change rather than with preventing anything. In fact, some of the participants even raised the question as to the appropriateness of applying public health models to community mental health in the absence of any evidence that the underlying assumptions of the public health approach could be translated into the areas of behavior and behavior pathology. Eventually agreement was reached that a multiplicity of models need to be tried, and that an unusually timely opportunity for creative thinking and experimentation exists.

Since it was agreed that community psychology encompasses more than community mental health, the conference members saw a need for a generalist kind of training, within which community mental health can be one appropriate area of specific functioning. The community psychologist should have the knowledge and skill to assess and modify the reciprocal relationships between individuals and the social systems with which they interact. He should utilize and integrate findings from psychology and the other social sciences which bear upon the individual-system variables. He must be acutely aware of the limitations of the current state of knowledge and art in the community psychology field and should therefore feel committed both to the generation of concepts and to the dissemination of knowledge in the field. The role of the community psychologist may therefore be seen as that of a "participant-conceptualizer." As such he is clearly involved in, and may be a mover of, community processes, but he is also a professional attempting to conceptualize those processes within the framework of psychological–sociological knowledge.

This attempt to visualize the role of community psychology led the Conference to recognize an important issue of personal choice for prospective entrants into this field. The consultation function, which has been the most important point of entry for psychologists in community mental health, is usually defined as a staff role in which line personnel receive service but retain control over policies and decisions. As one participant commented, this would seem to be the role of a knowledgeable and high status adviser to responsible decision-makers. The social change function implies, at least to many of the conference members, a more activist role with the psychologist retaining control and decision-making power. It was pointed out that the community psychologist frequently would be the person who is attentive to social system dysfunction or to the possibility of system improvement. The question of degree of activity in stimulating change processes is thereby posed and the division within the Conference reflects the personal and professional role conflicts which the community psychologist will have to resolve. It was agreed that we will need to develop a range of role models for students, as well as professional forums for the continued evaluation of the many ethical and value questions raised by these new possibilities for action.

Consensus was also reached that psychologists can live in both kinds of houses; that some can function in community mental health settings in the consultative role, but there will also be a need to develop social change settings where psychologists will have administrative responsibility.

In the development of social change settings, it was stressed that the dichotomy between university and field stations needs to be overcome. There is, the Conference felt, a profound underlying convergence of interests between these institutions once the goal of social change research is accepted, since both settings are in need of theory, research skill, and community action skills and sanctions. It was urged that a variety of bridging positions between the two systems be developed so that eventually personnel could move between them with complete flexibility.

It may be that the major work of the Boston Conference will turn out to be this attempt at a first articulation of the perspective of community psychology although the major questions of definition and training remain to be resolved through future experience. Many participants, in varied settings around the country, reported that their initial efforts toward a change agent role have been greeted by good will and an almost embarrassingly enthusiastic welcome. The challenge would seem to be how to keep the enthusiasm alive while striving for ways to respond responsibly, to reach mutually acceptable role definitions and role limits.

III

The 1970s

6

Preentry Issues in Consultation

Cary Cherniss

Three important issues confront "consultants" before initiating entry to a client setting. These are: Should one do consultation in this situation? Whose interests will the consultant serve? What will be the primary focus of consultation? Consultants can answer these questions in different ways, and the answers will be determined by a number of factors discussed in the paper. The main argument is that these issues are unavoidable and that consultation effectiveness will be improved if consultants carefully think through these issues early in the consultation process and remain aware of the stances adopted.

Long before the first approach to a potential client system, a consultant confronts several fundamental issues contained in the consultation process. The ways in which these issues are resolved will substantially influence the consultant's thinking and action throughout the consultation. The consultant's position on these issues also will determine how he or she will be regarded by consultees. These "preentry" issues are important because, if they are not thought through carefully (as they usually are not), frequently the result is unnecessary confusion and ambiguity around the consultant's role and mission. And as research has suggested, such ambiguity often is associated with less effective consultation (Mann, 1973). Finally, an adequate consideration of these preentry issues helps the consultant deal with subsequent issues and problems.

Originally published in the *American Journal of Community Psychology*, 4(1) (1976): 13–24.

A Quarter Century of Community Psychology: *Readings from the* American Journal of Community Psychology, edited by Tracey A. Revenson *et al.* Kluwer Academic/Plenum Publishers, New York, 2002.

As will be noted below, "consultation" can and is defined differently, depending on how the consultant answers the preentry questions. Generally, consultation may be defined as a process in which one or more individuals, possessing certain knowledge and skills, help individuals and groups within a particular social system work on one or more work-related problems. This definition of consultation includes the work of Caplan (1970), Argyris (1970), and Sarason, Levine, Goldenberg, Cherlin, & Bennett (1966).

The preentry issues of consultation include: Should one do consultation in this situation? Whose interests will the consultant serve? What will be the primary focus of consultation?

Unfortunately, few consultants have considered in any systematic way these fundamental questions. Most papers and books on the consultation process give scant attention to them. Much has been written about entry, but the equally important issues that temporally and conceptually *precede entry* have been relatively neglected. In this paper, I discuss these questions.

SHOULD ONE PROVIDE CONSULTATION IN THIS SITUATION?

There are always alternatives to consultation. The most experienced, effective consultants I have known consider the alternatives carefully each time they have an opportunity to provide consultation. They do not compulsively seize at any invitation they receive. Rather, they evaluate the situation according to a previously conceived set of criteria. Less effective consultants, on the other hand, do not seem to possess a set of criteria for deciding this question; in fact, in many instances, they do not even seem to see this question as worthy of consideration.

For instance, a short time ago, I participated in a meeting of a school consultation project. One of the consultants had had an opportunity to meet regularly with an administrator in a school system where mental health consultation was being delivered. Most members of the project seemed to feel that this was certainly a fortunate opportunity. However, the meetings with the consultee were considered by the consultant who attended them to be unproductive, and he thus raised the question: Why should we provide consultation to this person?

The initial response to the question was silence. The silence finally was broken by one individual's somewhat hesitant and confused explanation that consultation should be provided to the administrator because he had made himself available and because he had "high status in the system."

Agreeing to consult with someone in a system simply because he has "high status" does not seem to provide a clear, strong rationale for the consultation. This group of experienced, professional mental health consultants obviously had not given much thought to an important preentry question.

Why Is the Question Important?

The question, "to consult or not to consult," is important and useful because it forces the consultant to consider the "universe of alternatives." As Sarason (1971) has observed, carefully considering the possible alternatives to any course of action prevents one from acting in stereotyped, ineffective ways. It helps liberate one from the shackles of tradition, and it forces one to confront fundamental issues. Thus, by self-consciously asking whether or not to consult in a particular situation, the consultant will more likely become aware of *alternatives* to consultation. Then, after deciding to consult, it will be in the context of a careful examination of alternative ways of proceeding; such a stance ultimately will be liberating for both the consultant and the consultees.

The question of whether or not one should accept an invitation to consult is important not only because it seems to provide the basis for more effective consultation but also because of *economic considerations*. As Sarason (1969) pointed out in another context, we do not now have nor will we probably ever have enough consultants to help all of the social systems that are experiencing difficulty. Thus, a consultant who agrees to work within a system is tying up a substantial amount of professional time and energy. Agreeing to consult to one system limits a consultant's ability to consult to other systems. Of course, consultants can and do work in more than one system. However, their capacity to give help ultimately is limited, and they will have little time for future requests or opportunities to consult. Thus, for economic reasons, the question of whether or not a consultant should do consultation in a particular situation is an important one, and a socially responsible consultant will weigh this question carefully before making a major commitment of consultative time and energy.

A careful examination of this fundamental question suggests there really are two different types of alternatives suggested by the question. First, the question suggests that one may wish to intervene in a particular situation, but not through the method of consultation. As Caplan (1970) and others have suggested, it is only one of many different types of "social intervention" that can be employed (Hornstein, Bunker, Burke, Gindes, & Lewicki, 1971). Investigative reporting (e.g., Chu, 1973), the creation of alternative settings (Sarason, 1972), political action (Alinsky, 1971), or direct service delivery are other ways of confronting problems that exist in social systems. Thus, even when it is appropriate to intervene in a particular situation, consultation may not be the "method of choice."[1]

The question of whether or not one should consult also suggests that one may not wish to intervene at all in a particular situation. There will be many social systems and situations in which one could consult; and some will not be amenable to any constructive intervention at a particular time. Thus, one may decline to consult in a particular situation in favor of more promising ones.

Bases for Answering the Question

Value Congruence. Whether or not the consultant consciously raises and thinks through this basic question of consultation, it is answered in some way; and the answer will be influenced by a number of factors. One basis for answering the question is *value congruence*. For instance, Levine (1969) writes:

> *The goals or the values of the helping agent or the helping service must be consistent with the goals or the values of the setting in which the problem is manifested.* This postulate assumes that settings have important major purposes, and that the achievement of these purposes is vital to the continuance of the setting. It further assumes that the setting will act to expel or otherwise isolate or make ineffective those helping agents who promote goals or values at variance with the major goals and values of the setting (pp. 218–219).

During recent years, I have seen numerous examples in consultation practice that confirm Levine's premise. For instance, on more than one occasion I have witnessed individuals who were committed to a "radical–humanistic" conception of education assume the role of consultant in the public school system. In virtually every case I know of, the consultation failed, either with a "bang" (the consultants eventually were asked to leave in no uncertain terms) or with a "whimper" (the consultants—discouraged, hurt, and frustrated—eventually left without any sense of accomplishment). In such instances, it probably would have been better if the consultants initially had asked themselves if they should consult in these situations and had considered the congruence between their own values and those of the potential client system.

In many instances, consultants do answer the question negatively because of ethical or value considerations. For instance, despite Bard's eloquent pleas that mental health workers consult with police departments (Bard, 1971), I know of many consultants who will not do so because they

---

[1]In some cases, empirical research can help a consultant answer this and other preentry questions. For instance, future research could suggest the system or target characteristics that dictate consultation rather than another type of intervention.

believe the police represent values and purposes they regard as socially destructive or immoral. Thus, value congruence should be and often is an important consideration in deciding whether consultation should be provided in any given situation.

Resources. A second basis for determining whether one should consult in a situation is *the relationship between the consultant's resources of time and expertise and the resources required to consult effectively in the situation.* A consultant who is asked to provide consultation to an individual or system is, in effect, being asked to devote a certain amount of time and to call upon certain types of knowledge and skills. There will be instances when a consultant should decline to consult, lacking the time or technical resources necessary to help the people involved.

Unfortunately, consultants do not always consciously confront the problem of resources when deciding whether they should consult. Often, a request that one provide consultation to an individual or group flatters a consultant and generates a powerful sense of mission to alleviate suffering or to right some wrong. The sense of pride and desire to help are understandable. However, feeling flattered and wanting to save people may lead a consultant to ignore the problem of resources. Such a situation may result in a failure to assess the relationship between the resources required and the resources available. Or, in making the assessment, the consultant may *underestimate* the amount and type of resources that are required or *overestimate* the available resources. One way to prevent these problems is for would-be consultants always to be aware of and even make *known* and *explicit* their own particular knowledge, skills, and time constraints.

Consultee Characteristics. A third basis for deciding whether to consult in a particular situation is *the characteristics of the consultee.* Previous experience and writing on the consultation process suggest a number of characteristics that could be relevant. For instance, Caplan (1970) has observed that best results in mental health consultation seem to occur in consultees who are most upset by or concerned about their problems. Thus, the client's motivation to change could be an important consideration for Caplan in deciding whether he will consult in a particular situation.

Another writer on the consultation process, Chris Argyris (1970), will only consult to client systems that are "open to and capable of learning" and that provide the consultant access to "the power points in the client system that are the keys to the problem being studied." Argyris also will avoid situations in which proposals for change will be imposed on any part of the organization (Argyris, 1970, pp. 25–26). Not everyone will agree with Argyris's criteria, and exactly how one would assess a potential client system's "openness to learning" is not clear. Nevertheless, Argyris's criteria do suggest that one basis for deciding whether to consult is the presence or absence of certain characteristics in the client system. Undoubtedly, many experienced consultants do consider characteristics of the client system when deciding whether to consult. However, many others with whom I have worked do not seem to systematically consider client characteristics as a basis for answering the question. As a result, they often find themselves enmeshed in consultations that turn out to be of limited value and that tie up time and energy that could be better utilized in more promising situations.

The Influence of the Social Milieu. A basis for determining whether a consultant will work in a particular situation is provided by the *social milieu* in which consultants work. Consultants, like the rest of humanity, do not operate in a social vacuum. First, consultants always work in a particular *institutional context*; and the norms, traditions, policies, and economics of the consultant institution will influence when and where consultants intervene. For instance, university-based consultants are part of an institution that traditionally values teaching and research (Cherniss, 1972; Nisbet, 1971). These consultants will most likely consult in situations where there is an opportunity to pursue research of some sort and/or to involve students in some type of learning experience. For the individual working in a private, profit-oriented consulting firm, economic factors will play a large role in determining whether consultation is provided in a particular situation. Public sector consultants also are sensitive to financial considerations, since consultation frequently is a more institutionally marginal activity in their settings (e.g., community mental health centers) and thus must often "pay its own way" (Reiff, 1966; Cherniss, 1977).

In addition to their institutional context, consultants are influenced by *the ideas and social forces that shape the "spirit of the times."* The prevailing *zeit-geist* makes certain issues, problems, and even professional theories and methods seem more "important" and "timely" (Levine & Levine, 1970). Historical forces influence the consultant directly as an individual, and they also influence the institutional context in which the consultant works. For instance, when the Soviet Union launched its Sputnik in 1958, American pride was damaged, and concern with the quality of public education was aroused (Sarason, 1974). During the subsequent decade, growing numbers of professionals from education, mental health, and organizational science worked in public school settings. In the latter part of the 1960s, however, spurred in part by the Nixon administration's emphasis on the "law and order" issue and the growing unrest among inmates at Attica and other prisons, correctional settings increasingly were identified as targets for consultation (e.g., Reppucci, Sarata, Saunders, McArthur, & Michlin, 1973; Sarason, 1974; Katkin & Sibley, 1973; Levine, Gelsomino, Joss, & Ayer, 1973). Most recently, there has been growing pressure in a number of states to substantially reduce state mental hospital populations. To accommodate the growing numbers of discharged mental patients, various types of community living facilities have been created; and many community mental health professionals have become interested in providing consultation to these settings. Thus, the "spirit of the times" as well as the specific institutional context in which one works will influence a consultant's decisions about the desirability of consulting in any given situation.

In summary, the first important preentry question that a consultant faces is. "Should I consult in this situation?" Effective consultants recognize that there always are numerous possible alternatives, and consultation in a particular situation is but one of them. Also, they realize that their time and resources ultimately are limited and that the decision to provide consultation thus should be weighed carefully. In deciding whether to consult, one inevitably confronts issues such as one's own values and their congruence with those of the consultee, the relationship between the consultant's present resources and those required to consult effectively, certain consultee characteristics, and the consultant's own social milieu.

WHOSE INTERESTS WILL THE CONSULTANT SERVE?

All social settings are characterized by conflict and competition between diverse interest groups. These groups are aware of their differences, and when a consultant enters a setting, they are anxious to see whose interests the consultant seems to be representing. If consultants do not think through this issue before entering a setting, their behavior will appear ambiguous and confusing to consultees, trust between consultant and consultees will develop slowly at best, and consultation will be less effective.

The "constituency issue" also is important because its resolution will influence how consultants define their role, what immediate and long-term goals they will pursue, and what strategies and techniques they will use. Some potential implications of the question are discussed in the following example suggested by Seymour Sarason.

Suppose one has agreed to consult in an elementary school classroom where a number of conflicts and problems have occurred. Suppose further that the consultant is one who often helps consultees learn and use behavioral techniques to better manage problems in their work settings. Preliminary observation in the classroom suggests to the consultant that a modification of certain reinforcement contingencies will improve the situation. But whom will the consultant train in the use of the technique? This may seem to be an odd question, because most consultants would teach the techniques to the teacher without even thinking that there might be an alternative.

But recall the proposition that all social settings are characterized by conflict and competition between *diverse interest groups*. Waller (1967) argued that in the classroom, the teacher and the students represent different and usually antagonistic interests. They have different "agendas" and "priorities." Thus, in choosing to train the *teacher* in the use of behavioral technology, our hypothetical consultant has made an important decision (a decision that probably was made *before* entry with little awareness on the part of the consultant). The consultant could have chosen at least two other approaches in the situation: Training and consultation could have been offered to the *students* or to the students *and* the teacher. A recognition that competing interests were involved, and a careful consideration of the question, "Whose interests will I serve," could lead the hypothetical consultant to some very different decisions about role, strategy, and goals, and probably would facilitate development of the consultant–consultee relationship.

Unfortunately, consultants often ignore the "constituency issue." They seem unwilling to accept completely the existence of competing interests in social settings. Many consultants attempt to sidestep the issue by believing that "in the long run" everyone is interested in the same goals. In these cases, the consultants attempt to avoid taking a stand by asserting that they are "everybody's" agent or even that their constituency is "society." Such platitudes may help consultants to dismiss a sensitive and complex issue; and in "the long run," there may even be some truth to the claims. However, consultants working in the world of action never are dealing with the "long run"; they are facing various interest groups that are primarily concerned with very different goals. Unless consultants clarify their own stance *before* the entry phase begins and communicate that stance to the consultees, consultation may falter from ambiguity and mistrust.

WHAT WILL BE THE PRIMARY FOCUS OF THE CONSULTATION?

Prior to approaching a potential consultation, the consultant usually has selected a *primary focus*. The focus may not be articulated to others, and the consultant may not even be aware of having selected a focus that will guide future thinking and actions. However, choosing the primary focus is another important preentry issue which must be considered.

Four Areas of Focus in Consultation

The primary focus in most consultation work tends to be in one of four areas—organizational structure and process; technology; the mental health of individuals; and the group or organizational environment. To clarify how each of these can serve as a primary focus of consultation, let us examine them in the context of one possible client setting: a public elementary school.

Some consultants to a school setting will tend to focus on *organizational structure and process* (e.g., Argyris, 1970). They will be concerned with how well the internal social organization of the school is functioning. They will assess communication patterns, decision-making, interpersonal relations, morale, and performance. Their basic mission is to identify obstacles to adaptive organizational functioning and recommend modifications intended to rectify the problems. Consultants who take this focus may assume that an improvement in the school's organizational functioning will be beneficial for the mental health of individuals, for the educational process, and for the welfare of the entire community. However, they focus primarily on the organization and its properties, and a better internal climate and more effective problem solving are their primary goals.

Other consultants in this situation will focus on the *technology*. In a public school, this would be the educational process as it occurs within the classroom. A specific example would be a consultant who helps teachers transform their classes into "open classrooms." Such a consultant focuses on how the teacher thinks about, organizes, and conducts the educational process. The primary goals are to make the teacher a better teacher and the classroom a richer learning environment.

I refer to this primary focus as "the technology" with much misgiving. In human service settings, the term may be at best nondescript and at worst highly misleading. By "technology," I mean in part the skills, techniques, and processes required to perform a particular task, and this is the traditional definition of the term. However, in the case of educational, correctional, and mental health settings, "technology" as I am using it here also includes knowledge, values, and even personal feelings that are critical ingredients in performance of the teaching or helping process.

The *mental health of individuals* is yet another possible primary focus of consultation. When mental health is the focus, the consultant ultimately is concerned with the cognitive and affective functioning of particular individuals. Although the consultant may never see these individuals, the goal of the intervention is to bring about change that will facilitate either treatment or prevention of individual emotional problems. In the school setting, a mental-health-oriented consultant spends much time helping staff work more effectively with students who manifest some type of behavioral problem (cf. Caplan, 1970; Sarason *et al.*, 1966). When not concerned with a particular student, a mental-health-oriented consultant will tend to engage in activities closely related to student mental health (e.g., helping school staff set up an early identification program for "high-risk" students).

Still other consultants tend to focus on the *group or organizational environment*. In the school setting, such a consultant may be concerned with school–community relations and might attempt to help the school staff develop more effective community programs in the school. The ultimate goal is harmonious, mutually satisfying and beneficial relations between the school and its surrounding community. Staff morale, the quality of the teaching process, and student mental health are not of primary concern to this consultant. However, like the other consultants, this one may assume that the primary focus, better school–community relations, will improve functioning in other areas as well.

It can be argued that these areas of primary focus in practice are not mutually exclusive. A "mental health" consultant may (some would say "should") also become highly involved in organizational, technological, and community issues. In reality, one's primary focus is constantly shifting; and it should shift as the situation dictates in order to maximize the consultant's effectiveness. Some may also argue (e.g., Sarason *et al.*, 1966) that initially a consultant should avoid assuming a primary focus; the focus should be formulated in collaboration with the consultee(s) and based on a careful "assessment" of current needs and problems.

It is true that consultants often work on more than one type of concern, and, during the course of a consultation, the focus may shift. However, an individual consultant usually does assume some kind of primary *focus* as I have defined it, even though the specific activities may vary; and in one way or another this focus is communicated to the consultees. Thus, on both sides, consultants are identified with a particular concern: the mental health of individuals, the functioning of the organization, etc.

It should be noted that initially identifying a primary focus does not "hem in" consultants or make their roles too inflexible. Within each primary focus there is a wide latitude of possible activities in which the consultants may engage. For instance, a mental health consultant may work with individuals or with groups, with line staff or with administrators, around specific cases, around the consultee's own skills, or around programs. However, in all these instances, the consultant may retain a primary focus on the mental health of individuals.

Many consultants, in an effort to "keep their options open," attempt to avoid answering the question, "What will be the primary focus of the consultation?" In every case I know of, such a maneuver merely impeded the consultation, and eventually, if the intervention survived, the consultant became identified with the primary focus that might have been chosen anyway if the issue had been confronted in the very beginning. As with the other preentry questions, a consultant's failure to consider this one confuses the client about the nature of the consultant's role and thus interferes with consultation effectiveness. Flexibility in role is one of the unique advantages available to a consultant; however, role flexibility is different from the ambiguity, confusion, and manipulativeness that arise when a consultant attempts to avoid an identification with a primary focus.

Bases for Answering the Question

As was the case with the other questions I considered, there are many factors that will influence a consultant's choice of primary focus. For instance, a consultant's values and conception of society may lead to a favoring of one primary focus over another. Similarly, the policies and mission of a consultant's own institution may strongly influence the choice of focus. A consultant working out of a mental health agency will not only be expected to focus on mental health issues by colleagues and superiors; consultees also will expect the consultant to focus on mental health (Cherniss, 1977). Naturally, a consultant's previous training and experiences also will influence which primary focus is chosen. A school consultant who has extensively studied educational theory and practice will tend to focus on the technology, while a school consultant who has studied organizational and administrative theory will tend to focus on organizational functioning. Personal style and aptitude may be yet another factor influencing choice of focus.

The choice of primary focus has a number of implications for the consultation process. First, a consultant's primary focus may influence when and where the consultation occurs. It also may influence the entry process, the initial activities in which the consultant engages, and the initial "diagnostic questions" that are emphasized. In short, the decision concerning primary focus, made before contact with the consultee, influences a number of subsequent decisions and actions; and thus it is another important preentry issue in consultation.

CONCLUSION

I have argued in this paper that there exist certain basic questions of consultation. These questions should be confronted in some way by the consultant before "entry" and often before any contact is made with the client system. Observation of consultants at work suggests that these preentry questions are rarely articulated in any explicit way by consultants; and their failure to do so seems to impede consultant effectiveness. (Testing this particular notion would be a fascinating area of research.) Thinking through these questions helps a consultant make more rational, coherent choices about many of the issues that arise during the consultation and minimizes much of the ambiguity, conflict, and confusion that interfere with effective intervention.

Some of these questions can only be answered in the process of entry. For instance, deciding whether one should provide consultation in a particular situation requires some information about the situation. Much of this information can only be gathered during the entry process. Also, the nature of the contract negotiated between consultant and consultee during entry may resolve (or exacerbate) some of the preentry issues that have been discussed.

However, while many of these preentry issues cannot be resolved before entry, they should be and can be considered before entry begins. A consultant often must initiate entry to decide whether consultation would be appropriate; but the idea that "whether or not to consult" is an issue, and the criteria to be used in evaluating it, should be formulated *before* entry begins.

In conclusion, I believe there is a pressing need for well-thought-through models or theories of consultation that include clear, carefully arrived at answers to the preentry questions. In this sense I am endorsing Lewin's now famous statement that there is nothing so practical as a good theory. However, I also believe that, while formal models are necessary, they are not sufficient prerequisites for effective consultation. The effective consultants I have known are guided by theory, but they also are guided by a store of knowledge concerning *actual consultation experiences*. They have observed, both directly and indirectly, choices and actions actually made by consultants and the events that followed. In other words, effective consultants not only have studied the "preentry issues" in consultation; they also have devoted much time to the study of *the natural history of consultation practice*. However, as a way of understanding and making sense of this natural history, and as a necessary task in and of itself, thoughtful consideration of the preentry issues in consultation represents vitally important, unfinished business for most of us involved in the field.

ACKNOWLEDGMENTS

The author wishes to thank Richard Price, Ruth Schelkun, Deborah Cherniss, Susan Almazol Baker, and Octave Baker who looked over earlier drafts of this paper and provided useful comments.

REFERENCES

Alinsky, S. D. *Rules for radicals*. New York: Vintage, 1971.
Argyris, C. *Intervention theory and method*. Reading, Mass.: Addison-Wesley, 1970.
Bard, M. The role of law enforcement in the helping system. *Community Mental Health Journal*, 1971, 7, 151–160.

Caplan, G. *The theory and practice of mental health consultation*. New York: Basic Books, 1970.

Cherniss, C. *New settings in the University: Their creation, problems, and early development*. Unpublished doctoral dissertation, Yale University, 1972.

Cherniss, C. Creating new consultation programs in community mental health centers: Analysis of a case study. *Community Mental Health Journal*, 1977, *13*, 133–141.

Chu, F. Nader's raiders look at community mental health centers. Speech delivered before National Council of Community Mental Health Centers, February 26, 1973.

Hornstein, A. A., Bunker, B. B., Burke, W. W., Gindes, M., & Lewicki, R. J. *Social intervention: A behavioral science approach*. New York: Free Press. 1971.

Katkin, E. S. & Sibley, R. F. Psychological consultation at Attica State Prison: Post-hoc reflections on some precursors to a disaster. In I. I. Goldenberg (Ed.), *The helping professions in the world of action*. Boston: D. C. Heath & Co., 1973, 165–194.

Levine, M. Postulates of community psychology practice. In F. Kaplan & S. B. Sarason (Eds.), *The Yale Psycho-Educational Clinic: Papers and research studies*. Boston: Massachusetts Dept. of Mental Health (Community Mental Health Monograph), 1969.

Levine, M., Gelsomino, J., Joss, R. H., & Ayer, W. The "consumer's" perspective of rehabilitative services in a county penitentiary. *International Journal of Mental Health*, 1973, *2*(2), 94–110.

Levine, M. & Levine, A. *A social history of helping services*. New York: Appleton-Century-Crofts, 1970.

Mann, P. Student consultants: Evaluations by consultees. *American Journal of Community Psychology*, 1973, *1*, 182–193.

Nisbet, R. A. *The degradation of the academic dogma*. New York: Oxford University Press, 1971.

Reiff, R. Mental health manpower and institutional change. *American Psychologist*, 1966, *21*, 540–548.

Reppucci, N. D., Sarata, B. P. V., Saunders, J. T., McArthur, A. V., & Michlin, L. M. We bombed in Mountville: Lessons learned in consultation to a correctional facility for adolescent offenders. In I. I. Goldenberg (Ed.), *The helping professions in the world of action*. Boston: D. C. Heath & Co., 1973, 145–164.

Sarason, S. B. The creation of settings: A preliminary statement. In F. Kaplan & S. B. Sarason (Eds.), *The Yale Psycho-Educational Clinic: Papers and research studies*. Boston: Massachusetts State Dept. of Mental Health (Monograph Series), 1969, 197–207.

Sarason, S. B. *The culture of the school and the problem of change*. Boston: Allyn & Bacon, 1971.

Sarason, S. B. *The creation of settings and the future societies*. San Francisco: Jossey-Bass, 1972.

Sarason, S. B. *The psychological sense of community: Prospects for a community psychology*. San Francisco: Jossey-Bass, 1974.

Sarason, S. B., Levine, M., Goldenberg, I. I., Cherlin, D. L., & Bennett, E. M. *Psychology in community settings: Clinical, vocational, educational, social aspects*. New York: Wiley, 1966.

Waller, W. *The sociology of teaching*. New York: Wiley, 1967.

7

Social Stress and Community Psychology*

Barbara Snell Dohrenwend

Two questions that embrarrass community psychologists are: "What do community psychologists do?" "What's the difference between community psychology and clinical psychology?" A conceptual model is proposed to help to find answers to these questions. The model describes a process whereby psychosocial stress leads to psychopathology. The argument is developed that the apparently disparate activities of community psychologists are uniformly directed at undermining the stress process but, given the complexity of this process, vary because they tackle it at different points.

A question that seems to be a source of chronic embarrassment to community psychologists is "What do community psychologists do"? Since community psychology originated when a rebel band of discontented clinical psychologists got together at Swampscott, Massachusetts in the Spring of 1965, another version of this question is "What's the difference between community psychology and clinical psychology?" I will propose a conceptual model that I think may help us to find answers to these persistent and vexing questions.

*Presidential address, Division 27, 85th Annual American Psychological Association Convention, San Francisco, August 27, 1977. Originally published in the *American Journal of Community Psychology*, 6(1) (1978): 1–14.

A Quarter Century of Community Psychology: Readings from the American Journal of Community Psychology, edited by Tracey A. Revenson *et al*. Kluwer Academic/Plenum Publishers, New York, 2002.

Let me start by introducing some assumptions and a bias or two. The first assumption is that community psychology is concerned with reducing the amount of psychopathology in the population at large, an assumption with which I think you will all agree. The second assumption is that when community psychologists tackle this problem they are guided by a strong etiological hypothesis; specifically, that psychosocial stress is important in the causation of psychopathology. This assumption is, I think, also widely accepted.

As for my biases, I will present most of them packaged in a model specifying how psychosocial stress leads to psychopathology. I present this model, however, not because I want to be contentious about the causation of psychopathology but because I find that it provides a framework within which the apparently disparate activities of community psychologists take on a satisfying coherence and directedness. Our activities are, I will argue, uniformly directed at undermining the process whereby stress generates psychopathology but, given the complexity of this process, vary because they tackle it at different points. In order to present this argument, I will first discuss a stress model, which is described in the squared boxes in Figure 1.

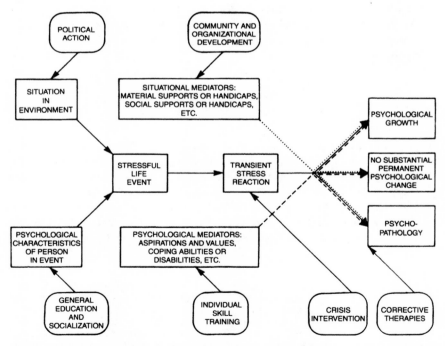

Figure 1. A model of the process whereby psychosocial stress induces psychopathology and some conceptions of how to counteract this process.

For the moment we will ignore the rounded boxes at the top and bottom of the figure.

A MODEL OF THE STRESS PROCESS

Let me note first that the process described in this model starts with a proximate rather than distant cause of psychopathology, with recent events in the life of an individual rather than with distant childhood experiences. It describes an episode that is initiated by the occurrence of one or more stressful life events and is terminated by psychological change, for good or ill, or by return to the psychological *status quo ante*.

Since the concept of a stressful life event is central to the model, let me start by taking up the issue of what defines a life event as stressful. One could, of course, rely on definition after the fact: A stressful life event is a life event that generates stress in the person who experiences it. This tautological definition is inappropriate, however, for a model concerned with understanding how stressful life events lead to psychopathology. For this purpose an independent definition of stressful life events is needed. We must, therefore, consider the argument between those who believe that change and the associated demands on the individual for readjustment are the critical conditions that make an event stressful (e.g., Holmes and Rahe, 1967) and those who believe that it is the undesirability of the event that makes it stressful (e.g., Gersten, Langner, Eisenberg, & Orzek, 1974; Vinokur & Selzer, 1975).

Although I may have been partly responsible for the development of this issue (B. S. Dohrenwend, 1973a), I now think that it is a false one, at least in its either/or form. Underlying my reasoning is the fact that, on the average, the undersirable events that have been studied entail considerably more change than the desirable events (Vinokur & Selzer, 1975, p. 334). For example, applying the change scores developed by Holmes and Rahe (1967) to a list of events used in our research in Washington Heights in Manhattan (B. P. Dohrenwend, 1974, pp. 281–282), I calculated that the average score for the undesirable events on our list was 413 while the average for the desirable events was only 225 (B. S. Dohrenwend, 1973a, p. 172). Given this kind of difference, one cannot argue that the effect of change has been excluded when one finds that, on the average, undesirable events have stronger effects on health than desirable events. There is the finding that change scores of undesirable events correlate with various outcomes while change scores of desirable events do not but the finding does not demonstrate that amount of change has no effect (cf. Gersten *et al.*, 1974; Vinokur & Selzer, 1975). In order to find out to what extent the stressfulness of events is a function of the amount of change they entail and to what extent it is a function of their undesirability, we will need to obtain equally refined measurements of these two dimensions, and examine their joint and separate effects. Meanwhile, on the basis of the evidence now available all we can say is that stressful life events seem to be events that involve change, the amount of change generally being greater when the event is undesirable than when it is desirable.

Turning now to the steps in the stress model, the first step specifies that stressful life events vary in the extent to which they are determined by the environment or by psychological characteristics of the central person in the event. For example, at one extreme, if a person is laid off from his or her job because a plant or office is closed, the event is clearly determined by environmental factors, probably largely economic, rather than by psychological characteristics of the laid off individual. In contrast, when an individual is fired for cause one infers, unless a grave injustice has been done, that the explanation of the event will be found to a large extent in some failing in the fired individual. By including this first step in the model I recognize the complexity of the causal relation between stressful life events and psychological outcomes. Specifically, this step implies that an individual may take part in creating the very events that appear later to cause him to undergo psychological change.

The next step in the model rests on a distinction emphasized by Selye (1956), and made by others as well (e.g., B. P. Dohrenwend, 1961), between a stimulus or event that initiates a stress response and the reaction to that stimulus or event. However, in making this distinction I do not want to imply agreement with Selye's well-known argument that "The pattern of the stress-reaction is very specific" (1956, p. 54). This argument, you will recall, rests on Selye's observations of a standard pattern of physiological reactions. However, there is now evidence suggesting that physiological reactions to stressful stimuli may vary considerably (Mason, 1975b, pp. 25–27). More important, the evidence concerning psychological responses to stressful events clearly indicates that they take many forms, including mood changes and a wide range of apparently pathological symptoms (e.g., B. S. Dohrenwend, 1973b; Markush & Favero, 1974; Myers, Lindenthal, & Pepper, 1974; Sheatsley & Feldman, 1964), even including some symptoms usually associated with serious psychotic disorders (Noyes & Kolb, 1963, p. 456).

What I do want to propose is that although the immediate psychological reaction to a stressful life event may resemble one or another type of psychopathology, a common characteristic of all these forms of stress reaction is that they are inherently transient or self-limiting. The evidence to support this proposition comes from studies of community reactions to disasters, which have shown repeatedly that most people who are exposed to these stressful events develop psychological symptoms, and that these symptoms are almost always transient, unless perpetuated by secondary gains (Dohrenwend & Dohrenwend, 1969, pp. 110–125).

In the next step of the model I suggest that what follows after the immediate, transient stress reaction depends on the mediation of situational and psychological factors that define the context in which this reaction occurs. Situational mediators are conditions in the environment that are external to but impinge on the individual and, I have suggested, include material supports or handicaps and social supports or handicaps. Let me note that for some theorists it is some of these relatively constant deprivations, particularly those associated with disadvantaged ethnic status and poverty, that are construed as the primary cause of stress reactions instead of passing stressful events (e.g., Langner & Michael, 1963). I am, however, not prejudging the relative importance of precipitating events as against situational constraints that mediate their impact, a question that can be answered empirically. Situational constraints may play the more important role in determining the nature of the outcome but, I am arguing, are not ordinarily sufficient by themselves to explain the occurrence of substantial changes in an individual.

One general hypothesis about situational mediators is then, that other things equal, an individual whose financial or other material resources are strained by the demands of a stressful life event is likely to have a worse outcome than a person with adequate material resources. Similarly, lack of social support is hypothesized to increase the likehood of a negative outcome (e.g., Gore, 1974; Kaplan, Cassel, & Gore, 1977; Nuckolls, Cassel, & Kaplan, 1972).

Psychological characteristics of the individual also mediate the impact of stressful events. These mediators, which include "values" and what I have labeled, generically, "coping abilities" have been the subject of extensive research by Lazarus (1966) and his colleagues, as well as Hinkle (1974), Horowitz (1976), and others. The results of this research indicate that intrapsychic predispositions and processes play an important role in determining the outcome of exposure to stressful events, but that the ways in which they interact with a stress reaction to determine the ultimate outcome are too complex to lend themselves to summary in one or two hypotheses (cf. Mason, 1975a, p. 11).

The final step in the model indicates that a transient stress reaction interacts with situational and psychological mediators to produce any of three general outcomes. First, a person who experiences stressful life events may undergo psychological growth as a result. That is, he may be judged to have matured or, in more general terms, to have changed his values and aspirations, or developed new capabilities in ways that are adaptive to and valued by others in the social setting in which he lives.

Another possibility is that the person resumes his life without notable change once the stressful life events and his immediate, transient stress reaction are over. The outcome is, then, that the events produce no substantial psychological change in the person.

Finally, an individual may develop psychopathology as a consequence of exposure to stressful life events. In the stress model that I am presenting, this outcome is defined as a dysfunctional reaction that contrasts with a transient stress reaction in that it is persistent and appears to be self-sustaining. Moreover, because the symptoms of persistent dysfunctional reactions and the symptoms of transient stress reactions often do not differ, the conception that psychopathology is self-sustaining and a stress reaction is not, is the critical distinction between them.

STRATEGIES FOR REDUCING THE RATE OF PSYCHOPATHOLOGY IN THE COMMUNITY

Clearly, we would all like to promote positive outcomes and prevent negative outcomes among individuals who are exposed to stressful life events. The value of this goal is indisputable. Disputes have developed, however, about what should be done to reduce the prevalence of psychopathology. Where one stands in these disputes depends, I suggest, on where one chooses to tackle the stress process. Let us, therefore, look at this process from the perspective of what to do about it, starting with the outcome and moving back through the model.

Treatment of Psychopathology

There is no disagreement that the individual who has developed self-sustaining psychopathology should be treated, with the aim of effecting a cure if possible. To this end, a wide range of psychological and psycho- pharmacological therapies have been developed. The relation of these therapies to the stress process is indicated in Figure 1 by showing that corrective therapies are designed to tackle established psychopathology.

These varied therapies are themselves a source of many disputes, with each type of therapy having its adherents as well as its critics. Even among the most dedicated adherents of particular methods, however, I think there are few who would argue that there is an established cure for psychopathology in general or for most particular types. Thus, in the face of considerable frustration and discouragement about the possibility of curing fully developed psychopathology, many psychologists have proposed that intervention be moved back to an earlier point in the stress process.

Crisis Intervention

Specifically, they have proposed that therapy be provided when the individual is experiencing a stress reaction, before self-perpetuating psychopathology has developed. As I have indicated in Figure 1, this approach is designated "crisis intervention." I should note that I am using this term in the narrow sense of providing brief psychotherapy during a life crisis (cf. Lindemann, 1944). I will come later to other types of aid that may be provided by various community agencies during a crisis, which are sometimes also called crisis intervention.

Therapy during a life crisis, it has been argued, is cost-effective compared to many kinds of traditional psychotherapy on two counts. First, clinicians believe that psychotherapy has greater impact on the client at the time of a stress reaction than later on, after the immediate crisis has passed (Bloom, 1975, pp. 134–138). Second, because therapy provided as crisis intervention can be relatively brief it is less costly than extended psychotherapy.

Note, however, that these arguments for the cost effectiveness of crisis intervention are put forth in the context of providing therapeutic services to persons who apply or are referred for them. What if we raise our sights and aim to provide crisis intervention for the entire community? The first problem is that we cannot assume that everyone who might need professional help in managing a life crisis will seek it. On the contrary, available evidence indicates that the great majority of people in psychological throuble never contact professionals trained to help them (e.g., Srole, Langner, Michael, Opler, & Rennie, 1962, p. 275).

Let us see, then, what might happen if an attempt is made to reach these people. Specifically, I will examine the results of a study of crisis intervention involving all persons in a community experiencing a particular stressful life event. In this experiment by Polak, Egan, Vandenbergh, and Williams (1975) families in one county who experienced a sudden death were identified through the coroner's office and assigned either to the experimental group, who were offered services, or to a control group, to whom services were not offered. An additional control was provided by studying families who were matched to the experimental and control groups on demographic characteristics but had not experienced a recent death.

The results of this study were not encouraging, since neither at the 6-month follow-up nor at 18 months (Bloom, 1975, p. 165) was there any evidence that the intervention had been effective. This study was flawed, however, by the investigators' inability to control precrisis levels of functioning in the families, so that the bereaved families were functioning more poorly than nonbereaved families before they entered the study as well as

after. Nor were the investigators able to control assignment of families to
the experimental and control groups, so that it turned out that the experimental group contained more families in which the death had been very
sudden or by suicide. Bloom (1975) argued on this basis that the study did
not provide an adequate test of the efficacy of crisis intervention in a general community population. Be that as it may, neither does the lack of evidence of improvement in the experimental group encourage adoption of
community-wide crisis intervention as a method of reducing the incidence
of psychopathology in the population.

Moreover, let me point out that if there were good evidence of the
effectiveness of crisis intervention as a method of community psychology, we
would still have at least two serious problems in implementing it. The first
concerns identification of persons in the community facing life crises.
Sometimes individuals' life crises arise from a community-wide disaster such
as a flood or tornado. Others occur in the context of a milestone event, such
as starting school, that occurs at the same time for each age cohort in the
community. However, many life crises do not result from such highly visible
or regularly occurring events but from events that are particular to the lives
of the affected individuals. Polak and his colleagues (1975) could, through
the coroner's office, identify families in their community who were experiencing one specific type of stressful life event. However, it is difficult to con-
ceive of equally effective ways of locating all the other people who, at any
particular time, are experiencing stressful events related to their work, their
family life, their friends, or any of their other life spheres. And if we could
locate them, a second problem would have to be faced. Could we really
afford to provide therapeutic aid to all of them? It seems unrealistic to suppose that we could, given the acknowledged insufficiency of mental health
services (e.g., Bloom, 1975, p. 221). Therefore, I conclude that, for lack of evidence of effectiveness, because of difficulties that would be encountered in
case-finding, and because the cost would probably be prohibitive, crisis
intervention holds little promise as a method of reducing the incidence of
stress-related psychopathology throughout a community population.

Although community psychologists have not explicitly arrived at such
a critical assessment of crisis intervention, they have clearly been searching
for other means of reducing the incidence of psychopathology. In looking
for alternative strategies, the general tactic of community psychologists has
been, as I see it, to tackle the stress process at still earlier stages.

Individual Skill Training

Moving back from crisis intervention at the time of the stress reaction,
Figure 1 shows that the next point of attack on the stress process is on

personal factors that mediate the impact of stressful life events. In abstract, what is wanted here is training that will develop a high level of ability to face and solve complex social and emotional problems. The necessary abilities have been described to some extent by the careful work on reactions to stressful stimuli and events by investigators such as Hinkle (1974), Horowitz (1976), and Lazarus (1966). Their work has not, however, been translated directly into training programs, nor am I sure that it lends itself readily to such translation. Instead, community psychologists are tackling this aspect of the stress process mainly through educational experiments with children. Often this work is done in schools with children who have exhibited more or less severely dysfunctional behavior in that setting (Cowen, 1973, pp. 450–453). From one perspective, this kind of school-based program is engaged in secondary prevention of psychopathology, since it aims to correct problems after they have become visible. My predecessor, Emory Cowen, made this point in his presidential address to Division 27 when he claimed that the Primary Mental Health Project, in which he and his colleagues provided special training aimed at maladapting primary school children, was misleadingly named (1977, p. 3). Looked at in this way, these programs belong with other treatment strategies at the end of the stress process. I think, however, that there is more to this strategy than Cowen's disclaimer allows. From the perspective of the stress model of psychopathology the Primary Mental Health Project and others like it can be seen as aiming to strengthen the personal skills with which the individual will confront stressful events later in life and thereby reducing the likelihood of his developing psychopathology on these later occasions. Moreover, some community psychologists who have implemented this kind of childhood intervention project have explicitly done so not only for the sake of children in trouble but also for the sake of the adults these children will become (e.g., Sandler, Duricko, & Grande, 1975, p. 31).

General Education and Socialization

Programs designed to help children who are in trouble have the advantage that the dysfunctional behavior of the child provides some guide as to what kind of help is needed. On the other hand, the weakness of this approach, conceived as primary prevention, is that it rests on the assumption that without intervention children who show identifiable problems will grow into ineffective adults and, conversely, that children who do not show such problems will very likely become effective adults. Moreover, selective intervention with problem children runs the danger of stigmatizing the children who receive special treatment. Considerations such as these have led to primary prevention programs which, instead of being aimed at children who are in trouble, are designed to improve the education and socialization either of children in general or of demographically defined high-risk groups, usually children starting life at the bottom of the socioeconomic system. Some of these programs are, like those aimed selectively at troubled children, designed to teach skills that may serve as coping mechanisms when stressful events are encountered later in life. In addition, however, particularly when the target population is a high-risk group, some of these programs seem to be intended to provide the child with skills needed to avoid occupational and interpersonal crises, such as job losses and family breakups, that might arise from their own failings as much as or more than from their life circumstances. As others (e.g., Zax & Spector, 1974) have noted, however, most of these programs are designed primarily to improve cognitive skills, with the explicit or implicit hope that there will be spillover into the kinds of general social competence that might prevent later crises in interpersonal relationships.

With programs of this kind we have, it seems, pushed back to the very origin of the stress process and have, therefore, moved as far as possible from treatment of individual cases of psychopathology into the realm of primary prevention. Indeed we have, so long as we focus on the skills and competence of the individual community member.

The stress model shows, however, that there is another path that can be taken in moving back through the stress process. We have seen that the outcome of the stress process is dependent not only on the individual's ability to cope with stressful events but also on the material and social supports that are available to him. Another preventive strategy that community psychologists have adopted, therefore, is to build or strengthen support systems in the community.

Development of Supportive Social Agencies

I noted earlier that the term "crisis intervention" has sometimes been given broader meaning than I gave it. Although I have limited this term to brief, professional therapeutic intervention at the time of a stress reaction, others have used it to designate any supporting services provided in the context of a stressful event (cf. Bloom, 1975, Chapter 8). I think it is useful, however, when describing the activities of community psychologists to distinguish between instances in which the psychologist, another professional, or someone under direct professional supervision provides therapeutic support to persons who have recently experienced stressful events, and instances in which the professional's role is to help community members build or strengthen their own support systems. In the latter situation the professional has no direct responsibility for the individuals who receive help from these systems. Moreover, his work with community members is not usually initiated by or limited to the time of particular stressful events.

One example of this strategy is the series of trainig projects developed by Bard with the New York City Police Department, the New York City Housing Authority Police, and a suburban police department. Each training project was based in part on what had been learned by the community psychologists from the previous project, and all were cumulatively designed to train the police to change their orientations and procedures so that they would function as effective agents of social support as well as social control on the frequent occasions when they are called on to deal with familial and other interpersonal conflicts (Bard, 1975).

Political Action with Disadvantaged Status Groups

In reporting their work, Bard and his colleagues pointed out that one reason for working with the police is that they are the agents that lower-class community members are most likely to call on during interpersonal crises (Bard & Berkowitz, 1969). Recall also that the status group often chosen as the target of programs designed to increase personal competence and coping ability is also the disadvantaged lower class, who are frequently minority group members. In general, the activities of community psychologists of the kinds that I have described up to now are most often directed at serving the poor, particularly poor minority groups.

Thus, despite the diversity of activities that characterizes community psychology one aim they have in common is helping the socioeconomic underdogs of our society. Noting this common aim, some community psychologists have taken the logical step of asking what we can do to eliminate the status of socioeconomic underdog (e.g., Rappaport, 1977, pp. 119–123). Viewed from the perspective of the stress process, they have asked how they can help this group get access to resources that would prevent avoidable stressful life events. Concretely, the questions are such as how to get stable jobs so as to avoid periodic unemployment, and how to get adequate health care so as to avoid unnecessary illnesses and deaths. Although the answers to these questions that have evolved from the experience of community psychologists are not simple (e.g., Heller & Monahan, 1977, pp. 371–411; Rappaport, 1977, pp. 188–213), at their core is the idea that political action by the disadvantaged groups is the *sine qua non* of programs designed to reduce the stressfulness of the lives of those who are impoverished and discriminated against in our society.

The stress model suggests, I think correctly, that with this strategy community psychologists have moved as far away as possible from the strategy of providing therapy for persons who have developed psychopathology.

With the strategy of political action, community psychologists have also moved into an area of maximum controversy, some of it among themselves. On the one hand, some have argued that political action, at least to the extent of supporting the existing distribution of wealth and power in the social system, is always implicit in the activities of the helping professions. From this premise it follows that community psychologists cannot avoid political action but can either, through indifference, opt for a policy of no social change, or, if concerned with the psychological problems generated by poverty and discrimination, engage in political action designed to promote social change. This position has been argued both by elder statesmen in our field, notably Robert Reiff (1971), and by more junior spokesmen such as Julian Rappaport (1977, pp. 4–5).

Other community psychologists have, however, taken a pessimistic view of the possibility of community psychologists becoming successful political activists, expressing the view that psychologists cannot and should not arrogate to themselves the responsibility for righting the social and economic wrongs of our society. Notable among these critics are Kessler and Albee in their *Annual Review of Psychology* article on primary prevention (1975, pp. 560, 577–578). From the perspective of the stress model, however, it seems possible to legitimize political action as an activity of community psychologists if it is clearly and explicitly directed at reducing the incidence of avoidable stressful life events. Perhaps, therefore, it will not be necessary to arrive at a full resolution of this controversy within community psychology, which would be difficult to do in any case, given its heavy ideological loading.

CONCLUSION

Let us return to the questions with which I started: What do community psychologists do? What is the difference between community psychology and clinical psychology? To answer the second question first, I suggest that the critical distinction that divides community from clinical psychology can be described by drawing a line through the model of the stress process between mediating factors and the stress reaction. Clinical psychologists come into the picture at the earliest when a reaction to stressful events has occurred. In treating the stress reaction or, more often, established psychopatholgy, they may aim to strengthen the individual's coping abilities and to prevent him from creating stressful life events for himself, but their task is basically to overcome current distress and dysfunction.

Community psychologists, I would argue, are distinguished from clinical psychologists by the fact that their strategies are directly concerned only with the earlier elements in the stress process, the preexisting mediating factors in the person or his environment and factors, again in the person or his environment, that tend to promote or prevent the occurrence of avoidable stressful life events.

Beyond suggesting this distinction between community and clinical psychology, my aim in presenting this stress model and its implications for action is to be descriptive rather than prescriptive. For the sake of providing an organizing scheme I have, I fear, presented a rather simplified description of the activities of community psychologists. I have not, for instance, explicitly included the fact that we do research designed to predict what strategies will be most effective with what persons or what type of potential psychopathology and to evaluate the effectiveness of strategies that have been implemented. In further explanation of the description based on the stress model, I should note that I do not mean to indicate that the categories of activities described in the domain of community psychology are mutually exclusive. The same program may be designed both to improve the quality of mediating factors, that is, individual coping skills or community supports, and to reduce the incidence of avoidable stressful life events. It seems, however, to be less common that a single program tackles these components in the stress process at the individual and at the organizational or community level at the same time.

With these qualifications, I hope that my schematic description of what community psychologists do, and do not do, is at least grossly accurate. I hope so, in part, because I would not want to misrepresent the field. In addition, however, I hope that it is accurate to say that the diverse activities of community psychologists are generated by strategies that complement each other in such a way that their effects will cumulate and multiply so as to reduce the amount of psychopathology in the communities we serve.

REFERENCES

Bard, M. Collaboration between law enforcement and the social sciences. *Professional Psychology*, 1975, *6*, 127–134.

Bard, M. & Berkowitz, B. A community psychology consultation program in police family crisis intervention: Preliminary impressions. *International Journal of Social Psychiatry*, 1969, *15*, 209–215.

Bloom, B. L. *Community mental health: A general introduction.* Monterey, Calif.: Brooks/Cole Publishing Company, 1975.

Cowen, E. Social and community interventions. *Annual Review of Psychology*, 1973, *25*, 423–472.

Cowen, E. Baby-steps toward primary prevention. *American Journal of Community Psychology*, 1977, *5*, 1–22.

Dohrenwend, B. P. The social psychological nature of stress: A framework for causal inquiry. *Journal of Abnormal and Social Psychology*, 1961, *62*, 294–302.

Dohrenwend, B. P. Problems in defining and sampling the relevant population of stressful life events. In B. S. Dohrenwend & B. P. Dohrenwend (Eds.), *Stressful life events*. New York: John Wiley & Sons, 1974.

Dohrenwend, B. P. & Dohrenwend, B. S. *Social status and psychological disorder: A causal inquiry*. New York: John Wiley & Sons, 1969.

Dohrenwend, B. S. Life events as stressors: A methodological inquiry. *Journal of Health and Social Behavior*, 1973, *14*, 167–175.

Dohrenwend, B. S. Social status and stressful life events. *Journal of Personality and Social Psychology*, 1973, *28*, 225–235.

Gersten, J. C., Langner, T. S., Eisenberg, J. G., & Orzek, L. Child behavior and life events: Undesirable change or change per se? In B. S. Dohrenwend & B. P. Dohrenwend (Eds.), *Stressful life events*. New York: John Wiley & Sons, 1974.

Gore, S. The influence of social support and related variables in ameliorating the consequences of job loss. *Dissertation Abstracts International*, 1974, *34*, (8-A, Pt. 2), 5330–5331.

Heller, K. & Monahan, J. *Psychology and community change*. Homewood, III.: Dorsey Press, 1977.

Hinkle, L. E., Jr. The effect of exposure to culture change, social change, and changes in interpersonal relationships on health. In B. S. Dohrenwend & B. P. Dohrenwend (Eds.), *Stressful life events*. New York: John Wiley & Sons, 1974.

Holmes, T. H. & Rahe, R. H. The social readjustment rating scale. *Journal of Psychosomatic Research*, 1967, *11*, 213–218.

Horowitz, M. J. *Stress response syndromes*. New York: Jason Aronson, 1976.

Kaplan, B. H., Cassel, J. C., & Gore, S. Social support and health. *Medical Care*, 1977, *15*, 47–58.

Kessler, M. & Albee, G. W. Primary prevention. *Annual Review of Psychology*, 1975, *26*, 557–591.

Langner, T. S. & Michael, S. T. *Life stress and mental health*. New York: Free Press of Glencoe, 1963.

Lazarus, R. S. *Psychological stress and the coping process*. New York: McGraw-Hill Book Company, 1966.

Lindemann, E. Symptomatology and management of acute grief. *American Journal of Psychiatry*, 1944, *101*, 141–148.

Markush, R. E. & Favero, R. V. Epidemiologic assessment of stressful life events, depressed mood, and psychophysiological symptoms: A preliminary report. In B. S. Dohrenwend & B. P. Dohrenwend (Eds.), *Stressful life events*. New York: John Wiley & Sons, 1974.

Mason, J. W. A historical view of the stress field: Part 1. *Journal of Human Stress*, 1975, *1*, 6–12.

Mason, J. W. A historical view of the stress field: Part 2. *Journal of Human Stress*, 1975, *1*, 22–36.

Myers, J. K., Lindenthal, J. J., & Pepper, M. P. Social class, life events and psychiatric symptoms: A longitudinal study. In B. S. Dohrenwend & B. P. Dohrenwend (Eds.), *Stressful life events*. New York: John Wiley & Sons, 1974.

Noyes, A. P. & Kolb, L. C. *Modern clinical psychiatry* (6th ed.). Philadelphia: W. B. Saunders, 1963.

Nuckolls, K. B., Cassel, J. C., & Kaplan, B. H. Psychosocial assets, life crisis and the prognosis of pregnancy. *American Journal of Epidemiology*, 1972, *95*, 431–441.

Polak, P. R., Egan, D., Vandenbergh, R., & Williams, W. V. Prevention in mental health: A controlled study. *American Journal of Psychiatry*, 1975, *132*, 146–149.

Rappaport, J. *Community psychology: Values, research, and action*. New York: Holt, Rinehart, & Winston, 1977.

Reiff, R. Community psychology and public policy. In G. Rosenblum (Ed.), *Issues in community psychology and preventive mental health*. New York: Behavioral Publications Inc., 1971.

Sandler, I. N., Duricko, A., & Grande, L. Effectiveness of an early secondary prevention program in an inner-city elementary school. *American Journal of Community Psychology*, 1975, *3*, 23–32.

Selye, H. *The stress of life*. New York: McGraw-Hill Book Company, 1956.

Sheatsley, P. B. & Feldman, J. The assassination of President Kennedy: Public reaction. *Public Opinion Quarterly*, 1974, *28*, 189–215.

Srole, L., Langner, T. S., Michael, S. T., Opler, M. K., & Rennie, T. A. C. *Mental health in the metropolis: The midtown study* (Vol. 1) New York: McGraw Hill Book Company, 1962.

Vinokur, A. & Selzer, M. L. Desirable versus undesirable life events; their relationship to stress and mental distress. *Journal of Personality and Social Psychology*, 1975, *32*, 329–337.

Zax, M. & Spector, G. A. *An introduction to community psychology*. New York: John Wiley & Sons, 1974.

IV

The 1980s

8

In Praise of Paradox: A Social Policy of Empowerment over Prevention*

Julian Rappaport

The thesis of this paper is that the most important and interesting aspects of community life are by their very nature paradoxical; and that our task as researchers, scholars, and professionals should be to "unpack" and influence contemporary resolutions of paradox. Within this general theme I will argue that in order to do so we will need to be more a social movement than a profession, regain our sense of urgency, and avoid the tendency to become "one-sided." I will suggest that the paradoxical issue which demands our attention in the foreseeable future is a conflict between "rights" and "needs" models for viewing people in trouble.

For those who are concerned with social/community problems the idea of prevention is the logical extension of a needs model which views people in difficulty as children; the idea of advocacy is an extension of the rights model of people as citizens. I will conclude that both of these are one-sided and propose an empowerment model for a social policy which views people as complete human beings, creates a symbolic sense of urgency, requires attention to paradox, and expects divergent and dialectical rather than convergent solutions.

*Presidential address, Division 27, Community Psychology, 88th Annual Meeting of the American Psychological Association, Montreal, Canada, September 3, 1980. Originally published in the *American Journal of Community Psychology*, 9(1) (1981): pp. 1–25.

A Quarter Century of Community Psychology: Readings from the American Journal of Community Psychology, edited by Tracey A. Revenson *et al.* Kluwer Academic/Plenum Publishers, New York, 2002.

THE PARADOXICAL NATURE OF
SOCIAL/COMMUNITY PROBLEMS

Basic to my argument is an assumption that unlike other (i.e., non-human, inanimate, or purely biological) systems, human social systems for living are paradoxical in nature. In order to make my case I will need to dabble in bits of philosophy and history, both social and psychological, and to define some terms. The terms are *paradox, antinomy, convergent and divergent reasoning*, and *dialectic*. I begin with a definition of paradox.

Paradox

A paradox, according to the Oxford English Dictionary (p. 450) is:

1. A statement or tenet contrary to received opinion or belief ... discordent with what is held to be established truth. 2. A statement or proposition which on the face of it seems self contradictory, absurd or at variance with common sense, though on investigation or when explained, it may prove to be well-founded ... often applied to a proposition or a statement that is actually self contradictory ... essentially absurd and false.

Notice that in this definition there are two possibilities when confronted with paradox: one is that we have discovered an essentially true phenomenon, a reality which at first seems to be self-contradictory but on investigation proves to be well founded. The second possibility is that the paradox is more apparent than real, or a false paradox. I am going to suggest in a moment that one of our tasks as social scientists is to discover the difference between true and false paradox. But first I need to introduce a related term: *antinomy*.

Antinomy

Basic to the idea of paradox is the notion of antinomy, "a contradiction in a law, or between two equally binding laws" This idea originates from conflict in authority or in canon or civil law wherein "whatever of the alternative solutions we adopt we are led to absurdity and contradiction" (Oxford English Dictionary, 1971, p. 371).

Antinomy is in many respects the rule rather than the exception in social and community life. As Schumacher (1977) points out, the frequently encountered opposites in education and politics, two major fields of social life, are freedom and equality. These are two equally positive values which, when mistakenly viewed one at a time, lead us to maximize one and ignore the other. Because they are intimately intertwined they constitute an antinomy and present us with phenomena that are true paradoxes. That is, the very nature of education and politics is paradoxical. The problems do not simply appear to be paradoxical; they actually are paradoxical problems because they are made up of real antinomies.

Using the example of freedom and equality in government: If we maximize one we find that the other is necessarily minimized. Allowing total freedom will lead the strong (in whatever form strength is found—social power, money, physical prowess) to dominate the weak and equality to be obliterated. Equality will require constraints on freedom, which will necessarily impose limits on certain people. This is of course a classical problem, but we tend to think that its solution will be similar to solutions in the physical sciences and can be found by convergent reasoning. The problem requires divergent thought. I will discuss the difference between convergent and divergent thought in a moment.

A crucial task for anyone interested in social/community problems is to look for paradox so as to discover antinomies, such as the one I have just described, in social and community relationships. Once discovered, we will often find that one side or the other has been ignored and its opposite emphasized. To discover which paradoxes of social life are founded on antinomy and which are founded on absurdity and false reasoning is part of our job. That is the understanding part. The action part of our job is then to confront the discovered paradoxes by pushing them in the ignored direction. To take this seriously means that those who are interested in social change must never allow themselves the privilege of being in the majority, else they run the risk of losing their grasp of the paradox. That is one reason why social change is not an end product but rather a process. This leads me to immodestly suggest, only in part facetiously, Rappaport's Rule: *When most people agree with you, worry.*

Dialectic

The idea of the dialectic is central to what this paper is about. The point is simply that much of what underlies the substance of our field requires us to recognize that we are being pulled in two ways at once and that we often need to pay attention to two different and apparently opposed poles of thought.

The picture of the dialectic which I like the best is one portrayed in a modest book called *The Simple Life* by Vernard Eller (1973). Eller likens the dialectic to a department store demonstration of a vacuum cleaner with its hose pointed upward and the machine turned to "blow." In the jet of air above the nozzle there is a Ping-Pong ball caught between two opposing forces. Gravity pulls it down to the air jet, which has the effect of blowing it up. As it goes up it gets out of the range of the force of the air and gravity pulls it back down. "Thought or action that operates out of this sort of dynamic tension, giving attention to one truth in such a way that attention must then immediately be given to its counterpart—this is what we mean by dialectic" (Eller, 1973, p. 11).

The tendency to become focused on one side of a dialectical problem, that is, to pay attention to one side of the truth so as to fail to take into account an equally compelling opposite, is what I refer to as being one-sided.

Joseph E. McGrath, current editor of the *Journal of Social Issues*, recently reviewed the history of that journal (Note 1) and came to the conclusion, rightly I think, "*that most of the social issues of our time are fundamentally of this form: a basic opposition of two or more 'valid'* (that is morally correct) *principles*" and that "*most social issues of this form have at least two 'decent' solutions* (i.e., morally justifiable) *sides to them (often more than two)*." (p. 36, italics in original).

An example from content in our domain of interest may help to demonstrate the dialectic. In order to implement a social policy decision one must confront the organizational level of analysis, yet as soon as we turn away from individual persons, either the target people or the administrators, we begin to lose our ability to be effective.

When we try to implement a social policy such as Public Law 94-142 (the right to education for all handicapped persons), unless we pay a great deal of attention to the individual teachers who implement such policy at the face-to-face level, we are likely to find the intention of the policy distorted in practice. On the other hand, to deal only with the individual teachers would be very ineffective as a means to alter public policy. Either strategy alone is one-sided.

Another example: the development of compensatory education in our public schools was a step which rejected the notion of stable IQ as the determinant of school performance in favor of direct instruction to enhance performance for high-risk, i.e., minority, children. Yet, as benign as was this intention, and indeed there is much reason to assume that direct instruction is useful and has its place, the development of a widespread policy of compensatory education led to what Herbert Ginsburg (1972) so rightly called "the myth of the deprived child." It became so one-sided that it sanctioned the belief that minority children lack not only the content of middle-class knowledge but the ability to learn, because it refused to acknowledge what they do know and how they acquire it (cf. Hunt, 1969). We, quite mistakenly, as Baratz and Baratz (1970) pointed out a decade ago, institutionalized our heretofore personalized racism. No one intended to do that; we simply paid attention to one side of the dialectic as opposed to the other. We forgot that just because these children could benefit from direct instruction in the content of middle-class knowledge it did not mean that they did not already have a great deal of knowledge and skill. We forgot that change in the schools as well as the children is essential. We allowed ourselves to be content to show a statistical gain on achievement test scores in second grade without bothering to ask if that meant real success in school or in the world. Most such programs have simply ignored the strengths and assets of the children and their families and failed to change the schools, or the opportunity structure of the society, so that program effects simply fade away (e.g., Gray & Klaus, 1970; Rappaport, 1977, Chapters 7 and 8). What we say is that the effects fail to generalize; what it means is that they don't make any difference in the real world of life.

The same may be said for desegregation. The national policy was intended to equalize educational opportunity. Busing children for racial balance in schools has, in many areas, effectively helped to destroy already decaying black neighborhoods. Respecting and fostering minority culture, preparing children for the majority culture, integration of minority and majority, strengthening local neighborhoods: these are equally compelling values with *opposite* poles. One does not necessarily lead to the other; one may hinder the other. It is by nature a dialectical problem and requires many divergent solutions.

Convergent and Divergent Reasoning

For a description of convergent and divergent reasoning I turn to the work of E. F. Schumacher, best known as the author of *Small is Beautiful* (1973). In his lesser known book, *A Guide for the Perplexed* (1977), Schumacher argues that there are two very different kinds of problems in the world. One type, convergent problems, are those characteristic of inanimate nature. For such problems many solutions are offered which gradually, over time, converge toward *the* right answer, one which turns out to be stable, if improvable, over time. Problems of this type are either solved or "as yet" unsolved. There is no reason, in principle, why unsolved convergent type problems should not one day be solved forever. It is obvious that this attitude is very effective in the material world, where by choice of problem, exact measurement, and quantification, all problems chosen can and will be solved. In fact, one selects only problems one believes to be solvable.[1] It is far from obvious that social problems are of this type.

What if, rather than converging, we find that equally clear, logical answers, which are exactly the opposite of one another, are developed by equally clear, logical people; that is, the solutions diverge rather than converge?

This is, in fact, the case in social science over time (Cronbach, 1975; Gergen, 1973). That is, as new solutions are developed and institutionalized they become one-sided and other solutions not seen before, and contradictory to the first, emerge (Takanishi, 1978). The juvenile court is one of my favorite examples (Note 2); originally developed as a means to divert children from the evils of the adult court, today we see many diversion programs aimed at diverting children from the evils of the juvenile court itself.

If we are dealing with problems that are dialectical by nature, then they will necessarily yield many divergent rather than one convergent solution, not only over time but even at the same moment in time. That may be one reason why social science seems to have no single dominant paradigm in the Kuhnian sense. Usually we lament this diversity of conflicting paradigms. It may be that the nature of the phenomena are such that diversity of paradigms is a true reflection of the things studied, which may be *best* understood in more than one way.

If by convergent reasoning we act as if there can be *the* solution we will become one-sided and necessarily create unintended negative consequences by ignoring the other side. This is exactly what we have done when we have tried to implement community mental health policy by taking people out of mental hospitals without paying attention to them, or to the people who would need to interact directly with them, as individuals. The results have often been not only disastrous but inhumane (cf. *N. Y. Times*, Note 3). Unfortunately, some will argue that this means we never should have allowed such people to leave the hospital. That is simply a one-sided solution in the other direction.

In fact, what is wrong is that we acted as if this were a convergent rather than a divergent problem, and we ignored its dialectual nature. The problem of chronic patient status has a variety of solutions, some of which are contradictory, and both sides of the contradiction need to have attention paid to them. This is an example of a problem with a paradoxical nature. When we pay attention to paradox we are more likely than otherwise to find ourselves being useful.

---

[1]Whether or not the physical sciences and engineering, fields more likely than ours to work on convergent problems, do solve all of their problems is actually irrelevant to my argument, which is less that social problems are not solvable and more that they are solvable in many different ways.

CONFRONTING PARADOX: TWO EXAMPLES
FROM OUR PAST

Perhaps one of the most important sources stimulating the origins of community psychology emerged from those who confronted the paradox that demand for human services infinitely expands to meet the services available and that we can never train enough professional mental health manpower to meet the needs (Albee, 1959; Cowen, Gardner, & Zax, 1967). Analysis of the paradoxical relationship between professional training, supply of services, demand and need, not only stimulated the nonprofessional movement, which gave vigor to both community mental health and community psychology, but also provided a kind of urgency to our work.

There are now enough studies of nonprofessionals (Rappaport, 1977) so that even if one is more conservative than to argue that they are better than professionals for certain problems (Durlak, 1979), neither can one argue that there is better evidence for the effectiveness of professionals. In fact, nonprofessional interventions have been subjected to more rather than less scrutiny than those of professionals, especially for service delivery other than psychotherapy per se. The fact that the American Psychological Association wishes to ignore this by exclusion and demanding licensing and credentialing is far more of a guild than an effectiveness issue (Gross, 1978; Koocher, 1979). But my aim here is not to convince you of that, it is rather to point out that confronting paradox led to more useful work and new ideas than most research programs.

Another outstanding example of confronting paradox is William Ryan's (1971) classic work, *Blaming the Victim*, and the brief but brilliant paper by Caplan and Nelson (1973) which pushes forward the implications of our individual "person blame" ideology. They presented us with an antinomy, a contradiction. It hurt our moral sensibilities and created a sense of urgency. It has served to fuel excitement in our field. When we see a glimpse of paradox we become charged with urgency because once the opposite to a one-sided solution is seen it burns to be said. Blaming the victim has been a major symbolic and ideological cry for community psychology as a social movement.

COMMUNITY PSYCHOLOGY AS A
SOCIAL MOVEMENT

Partly because community psychology has had the character of a social movement (Killian, 1964) it has been able to contribute to the pursuit of paradox, a task which involves emotionality, ideology, the symbolic, and the ideational (Zald, Note 4) as well as the logical and the concrete. As Lilly and Smith (1980) have recently shown for the field of special education, to the extent that a discipline becomes more a profession and less a social movement its practitioners are likely to become more defensive, conservative, and lose their sense of "urgency" (Hiller, 1975).

To hold on to urgency requires a cause that transcends ourselves, one that holds symbolic power. To burn with fervor for some higher purpose, be it expressed in understanding or in action, is to be alive and to push ourselves to create the possibilities for change. The most important contributions from community psychology have been fueled with a sense of urgency. To give up such urgency is to live with mediocrity.

A decade ago, in his presidential address to this Division, Jim Kelly (1980) proposed an "antidote for arrogance" as the ecological view of man and the role of the psychologist in the community rather than as simply a student of the community. Murray Levine's (1980) recent writing on investigative reporting pleads a similar case for the researcher who immerses one's self in the phenomena of interest. The psychologist of this variety is one who is deeply involved, "dotes" on the environment, and has a "love of community" (Kelly, 1970).

In the decade following Kelly's plea we have seen much of psychology become concerned with establishing itself as a legitimate profession. We have also seen a nation turn from a time of urgency in its search for corporate justice to a desire for individual protection of personal, especially economic, interests.

The context for doing community psychology has changed, and we are being affected by that change in a way which runs the risk of pushing us away from our sense of urgency about the really important questions in the life of the community, toward a consolidation of our own position and a temptation to settle for the security and the mediocrity of fitting in (Note 5).

If the antidote for arrogance is the ecological view of man the medicine for mediocrity is the pursuit of paradox. Pursuit of paradox means looking for the contradictions of life. It means finding those places in social and community institutions which have become what I have referred to as *one-sided* and trying to turn them around. When I say "have become one-sided" I am implying that there is more than one side to the ways in which our social institutions can operate to do their job. Partly because institutions have a tendency to become one-sided, many social problems are ironically and inadvertently created by the so-called helping systems—the institutions and organizations developed by well-meaning scientists and professionals—and often "solutions" create more problems than they solve.

I now see such problem-creation as a function of convergent reasoning about divergent problems which leads to an inability to think dialecticly and causes us to create one-sided monolithic and institutionalized solutions requiring the pursuit of paradox in order to make change possible. Such pursuit can be accomplished only by those who carry a sense of urgency into their work, because all the pressures of professionalism will ask one to ignore the paradox and to keep on doing what is "acceptable."

But fortunately there are always those who fight against such pressures. The anthropologist, Jules Henry (1963, p. 10) put it this way: "The strong inherent tendency of Homo Sapiens to search for solutions to problems he himself creates ranges from ... therapy ... to social revolution ... although culture is for man, it is also against him." This statement, presented as a characteristic of human nature, is the prototype. If it is correct that solutions create problems which require new solutions this should be of some interest to us, but not because we can expect to find a solution once and for all. Rather, it is the paradox itself that should be of interest because that should tell us something about the fact that *a variety of contradictory solutions will necessarily emerge* and that we ought not only expect but welcome this, because the more different solutions to the same problem the better, not the worse.

That social institutions and professions create as well as solve problems is *not* a call for working harder to find the single best technique or for lamenting the failure of our best minds to be creative. Quite the opposite. *It is a problem to be understood as contained in the basic nature of the subject matter of our field.* It will always be this way. There can never be a now and for all time single scientific "breakthrough" which settles and solves the puzzles of our discipline. Today's solution must be tomorrow's problem. And even today we need many different solutions to the same problem, not one monolithic answer. To seek *the* answer may be more than wrong, it may be dangerous. Thomas Merton (1968) put it this way:

> Knowledge expands man like a balloon, and gives him a precarious wholeness in which he thinks that he holds in himself all the dimensions of a truth the totality of which is denied to others. It then becomes his duty, he thinks, by virtue of his superior knowledge, to punish those who do not share his truth. How can he love others he thinks, except by imposing on them the truth which they would otherwise insult and neglect (p. 44)

This reality when pointed out by others such as Sarason (1978) has, I think, sometimes been misinterpreted to suggest that there are no solutions to social problems and that if we follow this view to its logical conclusion we must give up trying (Note 1). It is as if human problems can only be handled by positivistic convergent science or not at all. I do not believe that there are no solutions, only that given the nature of social problems there are no permanent solutions and no single "this is the only answer possible" solutions, even at any moment in time. Divergent, dialectical problems must have many solutions which, like the Ping-Pong ball in Eller's example, change with the currents. The challenge for our discipline is to continue to fuel the fires of urgency by seeking out the paradoxical, by finding those places where one-sided solutions have developed and pushing the institutions toward the other side. To do this requires that we pay some attention to social history.

SOCIAL HISTORY AND THE RIGHTS/NEEDS DIALECTIC

When the community mental health movement began to impact on psychology we believed that we were entering an era of exciting social change, and to some extent we may have been. What the community mental health movement did was to confront the fact that the mental health system had gone too far to one side and become an institutional warehouse for the poor and an existential philosophy for the wealthy. Confronting this one-sidedness was both necessary and useful. It had the character and urgency of a social movement, it pushed the dialectic within the mental health professions in an ignored direction, i.e., toward deinstitutionalization and extending the reach of viable services to the unreached.

For the profession of psychology the period between mid-1960 and mid-1970 was the community mental health decade, and many American psychologists were greatly influenced by and contributed to it; but taken out of historical time it is not well understood. To understand what we were experiencing requires historical context other than the purely professional.

Those in the community mental health movement may not have fully appreciated the extent to which they were riding on the cusp of a change between two essentially different eras—each on opposite sides of a dialectic formed between a "rights" and a "needs" view of dependent people. Community mental health was, I now believe, the last breath of a dying age which social historians call the Progressive Era (Bremner, 1956; Chambers, 1963; Davis, 1967; Gaylin, Glasser, Marcus, & Rothman, 1978; Lubove, 1969). I will rely heavily for my brief description of this era on the work of historian David Rothman (1971; 1980) and others in *Doing Good: The Limits of Benevolence* (Gaylin *et al.*, 1978).

The mainstream reform position in the United States between 1900 and 1965 was largely an attempt to translate the biological model of the caring parent into a program for social action. The prime moving rationale was belief in the state as parent, not simply as metaphor but literally. This belief informed both the questions and the answers. For the first two-thirds of this century the legislative, governmental, and administrative social policy makers built an apparatus to provide services to the needy with little concern about the possibility of abuse and loss of rights. In this scheme of things the helping professions were the frontline soldiers in an army that would benevolently care for the poor, the retarded, the mentally ill, and the downtrodden. Those in need were more or less like children, to be helped, told what to do, and kept off the streets. The liberal mind was captivated by this idea which Rothman (1980) sees as a union of "conscience and convenience."

By mid-1960, just as the Progressive Era was about to give way to a new ideology, the community mental health movement (together with the "war on poverty") began to emerge. The thrust of community mental health came as a last-ditch effort to parent the entire society by means of the noble ambition of extending the reach of services via catchment areas to the heretofore unreached. What is ironic is that the community mental health movement believed itself to be a new benevolence when in fact it was a dying twitch of a beheaded organism.

The helping professions themselves have been shaped out of the era of progressivism. Partly because the progressive era social programs and their community mental health offspring had promised too much and compromised too much; and partly because of the experience of the civil rights movement and the war on poverty, and partly because of economic factors and an overbloated beauracracy, and partly because of generalization from the perceived energy crisis and the movement toward conservation of material resources, there has now developed a seemingly strange alliance between fiscal conservatives and social reformers. The reformers want to break down what they see as the negative effects of the "helping" social control institutions; the fiscal conservatives want to save money (Note 6).

As the community mental health movement is transformed and dies out (of course I do not expect the words or the places named community mental health centers to die out so much as the intellectual vigor and social power of the idea) we are witnessing the rise of the idea of rights over needs. The paradox for the remaining years of this century will be encapsulated in a struggle between opposing views of the poor, the physically disabled, the mental patient, the retarded person, the juvenile, the elderly, and so on, as dependent persons to be helped, socialized, trained, given skills, and have their illnesses prevented, or as citizens to be assured of rights and choices. Symbols and imagery will be very important in this struggle. It makes a great deal of difference if you are viewed as a child or as a citizen, since if you believe it you are quite likely to act the part (Snyder & Swann, 1978; Swann & Snyder, 1980), and if those in power believe it they are likely to develop programs, plans, and structures that will help you to believe it.

The elderly are perhaps a case in point because of their relatively new status as either a "class to be represented" or as a population "at risk," depending on a rights or a needs point of view. There is already a struggle between those who see being old as a disease that requires services and those who see it as a period of life that requires assurance of citizen rights. While neither view is a panacea, the images they conjure up do have an impact on us as well as them. Likewise, for the physically and mentally handicapped there is a struggle between aims of normalization and protection.

Now is a time when there is great pressure for the courts and the legislatures, through law, social, and administrative policy, to offer fewer services and more rights. This has led to some strange bedfellows. We see them come together in the deinstitutionalization movements in mental health and child welfare, systems which are currently under fire on all sides, from radical noninterventionists through group-home advocates, from advocates of due process for children through advocates of benign neglect. The era of rights and fiscal conservatism is with us as its supporters compete with the more established help-centered agencies for symbolic, material, and social power (Glasser, 1978; Knitzer, 1980; Koocher, 1978; Webber & McCall, 1978).

Given our tendency to look for solutions as if we have convergent non-dialectical problems, we can expect to see two developments in the helping fields' reaction to the changing socio-political-economic atmosphere. Many of the helpers will try to maintain control and services, basically standing by the progressive era notion of the expert as parent giving benign treatments on an individualized basis to the downtrodden, albeit now outside the institution. We will see new and optimistic arguments for the effectiveness of therapy and other social services for the poor combined with economic arguments to refocus our gaze on doing treatment for those who want it and to ignore as "not our job" the social conditions under which many people live their lives (Buck & Hirschman, 1980).

Others, still unable to let go of the needs model of the progressive era, but dissatisfied with programs that only treat people after they are in obvious trouble, will maintain that our task is to assist high-risk populations to adjust to the reality of social institutions. We may now prefer to call this "teaching competencies" rather than doing psychotherapy, but the crucial element of "expert/helper," or the "doctor/patient relationship," or at least the "student/teacher relationship," will be maintained. There will be no question about who is "up" and who is "down." Even programs aimed at so-called structural change, when framed in terms of "prevention," create a metaphor that despite intentions, when adopted by our social institutions yields all the wrong symbols, images, and meta messages.

Frankly, I am beginning to suspect that as it grows in popularity among mental health professionals, even to the point where the National Institute of Mental Health makes it a training grant priority for clinical psychology training programs, the whole idea behind prevention will somehow lose out to the image it creates. Prevention programs aimed at so called high-risk populations, especially programs under the auspices of established social institutions, can easily become a new arena for colonialization, where people are forced to consume our goods and services, thereby providing us with jobs and money. Rothman (1980) observed that the progressives did not reduce the use of institutions; they added on new programs for more people while the supposed target groups continued to languish in institutions. Prevention programs may not change our current social institutions, but rather add on to them, and in turn to the therapeutic state (Kittrie, 1974); and I might add, with little evidence that they actually prevent anything.

This underlies much of what is called prevention: find so-called high-risk people and save them from themselves, if they like it or not, by giving them, or even better, their children, programs which we develop, package, sell, operate, or otherwise control. Teach them how to fit in and be less of a nuisance. Convince them that a change in their test scores is somehow the same as a change in their life. Operating our interventions through the professionally controlled educational and social agencies developed during the progressive era fosters this attitude, because it is consistent with the culture of these settings. Thus, we are consultants, not to people, but to agencies, schools, and other sanctioned social agents. Our role relationships to people need never change (Fairweather, 1972).

On the other side, equally convergent nondialectical in their thinking, stand both those who are saving money wasted on programs of unproven value and those who push for "freedoms" and "rights," including the right to be different to the point of missing the freedom to be the same as others, to obtain help, education, or services. Having rights but no resources and no services available is a cruel joke. While ostensibly motivated out of a great deal of respect for the individual right not to be socialized or controlled so long as one hurts no one but one's self and by the desire to limit the arbitrariness of the therapeutic state, or the arrogance of prevention programs which I have just criticized, this position easily becomes one of "benign neglect." Just as easily as helpers can slip from a real desire to prevent mental illness into a social control mentality that obliterates legitimate differences or to mistake change on test scores for change in the conditions of life, advocates and fiscal conservatives can slip from a critique of naive helpers and concern over the violation of the rights of dependent people into their own naive belief that help will somehow emerge from the private sector, or that it is not needed at all, or mistake a change in law for a change in the conditions of life. We can, in our overreaction to the failures of progressivism, be led to allow the state (i.e., the citizenry) to ignore its moral and social (as opposed to simply legal) obligations.

Stier (1978) calling on the work of Hart (1955) has recently suggested that if we rely on the courts to provide as "rights" conditions of living which are actually human "needs," we run the risk of confusing the rights of children with the moral duty of the state, and she reminds us that "inspiring society to meet its duties to children [I would say to all dependent persons] involves the creation of a sense of moral and social imperative" (p. 57). To the extent that we accept the notion that advocating for legal rights is *the* solution to problems in living we will settle for a one-sided solution that misses the dialectal relationship between rights and needs. What use is the right to treatment if treatment is neither available nor good? What good is the right to be in the community with no role, no respect, and no resources?

History seems to show that as society becomes more politically conservative we turn to a social science explanation favoring the intrapsychic as opposed to the environmental (Levine & Levine, 1970). It would be naive to think that in conjunction with our current swing toward conservative politics this will mean a simple return to older theoretical views of personality and psychodynamics, although that in part will be true. Rather, we will see an increased emphasis on *cognitive* (in-the-head) behavior modification and self-control, on socio-*biology*, on *individual* rights, and on changing the *person* side of person–environment fit as in so-called competency training as a form of socialization. These trends run counter to the behaviorism that helped to free us from our predetermined genetic background, the sociology that overturned the eugenics movement, the ecological view of context which has emphasized social change, and the civil liberties movement that sought corporate (class action) freedoms on the basis of moral imperatives.

There is now emerging a new kind of conservative intrapsychic and individual responsibility ideology that will blame victims in new and more clever ways. We will even be made to feel righteous about it. We will be asked to ignore the needs that do not fit into our social agencies, schools, and consulting rooms, as too costly a waste of resources on ineffective programs of unproven value. Those we ignore will be described as obtaining their right not to be coerced. This will salve our consciences as we collect money and prestige from the others. We will be told to become more of a profession (like real doctors) so we can qualify for certain social rewards by limiting our activities to those which are proper for licensed and accredited people and programs, i.e., those that are reimbursable by insurance or supportable by grants or by established social agencies.

Because this is a paradoxical, dialectical problem, they will be partly correct. There are people who benefit from a needs-oriented human service system and there are those who benefit from rights-oriented controls on that system; but there are a great many people, including the real social disasters of our society, who require both rights and needs. If we hope to be useful to them *we will need to find a renewed symbolic and ideational goal and a renewed sense of urgency.* We must be a social movement that confronts with divergent reasoning the antinomies in the paradox of helping others. Many of us have placed our bets on the ideology of prevention. It is my contention that this ideology has outlived its usefulness and is one-sided at its core. It is a product of our failed social history and it creates the wrong symbolism. In the final part of this paper I will make the case that empowerment rather than prevention is far more promising both as a plan of action and as a symbolic ideology for the social movement called community psychology.

By empowerment I mean that our aim should be to enhance the possibilities for people to control their own lives. If this is our aim then we will necessarily find ourselves questioning both our public policy and our role relationship to dependent people. We will not be able to settle for a public policy which limits us to programs we design, operate, or package for social agencies to use on people, because it will require that the form and the meta communications as well as the content be consistent with empowerment. We will, should we take empowerment seriously, no longer be able to see people as simply children in need or as only citizens with rights, but rather as full human beings who have both rights and needs. We will confront the paradox that even the people most incompetent, in need, and apparently unable to function, require, just as you and I do, more rather than less control over their own lives; and that fostering more control does not necessarily mean ignoring them. Empowerment presses a different set of metaphors upon us. It is a way of thinking that lends itself to a clearer sense of the divergent nature of social problems.

THE LOGIC AND THE IMAGERY OF EMPOWERMENT

There are at least two requirements of an empowerment ideology. On the one hand it demands that we look to many diverse local settings where people are already handling their own problems in living, in order to learn more about how they do it. This demand is obviously consistent with, indeed requires, divergent reasoning. On the other hand, it demands that we find ways to take what we learn from these diverse settings and solutions and make it more public, so as to help foster social policies and programs that make it more rather than less likely that others not now handling their own problems in living or shut out from current solutions, gain control over their lives.

Newbrough (1980) last year concluded his presidential address with a vision of what he called the participating society. He suggested, from a review of a variety of writers on justice, values, society, bureaucracy, politics, and community life, that "the public interest is the empowerment of people" (p. 15). Riger (Note 7) has also commented on the logic behind empowerment. I suggest that this be our call to arms and that it replace "prevention" as our aim because the connotations, the meta meanings, and the implications are different.

The idea of prevention is derived from a needs model of dependent people; it is a legacy of the progressive era and of the one-sided development of social service institutions. Within the context of social service agencies and a needs/dependency model, which views people as children, prevention is the most sensible logical alternative to clinical services for all the reasons of efficiency its adherents have argued (Caplan, 1964; Cowen, 1980; President's Commission on Mental Health, 1978).

Advocacy is an alternative based on a rights model of social responsibility (Webber & McCall, 1978). It is a logical approach based on the assumptions derived from a legal/due process ideology which views people as citizens rather than as children. It is just as logical as prevention and just as one-sided. Both advocacy and prevention suggest professional experts as leaders who know the answers and provide them for their clients. Despite many obvious differences this similarity in role relationships is striking.

What we require is a model which allows us to play within the dialectic and to pursue paradox, first to one side, then the other; one which allows us to welcome divergent reasoning that permits many simultaneous, different, and contradictory answers, rather than a single solution to every social problem. But we cannot afford to be dilettantes. We require social action and genuine involvement in the world. That, in turn, requires symbolic imagery to fuel the flames of urgency and to energize a movement. The imagery of empowerment has a very different feel than the imagery of prevention. Prevention suggests professional experts; empowerment suggests collaborators.

Empowerment implies that many competencies are already present or at least possible, given niches and opportunities. Prevention implies experts fixing the independent variables to make the dependent variables come out right. Empowerment implies that what you see as poor functioning is a result of social structure and lack of resources which make it impossible for the existing competencies to operate. It implies that in those cases where new competencies need to be learned, they are best learned in a context of living life rather than in artificial programs where everyone, including the person learning, knows that it is really the expert who is in charge (cf. Rappaport, Davidson, Wilson, & Mitchell, 1975).

If a problem is by nature divergent it must have many solutions. If a problem can have many solutions then it can have a diversity of people with a diversity of experiences who work out the solutions. Empowerment lends itself to the possibility of a variety of locally rather than centrally controlled solutions, which in turn fosters solutions based on different assumptions in different places, settings, and neighborhoods. The criterion shifts from a single one-sided standard of competence to genuine recognition that social problems have many different definitions as well as answers (Seidman, 1978), and that might (holding social power and material resources) does not necessarily make right, it simply allows one's solution to be acceptable.

As Illich (1976) has so well pointed out in the domain of physical health, the pervasive belief that experts should solve all of our problems in living has created a social and cultural iatrogenesis which extends the sense of alienation and loss of ability to control life even to one's own body. This is the path that the social as well as the physical health experts have been on, and we need to reverse this trend. We must begin to develop a social policy which gives up the search for one monolithic way of doing things according to *the* certified expert (i.e., the symbolic parent). Quality control from the central authority becomes a silly idea in this view. Rather than a top down or forward mapping of social policy it is a bottom up or backward mapping that starts with people and works backwards to tell officials what social policies and programs are necessary (Elmore, 1979). This means that empowerment will not only look different depending on what sort of problems in living one is confronting, but it may even look different in each setting that it operates. Diversity of form rather than homogeneity of form should dominate if the operating process is empowerment.

An Naparstek and Cincotta (National Commission on Neighborhoods, 1979) have suggested with regard to the problem of decaying cities:

> [One] reason for the persistent failure of … programs has been the tendency to perceive the problem on a grand scale. Virtually all efforts to halt the decline of our cities are marked by a failure to define national policy initiatives which serve the varied needs of differing neighborhoods. If we are to speak realistically of preconditions required for effective change, it must be recognized that the neighborhood—not the sprawling, anonymous metropolis—is the key. In real terms, people live in neighborhoods, not cities. In real terms, their investments, emotional as well as economic, are in the neighborhoods, not cities. And the city cannot survive if its neighborhoods continue to decline. (p. 1)

With regard to the poor, Berger and Neuhaus (1977) put it this way:

> Upper-income people already have ways to resist the encroachment of megastructures. It is not their children who are at the mercy of alleged child experts, not their health which is endangered by miscellaneous vested interests, not their neighborhoods which are made the playthings of

utopian planners. Upper-income people may allow themselves to be vic-
timized on all these scores, but they do have ways to resist if they choose
to resist. Poor people have this power to a much lesser degree ... empowering poor people to do the things that the more affluent can already do
aims at spreading the power around a bit more—and to do so where it
matters, in people's control over their own lives. (pp. 7–8)

It is not only the poor and the local neighborhoods that would benefit
from a public policy of empowerment. Even traditional clinical populations
stand to benefit from a goal which tends to foster more rather than less control over their own lives. There is no doubt that we lack a great deal of direct
experimental data on the wonderful mental health outcomes when we collaborate with grass roots people. However, there is also no doubt that the
same may be said for prevention programs (Novaco & Monahan, 1980) or
advocacy. On the other hand, programs which foster what I have called elsewhere (Rappaport, 1977) "autonomous alternative settings," obviously consistent with an empowerment ideology, such as the work of Fairweather
(1972, 1979; Fairweather, Sanders, Cressler, & Maynard, 1969; Fairweather,
Sanders, & Tornatzky, 1974) and of the Mendota group (Marx, Test, & Stein,
1973; Stein, Test, & Marx, 1975) with chronic patients, or the work of
Goldenberg (1971) with "hard core" delinquents, have presented data
which are as compelling as we are likely to find from programs for these
populations.

Moreover, it is not clear to me why the criterion should be a measure
of mental health in the narrow disciplinary sense. I am, frankly, willing to
argue that programs and policies which make it more possible for people to
obtain and control the resources that affect their lives are per se what
empowerment is all about. This is based, in part, on my social values, but
also in part on a variety of social science data bases.

There is ample psychological evidence from the study of normal (i.e.,
nonclinical) populations to safely conclude that the felt sense of internal
control or alienation (Phares, 1973; Phares & Lamiell, 1977; Rotter, 1975;
Seaman, 1972), learned helplessness (Seligman, 1975; Seligman & Maier,
1967; Sue & Zane, 1980), ascribed and achieved status (Sarbin, 1970),
expectancy for success (Gurin & Gurin, 1970; Seidman & Rappaport, 1974)
attributions (Strickland & Janoff-Bulman, 1980), the impact of perceived
labels (Rappaport & Cleary, 1980), and of the beliefs of powerful others
(Snyder & Swann, 1978; Swann & Snyder, 1980), matters a great deal to
people. It also seems safe to conclude that most people are likely to benefit psychologically from more rather than less control over their lives and
resources. In addition, laboratory studies and historical analysis of group
cohesiveness (Guttentag, 1970), as well as the obvious outcomes and popularity of self-help groups, labor unions, community organizations, and
community development projects (Hampden-Turner, 1975; National

Commission on Neighborhoods, 1979) must lead us to the same conclusion: Empowerment is a sensible social policy, but one which requires a breakdown of the typical role relationship between professionals and community people. Empowerment needs to be based on divergent reasoning that encourages diversity through support of many different local groups rather than the large centralized social agencies and institutions which control resources, use convergent reasoning, and attempt to standardize the ways in which people live their lives.

The implications of an empowerment ideology force us to pay attention to the mediating structures of society, i.e., those that stand between the large impersonal social institutions and individual alienated people. For Berger and Neuhaus (1977) these include the family, the neighborhood, the church, and voluntary organizations. These are the places where people live out their lives, and the more control they have over them the better.

As researchers, our obligations are to study and understand more about how such settings actually work to provide niches for people that enhance their ability to control their lives and allow them both affirmation and the opportunity to learn and experience growth and development. On the action side it is clear to me that we have been far too willing to intervene, label, and tell others how to cope with life without understanding how the diversity of settings in which people actually do live well, operate. Most of our advice is drawn from a very limited set of personal or professional experiences in settings designed and controlled *by* professionals *for* others.

It is now quite obvious that for many people their network of friends, neighbors, church relationships, and so on, provide not only support, but genuine niches and opportunities for personal development. How can we learn to help to create new settings, or to assist those who are isolated from such settings or those who are trapped in settings which are harmful rather than helpful, if we do not spend a great deal of time observing, describing, and collaborating?

The recent interest in so-called natural support systems (Gottlieb, 1976, 1979; Gottlieb & Todd, 1979; Hirsch, 1980; Riessman, 1976; Maton, Note 8, Note 9) and in social support as a moderator of stress (Cobb, 1976; Dohrenwend, 1978; Lin, Simeone, Ensel, & Kuo, 1979; Sandler, 1980) has the potential to serve as an impetus for research and action of a different variety than the traditional convergent, one-sided sort, which I have criticized in this paper, *only* if we are willing to see it as descriptive of how a variety of people are able to find a variety of means to solve their own problems in living. We can learn a great deal about how this works when it works well if we are willing to observe the process of empowerment when it is taking place, even if that is in settings which we typically ignore and over which we have no control. We need to recognize that many settings which are successful in the creation of opportunities, niches, and resources for empowerment will not concern themselves with mental health in our rather narrow disciplinary sense; and that not only are these genuine solutions of local people to their problems in living likely to be diverse, but the very behavior, attitudes, and life-styles which are useful to people will also differ from place to place. We need to learn from them what the range of solutions is really like and then to encourage social policies that enable more people to develop their own solutions.

Unfortunately, psychologists, and particularly mental health professionals, have a tendency to a priori exclude solutions to problems in living about which they know very little. For example, recent research comparing charismatic and mainline churches (McGaw, 1979) finds evidence that growth of so-called conservative congregations may be as much a function of a social structure which fosters a sense of community as is doctrinal appeal. Given what we know about the influence of organizational social structure on people in work settings (e.g., Hackman, 1976) or communes (Kanter, 1972), such findings in religious organizations are hardly surprising. Yet despite the fact that some two-thirds of Americans have formal membership in a church or synagogue (Jacquet, 1972) and that such settings provide a wide variety of important functions in people's lives (cf. Bergin, 1980; Pargament, 1982) these settings are likely to be either ignored by the mental health establishment, or conceptualized as if they were second-rate mental health agencies in need of psychological consultation, rather than as places for us to learn from. This, despite the fact that one of our professed goals is to enhance the psychological sense of community. The same may be said for a variety of other local groups and organizations in neighborhoods, voluntary associations, clubs, and so on.

This is not an argument for any single solution such as developing more churches, block organizations, or tenants' councils. It is an argument for our work, at both the local and the social policy level, to recognize and foster the legitimacy of more rather than fewer, different rather than the same, ways to deal with problems in living. To the extent that we try to force our understanding of community settings into a prevention of mental illness or a social adjustment model, or our preconceived notions of how people ought rather than how they do solve their own problems, we will misunderstand both the nature of social problems and the meaning and value of settings for living. We will thereby cut off the possibility that we can learn a variety of divergent solutions from them. As Jacob Bronowski (1956, p. 10) warned some 25 years ago: "Man masters nature not by force but by understanding. This is why science has succeeded where magic failed: because it has looked for no spell to cast over nature."

I conclude where I began. The most important and interesting aspects of community life are by their very nature paradoxical. Social problems, paradoxically, require that experts turn to nonexperts in order to discover the many different, even contradictory, solutions that they use to gain control, find meaning, and empower their own lives. From such study, which will require genuine collaboration fueled by a sense of urgency, we may be able to help develop programs and policies that make it possible for others to find niches for living and gain control over their lives. At this time in our history I believe that empowerment encapsulates the symbolic message required to bring a new sense of urgency and to transcend the rights/needs dialectic. Should empowerment become dominant as a way of thinking I have no doubt that it too will force one-sided solutions. I come, not to bury paradox, but to praise it.

ACKNOWLEDGMENTS

In a paper such as this one there are many intellectual debts. Those of which I am most aware are to the works of social historian David J. Rothman and economist and philosopher E. F. Schumacher. Perhaps less obvious but more direct is the influence of two colleagues whose papers (Sarason, 1978; Seidman, 1978) I deem to be among the more important written in this field, and which force me to see this one as a sequel. In addition, I am intellecutally indebted to my friend, Ronald Simkins, who quite directly gave me many of the ideas presented here, and to conversations with and the influence of many others including Thom Moore, Ken Maton, Fern Chertok, Bruce Rapkin, Ann Jolly, Kathy Roesch, and Arlene Rappaport.

REFERENCES

Albee, G. W. *Mental health manpower trends*. New York: Basic Books, 1959.
Baratz, S. & Baratz, J. C. Early childhood intervention: The social science base of institutional racism. *Harvard Educational Review*, 1970, *40*, 29–50.
Berger, P. L. & Neuhaus, R. J. *To empower people: The role of mediating structures in public policy*. Washington, D.C.: American Enterprise Institute for Public Policy Research, 1977.
Bergin, A. E. Psychotherapy and religious values. *Journal of Consulting and Clinical Psychology*, 1980, *48*, 95–105.
Bremner, R. *From the depths: The discovery of poverty in the United States*. New York: New York University Press, 1956.
Bronowski, J. *Science and human values*. New York: Harper, 1956.
Buck, J. A. & Hirschman, R. Economics and mental health services: Enhancing the power of the consumer. *American Psychologist*, 1980, *35*, 653–661.
Caplan, G. *Principles of preventive psychiatry*. New York: Basic Books, 1964.
Caplan, N. & Nelson, S. D. On being useful: The nature and consequences of psychological research on social problems. *American Psychologist*, 1973, *28*, 199–211.
Chambers, C. *Seedtime of reform: American social service and social action*. Minneapolis: University of Minnesota Press, 1963.

Cobb, S. Social support as a moderator of life stress. *Psychosomatic Medicine*, 1976, *38*, 300–314.

Cowen, E. L., The wooing of primary prevention. *American Journal of Community Psychology*, 1980, *8*, 258–284.

Cowen, E. L., Gardner, E. A., & Zax, M. (Eds.). *Emergent approaches to mental health problems*. New York: Appleton-Century-Crofts, 1967.

Cronbach, L. J. Beyond the two disciplines of scientific psychology. *American Psychologist*, 1975, *30*, 116–127.

Davis, A. F. *Spearheads for reform: The social settlements and the progressive movement*. New York: Oxford University Press, 1967.

Dohrenwend, B. S. Social stress and community psychology. *American Journal of Community Psychology*, 1978, *6*, 1–15.

Durlak, J. A. Comparative effectiveness of paraprofession and professional helpers. *Psychological Bulletin*, 1979, *86*, 80–92.

Eller, V. *The simple life: The Christian stance toward possessions*. Grand Rapids: Eerdmans, 1973.

Elmore, R. F. Backward mapping: Implementation research and policy decisions. *Political Science Quarterly*, 1979, *80*, 601–616.

Fairweather, G. W. *Social change: The challenge to survival*. Morristown, N.J.: General Learning Press, 1972.

Fairweather, G. W. Experimental development and dissemination of an alternative to psychiatric hospitalization: Scientific methods for social change. In R. F. Munoz, L. R. Snowden, & J. G. Kelly, (Eds.), *Social and psychological research in community settings*. San Francisco: Jossey-Bass, 1979.

Fairweather, G. W., Sanders, D. H., Cressler, D. L., & Maynard, H. *Community life for the mentally ill: An alternative to institutional care*. Chicago: Aldine, 1969.

Fairweather, G. W., Sanders, D. H., & Tornatzky, L. G. *Creating change in mental health organizations*. New York: Pergamon, 1974.

Gaylin, W., Glasser, I., Marcus, S., & Rothman, D. *Doing good: The limits of benevolence*. New York: Pantheon, 1978.

Gergen, K. J. Social psychology as history. *Journal of Personality and Social Psychology*, 1973, *26*, 309–320.

Ginsburg, H. *The myth of the deprived child: Poor children's intellect and education*. Englewood Cliffs, N.J.: Prentice Hall, 1972.

Glasser, I. Prisoners of benevolence: Power versus liberty in the welfare state. In N. Gaylin, I. Glasser, S. Marcus, & D. Rothman, *Doing good: The limits of benevolence*. New York: Pantheon, 1978.

Goldenberg, I. I. *Build me a mountain: Youth, poverty and the creation of new settings*. Cambridge, Mass.: MIT Press, 1971.

Gottlieb, B. H. Lay influences on the utilization and provision of health services: A review. *Canadian Psychological Review*, 1976, *17*, 126–136.

Gottlieb, B. H. The primary group as supportive milieu: Applications to community psychology. *American Journal of Community Psychology*, 1979, *7*, 469–480.

Gottlieb, B. H. & Todd, D. Characterizing and promoting social support in natural settings. In R. F. Munoz, L. R. Snowden, & J. G. Kelly (Eds.), *Social and psychological research in community settings*. San Francisco: Jossey-Bass, 1979.

Gray, S. W. & Klaus, R. A. The early training project. A seventh year report. *Child Development*, 1970, *41*, 909–924.

Gross, S. J. The myth of professional licensing. *American Psychologist*, 1978, *33*, 1009–1016.

Gurin, G. & Gurin, P. Expectancy theory in the study of poverty. *Journal of Social Issues*, 1970, *26*, 83–104.

Guttentag, M. Group cohesiveness, ethnic organization and poverty. *Journal of Social Issues*, 1970, *26*, 105–132.

Hackman, R. J. Group influences on individuals. In M. P. Dunnette (Ed.), *Handbook of industrial and organizational psychology*. New York: Rand McNally, 1976.

Hampden-Turner, C. *From poverty to dignitiy*. Garden City, N. Y: Anchor Press/Double-day, 1975.

Hart, H. L. A. Are there any natural rights? *The Philosophical Review*, 1955, *44*, 289–298.

Henry, J. *Culture against man*. New York: Random House, 1963.

Hiller, H. H. A reconceptualization of the dynamics of social movement development. *Pacific Sociological Review*, 1975, *18*, 342–360.

Hirsch, B. J. Natural support systems and coping with major life changes. *American Journal of Community Psychology*, 1980, *8*, 159–172.

Hunt, J. McV. *The challenge of incompetence and poverty*. Urbana: University of Illinois Press, 1969.

Illich, I. *Medical nemesis: The expropriation of health*. New York: Pantheon, 1976.

Jacquet, C. H. (Ed.). *Yearbook of American churches*. Nashville: Abingdon, 1972.

Kanter, R. M. *Commitment and community: Communes and utopias in sociological perspective*. Cambridge, Mass.: Harvard University Press, 1972.

Kelly, J. G. Antidotes for arrogance: Training for a community psychology. *American Psychologist*, 1970, *25*, 524–531.

Killian, L. M. Social movements. In R. E. L. Faris (Ed.), *Handbook of modern sociology*. Chicago: Rand-McNally, 1964.

Kittrie, N. *The right to be different: Deviance and enforced therapy*. Baltimore: Johns Hopkins Press, 1974.

Knitzer, J. Advocacy and community psychology. In M. S. Gibbs, J. R. Lachenmeyer, & J. Sigal, *Community psychology: Theoretical and empirical approaches*. New York: Gardner, 1980.

Koocher, J. *Children's rights and the mental health professionals*. New York: Wiley, 1978.

Koocher, J. Credentialing in psychology: Close encounters with competence? *American Psychologist*, 1979, *34*, 696–702.

Levine, M. Investigative reporting as a research method: An analysis of Bernstein and Woodward's *All the president's men. American Psychologist*, 1980, *35*, 626–638.

Levine, M. & Levine, A. *A social history of helping services: Clinic, court, school and community*. New York: Appleton-Century-Crofts, 1970.

Lilly, M. & Smith, P. Special education as a social movement. *Education Unlimited*, 1980, *2*(3), 7–11.

Lin, N., Simeone, R. S., Ensel, W. M., & Kuo, W. Social support, stressful life events, and illness: A model and an empirical test. *Journal of Health and Social Behavior*, 1979, *20*, 108–119.

Lubove, R. *The professional altruist: The emergence of social work as a career, 1880–1930*. New York: Antheneum, 1969.

Marx, A. M., Test, M. A., & Stein, L. I. Extrohospital management of severe mental illness. *Archives of General Psychiatry*, 1973, *29*, 505–511.

McGrath, J. E. *Social science and social action: A retrospective look through the pages of the Journal of Social Issues*. Mimeograph, University of Illinois at Urbana-Champaign, 1978.

McGaw, D. B. Commitment and religious community: A comparison of a charismatic and a mainline congregation. *Journal for the Scientific Study of Religion*, 1979, *18*, 146–163.

Merton, T. *Conjectures of a guilty bystander*. Garden City, N.Y.: Doubleday-Image, 1968.

National Commission on Neighborhoods. *Report to the President*. Washington, DC: U.S. Government Printing Office, 1979.

New York Times. Story reported on October 20, 1974.

Maton, K. I. *Participant inhabitant observation, empirical investigation and social ecology.* Paper presented at the annual meeting of the American Psychological Association, New York, September 1979.

Maton, K. I. *Empowerment in a religious setting: An exploratory study.* Masters thesis, University of Illinois at Urbana-Champaign, 1980.

Newbrough, J. R. Community psychology and the public interest. *American Journal of Community Psychology,* 1980, *8,* 1–17.

Novaco, R. W. & Monahan, J. Research in community psychology: An analysis of work published in the first six years of the *American Journal of Community Psychology. American Journal of Community Psychology,* 1980, *8,* 131–146.

Oxford English Dictionary (Compact ed.). New York: Oxford University Press, 1971.

Pargament, K. The interface among religion, religious support systems, and mental health. In D. E. Biegel and A. J. Naparstek (Eds.), *Community support systems and mental health: Research, policy and practice.* New York: Springer, 1982, pp. 161–174.

Phares, E. J. *Locus of control: A personality determinant of behavior.* Morristown, N.J.: General Learning Press, 1973.

Phares, E. J. & Lamiell, J. T. Personality. *Annual Review of Psychology,* 1977, *28,* 113–140.

President's Commission on Mental Health. *Report of recommendations* (Vol. 1). Washington, DC: U.S. Government Printing Office, 1978.

Rappaport, J. *Community psychology: Values, research and action.* New York: Holt, Rinehart & Winston, 1977.

Rappaport, J. *Standards for juvenile justice as an example of fundamental change in social attitudes, law and social policy: Opportunities and dangers for psychologists.* Mimeograph, University of Illinois at Urbana-Champaign, 1980.

Rappaport, J. & Cleary, C. P. Labeling theory and the social psychology of experts and helpers. In M. S. Gibbs, J. R. Lachenmeyer, & J. Sigal (Eds.), *Community psychology: Theoretical and empirical approaches.* New York: Gardner, 1980.

Rappaport, J., Davidson, W. S., Wilson, M. N., & Mitchell, A. Alternatives to blaming the victim or the environment: Our places to stand have not moved the earth. *American Psychologist,* 1975, *30,* 525–528.

Report of a panel on public policy contributions to the institutionalization and deinstitutionalization of children and youth. National Academy of Sciences, in preparation. This project is a 3-year study to be completed in 1981, under the Chairmanship of law professor Joel F. Handler. The interdisciplinary panel, of which this author is a member, is reviewing the deinstitutionalization experience for status offenders in seven states.

Riessman, R. *The inner-city child.* New York: Harper & Row, 1976.

Riger, S. *Toward a community psychology of empowerment.* Paper presented at a symposium, "Community Psychology in Times of Scarcity," Midwestern Psychological Association meeting, St. Louis, May 1980.

Rist, R. C. Student social class and teacher expectations: The self-fulfilling prophecy in ghetto education. *Harvard Educational Review,* 1970, *40,* 411–451.

Rothman, D. J. *The discovery of the asylum.* Boston: Little, Brown, 1971.

Rothman, D. J. *Conscience and convenience: The asylum and its alternatives in progressive America.* Boston: Little, Brown, 1980.

Rotter, J. B. Some problems and misconceptions related to the construct of internal versus external control of reinforcement. *Journal of Consulting and Clinical Psychology,* 1975, *43,* 56–57.

Ryan, W. *Blaming the victim.* New York: Random House, 1971.

Sandler, I. N. Social support resources, stress, and maladjustment of poor children. *American Journal of Community Psychology,* 1980, *8,* 41–52.

Sarason, S. B. The nature of problem solving in social action. *American Psychologist*, 1978, *33*, 370–380.

Sarbin, T. R. A role theory perspective for community psychology: The structure of social identity. In D. Adelson & B. L. Kalis (Eds.), *Community psychology and mental health: Perspectives and challenges.* Scranton, Pa.: Chandler, 1970.

Schumacher, E. R. *Small is beautiful.* New York: Harper & Row, 1973.

Schumacher, E. F. *A guide for the perplexed.* New York: Harper & Row, 1977.

Seaman, M. Social learning theory and the theory of mass society. In J. B. Rotter, J. Chance, & E. J. Phares, *Applications of a social learning theory of personality.* New York: Holt, Rinehart & Winston, 1972.

Seidman, E. Justice, values and social science: Unexamined premises. In R. J. Simon (Ed.), *Research in law and sociology* (Vol. 1). Greenwich, Conn.: JAI Press, 1978.

Seidman, E. & Rappaport, J. You have got to have a dream, but its not enough. *American Psychologist*, 1974, *29*, 569–570.

Seligman, M. E. P. *Helplessness: On depression, development and death.* San Francisco: W. H. Freeman, 1975.

Seligman, M. E. P. & Maier, S. F. Failure to escape traumatic shock. *Journal of Experimental Psychology*, 1967, *74*, 1–9.

Snyder, M. & Swann, W. B. Behavioral confirmation in social interaction: From social perception to social reality. *Journal of Experimental Social Psychology*, 1978, *14*, 148–162.

Special issue on licensing and accreditation. *Division of Community Psychology Newsletter*, Summer 1979, *12*, 1–16.

Stein, L. I., Test, M. A., & Marx, A. J. Alternative to the hospital: A controlled study. *American Journal of Psychiatry*, 1975, *132*, 517–522.

Stier, S. Children's rights and society's duties. *Journal of Social Issues*, 1978, *34*, 46–58.

Strickland, B. R. & Janoff-Bulman, R. Expectancies and attributions: Implications for community mental health. In M. S. Gibbs, J. R. Lachenmeyer, & J. Sigal (Eds.), *Community psychology: Theoretical and empirical approaches.* New York: Gardner, 1980.

Sue, S. & Zane, N. Learned helplessness theory and community psychology. In M. S. Gibbs, J. R. Lachenmeyer, & J. Sigal (Eds.), *Community psychology: Theoretical and empirical approaches.* New York: Gardner, 1980.

Swann, W. B. & Snyder, M. On translating beliefs into action: Theories of ability and their application in an institutional setting. *Journal of Personality and Social Psychology*, 1980, *38*, 879–888.

Takanishi, R. Childhood as a social issue: Historical roots of contemporary child advocacy movements. *Journal of Social Issues*, 1978, *34*, 8–28.

Webber, G. H. & McCall, G. J. (Eds.). *Social scientists as advocates: Views from applied disciplines.* New York: Sage, 1978.

Zald, M. *The federal impact on the deinstitutionalization of status offenders: A framework.* Working paper commissioned by a Panel on Public Policy Contributions to the Institutionalization and Deinstitutionalization of Children and Youth. National Academy of Sciences, 1980.

9

Primary Prevention During School Transitions: Social Support and Environmental Structure

Robert D. Felner, Melanie Ginter, and Judith Primavera

The nature and evaluation of a primary prevention project for students during the transition to high school are presented. In order to facilitate students' coping efforts during this transition, the project sought to increase the level of social support available as well as to reduce the degree of flux and complexity in the school setting. Midyear and end of ninth-grade assessments were done of Project and matched Control students' self-concepts, their perceptions of the school environment, and their eighth- and ninth-grade attendance and grade averages examined. By the end of ninth grade, Project participants showed significantly better attendance records and grade point averages as well as more stable self-concepts than controls. Further, by the final evaluation point, Project students also reported perceiving the school environment as having greater clarity of expectations and organizational structure and higher levels of teacher support and involvement than did nonproject Controls.

Individuals experiencing stressful life events or life transitions have been pointed to as potentially important groups toward which to target primary

Originally published in the *American Journal of Community Psychology, 10*(3) (1982): 277–290.

A Quarter Century of Community Psychology: Readings from the American Journal of Community Psychology, edited by Tracey A. Revenson *et al.* Kluwer Academic/Plenum Publishers, New York, 2002.

preventive efforts (Bloom, 1979; Dohrenwend, 1978; Felner, Farber, & Primavera, 1980). During normative life transitions or "milestones" (Bloom, 1978), such as entering a new school, getting married, or retirement, individuals may experience increased stress and heightened susceptibility to enduring adaptive or maladaptive changes in adjustment (Goldston, 1978). Thus, several authors (Bloom, 1979; Goldston, 1978; Felner *et al.*, 1980) have suggested that preventive efforts be organized around stressful life events or life transitions which have a relatively high base-rate of occurrence in the general population and which have been shown to place the individuals who experience them at heightened risk for the development of maladaptation. One life transition generally experienced by children and adolescents, around which the organization of preventive programming may be appropriate, is the experience of transferring to a new school.

A number of studies have found both cumulative and single school transfers to be related to poorer academic achievement (Felner, Primavera, & Cauce, 1981; Levine, Wesolowski, & Corbet, 1966; Schaller, 1975), increased classroom behavior problems (Kemme, 1971), and heightened anxiety, particularly over gaining peer acceptance and meeting school expectations (Levine, 1966; Rakieten, 1961). Although some studies have failed to find an association between poor school adjustment and either cumulative school transfers (Collins & Coulter, 1974; Cramer & Dorsey, 1979; Goebel, 1978) or any single school change precipitated by residential mobility (Felner *et al.*, 1981), the normative transition into high school has been clearly demonstrated to be a time of increased vulnerability to school maladjustment (Felner *et al.*, 1981).

In a recent work, Felner *et al.* (1981) examined changes in the academic adjustment of students during the transition to high school. Overall, significant decreases in academic performance and increases in absenteeism were found. These findings have broader adaptive implications as well. Both low grades and high rates of absenteeism have been found to be strong predictors of later school failure, "dropping-out" (U.S. Department of Health, Education & Welfare, 1975), and the more serious emotional maladjustment associated with these difficulties (Bachman, Green, & Wirtanen, 1971; Cowen, Pederson, Babigian, Izzo, & Trost, 1973). Moreover, further exploration of factors mediating the relative vulnerability of students during this transition found that those students typically seen as being at heightened risk for school failure, i.e., minorities and those with histories of higher levels of mobility (U.S. Department of Health, Education & Welfare, 1975), were particularly vulnerable during this transition.

A number of potentially important mediators of an individual's ability to cope with life transitions have been identified. Psychological characteristics of the individual, such as personal competences and coping style (Bogat,

Jones, & Jason, 1980; Caplan, 1965; Cumming & Cumming, 1962; Kobasa, 1979), as well as such situational or environmental factors as the difficulties and complexities of the tasks confronting the individual (Lazarus & Launier, 1978) or the availability and accessibility of instrumental and affective social support (Caplan, 1974; Gottlieb, 1981) may differentially facilitate adaptation to such an event (Dohrenwend, 1978; Felner et al., 1980).

Several previous studies of efforts to enhance the adaptive efforts of students experiencing school change have sought to augment their coping skills or cognitive understanding of the situation (Bogat et al., 1980; Hirshowitz, 1976). However, studies of attempts to influence the social environment to facilitate students' successful adaptation during this transition, either by reducing the difficulty of mastering the transitional tasks accompanying such change or by facilitating the individual's access to important coping resources in the environment, are lacking. The importance of such an approach has been suggested by several authors. Bronfenbrenner (1979) has suggested that students changing schools are confronting "ecological transitions" which involve adapting to both role and setting changes and that adjustment may be facilitated or impeded by characteristics of the setting being entered. More specifically, it has been argued that the nature of the social setting confronting the adolescent during the transition to high school may, in part, account for the heightened vulnerability to maladjustment and school failure associated with this particular school change (Felner et al., 1981). Thus, it may be particularly important in the development of preventive efforts targeted at those entering high school to attend to key aspects of the social environment which may be modified to facilitate students' adaptation during this transition.

One feature of the school setting which may exacerbate students' difficulties in coping with the transition into high school is that the entire local social system is in a state of flux with all incoming students (generally from several different "feeder" elementary or junior high schools) attempting to adapt to the new setting at the same time. All students in the entering class are simultaneously confronted by a new physical environment and a larger and generally unfamiliar set of peers and school personnel. Such broad systemic flux may interfere with a student's adaptive efforts in several ways. A student's mastery of transitional tasks, such as gaining an understanding of the school's expectations and regularities (Bogat et al., 1980) or reconstructing and reorganizing his or her formal and informal support systems (Dohrenwend, 1978; Felner et al., 1980) may be made more difficult by the social setting context. Similarly, teachers and guidance staff are confronted with getting to know and providing information and support for large numbers of new students. Thus in addition to those tasks typically confronted by a student transferring into a new school, the students entering high school are also confronted by a less stable, less predictable environment in which the resources available to aid them in their coping efforts may be seriously taxed.

The present work reports the structure and evaluation of a multi-element primary prevention program for students entering high school. The program includes elements aimed at reducing the degree of flux and complexity of the social setting the student is entering, as well as increasing the instrumental and affective social support from teachers and peers.

METHOD

Subjects

During the summer preceding their freshman year, students were randomly selected for participation in the Transition Project (Project) from among approximately 450 students entering a large urban high school (total enrollment of approximately 1,700). The school serves adolescents from predominately non-white, lower income backgrounds with the ethnic composition of the school population being approximately 57% black, 19% white, 22% Hispanic, and 2% other. A total of 65 students participated in all phases of the project and its assessment. The Project was designed to be primary preventive in its focus; thus, two general constraints were placed on the pool of subjects from which the sample of students were drawn. That is, only those students who were, at that point, showing generally satisfactory school adjustment (i.e., meeting all grade and attendance requirements in eighth grade for promotion into high school) and those not considered in need of any special mental health programming were eligible for Project participation. Students included in the Transition Project were matched by sex, age, and ethnic background with 120 nonproject (Control) freshmen from the same school who also met the inclusion critiera. These latter students were unaware of their status as control for this project and, except for the administration of the assessment instruments at the two evaluation points, experienced no differences in school routine or procedures from other incoming nonproject freshmen. Evaluation procedures were explained as being part of a general study of school attitudes and adjustment of high school freshmen.

Some Project and Control students did not fully complete all the assessment instruments or incorrectly completed certain sections. Thus, the full samples on which all analyses were performed consisted of 59 Project students and 113 Control students. Chi-square analyses showed these groups to be matched on the aforementioned demographic variables.

Transition Project

The Transition Project sought to increase levels of peer and teacher support during the transition to high school and to reduce the difficulties of mastering the transitional tasks they encountered. Based on the prior literature, it was posited that if the Project was successful in addressing these concerns, students' vulnerability to the development of academic and emotional difficulties during the transition to high school would be reduced and the development or maintenance of positive perceptions of the school environment would be facilitated.

The Project had two primary components: (a) restructuring of the role of homeroom teachers; (b) reorganizing the regularities of the school environment to reduce the flux of the social setting confronting the student. For the first component, all Project freshmen were assigned to one of four Project homerooms. The student population of these homerooms consisted solely of project participants. Roles were redefined so that the homeroom teacher served as the primary administrative-counseling link between the students, their parents, and the rest of the school, performing many guidance and administrative duties usually done by guidance counselors and other school personnel. For example, homeroom teachers, rather than guidance staff, aided Project students in choosing classes and counseled them regarding school or personal difficulties or concerns. Moreover, when a student was absent, the homeroom teacher, not other school personnel (as is usually the case), contacted the family and handled excuses. Finally, before the school year began, Project homeroom teachers contacted the parents of Project students, explained the nature of the program to them, and encouraged participation and contact with the Project teachers. The intent of these changes were threefold: (a) to increase the amount of instrumental and affective social support from a school-based source (i.e., teachers) the students perceived as present in their daily school environment; (b) to increase students' feelings of accountability and decrease their sense of anonymity; and (c) to reduce the difficulty with which students could gain access to important information about school expectations, rules, and regularities.

The second component of the project involved a partial reorganization of the social system the student was entering. Primary goals of this component were to reduce the degree of flux the students confronted upon entering high school and to facilitate the restructuring and establishment of a stable peer support system. Toward these ends, all Project students were assigned to classes so their four primary academic subjects (English, Mathematics, Social Studies, and Science) were taken only with other Project students. Thus, there was no longer a constantly shifting peer group in each of the student's classes across the school day, as would occur if students were assigned to classes from among the full set of incoming freshmen. Now, in at least four classes as well as homeroom, there was a high degree of overlap and consistency among the students in the class. Again, it was hoped that this change in the social ecology of the system would facilitate the development of peer support and enhance the students' sense of belonging as well as result in a perception of the school environment as a stable, well-organized/understandable, and cohesive place.

Teachers were selected to participate in the project as follows: Volunteers to serve as Project teachers were sought from among all instructors of freshman academic subject classes. With few exceptions, eligible teachers expressed interest in participating as Project teachers. The final selection of Project teachers was based on two additional criteria. The first consideration was that there be only one teacher from each of the four primary academic subjects. (Academic subject teachers also served as Project homeroom teachers.) Second, to further reduce the complexity of the school environment for students, teachers from within each area were selected based on the degree to which their classroom/homeroom was in physical proximity in the building to the other participating teachers. It was hoped that minimizing the distance between classes would facilitate the students both feeling more familiar with, and comfortable in, the school as well as engaging in greater informal interaction with classmates between classes.

Two additional details of the project's operation should also be noted. First, in addition to teaching the Project classes the selected teachers also taught other freshmen classes in their subject area throughout the remainder of the day. Thus, Control students may have taken several classes with Project teachers as well as with teachers who volunteered but were not selected to participate for the above reasons. Second, although there was no specific formal training regime per se for Project teachers, prior to the inception of the project teachers met several times with school guidance personnel to discuss concerns and gain further information about the issues noted. Moreover, throughout the course of the project, consultation was available to teachers from school guidance personnel.

Procedures

All Project and Control students were evaluated at the midpoint of the academic year and again, as recommended by Lorion and Lounsbury (1981), at a later, end of school-year follow-up on three sets of criterion measures: (a) a self-concept scale; (b) a measure of the students' perception of various dimensions of the social climate of the school; and (c) the students' eighth- and ninth-grade attendance records and grade point averages

(GPAs). No preintervention data are available other than for grades and absences. However, Campbell and Stanley (1963) have argued than such pretesting is not essential in assessing whether an intervention had an effect if, as in the present work, care has been taken to use randomization procedures in assigning subjects to treatment and control group assignment.

Instruments

Self-Appraisal Inventory (SAI). The SAI (Frith & Narikawa, 1972) consists of 36 yes-no items assessing four aspects of a school-age child's self-concept: Scholastic, Peer, Family, and General self-concept. In the present study items were modified as recommended by Popham (note 1) to make them more appropriate for an adolescent population (e.g., "Are you a good child?" was changed to "Are you a good person?") and the Family subscale was omitted. An overall Total self-concept score was obtained by summing the scores on the remaining subscales as recommended by Frith and Narikawa (1972). Higher subscale and overall scores indicate a more positive self-concept.

High School Environment Scale (HES). The HES used in the present study consists of a modification of the Trickett and Moos (1973) Classroom Environment Scale (CES) Short Form plus eight additional items from the CES which load on subscales of particular concern for this work, i.e., Teacher Support and Affiliation. CES questions were modified to refer to the school environment in general rather than the specific classroom environment. The HES provides information about a student's perceptions of three general dimensions of a school's social climate on nine subscales. The general social environment dimensions and the subscales which comprise them are (a) a Relationship dimension which includes the Involvement (4 items), Affiliation (8 items), and Teacher-support (8 items) subscales; (b) a Personal development dimension consisting of Task orientation (4 items) and Competition (4 items) subscales; and (c) a System maintenance and System change dimension comprised of the Order and organization, Rule clarity, Teacher control, and Innovation subscales (4 items each). Subscale scores are obtained by summing the number of items answered in the scored direction. Again, higher scores are indicative of a student's perception of that social climate dimension being more characteristic of the social climate of the school.

Academic Adjustment Measures. The student's permanent record served as the primary source of data. Eighth- and ninth-grade attendance and grade records were obtained. Overall cumulative eighth- and ninth-grade GPAs (A = 4 points, F = 0 point) were calculated for each student based on academic grades in English, Mathematics, Science, and Social

Studies. Cumulative eighth- and ninth-grade attendance figures were also computed for each student.

RESULTS

Academic Adjustment

The cumulative eighth- and ninth-grade GPAs and absences of Project and Control students were compared using a repeated measure analysis of variance (ANOVA). There were significant group differences both on GPA and attendance, $F(1, 172) = 53.2, p \leq .05; F(1, 172) = 5.46, p \leq .05$, respectively, as well as significant time, $F(1, 172) = 3.71, p \leq .05$, and group by time interactions, $F(1, 172) = 5.20, p \leq .05$, for grades.

To further clarify these findings and insure the initial comparability of the group on GPA and absenteeism, subsequent t tests were done. There were no significant differences between Project and Control students on their preproject, i.e., end of eighth grade, levels of absenteeism, $t \leq 1$. However, Control students were absent significantly more often in ninth grade than were Project students (M = 25.1 and 16.7 days/year, respectively), $t = 2.54, p \leq .02$. Examination of group GPAs revealed a similar pattern of results. While Project and Control students had almost identical cumulative eighth grade GPAs (M = 2.64 and 2.61, respectively), $t \leq 1$, at the end of ninth grade, Project students had significantly higher GPAs (M = 2.78 and 2.29, respectively), $t = 2.59, p \leq .01$.

Self-Concept

Repeated measure ANOVAs examined differences between Project and Control students on midyear and end-of-year self-concept scores. The results of these analyses are presented in Table 1. Significant main effects for group and time were found on all three SAI subscales, as well as significant group by time interactions on all but the Peer scale, on which the interaction approached significance ($p \leq .10$). Significant group and group by time effects were also found on SAI Total scores with the time effect approaching significance ($p \leq .10$).

Examination of group means on the subscales and overall self-concept scores indicate that while Project students' self-concepts generally remained stable, Control students showed marked declines in these adjustment indices across the school year.

Table 1. Comparison of Project and Control Group Self-Concept Scores: Midyear Versus End-of-year

SAI self-concept scale	Groups	Means		F		
		Midyear	End-of-year	Group	Time	Group × Time
Total	Project	16.19	15.85	4.72^b	6.78^a	4.59^b
	Controls	15.44	11.85			
Scholastic	Project	4.76	4.64	14.95^c	6.03^b	2.47
	Controls	4.20	3.31			
Peer	Project	4.96	4.62	10.22^c	15.08^c	2.79^a
	Controls	4.62	3.52			
General	Project	6.66	6.69	8.54^c	11.72^c	6.55^c
	Controls	6.55	5.01			

$^a p \leq .10.$
$^b p \leq .05.$
$^c p \leq .01.$

Social Environment

A series of multiple analyses of variance (MANOVAs) and ANOVAs were done to test differences between Project and Control students' perceptions of the school environment, based on mid- and end-of-year HES ratings of school social climate. The nine HES scales were assigned to one of three MANOVAs as a function of their relationship to the three general dimensions of the social environment (Trickett & Moos, 1973). Thus, three separate MANOVAs included the scales comprising HES' Relationship, Personal growth, and System maintenance and change dimensions, respectively.

All three MANOVAs revealed significant main effects for group membership. The results of these analyses are summarized in Table 2. Most of those differences were attributable to Project students reporting more positive feelings than Controls concerning the social climate dimension. Within each general dimension, ANOVAs examining the ratings on the component scales followed much the same pattern. Further, on several ANOVAs on individual scales as well as the overall MANOVA on the Personal growth dimension significant group by time or time effects were found.

Project students responded more positively than Controls on the Relationship dimension. Individual ANOVAs showed that Project students reported significantly higher levels of Teacher support, Teacher affiliation, and Involvement than Controls. There were also significant time effects on the Involvement and Teacher affiliation subscales and a group by time interaction on Teacher support. Generally, mean scores of Project students

Table II. MANOVA and ANOVA Comparisons of Project and Control Group HES Dimensions and Subscales

HES dimensions/subscales	Groups	Means Midyear	Means End-of-year	F Group	F Time	Group × Time
Relationship						
MANOVA				3.43^b	2.23^a	0.67
Involvement	Project	1.93	1.71	10.53^c	6.53^c	1.21
	Controls	1.69	1.22			
Teacher affiliation	Project	2.95	2.84	28.06^c	7.56^c	2.06
	Controls	2.40	1.90			
Teacher support	Project	3.83	4.15	31.04^c	2.15	4.45^b
	Controls	3.15	2.59			
Personal growth						
MANOVA				5.04^c	1.60	3.14^b
Task orientation	Project	4.03	3.78	16.51^c	7.12^b	0.83
	Controls	3.43	2.83			
Competition	Project	2.16	2.22	10.60^c	11.41^c	7.56^c
	Controls	2.10	1.47			
System maintenance and change						
MANOVA				4.04^c	1.51	1.00
Order and organization	Project	1.61	1.64	17.82^c	8.75^c	5.67^b
	Controls	1.41	0.94			
Rule clarity	Project	3.08	2.74	28.46^c	21.12^c	1.75
	Controls	2.54	1.88			
Teacher control	Project	3.08	2.74	6.62^c	10.12^c	2.89^a
	Controls	2.54	1.88			
Innovation	Project	2.47	2.27	33.04^c	7.35^c	0.54
	Controls	1.84	1.45			

$^a p \leq .10.$
$^b p \leq .05.$
$^c p \leq .01.$

remained fairly stable on these dimensions between the midyear and end-of-year testing while, in all cases, Control student ratings were lower at the end-of-year assessment than at midyear.

Project and Control students also significantly differed in their perceptions of the Personal growth-enhancing dimensions of the school environment, with a significant group by time interaction also present. Project students rated this social climate dimension as being more characteristic of the school environment than did Controls, particularly at the end of the year. ANOVAs on both the Task orientation and Competition scales revealed similar group effects and a significant group by time interaction on the competition scale, due primarily to stable perceptions by Project students as opposed to marked declines in end-of-year ratings by Controls.

Project students also rated the environment significantly more positively than Controls on the Systems maintenance and change dimension. All four individual ANOVAs on the subscales showed significant main effects for group membership in that same direction. Further, main effects for time were also found on all four scales. In addition, on the Order and organization scale there was also a significant group by time interaction while for Teacher control this interaction approached significance ($p \leqslant .10$). Time and interaction effects in these analyses were due less to changes in Project student's responses and more to declines in the ratings of the school environment by Controls.

DISCUSSION

The present data suggest that Project students were more successful in coping with the transition to high school than Controls. Project students generally showed little change in either their academic performance from eighth to ninth grade or in their midyear vs. end-of-year self-concept and school environment ratings. By contrast, Control students did significantly less well in academic adjustment in ninth grade compared to eighth grade and declined sharply both in their self-concept scores and ratings of the school climate. Hence, by the end of ninth grade, Project students compared to Controls had significantly better GPAs and attendance records, more positive self-concepts, and saw the school environment as having clearer expectations and organizational structure and higher levels of teacher support.

Several factors limit interpretation of the results. For example, it could be argued that differences in ninth grade GPAs between Project and Control students were due to expectations on the part of teachers that Project students would do better. Although that is theoretically possible, certain of the data support the alternative view, i.e., that these differences do, in fact, reflect better performance by Project students. First, although Project students had significantly higher ninth grade GPAs than Controls, the difference was due primarily to drops in the grades of Controls. Second, and perhaps more important, Controls' poorer GPAs in ninth grade are accompanied by a significantly higher rate of absenteeism than that of Project students. Absenteeism strongly predicts school failure (U.S. Department of Health, Education, & Welfare, 1975) and is not directly influenced by teacher expectancies. The pattern of declining GPA and increasing absenteeism among Controls is similar to findings reported by

Felner *et al.* (1981) suggesting the heightened potential for the development of academic difficulties in innercity students accompanying high school entry. In summary then, GPA differences between the groups may well reflect *actual* differences in academic adjustment.

Additionally, Project students' expectancies and perceived response-demand because of the special treatment they had conceivably could have led to a response bias inflating their self-concept and social climate ratings. Hence, group differences on these measures might be interpreted as due either to (a) response biases or (b) actual program effects. Examination of the patterns of the groups' mean self-concept and social climate ratings suggest the latter may be the more defensible explanation. Although Project students did show slightly higher scores than Controls on most measures by the midyear evaluation, those differences were generally small and non-significant. In most cases, significant group differences on these variables did not emerge until the second (end-of-year) evaluation point, and were due primarily to marked declines in Controls' self-concept and social climate ratings rather than higher ratings by Project students.

One might also question whether the observed Project versus Control differences were due to the intervention program or to special characteristics of participating teachers. It could, for example, be argued that especially talented, compassionate teachers could affect students in ways similar to the reported program effects in this paper. Moreover, the fact that Project teachers were volunteers suggests that they were more than minimally involved in their jobs. Examination of the recruitment procedures and teaching patterns, however, suggests that the results of the intervention cannot be explained solely by teacher effects. First, although all Project teachers were, indeed, volunteers, other ninth-grade teachers (as noted above) also expressed a willingness to participate, but were not selected either because of classroom location or because only one teacher in each subject area was used. Thus, although Project teachers were surely invested in their jobs, they were not necessarily more invested than other, non-Project ninth-grade teachers. Participation criteria other than those already noted were not used and there was no attempt to pick particularly "talented" teachers for the project. Indeed, any such effort might well have led to negative reactions by excluded teachers which would have seriously jeopardized the program and its evaluation. Second, although Project teachers carried academic and homeroom responsibilities for program participants as a major part of their teaching load, they also taught non-Project classes in which many Control students were enrolled.

In summary, this study demonstrates that low-cost changes in the roles of school personnel and the social ecology of the high school environment can effectively prevent academic and personal difficulties associated with school change by increasing the levels of social support available to students and decreasing the confusion and complexity of the setting being entered. Project students' attitudes toward the school environment and school personnel, as well as their personal and academic adjustment, were more positive than those of Controls. Given the absence of long-term follow-up data, caution should be exercised in arguing for lasting preventive efforts for the program. However, as noted elsewhere (Felner *et al.*, 1981; U.S. Department of Health, Education, & Welfare, 1975), because significant declines in academic performance and increases in absenteeism found for Control students are often associated with the development of enduring school problems and higher dropout rates, Control students are at greater risk for future school difficulties than Project students.

Overall, these findings support the arguments that attempts to understand and modify social environments (Bronfenbrenner, 1979; Moos, 1976) can be adapted fruitfully to preventive programs designed to increase people's ability to cope with the adaptive tasks of life transitions. To refine such preventive efforts, additional research is needed to elaborate both the tasks and difficulties encountered by individuals during such times and the ways in which key aspects of the social environment mediate adaptation. A fuller understanding of these issues will aid in the targeting and design of future attempts to modify social environments to facilitate successful coping during life transitions.

ACKNOWLEDGMENTS

The authors would like to thank Edison Trickett and Stephanie S. Farber for their helpful comments on earlier drafts of this paper and Lisa G. Martin for her aid in the preparation of this manuscript. Appreciation is also due to Martin Klotz for his contributions in all phases of this work. This project was supported by grants from the Edward W. Hazen Foundation and the New Haven Foundation. An earlier version of this paper was presented at the 87th annual convention of the American Psychological Association, New York, 1979.

REFERENCES

Bachman, J. G., Green, S., & Wirtanen, I. D. *Youth in transition* (Vol. 3). Ann Arbor: Survey Research Center, Institute for Social Research, 1971.

Bloom, B. L. Marital disruption as a stressor. In D. G. Forgays (Ed.), *Primary prevention of psychopathology* (Vol. 2). *Environmental influences.* Hanover, N.H.: University Press of New England, 1978.

Bloom, B. L. Prevention of mental disorders: Recent advances in theory and practice. *Community Mental Health Journal*, 1979, *15*, 179–191.

Bogat, G. A., Jones, J. W., & Jason, L. A. School transitions: Preventive intervention following an elementary school closing. *Journal of Community Psychology*, 1980, *8*, 343–352.

Bronfenbrenner, U. *The ecology of human development: Experiments by nature and design.* Cambridge: Harvard University Press, 1979.

Caplan, G. Opportunities for school psychologists in the primary prevention of mental disorders in children. In N. M. Lambert (Ed.), *The protection and promotion of mental health in schools* (U.S. Department of Health, Education & Welfare, Public Health Service Publication No. 1226). Washington, DC: U.S. Government Printing Office, 1965.

Caplan, G. *Support systems and community mental health: Lectures on concept development.* New York: Behavioral Publications, 1974.

Campbell, D. T. & Stanley, J. C. *Experimental and quasi-experimental designs for research.* Chicago: Rand McNally College Publishing, 1963.

Collins, J. M. & Coulter, F. Effects of geographical movement on the social and academic development of children of army personnel. *Australian and New Zealand Journal of Sociology,* 1974, *10,* 222–223.

Cowen, E. L., Pederson, A., Babigian, H., Izzo, L. D., & Trost, M. A. Long-term follow-up of early detected vulnerable children. *Journal of Consulting and Clinical Psychology,* 1973, *41,* 438–446.

Cramer, W. & Dorsey, S. Are movers losers? *Elementary School Journal,* 1979, *70,* 387–390.

Cumming, J. & Cumming, E. *Ego and milieu: Theory and practice of environmental therapy.* New York: Atherton, 1962.

Dohrenwend, B. S. Social stress and community psychology. *American Journal of Community Psychology,* 1978, *6,* 1–15.

Felner, R. D., Farber, S. S., & Primavera, J. Children of divorce, stressful life events and transitions: A framework for preventive efforts. In R. H. Price, R. F. Ketterer, B. C. Bader, & J. Monahan (Eds.), *Prevention in mental health: Research, policy and practice.* Beverly Hills: Sage, 1980.

Felner, R. D., Primavera, J., & Cauce, A. M. The impact of school transitions: A focus for preventive efforts. *American Journal of Community Psychology,* 1981, *9,* 449–459.

Frith, S. & Narikawa, O. *Attitudes toward school.* Los Angeles: Instructional Objective Exchange, 1972.

Goebel, B. L. Mobility and education. *American Secondary Education.* 1978, *8,* 11–16.

Goldston, S. E. A national perspective. In D. G. Forgays (Ed.), *Primary prevention of psychopathology* (Vol. 2). *Environmental influences.* Hanover, N.H.: University Press of New England, 1978.

Gottlieb, B. H. Social networks and social support in the design of preventive intervention. In B. H. Gottlieb (Ed.), *Social networks and social support in community mental health.* Beverly Hills: Sage, 1981.

Hirschowitz, R. B. Groups to help people cope with the tasks of transitions. In R. D. Hirschowitz & B. Levy (Eds.), *The changing mental health scene.* New York: Spectrum Press, 1976.

Kemme, M. L. Factors relevant to the mobile child's management of entry into a new school. *Dissertation Abstracts International,* 1971, *32,* 1849.

Kobasa, S. C. Personality and resistance to illness. *American Journal of Community Psychology,* 1979, *7,* 413–424.

Lazarus, R. S. & Launier, R. Stress-related transactions between person and environment. In L. A. Pervin and M. Lewis (Eds.), *Perspectives in interactional psychology.* New York: Plenum Press, 1978.

Levine, M. Residential change and school adjustment. *Community Mental Health Journal,* 1966, *2,* 61–69.

Levine, M., Wesolowski, J. C., & Corbett, F. J. Pupil turnover and academic performance in an inner city elementary school. *Psychology in the Schools,* 1966, *3,* 153–156.

Lorion, R. P. & Lounsbury, J. W. Conceptual and methodological considerations in evaluating preventive interventions. In W. R. Tash & G. Stahler (Eds.), *Innovative approaches to mental health evaluation*. New York: Academic Press, 1981.

Moos, R. H. *The human context: Environmental determinants of behavior*. New York: Wiley, 1979.

Popham, W. J. (1972, November). *Empirically based revision of an affective measuring instrument*. Paper presented at the annual meeting of the California Educational Research Association, San Jose, CA.

Rakieten, H. *The reactions of mobile elementary school children to various elementary school induction and orientation procedures*. Unpublished doctoral dissertation, Teachers College, Columbia University, 1961.

Schaller, J. The relationship between geographic mobility and school behavior. *Man-Environment Systems*, 1975, *5*, 185–187.

Trickett, E. J. & Moos, R. H. The social environment of junior high and senior high school classrooms. *Journal of Educational Psychology*, 1973, *65*, 93–102.

U.S. Department of Health, Education & Welfare. *Dropout prevention*. Washington, DC : Educational Resources Information Center, 1975 (ERIC Document Reproduction Service No. ED105 354).

10

The Fidelity–Adaptation Debate: Implications for the Implementation of Public Sector Social Programs

Craig H. Blakely, Jeffrey P. Mayer, Rand G. Gottschalk, Neal Schmitt, William S. Davidson, David B. Roitman, and James G. Emshoff

The modified Research, Development, and Diffusion (RD&D) model, as exemplified by change agents in federal organizations, was examined as a viable strategy for disseminating social program innovations. This study of seven nationally disseminated education and criminal justice projects was designed to refine the methodology for measuring innovation implementation. We measured program fidelity, reinvention, and effectiveness in a diverse set of program settings. Results of the research suggested that high-fidelity adopters tended to produce more effective implementations than low-fidelity adopters. Local modifications to the model were unrelated to effectiveness, whereas local additions to the model tended to enhance effectiveness. Findings supported the utility of the modified RD&D model of innovation dissemination with public sector social programs.

Throughout its brief history, community psychology has been concerned with interventions focused at multiple levels of society (e.g., Cowen,

Originally published in the *American Journal of Community Psychology, 15*(3) (1987): 253–268.

A Quarter Century of Community Psychology: Readings from the American Journal of Community Psychology, edited by Tracey A. Revenson *et al.* Kluwer Academic/Plenum Publishers, New York, 2002.

Gardner, & Zax, 1967; Heller, Price, Reinharz, Riger, & Wandersman, 1984; Rappaport, 1977). To this end, the field has focused on the development of innovative social programs as the preferred model of change (Fairweather & Tornatzky, 1977). However, organizational change is a very slow process. Often, newly developed programs, rigorously evaluated as demonstration projects, are not implemented on a large scale and, consequently, never have a significant effect on the broader social problem of interest (Fairweather, Tornatzky, Fergus, & Avellar, 1980; Rappaport, 1977). The current research effort was undertaken to begin to gain a better understanding of the processes inherent in organizational change in general and of the Research, Development, and Diffusion (RD&D) model of change in particular.

HISTORICAL PERSPECTIVE

The classical RD&D model was extremely popular among federal policy-makers in the 1960s and 1970s (Havelock, 1969). At the heart of the RD&D model was the development of programs that were subjected to rigorous validation efforts (demonstration projects). The RD&D model was in part inspired by the success of the federally sponsored R&D efforts in space exploration (House, 1981). In this model, laboratories and research groups specializing in R&D would develop new social technologies. These technologies would then be subjected to rigorous evaluation prior to dissemination to potential users. Program adopters (e.g., schools, service agencies, local municipalities) were assumed to value evaluation results highly and act as relatively passive consumers in the dissemination process (Tornatzky, Fergus, Avellar, Fairweather, & Fleischer, 1981).

Some of the assumptions of this paradigm have been questioned by recent research (e.g., Berman & McLaughlin, 1978; Farrar, deSanctis, & Cohen, 1979; Fullan & Pomfret, 1977; House, 1975; Rappaport, Seidman, & Davidson, 1979). It was argued that adopting organizations were far from the passive recipients the classical RD&D model would have us believe. Rather, numerous organizational factors combined to influence the degree to which adopting sites faithfully implemented a model program. Further, research by Rogers and his colleagues (Eveland, Rogers, & Klepper, 1977; Rogers, 1978) indicated that local adopters changed ("reinvented") innovative model programs to fit their local needs and provide a sense of ownership.

These research findings led to some changes in the conceptualization of the classical RD&D model to account for the importance of local organizational influences. Retaining the major underlying tenet of the classical model, the new RD&D model still called for the development of programs using scientifically rigorous research and evaluation methodology and initial funding channeled to innovation developers. However, a more active model of dissemination efforts emerged that involved potential adopters site visiting developers' programs, the placement of state-level change agents, developer-sponsored training sessions, and innovation "awareness" conferences. This new model, appropriately labeled by many "the modified RD&D model," bears a great similarity to the Linkage Model outlined by Havelock (1969).

Although these modifications to the classical RD&D model were based on research findings, they were seen as only one alternative to the classical position. In fact, many argued for completely abandoning the RD&D model in favor of a "decentralized," local problem-solving approach (Berman, 1981; House, 1975).

CURRENT PERSPECTIVE

The field of social innovation and organizational change can be seen as divided into two opposing camps. Those advocating the "profidelity" position have viewed innovations as consisting of a number of relatively well-specified program components. They have argued that validated innovative programs should be adopted with close correspondence (fidelity) to the original model (Boruch & Gomez, 1977; Calsyn, Tornatzky, & Dittmar, 1977). Altering or diluting the program was expected to lead to decreased effectiveness. A more moderate fidelity perspective has been outlined by Hall and his associates (e.g., Hall & Loucks, 1978). Hall argued that adaptation or reinvention was acceptable up to a "zone of drastic mutation," beyond which continued dilution compromised the program's integrity and effectiveness.

On the other hand, those supporting a "proadaptation" or decentralized perspective have argued that differing organizational contexts and practitioner needs have almost always demanded on-site modification of disseminated program models (Berman & McLaughlin, 1978). The more a program user was free to modify the model to fit local needs, the greater the likelihood of positive results. Further, given the greater degree of flexibility, the program user's sense of program ownership should increase, resulting in longer program life. An even more radical implication of the proadaptation perspective suggested that the channeling of initial program development funds to centralized developers or RD&D labs should cease. Rather, one could infer from this position that organizations should be given funds to build local capacities allowing for the independent development of innovations.

Although the proadaptation position has attracted an increasing number of adherents in recent years, Datta (1981) has suggested that the momentum of the proadaptation movement may be impelling us to throw out the "R&D baby" with the bath water. Datta has criticized the empirical base of the pro-adaptation perspective. For example, a frequently cited Rand report on federal programs supporting educational change (Berman & McLaughlin, 1978) found three dominant patterns of implementation: (a) cooptation, adapting a program model without any accompanying changes in organizational behavior; (b) mutual adaptation, adapting a program model with accompanying changes in organizational behavior; and (c) nonimplementation, failure to adopt and implement an innovative program model. Berman and McLaughlin (1977) reported that mutual adaptation was the only situation in which actual changes occurred in organizational behavior. They also reported that mutually adapted projects were more likely to be effective than were coopted projects. More importantly, they noted a striking absence of high-fidelity implementation.

Closer inspection of their fidelity instrument revealed a predisposition toward findings of reinvention or adaptation, rather than fidelity. The measure of implementation was "the extent to which projects met their own goals, different as they might be for each project" (Berman & McLaughlin, 1977, p. 50). Thus, they incorporated no bona fide measure of component-specific fidelity, and there was no conclusive way to determine the extent to which programs were modified. Further, Datta (1981) noted that the program models studied were for the most part loosely defined policy statements rather than highly specified social programs. Thus, it was impractical from the outset to measure fidelity.

In fact, Berman (1981) advanced the fidelity–adaptation debate considerably when he proposed a contingency model of implementation strategies. The implications of this model suggested that different strategies were appropriate in different settings. He argued that either strategy, profidelity or proadaptation, can be effective when applied to the appropriate policy situation: There exists no global, best strategy. He argued that the profidelity perspective is likely to function best with relatively structured and well-specified innovations, whereas adaptive strategies are more appropriate with relatively unstructured innovations. However, many situations are so complex that some combination of the two strategies might prove to be most successful.

Despite the rational positions outlined by Berman (contingency model) and Hall (zone of drastic mutation), the debate rages on and the policy trend toward a decentralized position continues relatively unchecked. The research reported here attempted a further examination of the modified RD&D model. In short, the current research effort was intended to determine the viability of the modified RD&D model as a vehicle for the dissemination of relatively well-specified social technologies in organizational settings.

To test the viability of the modified RD&D model, it was necessary to identify several innovative social technologies that had been developed and subjected to a rigorous evaluation effort and then disseminated nationally. The modified RD&D approach has been used extensively in two major policy areas, the National Diffusion Network (NDN) in education and the Exemplary Projects Program (EPP) in criminal justice. The mission of these organizations has been to develop highly specific descriptions of effective programs to encourage their replication. Within this setting, this research addressed three major questions: (a) Can programs that have been developed and defined in relatively unambiguous terms be implemented with acceptable fidelity? (b) Will initially successful programs prove to be effective at a replication site if implemented with fidelity? (c) What is the relative importance of fidelity and reinvention in determining program effectiveness?

METHOD

Sample of Organizations

The National Diffusion Network and the Exemplary Projects Program provided two excellent examples of the modified RD&D model in practice. The nearly 200 innovations disseminated by these two organizations served as the source from which the final set of disseminated innovations were selected. Two major selection criteria were used: (a) for sample purposes, innovation models had to have at least 20 adopters in operation nationally that could serve as sites to be studied, and (b) innovations had to incorporate an organization-wide quality. Since the focus of the study was organizational change and organizational characteristics might interact in this process, innovations that could be independently adopted and implemented by a single teacher, police officer, etc., were excluded.

Written materials available on the 200 programs disseminated through these two agencies were reviewed with respect to the above criteria. Initial cuts yielded a pool of 15 programs. Additional information was gathered from phone interviews at each of the 15 developers' sites, and seven innovations (listed in Table 1) were ultimately selected for research purposes.

Within each innovation, the effective sampling pool was constrained by the following criteria: (a) sites had to be currently operating the program; (b) the implementation had to be in place for at least 2 years; and

Table 1. Social Innovations Selected for Study

Education

1. Host (help one student to succeed): A diagnostic, prescriptive, tutorial reading program for grades 2–6. Daily 1/2-hour pull-out tutoring program. Tutors are community volunteers and cross-aged students.
2. EBCE (experience-based career education): Program provides students with career experiences outside of school at volunteer field sites. Utilizes individualized learning plans which integrate career experiences and academic learning. Programs typically take students from Grades 11–12.
3. FOCUS (focus dissemination projects); A "school within a school" for disaffected junior and senior high school students. Behavioral contracting and a governing board with student representatives are important features. Classes involve individualized, self-paced instruction.

Criminal justice

4. ODOT (one day/one trial): A jury management system that calls in a certain number of potential jurors per day. Potential jurors come in for that day and, if not selected to serve in a trial, have completed their annual obligation.
5. CAP (community arbitration project): Juvenile offenders are sent to a formal arbitration hearing run by the court intake division, rather than to courts. Juveniles have the specific consequences of their actions explained. Parents and victims are frequently present at hearing. Youths are typically assigned hours of work in the community. Restitution is also frequently required.
6. SCCPP (Seattle community crime prevention program): A three-phase attack on residential burglary. It involves the establishment of a neighborhood block watch through proactive targeting of neighborhoods. property marking and inventory, and home security inspections.
7. MCPRC (Montgomery County prerelease center): Involves prisoners in a residential setting separate from the prison. This facility should be in the community from which most of the inmates are drawn. Inmates are encouraged to work so that they will have a job upon release. Counseling, social awareness instruction, and behavioral contracting are also part of the program.

(c) there had to be a reasonably high probability that at least some outcome effectiveness data would be available. Seventy sites, 10 per innovation, were selected for site visits using these criteria.

Strategy of Measurement

The concept of *fidelity* (adherence to a program model) is not new. However, the development of a methodology to quantify the degree of adherence to an original program model is a recent phenomenon. Hall and his associates at the Texas R&D Center developed such a pioneering strategy (Hall & Loucks, 1978; Heck, Steigelbauer, Hall, & Loucks, 1981). They

conceptualized social programs as consisting of a finite number of components or parts. Program fidelity could then be defined as the number or proportion of finite program components that were implemented. Hall and his
colleagues also allowed for the quantification of the degree of presence of
each element. They viewed these component variations as ideal, acceptable,
or unacceptable.

This general approach required the development of detailed "process"
measures that identified specific program components which could then be
observed at adopting/implementing sites to determine adherence to the
model, or fidelity. The current research effort used this method of defining
fidelity, with minor modifications to suit the scope and intent of the
research questions addressed. Rather than allowing first-generation
adopters to influence the development of instruments to measure fidelity,
as in Hall and Loucks' initial approach, fidelity was defined solely in terms
of the developer's innovation model. Although any perspective on fidelity
is somewhat arbitrary, selecting the developer's perspective provided a
conservative test of the RD&D model.

The term *reinvention* was introduced by Rogers and his colleagues to
capture the nature of the active change process that occurs at an adopter
site. As noted above, it was viewed as instrumental in a site's reaction to the
"not invented here" syndrome often considered a threat to program
longevity (e.g., Eveland *et al.*, 1977; Rice & Rogers, 1979). Fidelity alone can
be viewed as the most parsimonious indicator of the degree of implementation, suggesting that *reinvention* is an unnecessary synonym for
low-fidelity implementation. However, we considered more closely the
implications of reinvention for the modified RD&D process. As a result,
two alternative definitions of reinvention were developed. The first type of
reinvention is characterized by the addition of something new to the program model. This would occur if a site added new components to the program. The second type of reinvention is characterized by the change or
modification of existing components. Thus, reinvention could occur either
as an addition to the original model or as a modification of existing program components. However, if a component was deleted altogether, it was
viewed as an unacceptable variation or a simple lack of fidelity. Thus, omis-
sions of components did not contribute to increased reinvention scores.

Fidelity

The five-step model of assessing fidelity developed by Hall and his colleagues was modified slightly to suit the scope and intent of the current
research (Hall & Loucks, 1978). This strategy involved extensive interviews

and in-person observations of a particular model program in place at the developer's site as well as at user sites. Our desire was to determine the degree to which sites implemented programs with fidelity to the disseminated model. Therefore, we restricted the frame of reference to observations at the dissemination site(s), material published by the developer, and interviews with staff at the developer site.

Two of the authors visited each developer site, conducted in-person observations of programs in practice, and interviewed developer staff. Audio tapes of staff interviews and observation notes were then content analyzed to identify innovation components for each of the seven innovations studied. Components were required to conform to the following criteria:

1. A component should be an observable activity, material, or facility. If not observable, the implementation of the component should be verifiable through interviews with staff members and clients of the implementing organization.
2. Each component should be logically discrete from other components. If not, the implementation of a component should not depend on the implementation of another component.
3. Components should be innovation specific. Activities, materials, or facilities that are common to other programs in the developing organization should not be considered innovation components.
4. The list of components should exhaustively describe the innovation.

The methodology required the identification of component variations scaled as ideal, acceptable, and unacceptable. Variations were identified by research team staff following initial innovation developer site visits. Both the initial list of innovation components and their related variations were then submitted to developer staff for review and modification. Final lists of components for each of the seven innovations ranged from approximately 60 to just over 100 components. Table 2 presents several examples of fidelity items.

Site visits were conducted by two research staff pairs who spent 2 days at each site observing activities, materials, and facilities, and talking with program staff and "clients." Block watch meetings, juror orientation sessions, arbitration hearings, classroom reading laboratories, etc., were observed firsthand. Archival records, fiscal information, training manuals, and other materials were either collected or carefully reviewed during visits. Immediately following each day's sessions, site visitors rated each innovation fidelity component as ideal, acceptable, or unacceptable (see Table 2).

Interrater reliability was assessed at 20% of the sites. Each of the two site visit teams conducted a reliability check at one randomly selected site

Table 2. Examples of Fidelity Items[a]

Example 1: Component 48: Experience-based career education (EBCE)

48. Career site: Resource person (employer) commitment.
   - I   Resource people are asked to make specific commitments regarding the specific learning experiences offered at the career site.
   - A   Resource people are asked to make more general commitments regarding the general kinds of learning experiences offered at the career site.
   - U   Resource people are not asked to make any commitments regarding the learning experiences offered at the career site.

Example 2: Component 38: Community arbitration project (CAP)

38. Victims reports on the incident and what s/he would like the hearing outcome to be.
   - I   Victim reports on what s/he saw and what s/he would like the hearing outcome to be.
   - A   Victim reports only on what s/he saw or on what s/he would like the hearing outcome to be.
   - U   Victim reports neither what s/he saw nor what s/he would like the hearing outcome to be.

Example 3: Component 58: FOCUS educational program for disaffected youth

58. Hourly attendance is taken.
   - I   Hourly attendance is taken for all students.
   - A   Hourly attendance is taken only for those students who the teacher feels are an attendance problem.
   - U   Hourly attendance is not taken for any students.

Example 4: Component 65: Montgomery County prerelease center (MCPRC)

65. Teams discuss both new and continuing cases at meetings.
   - I   At regular team meetings, staff review all current cases and all starts of new cases in depth.
   - A   At regular team meetings, staff review all starts of new cases, all continuing cases with significant changes, and as many other continuing cases as time allows.
   - U   At regular team meetings, staff spend little time reviewing current cases with significant changes and focus primarily on new cases.

[a]I = ideal; A = acceptable; U = unacceptable.

for each of the seven innovations. At each site where reliability checks were taken, the two research team staff *together* observed all activities, checked available archival data, and conducted all interviews. Following the site visit, the two independently coded fidelity instruments. The two sets of scores were then compared. Summed across the total set of reliability checks (i.e., the seven sites, one per innovation, where reliability checks were completed), an exact agreement figure of .81 was achieved. Other indices, such as kappa, are frequently useful in such situations. Although the intent of the kappa statistic is to account for the baseline of responses, kappas were misleadingly low in this case because of the relatively consistently high fidelity scores observed. Thus, percentage exact agreement was viewed as the most easily interpreted index of agreement.

Validity was examined by comparing data across sources (e.g., respondents from different organizational roles, multiple observations of events, and examinations of archival records). The convergence of item-level fidelity scores was used as an assessment of the validity of the method. For example, where reports from or observations of two different program actors resulted in an identical coding of a fidelity item, it was viewed as an indicator of the validity of the measurement scheme (convergence of source). On the other hand, differing codings detracted from the validity index. Multiple sources of fidelity data were available, on the average, for more than 75% of the items at each site. This between-source comparison strategy, summed across all 70 sites, produced an exact-agreement convergence rating of .96.

Reinvention

The current state of the art with respect to the measurement of reinvention could best be viewed as a state of infancy. Therefore, systematic guidelines rather than closed-ended questions were used to collect reinvention data. Data collection consisted of audio recordings of site visitors' observations about local program implementations that might be viewed as examples of reinvention. These audio tapes were then transcribed and content analyzed by project staff. In coding the transcribed data, three levels of decision were made. First, a determination was made concerning whether or not the activity in question was a legitimate instance of reinvention and not a simple presence or lack of fidelity. If the activity in question was determined to be an instance of reinvention, two additional coding decisions were made. The first focused on the type of reinvention occurring (see below). The second was a quantification of the magnitude of the reinvention based on departure from the developers program philosophy.

In judging the type of reinvention, an instance could be categorized as an *addition* or a *modification* to the developed innovation. In the case of an addition, the instance (e.g., activity, material, or facility) would not fall within the activities, materials, facilities, etc., defined by any of the existing fidelity components. For example, a teacher implementing the HOSTS reading program required the students to line up before leaving the classroom at the end of the period. The teacher then queried each student in turn with an individualized question designed to provide positive feedback at the end of the session. This was clearly an additional program component created by this teacher.

An instance of reinvention that was categorized as a modification would fall within the realm of activities defined by an existing fidelity component but outside the bounds defined by prescribed variations. For example, the Community Arbitration Project required the victims of youth crimes to attend hearings and make their own suggestions concerning the hearing outcomes. One program that did not require the victim to be present at the hearing did require a written statement from the victim concerning hearing outcomes. This represented a modification of an existing program component. In other words, modification implied that the local site had implemented the activity, material, or facility required by the innovation, but had done so in a novel way. This dimension deals with the substance of the change by assessing what is changed within or outside the realm of existing components.

As noted above, magnitude represents a simple quantification of the degree of departure from fidelity. A large number of the instances of reinvention identified were relatively insignificant departures from the original model. We wanted to distinguish these from more substantial deviations. A three-point rating scale (i.e., minor, moderate, and substantial levels of degree of departure) was devised to measure the extent of reinvention reflected by each reinvention instance. These judgments were based on the importance and amount of the change to the developer's program model. Thus, the addition score was the sum of all "degree of departure" weighted instances that were judged to be additions.

To assess intercoder reliability, each instance was classified as "reinvention" or "not reinvention" by each pair of site visit staff, independently. All codings were compared to check reliability. For judgments that classified an instance as reinvention or not reinvention, the percentage agreement between pairs was .80 across all instances. In cases of disagreement, a consensus decision was reached and used as the final data point. A similar strategy was used to assess the reliability of addition–modification judgments, for which agreement rates were .82. Agreement figures for magnitude judgments were .80.

Effectiveness

Each of the seven innovation developers was required to submit evaluation results to the NDN or EPP prior to acceptance for dissemination activities. Most of the programs we visited (65 of 70) had effectiveness data available that included several outcome variables. These same variables served as the basis for effectiveness evaluations in the current research effort. Examples included recidivism data for the Prerelease Center and Community Arbitration Project, standardized reading scores and grade equivalents for the HOSTS program, several juror usage indices for the One Day/One Trial jury management program, and burglary rates for Crime Prevention Programs.

The quality, format, and type of outcome effectiveness data varied somewhat, both between and within programs. Consequently, a procedure of rank ordering sites within innovation on relevant effectiveness criteria was employed. For each innovation, the ranks could potentially range from 1 to 10 (one rank berth per visited site), based on staff judgments from archival data (e.g., reports, records, personnel files) that best matched the developer's validation measures (e.g., reading scores). The timing of fidelity and outcome measurement was, in most cases, contiguous. Two pairs of independent research staff rankings of the 65 sites with useful effectiveness data were then correlated to estimate the reliability of the ranking procedure. An overall rank-order correlation of .90 (Spearman rho, with Spearman-Brown correction for two sets of raters) was obtained, indicating that the procedure was reliable.

RESULTS

The first research issue addressed was the extent to which programs disseminated through the modified RD&D model were implemented with acceptable degrees of fidelity. Figure 1 presents the mean fidelity scores for each of the disseminated programs. Recall that fidelity components were scored as ideal, acceptable, or unacceptable. All seven scores fell within the acceptable range; four actually exceeded scores of 1 (= acceptable).

Despite the fact that program differences were noted ($F(6, 63) = 11.45$, $p < .001$, $W^2 = .47$), programs with the lowest mean fidelity scores were implemented within developer-defined levels of acceptability. Given the conservative nature of the fidelity measure, it appears that all innovations were disseminated with a respectable degree of fidelity.

The second research issue involved the association between program fidelity and effectiveness. Prior to conducting analyses across programs, the fidelity and effectiveness scores were standardized. The Pearson correlation between fidelity and effectiveness was .38 ($p < .01$; $r = .44$ when corrected for attenuation).

The third research issue surrounded the relative importance of fidelity and reinvention in producing effective replicates of disseminated social programs. As noted above, the correlation between fidelity and effectiveness was .38 ($p < .01$). The correlation between reinvention and effectiveness was .33 ($p < .05$). At first glance, the data suggested that fidelity was no more critical in producing effective replicates than was reinvention.

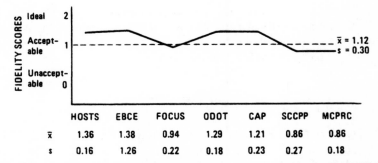

Figure 1. Across-site means of average item fidelity scores. HOSTS, help one student to succeed; EBCE, experience-based career education; FOCUS, program for disaffected school youth; ODOT, one day/one trial jury management program; CAP, community arbitration project; SCCPP, Seattle community crime prevention project; MCPRC, Montgomery County prerelease center.

However, holding reinvention constant did not substantively affect the correlation between fidelity and effectiveness ($r = .26, p < .05$). The partial correlation between fidelity and effectiveness was essentially of the same magnitude as the zero-order correlation. On the other hand, when the effect of fidelity was held constant, the relationship between reinvention and effectiveness was not significantly different from zero ($r = .17$, ns). In other words, fidelity appeared to be operating as a moderator variable in the reinvention–effectiveness relationship.

A second set of partial correlational analyses shed additional light on the reinvention–effectiveness relationship by looking directly at the reinvention subindices of addition and modification. These findings suggested that additions contributed to the effectiveness of programs whereas modifications did not. The partial correlation between addition and effectiveness while holding modification constant was .38 ($p < .01$). The partial correlation between modification and effectiveness while holding addition constant was $- .09$ (ns).

In order to truly determine the unique contribution of additive components of reinvention to the effectiveness of replicates of model programs, a third partial correlation between addition and effectiveness while holding fidelity constant was computed. The result ($r = .26, p < .02$) indicated that additions to the program replicate did contribute to the effectiveness of the implementation. Instances of modification, when controlling for shared variance with fidelity, were not related to greater program effectiveness ($r = - .01$, ns).

These analyses suggested that additions were positive in character and contributed to overall effectiveness. Thus, the broad picture that emerged suggested that effective programs tended to exhibit higher fidelity and tended to augment critical program model components with additional components that were related to positive outcomes. Instances of modification appeared to be unrelated to effectiveness.

DISCUSSION

The work of Gene Hall and his associates (e.g., Hall & Loucks, 1978) led to a method of identifying and measuring specific innovation components. These methods were utilized within the current research effort and found to be extremely useful in the identification and monitoring of implementation components at adopting organizations. This process led to a quantification of site-specific fidelity assessment across both programs and sites.

Reinvention was defined such that it could occur simultaneously with fidelity; that is, both could be observed and quantified at the same site. This measurement scheme allowed added insight concerning the fidelity–adaptation debate prominent in the literature because it was possible to identify and quantify different types of reinvention.

In addition, a methodology was developed to gather and quantify effectiveness data in a manner that allowed direct comparisons across innovations. Considerable variability existed in both the quantity and quality of outcome data. However, through the construction of outcome data grids and a rank-ordering process, reliable ranks were computed that were directly comparable across innovation types. Although some precision was lost in the move from interval or ratio data to ordinal data, the compatibility of outcome rankings across diverse program content areas provided an invaluable ability to generalize beyond a single innovation type (Tornatzky & Klein, 1982).

Because they indicated generally high levels of fidelity at adopting sites, these results contrast with much of the recent literature that suggests that it is generally impossible, dangerous, or foolhardy to promote high-fidelity implementations at adopting sites (e.g., Farrar *et al.*, 1979). However, considerable across-program variation was observed. Therefore, these results do not warrant the institution of efforts to ensure that all adopters implement programs with high fidelity. Variability in fidelity scores, both among and within innovation types, was apparently linked not only to characteristics of the innovation but also to the proactive, fidelity-linked perspective of the innovation developer exhibited during the dissemination process (e.g., HOSTS vs. FOCUS or MCPRC, see Figure 1), and to the characteristics of the adopting organizations (e.g., local constraints imposed on implementation). But these findings do suggest that a blanket move toward a decentralized RD&D policy, indicative of current federal policy and based on the belief that good replication is not possible, is also short-sighted.

To some extent, fidelity did contribute to the effectiveness of the innovative programs. Although neither the authors nor the program developers would argue that the seven innovations studied were beyond improvement, local reinvention tended to contribute to the effectiveness of a program only when the reinvention took the form of additions to the model. That is, local improvements that took the form of expansion tended to improve local effectiveness. Reinvention that modified existing program components was not related to the effectiveness of the program. Again, this finding should not be interpreted as an indication that components could not be improved on. Rather, it appears that the greater the number of modifications present, the greater the likelihood that key components linked to effectiveness were changed. In short, fidelity and additions to the model were positively related to local effectiveness whereas modification of developer-defined program components was at best unrelated to effective local implementations.

These results lend considerable support to the use of the modified RD&D model of dissemination. However, they must be interpreted within the context of the study. The key fact is that the programs studied here were relatively well-specified innovations. Relatively complex, all-encompassing, well-specified innovations are very amenable to dissemination through the modified RD&D model. With less well-specified programs, such a proactive dissemination effort is less likely to produce high-fidelity implementations. Consequently, generalization to dissemination efforts involving broad-based, less well-specified innovations should not be attempted. Given the earlier comments concerning the Berman and McLaughlin research (1978), there is no contradiction between their results and ours. Rather, the contradiction lies in the interpretation of their findings (e.g., Datta, 1981) in light of these results. The lack of specificity in the program models they studied and the measures they used probably account for the different findings. Hollisfield and Slavin (1983) labeled this problem specification failure. In fact, both sets of results, when considered together, support Berman's more recent proposal of a contingency model of implementation (Berman, 1980). Highly specified innovations may require fidelity-supportive approaches, whereas broad policy innovations imply the use of decentralized strategies.

Another major implication of these findings for future research is that community psychologists involved in the development of applied programs should determine which program components are actually empirically linked to effectiveness at the developer sites. With this additional information in hand, those involved in dissemination efforts, as well as potential adopters, can more directly determine the feasibility of producing effective replicates, and also determine the boundaries of the "zone of drastic mutation."

Finally, these findings support Fairweather's Experimental Social Innovation (ESI) model of the community psychologist's role in the development of social programs (Fairweather, 1967). The final steps of the ESI model call for an active role in the dissemination of a successfully validated innovation. These findings suggest that the developer should be obligated to determine the core components that are directly linked to program effectiveness and actively seek high-fidelity implementations of those specific components.

ACKNOWLEDGMENTS

This work was completed under a grant from the National Science Foundation #ISI-7920576-01. The opinions represent the views of the authors and do not necessarily reflect the position of the National Science Foundation.

REFERENCES

Berman, P. (1980). Thinking about programmed and adaptive implementation: Matching strategies to situations. In H. M. Ingram & D. E. Mann (Eds.), *Why policies succeed or fail* (pp. 205–227). Beverly Hills: Sage.

Berman, P. (1981). Educational change: An implementation paradigm. In R. Lehming & M. Kane (Eds.), *Improving schools: Using what we know* (pp. 253–286). Beverly Hills: Sage.

Berman, P. & McLaughlin, M. W. (1977). *Federal programs supporting educational change: Vol. 7. Factors affecting implementation and continuation* (Contract No. R-1589/7). Washington, DC: U.S. Office of Education.

Berman, P. & McLaughlin, M. W. (1978). *Federal programs supporting educational change: Vol. 8. Implementation and sustaining innovations* (Contract No. R-1589/8). Washington, DC: U.S. Office of Education.

Boruch, R. R. & Gomez, H. (1977). Sensitivity, bias, and theory in impact evaluation. *Professional Psychology, 8*(4), 411–433.

Calsyn, R., Tornatzky, L. G., & Dittmar, S. (1977). Incomplete adoption of an innovation: The case of goal attainment scaling. *Evaluation, 4,* 128–130.

Cowen, E. L., Gardner, E. A., & Zax, M. (1967). *Emergent approaches to mental health problems.* New York: Appleton Century Crofts.

Datta, L. E. (1981). Damn the experts and full speed ahead: An examination of the study of federal programs supporting educational change, as evidence against directed development for local problem-solving. *Evaluation Review, 5*(1), 5–32.

Eveland, J. D., Rogers, E., & Klepper, C. (1977). *The innovation process in public organizations: Some elements of a preliminary model.* Springfield, VA: NTIS.

Fairweather, G. W. (1967). *Methods for experimental social innovation.* New York: Wiley.

Fairweather, G. W. & Tornatzky, L. G. (1977). *Experimental methods for social policy research.* New York: Pergamon.

Fairweather, G. W., Tornatzky, L. G., Fergus, E., & Avellar, J. (1982). *Innovation and social process*. New York: Pergamon.

Farrar, E., deSanctis, J. E., & Cohen, D. K. (1979). *Views from below: Implementation research in education*. Cambridge, MA: Huron Institute.

Fullan, M. & Pomfret, A. (1977). Research on curriculum and instruction implementation. *Review of Educational Research, 47*(2), 335–397.

Hall, G. E. & Loucks, S. F. (1978, March). *Innovation configurations: Analyzing the adaptation of innovations*. Paper presented at the annual meeting of the American Educational Research Association, Toronto, Ontario, Canada.

Havelock, R. G. (1969). *Planning for innovation through dissemination and utilization of knowledge*. Ann Arbor, MI: Institute for Social Research.

Heck, S., Steigelbauer, S., Hall, G. E., & Loucks, S. F. (1981). *Measuring innovation configurations: Procedures and applications*. Austin: Research and Development Center for Teacher Education, University of Texas.

Heller, K., Price, R., Reinharz, S., Riger, S., & Wandersman, A. (1984). *Psychology and community change* (2nd ed.). New York: Dorsey Press.

Hollisfield, J. H. & Slavin, R. E. (1983). Disseminating student team learning through federally funded programs. *Knowledge: Creation, Diffusion, Utilization, 4*, 576–589.

House, E. R. (1981). Three perspectives on innovation: Technological, political, and cultural. In R. Lehming & M. Kane (Eds.), *Improving schools: Using what we know* (pp. 17–41). Beverly Hills: Sage.

House, E. R. (1975). *The politics of educational innovation*. Berkeley, CA: McCutchan.

Rappaport, J. (1977). *Community psychology: Values, issues & action*. New York: Holt, Rinehart & Winston.

Rappaport, J., Seidman, E., & Davidson, W. S. II. (1979). Demonstration research and manifest versus true adoption: The natural history of a research project to divert adolescents from the legal system. In R. S. Muñoz, L. R. Snowden, J. G. Kelly, and Associates. *Social and psychological research in community settings*. San Francisco: Jossey Bass, Inc. (pp. 101–144).

Rice, R. E. & Rogers, E. M. (1979). Reinvention in the innovation process. *Knowledge: Creation, Diffusion, Utilization, 1*, 499–514.

Rogers, E. M. (1978). Reinvention during the innovation process. In M. Radnor *et al.* (Eds.), *The diffusion of innovations: An assessment* (Contract No. PRA-7680388). Washington, DC: National Science Foundation.

Tornatzky, L. G., Fergus, E. O., Avellar, J. W., Fairweather, G. W., & Fleischer, M. (1981). *Innovation and social process: A national experiment in implementing social technology*. New York: Pergamon.

Tornatzky, L. G. & Klein, K. J. (1982). Innovation characteristics and innovation adoption-implementation: A meta-analysis of findings. *IEEE Transactions on Engineering Management, 29*, 28–45.

11

Back to the Future, Community Psychology: Unfolding a Theory of Social Intervention*

Edward Seidman

Join me in my flux capacitor; it makes time travel possible. Let's go back just over two decades. Date: May 4–8, 1965; Place: Swampscott, Massachusetts; Event: the Conference on Education of Psychologists for Community Mental Health.

What happened there? Quoting directly from the conference proceedings,

> A deep stirring and metamorphosis was seen as being in process. The conference participants, while holding diverse views on how to interpret these changes, decided to expand the conference mandate and move toward the conception of a new field tentatively labeled "Community Psychology." (Bennett *et al.*, 1966, p. 4)

The diverse views that were noted at the conference have continued throughout the short history of Community Psychology and serve as a sign of the discipline's ultimate vitality. For too many, the deep stirrings have become quiescent. But, I sense the reemergence of these stirrings on a larger scale. For those of you who attended the First Biennial Conference on Community Research and Action this spring, for those of you who heard or read Rappaport's (1987) call for theory last year, these stirrings will be obvious.

*Presidential address presented to the Division of Community Psychology at the annual convention of the American Psychological Association in New York, NY, August 30, 1987. Originally published in the *American Journal of Community Psychology*, *16*(1) (1988): 3–24.

A Quarter Century of Community Psychology: Readings from the American Journal of Community Psychology, edited by Tracey A. Revenson *et al.* Kluwer Academic/Plenum Publishers, New York, 2002.

As we travel backward and forward in time, I use the past to illustrate that the call for an action-oriented discipline has existed for some time. More importantly, I highlight ideas from the past that provide the rudiments of a theory of social intervention and change. Finally, I endeavor to develop each of these ideas, link them, and unfold them as an initial statement of a theory of social intervention and change unique to Community Psychology. Hopefully, the unfolding of such a theory can set us upon a different trajectory.

The delineation of a focal construct or phenomenon of interest is an essential first step in this process; it is essential to drive theory, action, and research. But prior to enumerating what the focal construct should be, I want to address our continuing ambivalence about action as a profession and science. In short, I see this continuing ambivalence about being an action science as a perpetual stumbling block. We must take a position if we are to grow as a field or contribute to human and social betterment, even at the cost of reducing our diversity.

THE AMBIVALENCE TOWARD THE CONJUNCTION OF SCIENCE AND ACTION

At the Swampscott conference, participants

> described current activities as helping school administrators to restructure the communication patterns within their school systems so as to ease the transition to junior high school for elementary school children; advising the administrators of cooperative housing projects on the design and evaluation of the governmental and social structures which tenants in such structures evolve; advising governors of states and legislative committees on a wide range of public policy decisions; and in some instances taking the initiative toward starting new public programs. (Bennett *et al.*, 1966, pp. 4–5)

As one can tell, the conference participants discussed many innovative and exciting intervention endeavors. Many at the Swampscott conference argued for what Argyris, Putnam, and Smith (1985) have since labeled "action science." Action science is interested in research that generates and tests propositions concerning both the variables embedded in the status quo and variables involved in changing the status quo. Action science challenges the status quo; basic and applied sciences do not.

Despite the Swampscott participants' activities and agenda, they remained ambivalent about the role of action. Some felt action was not a legitimate part of our professional role, that it was unscientific to engage in

such interventions as a community psychologist! For some of you – I suspect many of you – this ambivalence remains.

It is precisely in the role of an action science that Community psychology's uniqueness can be realized. Herein lies our potential contributions to
both social change and social science. In my judgment, we must put this
ambivalence behind us once and for all, or we will fail to bring to fruition
our own distinct and mature identity.

Let us reenter the flux capacitor and travel back another three decades
to the 1940s, where we can witness the creation of SPSSI – the Society for the
Psychological Study of Social Issues. It was born during an earlier period of
social turmoil. Then and now, SPSSI shares a common set of social values and
concerns with Community Psychology. (In fact, many of us belong to both
divisions.) Though many would argue vociferously with me, as I see it, SPSSI's
resolution of the ambivalence toward action, for the most part, has been to
observe and describe from the sidelines, despite their intellectual allegiance
to Kurt Lewin. Lewin (1947/1951), too, had mapped the outlines of an action
science, 20 years before Swampscott. Ambivalence over the scientific legitimacy of direct action has constrained the activities and contributions of
many of Lewin's descendants, as well as SPSSI as an organization.

During the 1940s and the two previous decades, John Dewey (1946)
also articulated an action science in the public interest.

> The very foundation of the democratic procedure is dependence upon
> experimental production of social change; and experimentation directed
> by working principles that are tested and developed in the very process of
> being tried out in action. (p. 157)

Thus, both Dewey and Lewin, with well-formulated arguments, called for
the development of action science several decades before the historic
Swampscott meeting. During the short history of Community Psychology,
Fairweather (1972), through his model of experimental social innovation,
has also consistently advocated for a science of action. Nevertheless, on a
larger scale, the practice of Community Psychology has remained ambivalent with regard to the conjunction of science and action. I often wonder
what the present would be like if the founders of Community Psychology
had succeeded in decisively resolving this ambivalence in favor of an action
science.

To this point, my intent has been twofold: to demonstrate the existence
of the ambivalence toward the integration of science and action despite the
voices of strong intellectual figures of the past, and simultaneously to highlight its importance for our future. The challenge is to put this ambivalence
behind us, to further develop the historical legacy of Dewey and Lewin, and
to develop Community Psychology as a genuine action science.

CENTRALITY OF THEORY AND A PHENOMENON OF INTEREST

Dewey, Lewin, and others have made the case for theory as vital to the development of both action and science. If, we are – or hope to become – an action science, we must have a theory of action, or more accurately, a theory of social intervention and change.

Join me once again in the flux capacitor as we catapult forward to the very recent past. Just 1 year ago, Julian Rappaport (1987) underscored the critical need for the development of a theory and an orienting phenomenon of interest for Community Psychology. In his Distinguished Contribution address he argued,

> The point of a theory is, among other things, to explain, predict, create, stimulate, and encourage understanding of certain phenomena of interest. If a theory is not about the phenomena of interest it is useless in guiding the scientist's work. (p. 123)

Twenty years earlier, at the Swampscott conference, Jack Glidewell (1966) also discussed the centrality of a phenomenon of interest in his keynote address. He said:

> I have come to accept the notion that it is quite clearly possible to specify the particular phenomena of interest... I have also come to accept the notion that it is quite clearly difficult to be clear and simple and precise in constructing such a specification. It seems to me, however, that we must, for our own self-respect, keep trying to accomplish this difficult job. (p. 33)

Our professional and scientific ambivalence about the rightful place of action has inhibited our development of a theory of social intervention and change. "Unless, however, one can develop some means of adequately describing the structure of a system, one can hardly turn to what is perhaps a more fascinating problem of describing structural change in that system" (Laumann & Pappi, 1976, p. 5). I find it difficult to imagine the long-term future of the discipline of Community Psychology without such theoretical development.[1] Furthermore, as both Glidewell (1966) and Rappaport (1987) have suggested – 20 years apart – a theory's underlying phenomena

---

[1] It should be noted that Murrell (1973), Trickett, Kelly, and their colleagues (e.g., Trickett, Kelly, & Todd, 1972), Rappaport (1977, 1987), and Heller and Monahan (1977) have endeavored to provide a theoretical foundation for Community Psychology. These undertakings have and continue to serve the discipline well; individually and collectively, these theoretical statements have important and useful implications for action. In this paper, however, I wish to move these theoretical advances a step further, toward an avowed, and more prescriptive, theory of action.

of interest must be specified. It is this difficult task that I attempt to tackle in the remainder of this paper.

During the last two decades several concepts have been offered as *the* phenomenon of interest, orienting or focal construct for Community Psychology. These include the psychological sense of community (Sarason, 1974), social competence (Spivak & Shure, 1974), psychological wellness (Cowen, 2000), the competent community (Iscoe, 1974), prevention (Felner, Jason, Moritsugu, & Farber, 1983), and empowerment (Rappaport, 1981, 1987). Each of these constructs has utility for Community Psychology, though several remain trapped in an individual and asocial mindscape (Maruyama, 1983; Sarason, 1981; Seidman, 1978; Seidman & Rappaport, 1986). Even those constructs that have the potential to move beyond an individual level of analysis, particularly the constructs of prevention and empowerment, do not provide us sufficient direction in how to choose targets of intervention. Nor do they suggest how we might accomplish such changes. If there is to be an over-arching phenomenon of interest for an action science of Community Psychology, it must, at a minimum, steer us to look in the appropriate place and, as a result, suggest specific strategies and tactics of intervention.

Too often our unit of analysis and target of intervention continue to be the individual or an aggregate of individuals, frequently in the guise of a systems-oriented intervention (Seidman, 1987). At the same time, our rhetoric expresses the notion that we do not wish to do "more of the same" – that is, make things function more efficiently without any fundamental alterations of the status quo. We wish to go beyond first-order change (Watzlawick, Weakland, & Fisch, 1974). Yet, we talk, myself included, about second-order change without a precise description of what is to be changed or how to change it. As you will recall from Argyris *et al.*'s (1985) criteria for an action science described earlier, the status quo may be the crux of our search for the phenomenon of interest. Thus, what is to be changed – the status quo – must become the phenomenon of interest.

SOCIAL REGULARITIES

The initial steps in constructing any theory[2] are to (a) define the construct or phenomenon of interest – in this case, social regularities;

---

[2]Space limitations preclude me from unfolding a complete theory. Only the key concepts, processes, and issues pertinent to social intervention and change are highlighted. These ideas are more fully embedded in the extensive body of ecological, transactional, and general systems' theories.

(b) specify its monological network; and (c) suggest possible ways to operationalize it.

In searching to define our focal construct of social regularities, we begin our journey by returning once again to Swampscott. Here, we find our founders defining the field by discussing the centrality of assessing and modifying "the reciprocal relationships between individuals and the social systems with which they interact" (Bennett *et al.*, 1966, p. 7). What emerges from this definition is much more than a simple focus on community or individual variables, or on individuals in context. It is the reciprocal relationships and interdependencies between individuals and social systems that represent a unique and emergent synthesis of community and psychology.

Similarly, ecology, which most of us consider the theoretical underpinning of Community Psychology, is defined as the relationship between the organism and its environment. Again, the key is the relational dimension, and for a social ecology, social relations. Once again, a focus on the emergent patterns of social relations is quite similar to what Dewey and Bentley described in 1949 as the transactional viewpoint. In the *Handbook of Environmental Psychology*, Altman and Rogoff (1987) have provided an excellent discussion of transactional approaches: "Transactional approaches begin with the phenomenon – a confluence of psychological processes, environmental qualities, and temporal features – and employ all necessary principles and combination of principles, including emergent ones, to account for it" (p. 28). Although selected operationalizations of this emergent construct of social relations, viewed temporally, have been investigated occasionally, it has not been fully developed as a construct. Moreover, it has not been seen as the central phenomenon of interest to guide the action, theory, and research of Community Psychology. It is in these respects that I believe this temporally oriented social relations construct – social regularities – has a great deal of promise for the future development of the discipline.

Return with me to 1947 and listen to Kurt Lewin:

> structural properties of a dynamic whole are different from the structural properties of subparts .... Structural properties are characterized by *relations* between parts or elements themselves ... throughout the history of mathematics and physics problems of constancy of relations rather than of constancy of elements have gained importance and have gradually changed the picture of what is essential. The social sciences seem to show a very similar development. (1947/1951, p. 192)

From my knowledge, the social sciences, and more specifically, the study of social intervention and change, have yet to incorporate this development – studying constancy of relations – in any significant fashion into practice or the corpus of knowledge. Floyd Allport (1962) offered a similar perspective:

> Wholeness, or totalities, must be sought not in "things" or "agents"....
> instead, in...structures of ongoings and events. Actually, we live in and
> through *structuring* at all levels; and it behooves us to try to understand its
> general forms and laws.... Causation, in the structural view, is not histori-
> cal nor linear, but continuous, time independent, and reciprocally cyclical.
> One looks for it neither in society *nor* in the individual...but in the com-
> pounded patterns of structuring which are the essential reality underlying
> both. (pp. 18–19)

These perspectives from social psychology are consistent with much of Gregory Bateson's writing (1972, 1979). Bateson enabled us to see that meaning is carried not by "entities" or "things" (parts or elements in Lewin's terms), but by the "connections that unite" the entities or elements – what he referred to as the "relata" or patterns of relations. At this point Bateson's abstractness, compounded with my own proclivity toward obtuseness, must be mind boggling. An illustration is necessary.

In Bateson's terminology, a person or an attribute of a person is an entity or thing. Two elements could be a teacher and her pupils, to use a well-known example of Seymour Sarason's (1982). What Lewin, Allport, Bateson, and Sarason are all suggesting is that by simply studying attributes of the students or attributes of the teacher we learn very little that helps us to understand the behavior or phenomenology of either party in the context of the classroom. Instead, observing the frequency and pattern of behavior or communication between the two over time suggests not only potentially important social regularities but carries meaning about self and other, at least in context, for both parties. More specifically, the fact that teachers ask the overwhelming majority of questions – often, questions of a simple "spit back the facts" nature – while students ask hardly any questions allows us to understand an important social regularity about the classroom. Furthermore, this regularity may very well suggest to the pupils that school is not enjoyable, that they cannot think for themselves, that teachers know everything, and so forth. At the same time, it may suggest or reinforce prior beliefs of the teachers that students are not motivated, that they need to be spoon-fed (thus, "blaming the victim"), or that teaching is a chore. Thus, this social regularity is a key to understanding a great deal about the ecology and meaning of classroom behavior and the behavior of classroom participants. Any information about the pupils or teacher alone, without its connection or linkage to the context (and here students and teachers represent an important element of each others' context), provides only a minimal under-standing and even fewer hints on how to alter the situation.

I refer to these patterns of social relations, connections, or linkages as social regularities; they are the phenomena of interest in a theory of social intervention. Yes, social regularities bear a striking resemblance to the concepts of programmatic and behavioral regularities introduced by Seymour Sarason in *The Culture of the School and the Problem of Change* (1971, 1982). However, the construct of social regularities – as I am using it – is both encompassing of behavioral and programmatic regularities and more specific. It is more specific because it is restricted to regularities that are directly or indirectly social; it is these social interdependencies that link community and psychology, environment and individual.

Social regularities are defined jointly by the ideas of social relations and temporal patterning. Social relations can be represented by differences and ratios along one or more substantive dimensions.[3] Differences occur *between* social units – groups, populations, or organizational entities; ratios represent a group or population in relation to a larger organizational unit. More specifically, these social units might include men vs. women, ethnic groups, age groups, the "haves" vs. the "have nots," management vs. the rank and file, patients vs. service delivery personnel, and complex combinations of these.

The social interdependencies may center on clear-cut social relations, such as power, roles, status, participation, and communication, or on resources that are indirectly social, such as income, services, education, health, well-being, and leisure. As previously illustrated, the difference between the number of questions asked by students versus teachers is a social regularity. In schools with large student bodies, there are fewer roles or niches available for each student; this is a ratio indexing a social regularity.

Temporal patterning refers to the form of the difference or ratio over time. Bateson (1979) believes that is precisely this patterning through time that carries meaning: "To produce news of difference, i.e., *information*, there must be two entities (real or imagined) such that the difference between them can be immanent in their mutual relationship" (p. 76). Critical social regularities are indexed by patterns of constancy in relations or, in quantitative terms, when the temporal variability of the pattern is low and/or its cycles essentially repeat themselves. Returning to the classroom example, if the balance of questions asked by teacher and students remains similar from day to day, a social regularity is suggested. This social regularity not only communicates and symbolizes information and meaning to the school's inhabitants but suggests a potential target of intervention.

---

[3]Linney (1986) has made one of the few innovative efforts to operationalize and statistically analyze the construct of social regularities in an evaluation of a court-ordered desegregation plan.

The construct of social regularity is essentially equivalent to concepts that are derived primarily from General Systems' Theory (see, for example, Buckley, 1968); these include the status quo, bias, calibration, setting, home-ostasis, equilibrium, or perhaps more appropriately, quasi-stationary equi-librium (as defined by Lewin, 1947/1951), "rule of the game" or first-order change (Watzlawick *et al.*, 1974), and functional outcome. A prelude, or at the least a corollary, to intervention is the identification of the critical social regularities. How beneficial or negative the effects of these regularities are is a separate question; this question is value-driven and includes aspects that are concerned with asking for whom, for what purposes, and when?

By traveling backward through time, we can find early examples of operationally defined social regularities. Returning once again to 1947, we find Kurt Lewin writing about racial discrimination. He defined the degree of discrimination as the:

> number of refusals and permissions, orderings and yieldings, which indi-
> cate open and closed possibilities for various individuals in their daily liv-
> ing.... We are dealing with a process, which like a river, continuously
> changes its elements even if its velocity and direction remain the same.
> (1947/1951, p. 202)

Around the time of Community Psychology's beginnings, Barker (1968), a student of Lewin, developed an intriguing operationalization of a social regularity: the concept of manning. It should more appropriately be referred to as personning. This operationalization describes an important social regularity for the field of Community Psychology. It refers to the ratio of available roles for the settings' inhabitants. Recall the illustration I alluded to previously concerning students in large schools. Any setting has a finite number of roles, and if there are a large number of students in a school, we have an overpersonned setting, where students find fewer roles and niches from which to derive meaning and satisfaction, and the setting often fails to meet its avowed goals.

Traveling forward to the present, we find the field of Community Psychology steeped in social network research. As used by some investiga-tors, social networks assess the nature and form of social connections; in this way, social network measures too can serve as profitable operational-izations of a social regularity. An example of a social regularity, from a larger societal perspective, is the pattern and distribution of income between the haves and have nots. If one looks at the percentage of income of the wealthiest 5% of the population one finds that they earn over 19% of all income in this country, while the lowest 20% earn a minuscule 3.8% of all income (U.S. Bureau of the Census, 1986). Furthermore, examining these data annually for the last 20 years one finds very little change in these proportions. Hence the maxim: The more things seem to change, the more they stay the same. The inequities of our economic system continue unabated, despite policies and rhetoric to the contrary. As a social regularity this pattern of inequity conveys a great deal of meaning to the have nots, and is not incidentally related to their higher rates of psychosocial dysfunction (see, for example, Seidman & Rapkin, 1983). Moreover, it represents a social regularity of our society that should become a central focus for intervention and change.

In traveling backward through time, we have been able to identify the kernels of the construct of social regularities in the writings of our predecessors. The trip has enabled us to see that a phenomenon of social regularity is crucial for a Community Psychology that aspires to be an action science. Greater articulation of its nomological net is needed before it has maximum utility (though these "waters" may be loaded with hidden mines, as construct validation has been an activity directed primarily toward static constructs). Nevertheless, its existence can guide both our future interventions and evaluations of their impact.

UNIT OF ANALYSIS

Where and how does the construct of social regularity interface with level or unit of analysis? Notions regarding level of analysis have been central to the concerns of Community Psychology (see, for example, Rappaport, 1977). In order to fully address the interface of social regularity and level of analysis, I present a modified version of a levels of analysis schema that I recently described (Seidman, 1987). Table 1 presents a framework for understanding social intervention and change at each of four levels of analysis: individual, population, setting, and mesosystem.

Individual

There is no need for an elaborate explanation for the individual as the unit of analysis. When we conceptualize the individual as the unit of analysis, we are referring to the person or a psychological attribute of the person, such as intelligence, locus of control, or adjustment. For most of Community Psychology's short history our interventions and research questions have rested primarily at this level, under the rubric of secondary prevention. This is our legacy from Clinical Psychology.

In Bateson's framework the nature of an individual focus is entity- or thing-oriented. Individuals are seen as having agency and capable of altering

Table 1. Framework for Understanding Social Intervention and Change

| Unit of analysis | Epistemological underpinnings | | | |
	Nature of phenomenon	Causal assumptions	Disciplinary legacy	Processes of system change
Individual	Element, part, or attribute	Unidirectional and linear	Clinical psychology	—
Population	Aggregate of, elements parts, or attributes	Unidirectional and linear	Public health and epidemiology	Tuning Incremental
Setting	Relational (within setting)	Transactional and recursive	Community psychology	Restructuring
Mesosystem	Relational (between settings)	Transactional and recursive	Community psychology	Restructuring

themselves or external circumstances in a unidirectional causal fashion. The premise of individualism is a Western mindscape that has been with us for a long time and severely restricts our vision (Seidman & Rappaport, 1986). Yet, it is the most traditional level of analysis for psychology and, I suspect, the one with which we are still most comfortable.

Population

When we consider population as the unit of analysis, we are simply referring to an aggregate of individuals not united by any particular relationship or shared set of goals. What they have in common is a demographic attribute (e.g., gender, race, age), an event or experience (e.g., job loss, physical disability), or a setting that they inhabit (e.g., school, hospital, jail). We have seen an increasing number of interventions that are population-based rather than individual-focused: for example, classroom-based interpersonal problem solving and social skills training interventions. Although population-centered interventions represent a welcome and positive step in the scope of potential effects, they remain functionally identical to an individual-level approach, in that they are also entity-centered and based on assumptions of linear causality. Population-level interventions are our legacy from Public Health and Epidemiology.

Both the individual and population levels of analysis fail to come to grips with a transactional-ecological model, either practically or with regard to their underlying epistemological assumptions, that is, being entity-centered and assuming linear causality. In fact, it is futile to look within either of these levels to identify social regularities; they emerge only when we look *between* elements for a contextual understanding.

Setting

Social regularities are an emergent construct at both the setting and mesosystem levels. Both levels of analysis focus on Bateson's notion of relata or the pattern and structure of social relations. Both setting and mesosystem levels of analysis implicitly assume a recursive model of causality concerned with mutuality of influence.

A setting, in part paraphrasing and in part modifying Sarason's (1972) definition, is two or more sets of people in a relationship over a sustained period of time in order to achieve certain goals. Each set of people consti-tutes a group by virtue of one or more common characteristics (e.g., demo-graphic, role, or status). The relationship, shared goals, and continuity define setting as the unit of analysis and differentiate it from the individual and population levels. Collectively, these three criteria – relationship, shared goals, and continuity – describe temporal social interdependencies and thus help to define the setting's social regularities or rules of the game. My use of the concept of setting is similar to Bronfenbrenner's (1979) notion of microsystems or Berger and Neuhaus's (1977) term "mediating structures." It differs from Barker's (1968) definition of behavior settings in that it is not time- or place-bound. Examples of settings include peer net-works, the workplace, school, and religious, neighborhood, and voluntary organizations. The goal of setting interventions is to alter the *within-setting* social regularities.

Early in the history of Community Psychology, there were a number of interventions aimed at altering a setting's fundamental social regularity, though they were not conceptualized in precisely this manner. In retro-spect, two of these endeavors stand out as classic exemplars of an action sci-ence built upon social regularities. One is Fairweather, Sanders, Cressler, and Maynard's (1969) creation of a "community lodge" for long-term chronically ill mental patients. The other is Ira Goldenberg's (1971) cre-ation of an innovatively organized Residential Youth Center (RYC) for "hard core" delinquent youth. For the sake of brevity, I describe briefly Goldenberg's RYC.

The RYC was created as an alternative to traditional prison-like set-tings for delinquent youth where the social organization was (and is) verti-cal in nature. That is, the staff made all the decisions (and there was even an elaborate hierarchy among the staff) and the youth were obligated to com-ply. This rigid and unchanging organizational structure was seen as the fun-damental, and problematic, social regularity. The social regularity of this and similarly organized "treatment" settings communicates meaning to both staff and residents, not only about their current status but also about their future psychological capabilities and social prospects. This bleak picture for residents is validated most often by their repeated recidivism. Thus, Goldenberg developed an alternative setting based on a horizontal organizational structure – one in which residents and staff engaged in collaborative decision making. For example, all setting inhabitants, regardless of their official job, status, or educational background, performed all roles in the setting (e.g., cook, accountant, case worker). In sum, a new setting was created with a fundamentally antithetical social regularity.

Stepping off our flux capacitor into the 1980s, we discover two other exemplary setting-level interventions in which changing the social regularities are foremost in accounting for their success. The first was developed by Felner, Ginter, and Primavera (1982) to smooth the turbulence of the transition to high school. The academic and psychosocial functioning of many adolescents deteriorate as they enter high school. Putting Sarason's writings (1971) into action, Felner and his colleagues observed that one social regularity is the abrupt change in social networks that occurs within the school setting at the time of the transition to high school. Both in-school peer networks as well as ties to teachers and administrators in the school are dramatically altered. Students no longer have a set of peers with whom they move through many of their classes and have a different teacher in every class. Thus, there is little consistency in the peers or adults whom they encounter from hour to hour.

Consequently, the intervention had two components: (a) a partial reorganization of the social system by assigning experimental students to classes in their four primary academic subjects with other project students; and (b) restructuring the role of the homeroom teacher by redefining her/his role and responsibilities to serve as the primary administrative-counseling link between students, their parents, and the rest of the school. The objective of the reorganization was to decrease the flux that new high school students encounter – a social regularity – and to establish a stable support system. Restructuring the role of the homeroom teacher was intended to increase students' perception of social support, feelings of involvement, and knowledge of expectations and roles. In a broader and long-term sense, the intervention was intended to promote academic success and well-being and to avert psychosocial dysfunction for the participating students, which it did (R. D. Felner, personal communication, May 1987).

The other contemporary project I discuss is the collaborative work that I, Julian Rappaport, and our students have done with GROW, a mutual help organization for the "mentally ill" (see, for example, Rappaport et al., 1985; Salem, Seidman, & Rappaport, 1987). GROW serves as an alternative to the traditional mental health system. A social regularity that the founders of GROW observed, being former or current recipients of mental health services, was that they were always in a "one down" position; things were being done "to" or "for" them and never "with" them. (This echoes Goldenberg's, 1971, distinction between vertical and horizontal organizational structure in residential treatment settings.) This social regularity carried a great deal of information and meaning that affected members' attitudes, behavior, and skills on a long-term basis, and not in a particularly positive manner. The GROW founders recognized that one of the most effective ways to relate with others was as equals; this led to their own development of a comprehensive mutual help organization, or what they refer to as a "caring and sharing community." Thus, their intervention was to replace the to and for style of delivery of human services with voluntary, ongoing mutual support linkages. This was achieved, initially in Australia with over 400 groups, and most recently in Illinois with over 100 groups. Another more subtle, but perhaps more important, aspect of the social regularity that they altered was to create niches and roles for their members consistent with their level of functioning at the time, where few had existed. These, in fact, give meaning and value to people who previously had precious little. Thus, they create underpersonned settings (Zimmerman *et al.*, 1985).

As should be apparent, the construct of social regularity is vital to both a full comprehension of the ecology of a setting and setting-based intervention and change.

Mesosystems

Settings exists in a much larger context. Each setting or subsystem has ongoing transactions and social relations with both other subsystems and the larger environment; these relationships and effects are reciprocal. I adopt the term "mesosystem" from Bronfenbrenner (1979) to refer to this complex arena and to the *between-system* relations or intrasocietal relationships (Seidman, 1983a) in particular. We cannot ignore issues at the level of the mesosystem; they influence whatever happens at the setting level. Moreover, mesosystem interventions offer Community Psychology an even greater challenge for the future.

The mesosystem is the most complex unit of analysis. In the *Handbook of Social Intervention*, I presented a social systems' framework depicting the transactions between societal systems, portraying donor, administrative, delivery, recipient, macro- and microsystems (or settings) (Seidman, 1983a). The mesosystem refers to these intrasocietal relationships – to connections *among* these systems. The foci of mesosystems, as it was for settings, is once again the connections, relations, or interdependencies, but at a higher level of social complexity. Here, the social regularity is located *between* settings in contrast to *within* settings. Thus, the construct of social regularities undergirds both the mesosystem and setting levels of analysis.

Strategies of impacting mesosystem regularities are often policy initiatives. To be effective, however, they must be aimed at altering the connections or relationships between systems or settings. Thus, a policy initiative must be very specific; most often, they have not been.

Let me provide an illustration of a social regularity at the mesosystem level. There is often a predictable pattern or social regularity in which alleged juvenile offenders are handled by different components of the juvenile justice system. Status offenders (youth who would not be charged with a crime if they were an adult, e.g., chronic truancy, incorrigibility) are often processed by the system in a manner very similar to youth accused of serious crimes. Consequently, status offenders – members of the recipient system – are entered into the juvenile justice system by police who have a great deal of discretion with regard to the disposition of their cases.

In work done with Julian Rappaport and Bill Davidson (Rappaport, Seidman, & Davidson, 1979; Seidman, 1981), the police – here, the delivery system – would file a petition with the court – the administrative system. The court would ask the probation department – another component of the delivery system – to do an investigation. Inevitably, the probation department would recommend a probationary status which the judge would just as inevitably agree to. The probation department would pick up the case, but in actuality, the youth was provided with minimal surveillance, counseling, or any other form of assistance. In all fairness, each probation officer was already carrying an unmanageably large caseload. Not surprisingly, these processed status offenders would tend to recidivate. This illustrates a pattern of between system regularities that are essential to observe and understand, and must become a central target of any effective community intervention, preventive or otherwise.

In the process of developing a secondary preventive intervention for more serious alleged offenders, we convinced the police *not* to process status offenders in the same way that they had been, but instead to "warn and release" them; that is, to alter the constant pattern of social interdependencies between referred status offenders and police dispositional decisions (Seidman, Rappaport, & Davidson, 1980). During the years of our actual involvement, there was a substantial decrement in the number of status offenders on whom court petitions were filed. But after we left, the gains were lost. We had not successfully altered the social regularity in a permanent fashion.

These efforts were an attempt to alter the mesosystem regularities from the bottom-up. Turning to a top-down example of a policy initiative, the state of Virginia attempted to resolve the issue of status offenders' continual penetration of the juvenile justice system by a legislative initiative. Virginia passed model legislation decriminalizing status offenses. There was a dramatic decrement in the number and rate of status offenses subsequent to the implementation of that legislation. However, the legislative change also led to an increase in the rate of youth charged with more serious delinquent offenses (Mulvey & Hicks, 1982). It appeared that many of those previously labeled as status offenders were relabeled, thus subverting both the statute's intent and a genuine change in the critical social regularity of the social system.

Summary

Social regularities only arise as a meaningful and salient construct when the unit of analysis is the setting or mesosystem. It is not salient when the underlying epistemology suggests an individual or a population as the target of intervention or unit of analysis. The identification of a setting or a mesosystem's social regularity is an essential first step in either theory development or the actual process of social intervention. Community Psychology will profit by beginning to explicitly identify the critical social regularity(ies). The social regularity yields information concerning the setting or mesosystem rule and ultimate functional outcomes. One needs to determine whether these are the intended and desired outcomes, as well as what is the possible universe of alternative regularities (Sarason, 1972). If the existing social regularity is not the desired and intended one, the desired social regularity should serve to focus the nature and type of intervention. In any case, identification of the within- or between-setting social regularity both provides information about the current state of affairs and helps guide future actions. Thus, identifying and changing within- or between-setting social regularities can serve as a foundation on which Community Psychology must stand.

PROCESSES AND FORMS OF CHANGE

Changing the social regularity – within a system at a setting level, or between systems at a mesosystem level – can occur by employing any one or more of a wide variety of strategies and tactics of social intervention, such as policy initiatives or community organization. What needs to precede selection of specific strategies and tactics is deliberation about the particular form of the desired change process. The match between the desired level, type, nature, and intended outcome of the change process may foreclose on the utility or appropriateness of certain strategies. There are three forms of the change process that aspire to achieving system-oriented change: tuning, incremental change, and restructuring. I discuss each briefly.

Tuning

Tuning represents a form of system change that occurs through accommodation or adaptation of the various people, groups, or settings. Barker (1968) described two tuning tactics or ways of restoring a setting's balance: correcting and removing troublesome elements, respectively referred to as deviation-countering and vetoing. Thus, the goal is to help the system function "better," that is, more effectively, efficiently, harmoniously, within existing structural arrangements. In other words, its aim is to maintain the status quo. The basic structural arrangements remain unaltered. Maruyama (1963) has referred to this as "morphostatic change."

A number of years ago Julian Rappaport and I were called upon to consult with a high school following a racial disturbance. We were asked to run "rap" sessions among the different groups of students. The goals, implicit in the request, were those of tension reduction. If we had engaged in the requested tactics, the setting's fundamental social regularities – the genuine target of second-order change – would have had no chance of being altered. Although tuning is probably the most prevalent form of change endeavor in which social scientists find themselves engaged, it can only hinder (via distraction and delusion) our quest to change fundamental social regularities at the setting or mesosystem levels.

Incremental Change

Incremental or remedial change occurs over time by the gradual increase in some attribute, for example, more resources or services for individuals or populations. Many social reforms possess these characteristics. Often a group or population is given, or attains, an increased number of services or resources. However, a frequent concomitant change is the gain in the quantity of resources or services received by other groups. As a result, the social relationship of the target group to the rest of the population often remains the same; there is not a differential change between the targeted group and the larger population over time. When incremental forms of change are employed, the target of the intervention is usually at the population level. Consequently, changing the fundamental social regularity of the system is not clearly envisioned, and rarely achieved, despite the best of intentions.

For example, one of Sesame Street's original objectives was to increase the academic readiness and achievement of "underclass" children. This creative mass media intervention – a population-centered intervention – did increase these skills in underclass children. However, it also increased the skills of students from higher social strata, in fact, to a greater degree (Cook *et al.*, 1975). As an unintended result, the discrepancy in skills between classes of children increased. I am not suggesting that this was a "bad" intervention. It was successful in achieving incremental change but unsuccessful in altering the salient social regularities.

Restructuring

Unlike the objectives of tuning and incremental forms of change, restructuring clearly envisions a fundamental alteration of the existing social regularities or the creation of new sociostructural regularities. These change processes are often discontinuous as opposed to continuous.

There are three very general forms of intervention that could accomplish restructuring: altering the existing social regularity, creating a new or alternative social regularity, and possibly, making the existing social regularity known. To alter the existing social regularity, a variety of different strategies could be employed. But the level of intervention would need to be either the setting or mesosystem, and the fundamental social regularity would have to be clearly indentified and targeted.

In Felner *et al.*'s work (1982), described earlier, fundamental social regularities of the school setting were altered, in a relatively simple and straightforward fashion. However, changing the fundamental social regularity within or between settings is often considered impossible or too costly. In these situations, a new setting is often created. This was the case in several of my prior illustrations: Fairweather's community lodge, Goldenberg's Residential Youth Center, and the creation of GROW. These new and alternative settings, when dramatically successful, may ultimately lead to a change in the social regularity at the larger mesosystem level.

Finally, making the existing social regularity known is most often, and more colloquially, referred to as consciousness raising. This can only lead to a discontinuous change in the existing social regularities over a long period of time. In the short-term, the nature of change is incremental in form, and may be all that is possible. However, it allows for the possibility of restructural change over the long-term. Many have argued vociferously that this is the only way to go on many important social issues. The woman's movement has followed this course. But have those incremental changes led us to a point where restructural change is possible (and likely) or that a redefinition in theory and practice of the role relationships between men and women, on a societal scale, will be achieved?

Summary

Tuning forms of change are not congruent with the intention of changing social regularities; restructuring types of change processes are congruent. Although incremental forms of change per se are incongruent with our avowed objectives of altering the fundamental social regularities at the setting and mesosystem levels, the jury is still out on their long-term compatibility. This stems primarily from the question of whether one can have a long-term plan of changing salient social regularities by initially employing incremental processes as tactics that will ultimately lead to a threshold that makes the likelihood of restructural change more possible. In general, incremental forms of change fail to alter salient social regularities, though such outcomes may be possible as part of a long-term plan that eventuates in a change in the social regularity.

TRAVELING ITINERARY

There are many parallels with the present in the past; events keep repeating with new characters. With just minor changes in the events that occurred, today could have been very different for Community Psychology and, perhaps even for the social good. If we were able to travel back in time, or for some of us, to return to Swampscott, I would give this advice: "Remember anything you do could have serious repercusions on future events" (Spielberg, Gale, Canton, & Zemeckis, 1985).

This time I plan to reenter the flux capacitor to travel into the future. Before I leave, let me describe to you, in brief, what I plan to do there:

1. Identify important social regularities related to social issues and problems.
2. More fully develop the construct of social regularities in terms of its nomological network and operational definitions.
3. Try to understand the role that social regularities play in the ecology of settings and mesosystems.
4. Perhaps, most importantly, try to change[4] these social regularities by matching the forms of change to our objectives and values.
5. And last, but of course not least, evaluate these interventions, in terms of the processes themselves as well as the outcomes at multiple

---

[4]The development, implementation, and evaluation of social interventions are not imposed on people and communities by an "outsider." Instead, the action scientist is in close collaboration with the involved individuals at every stage of the process (see, for example, Chavis, Stuckey, & Wandersman, 1983; Kelly, 1986; Serrano-García, 1984; Tyler, Pargament, & Gatz, 1983).

levels – including the individual – as they relate to other important phenomena of interest. If we are to genuinely embrace an ecological-transactional model, new methods of research design and quantitative methods will need to be derived from these different epistemological assumptions (Seidman, 1983b, 1987).

And doing so, if my flux capacitor still works, I will travel back to the present, hoping that reentry is not too bumpy, replete with that knowledge so we can reformulate a better theory to help change the future.

ACKNOWLEDGMENT

I wish to express my appreciation to the many former graduate students and my friend and colleague, Julian Rappaport, at the University of Illinois at Urbana-Champaign, who over the last 15 years, helped me develop the seeds of many of the ideas expressed in this address (see, for example, Seidman & Rappaport, 1979). During 1987, the students in my graduate seminar on Intervention and Social Change, both at New York University and the University of Hawaii, gave me substantial assistance in clarifying these evolving notions. Finally, I am indebted to Tracey A. Revenson who labored over multiple iterations of this manuscript enabling me to crystallize these ideas in a more compelling and understandable fashion. Preparation of this manuscript was facilitated by grants from the National Institute of Mental Health (43084) and the Carnegie Foundation.

REFERENCES

Altman, I. & Rogoff, B. (1987). World views in psychology: Trait, interactional, organismic and transactional perspectives. In D. Stokols & I. Altman (Eds.), *Handbook of environmental psychology* (pp. 7–40). New York: Wiley.

Allport, F. H. (1962). A structuronomic conception of behavior: Individual and collective. I. Structural theory and the master problem of social psychology. *Journal of Abnormal and Social Psychology, 64*, 3–30.

Argyris, C., Putnam, R., & Smith, D. M. (1985). *Action science: Concepts, methods, and skills for research and intervention.* San Francisco: Jossey-Bass.

Barker, R. G. (1968). *Ecological psychology: Concepts and methods for studying the environment of human behavior.* Stanford, CA: Stanford University Press.

Bateson, G. (1972). *Steps to an ecology of the mind.* San Francisco: Chandler.

Bateson, G. (1979). *Mind and nature: A necessary unity.* New York: Bantam.

Berger, P. & Neuhaus, R. J. (1977). *To empower people: The role of mediating structures in public policy.* Washington, DC: American Enterprise Institute.

Bennett, C. C., Anderson, L. S., Cooper, S., Hassol, L., Klein, D. C., & Rosenblum, G. (Eds.). (1966). *Community psychology: A report of the Boston Conference on the Education of Psychologists for Community Mental Health.* Boston: Boston University Press.

Bronfenbrenner, U. (1979). *The ecology of human development*. Cambridge, MA: Harvard University Press.

Buckley, W. (Ed.). (1968). *Modern systems research for the behavioral scientist: A sourcebook*. Chicago: Aldine.

Chavis, D. M., Stuckey, P. E., & Wandersman, A. (1983). Returning basic research to the community: A relationship between scientists and citizens. *American Psychologist, 38*, 424–434.

Cook, T. D., Appleton, H., Conner, R., Shaffer, A., Tamkin, G. & Weber, S. J. (1975). *Sesame Street revisited: A study in evaluation research*. New York: Russell Sage Foundation.

Cowen, E. L. (2000). Community psychology and routes to psychological wellness. In J. Rappaport & E. Seidman (Eds.), *Handbook of community psychology* (pp. 79–99). New York: Plenum Press.

Dewey, J. (1946). *Problems of men*. New York: Philosophical Library.

Fairweather, G. W. (1972). *Social change: The challenge to survival*. Morristown, NJ: General Learning Press.

Fairweather, G. W., Sanders, D. H., Cressler, D. L., & Maynard, H. (1969). *Community life for the mentally ill: An alternative to institutional care*. Chicago: Aldine.

Felner, R. D., Ginter, M., & Primavera, J. (1982). Primary prevention during school transitions: Social support and environmental structure. *American Journal of Community Psychology, 10*, 277–290.

Felner, R. D., Jason, L. A., Moritsugu, J. N., & Farber, S. S. (Eds.). (1983). *Preventive psychology: Theory, research and practice*. New York: Pergamon.

Glidewell, J. C. (1966). Perspectives in community mental health. In C. C. Bennett, L. S. Anderson, S. Copper, L. Hassol, D. C. Klein, & G. Rosenblum (Eds.). (1966). *Community psychology: A report of the Boston Conference on the Education of Psychologists for Community Mental Health* (pp. 33–49). Boston: Boston University Press.

Goldenberg, I. I. (1971). *Build me a mountain: Youth, poverty, and the creation of new settings*. Cambridge, MA: MIT Press.

Heller, K. & Monahan, J. (1977). *Psychology and community change*. Homewood, IL: Dorsey.

Iscoe, I. (1974). Community psychology and the competent community. *American Psychologist, 29*, 607–613.

Kelly, J. (1986). Context and process: An ecological view of the interdependence of practice and research. *American Journal of Community Psychology, 14*, 581–589.

Laumann, E. O. & Pappi, F. U. (1976). *Networks of collective action: A perspective on community influence systems*. New York: Academic Press.

Lewin, K. (1951). Frontiers in group dynamics. In D. Cartwright (Ed.), *Field theory in social science: Selected theoretical papers by Kurt Lewin*. Chicago: The University of Chicago Press. (Reprinted from *Human Relations*, 1947, *1*, 2–38)

Linney, J. A. (1986). Court-ordered school desegregation: Shuffling the deck or playing a different game. In E. Seidman & J. Rappaport (Eds.), *Redefining social problems* (pp. 259–274). New York: Plenum Press.

Maruyama, M. (1963). The second cybernetics: Deviation amplifying mutual causal processes. *American Scientist, 51*, 164–179.

Maruyama, M. (1983). Cross cultural perspectives on social and community change. In E. Seidman (Ed.), *Handbook of social intervention* (pp. 33–47). Beverly Hills: Sage.

Mulvey, E. P. & Hicks, A. (1982). The paradoxical effect of a juvenile code change in Virginia. *American Journal of Community Psychology, 10*, 705–721.

Murrell, S. A. (1973). *Community psychology and social systems*. New York: Behavioral Publications.

Rappaport, J. (1977). *Community psychology: Values, research and action*. New York: Holt, Rinehart, & Winston.

Rappaport, J. (1981). In praise of paradox: A social policy of empowerment over prevention. *American Journal of Community Psychology, 9,* 1–25.

Rappaport, J. (1987). Terms of empowerment/exemplars of prevention: Toward a theory of community psychology. *American Journal of Community Psychology, 15,* 121–148.

Rappaport, J., Seidman, E., & Davidson, W. S. (1979). Demonstration research and manifest versus true adoption: The natural history of a research project to divert adolescents from the legal system. In R. F. Munoz, L. R., Snowden, & J. G. Kelly (Eds.), *Social and psychological research in community settings* (pp. 101–132). San Francisco: Jossey-Bass.

Rappaport, J., Seidman, E., Toro, P. A., McFadden, L. S., Reischl, T. M., Roberts, L. J., Salem, D. A., Stein, C. H., & Zimmerman, M. A. (1985). Collaborative research with a mutual help organization. *Social Policy, 15,* 12–24.

Salem, D., Seidman, E., & Rappaport, J. (1987). *Community treatment of the mentally ill.* Manuscript submitted for publication.

Sarason, S. B. (1971). *The culture of the school and the problem of change.* Boston: Allyn & Bacon.

Sarason, S. B. (1972). *The creation of settings and the future societies.* San Francisco: Jossey-Bass.

Sarason, S. B. (1974). *The psychological sense of community: Prospects for a community psychology.* San Francisco: Jossey-Bass.

Sarason, S. B. (1981). Psychology misdirected. New York: Free Press.

Sarason, S. B. (1982). *The culture of the school and the problem of change* (2nd ed.). Boston: Allyn & Bacon.

Seidman, E. (1978). Justice, values and social science: Unexamined premises. In R. J. Simon (Ed.), *Research in law and sociology* (pp. 175–200). Greenwich, CT: JAI.

Seidman, E. (1981). The route from the successful experiment to policy formation: Falling rocks, bumps and dangerous curves. In R. Roesch & R. Corrado (Eds.), *Evaluation and criminal justice policy* (pp. 81–102). Beverly Hills: Sage.

Seidman, E. (1983a). Introduction. In E. Seidman (Ed.), *Handbook of social intervention* (pp. 11–17). Beverly Hills: Sage.

Seidman, E. (1983b). Unexamined premises of social problem solving. In E. Seidman (Ed.), *Handbook of social intervention* (pp. 48–67). Beverly Hills: Sage.

Seidman, E. (1987). Toward a framework for primary prevention research. In J. A. Steinberg & M. M. Silverman (Eds.), *Preventing mental disorders: A research perspective* (pp. 2–19). Washington, DC: U.S. Government Printing Office.

Seidman, E. & Rapkin, B. (1983). Economics and psychosocial dysfunction: Toward a conceptual framework and prevention strategies. In R. D. Felner, L. A. Jason, J. N. Moritsugu, & S. S. Farber (Eds.), *Preventive psychology: Theory, research and practice* (pp. 175–198). New York: Pergamon.

Seidman, E. & Rappaport, J. (1979, March). *The search for alternative social change conceptions, methods, and interventions: A dialogue.* Invited address in the Community and Social Change Public Lecture Series, University of Michigan, Ann Arbor, MI.

Seidman, E. & Rappaport, J. (1986). Framing the issues. In E. Seidman & J. Rappaport (Eds.), *Redefining social problems* (pp. 1–8). New York: Plenum Press.

Seidman, E., Rappaport, J., & Davidson, W. S. (1980). Adolescents in legal jeopardy: Initial success and replication of an alternative to the criminal justice system. In R. R. Ross & P. Gendreau (Eds.), *Effective correctional treatment* (pp. 103–123). Toronto: Butterworths.

Serrano-Garciá, I. (1984). The illusion of empowerment: Community development within a colonial context. *Prevention in Human Services, 3,* 173–200.

Spielberg, S., Gale, B., & Canton, N. (Producers), & Zemeckis, R. (Director). (1985). *Back to the future* [Film]. Hollywood, CA: Universal.

Spivak, G. & Shure, M. B. (1974). *Social adjustment of young children.* San Francisco: Jossey-Bass.

Trickett, E. J., Kelly, J. G., & Todd, D. M. (1972). The social environment of the high school: Guidelines for individual change and organizational redevelopment. In S. E. Golann & C. Eisdorfer (Eds.), *Handbook of community mental health* (pp. 331–406). New York: Appleton-Century-Crofts.

Tyler, F. B., Pargament, K. I., & Gatz, M. (1983). The resource collaborator role: A model for interactions involving psychologists. *American Psychologist, 38*, 388–398.

U.S. Bureau of the Census. (1986). *Current Population Reports: Money income of households, families and persons in the United States: 1984* (Series P-60, No. 151). Washington, DC: U.S. Government Printing Office.

Watzlawick, P., Weakland, J. H., & Fisch, R. (1974). *Change: Principles of problem formation and problem resolution.* New York: Norton.

Zimmerman, M. A., McFadden, L. S., Toro, P. A., Salem, D. A., Reischl, T. M., Rappaport, J., Seidman, E., & Berggren, D. (1985, May). *Expansion of a mutual help organization: The "Johnny Appleseed" approach.* Paper presented at the annual meeting of the Midwestern Psychological Association, Chicago, IL.

12

Community Settings as Buffers of Life Stress? Highly Supportive Churches, Mutual Help Groups, and Senior Centers

Kenneth I. Maton

Examined the stress-buffering potential of community settings in three studies. The first study focused on economic stress among 162 members of three churches, the second on bereavement stress among 80 members of eight mutual help groups for bereaved parents, and the third on bereavement stress among 85 members of six senior centers. In each study, high and low support settings were defined by aggregate measures. For churches and mutual help groups, high life stress individuals reported greater well-being in high support than low support settings while low life stress individuals did not differ across settings. Tangible aid receipt (churches) and friendship development (mutual help groups) contributed to the stress-buffering findings. For senior centers, aggregate setting support was related to well-being in main effect fashion. The implications for inquiry and action at the community setting level of analysis are discussed.

Shinn (1987) recently challenged community psychologists to expand their domains of inquiry and action through increased focus on community settings such as religious congregations, voluntary associations, work sites,

Originally published in the *American Journal of Community Psychology, 17*(2) (1989): 203–232.

A Quarter Century of Community Psychology: *Readings from the* American Journal of Community Psychology, edited by Tracey A. Revenson *et al.* Kluwer Academic/Plenum Publishers, New York, 2002.

government, and schools. Such community settings are important as sites of research and intervention in part because they present psychologists the opportunity to focus on the organizational level of analysis (Keys & Frank, 1987). Traditionally, community-based work by psychologists has been limited to the individual or small-group level, including most of the recent research generated by the stress-buffering paradigm (e.g., Cohen & Wills, 1985). The stress-buffering paradigm asserts that key psychological moderator variables (e.g., perceived social support, coping ability) protect high life stress individuals from the deleterious effects of stress, while having significantly smaller or no impact on low life stress individuals. As an expansion of this paradigm, one important question at the organizational level of analysis is whether community settings (within and across domains) differ in their ability to buffer members from the deleterious effects of disruptive life stress. If community settings do differ in their potential to serve a stress-buffering function, and we can discover why, then researchers and policy makers will have an expanded and potentially far-reaching point of entry for community-based prevention and empowerment efforts.

To date, there has been little organizational-level focus on the role of community settings as potential buffers of life stress. Most of the work on stress-buffering effects has focused on personological (e.g., coping, hardiness) and interpersonal (e.g., social support) variables. Concepts such as sense of belonging or social integration in the community are sometimes discussed as important components of social support. However, the research in these areas has often focused on family and friendship contexts, to the exclusion of settings such as congregations and voluntary associations. In addition, when research samples are obtained from work, school, and neighborhood settings, attention tends to focus, for instance, on social support from coworkers, problem-solving training from teachers, or level of neighboring. Little or no attention is paid to the setting-level processes within the work site, school, or neighborhood that facilitate high levels of social support, problem solving, or neighboring. The current research adds an organizational-level focus to the stress-buffering paradigm, by examining whether aggregate setting-level support interacts with level of individual life stress in stress-buffering fashion. Although the current research is cross-sectional in nature, and thus cannot depict causal processes, findings suggestive of stress-buffering effects set the stage for future, longitudinal research programs.

Settings that facilitate higher levels of social support, adaptive coping skills, and meaningful roles may be expected to better protect members from deleterious effects of stress than settings lacking these capabilities. Social support may be experienced directly, through relationships with friends or acquaintances in the setting, or indirectly, through a general sense that the setting has a high sense of cohesiveness and that support is generally available.

Adaptive coping strategies may be learned formally, as in small-group work-shops, informally, through discussions with setting members, or indirectly, through observing respected role models. Finally, involvement in meaningful, valued roles may enhance self-esteem, provide distraction, and generally facilitate a sense of meaning and purpose. These benefits may prove especially adaptive for individuals under high levels of stress (Maton, 1989).

In the present research, settings high and low on perceived levels of support were compared on their stress-buffering potential. Level of setting support was chosen as the key variable on which to categorize settings since empirical findings consistent with a stress-buffering effect for social support have accumulated in recent years (Cohen & Wills, 1985). It was hypothesized that among individuals experiencing high levels of life stress, those who reside in settings with significantly higher levels of aggregate perceived support will report greater well-being than those in settings with lower perceived support. Smaller or no differences in well-being should obtain for low life stress individuals in high- versus low-support settings. This stress-buffering hypothesis was examined through cross-level analyses. Life stress and well-being were assessed at the individual level, while setting support was defined as a setting-level variable (in this research, based on aggregate individual perceptions).

There are two primary advantages to cross-level analyses involving organizational and individual variables. First, an explicit organizational perspective is encompassed. If significant findings emerge across settings, interpretation will naturally focus on the organizational context that facili-tated the setting differences in potential stress-buffering impact—future work at the organizational level of analysis follows logically. Second, it is possible to carry out direct comparisons of the contributions of setting-level variables with and without potential stress-buffering individual-level vari-ables included in the analysis. Examination of the differing results from these analyses allows determination of the extent to which setting-level findings are explained by, or are independent of, stress-buffering variance tapped by individual-level variables (Shinn, 1990).

In the first study reported below, aggregate levels of support providing and support receiving differed significantly across settings and were used to assign settings to high- versus low-support categories. In the second and third studies, aggregate scores on the social climate measure of setting cohe-sion differed significantly across settings and were used to assign settings to high- versus low-support categories. The latter measure, perceived cohesion, has been used as a measure of perceived support in individual-level studies of family and workplace, and generally found to be related to well-being (e.g., Holahan & Moos, 1981; Moos & Moos, 1983). In addition, relationships between setting-level cohesion and criterion measures have emerged in studies of diverse community settings, including block associations

(Giamartino & Wandersman, 1983), religious congregations (Pargament, Silverman, Johnson, Echemendia, & Snyder, 1983), college residences (Moos & Van Dort, 1979), and various community treatment facilities (e.g., Cronkite, Moos, & Finney, 1983).

Each of three studies in the current research focused on a different type of community setting. The first study focused on religious congregations, a community setting to which 140 million Americans belong, and which 40% of Americans frequent on any given Sunday (Jacquet, 1984). The life stress variable assessed was perceived economic stress, and the criterion variable was life satisfaction. Although it has often been suggested that religion (e.g., Fichter, 1981) and religious congregations (Maton & Pargament, 1987) serve a stress-buffering role for individuals, no research has explicitly compared religious congregations on their stress-buffering potential. Provision of meaning, hope, a world view, daily practices, and social support are among the elements of involvement in religious congregations which have been hypothesized as stress-buffering (Maton & Pargament, 1987). Previous research by the investigator, focused on a single congregational sample, found a relationship between life satisfaction and tangible support bidirectionality (high levels of tangible support providing and receiving with congregational members). Perceived economic stress for self/family was included as a covariate (Maton, 1987). The current research included the original congregational sample and two other congregations ($N = 162$). It examined whether setting-wide level of tangible support interacted in a stress-buffering fashion with perceived economic stress in predicting life satisfaction.

The second study focused on mutual help groups for bereaved parents. Although it is generally assumed that mutual help groups serve a stress-buffering function for their members, little outcome research on their effectiveness has been carried out. Receipt of social support, development of coping skills, information sharing, and the opportunity to help others are among the components of mutual help group involvement which may contribute to member well-being (Levy, 1976; Powell, 1987). Previous research by the investigator on three different types of mutual help groups, including five groups for bereaved parents, indicated that individuals who provided and received emotional support reported greater well-being than those who did not (Maton, 1988). Recency of the death of the child, an index of bereavement stress, was included as a covariate in that study. The current research included the five bereaved parent groups from the earlier study plus three additional bereaved parent groups ($N = 80$). It examined whether setting-wide level of emotional support interacted with level of bereavement stress in predicting depression and self-esteem.

The third study focused on senior centers for the elderly, of which there are currently more than 8,000 in American communities (Lowy,

1985). Historically, senior centers have been conceived of as important sites for the development of socially supportive relationships and activities for the elderly (Gelfand, 1984; Lowy, 1985). For elderly citizens under high levels of stress, and perhaps especially for those whose support systems are disrupted due to deaths of family or friends, the support received at such community centers can potentially serve a stress-buffering function (Gelfand, 1984). Companionship, sharing of common stressful experiences, the chance to be helpful to others, and tangible aid are some of the stress-buffering mechanisms that might prove especially important in the senior center context. To date, there has been little research on the relationship between involvement in senior centers, life stress, and well-being. The current research included members from six senior centers ($N = 85$), and examined whether setting-wide level of emotional support interacted with level of bereavement stress in predicting mood disturbance and depression.

The present research appears to be the first test of the stress-buffering potential of high- versus low-support community settings. The three studies were conceptualized as parallel tests of the same stress-buffering research hypothesis. Comparison of results across the studies can provide preliminary information about commonalities and differences in stress-buffering potential, and possible mechanisms of influence, across three types of community settings.

STUDY 1

Method

Sample and Procedure

As part of a larger study on patterns and correlates of economic sharing within religious settings, members of three congregations completed economic sharing logs and research questionnaires over a 9-month period. The primary setting for the larger study was a nondenominational Christian Fellowship of about 200 members which had been the site of ongoing research by the investigator (Maton, 1987; Maton & Rappaport, 1984). The setting was distinctive in the depth of members' religious commitment, economic sharing among members, and the emphasis on family-like community. A second congregation studied, an Assembly of God congregation of about 300 members, was somewhat similar to the Fellowship in terms of religious commitment, economic sharing, and focus on community, but also contained some of the features of more mainline Protestant congregations. The third congregation chosen for study was a relatively traditional, mainline Protestant congregation, a Church of Christ congregation of approximately

175 members. This setting was included in the research because a number of the leaders and members in the nondenominational Fellowship had formerly been highly involved in the Church of Christ denomination. Although not necessarily representative of religious settings in general, the three settings represented three theoretically important types of midwestern Protestant congregations.

Stratified random procedures based on sex, living situation (single, couple without children, parents with children), and number of years involvement in the congregation were used to select individuals from each setting to participate in the research (with 50% of the population of the Fellowship, and 20% from each of the two other congregations, set as target goals).[1] Of the 389 individuals contacted by phone, 240 agreed to take part (61.7% acceptance rate). Each research participant was to complete a 7-day activity log once every 4 weeks, and a questionnaire once every 8 weeks, throughout the 9-month study. Of those who agreed to take part, 162 completed all research forms (67.5% completion rate). There were no significant differences in age, sex, number of years in congregation, or occupational level between those who successfully completed the study and those who did not.

The final sample comprised 103 members from the Fellowship, 34 members from the Assembly of God congregation, and 25 members from the Church of Christ congregation. The average age of participants was 30.9, 57% were female, the average occupational status was 71.5 (where 33 is a waitress, 66 a bookkeeper, and 99 a physician; Nam & Powers, 1968), 49% had one or more children living in the home, and the average length of congregational membership was 3.25 years.

Measures

On the 7-day activity logs each participant listed all members of their congregation they had contact with each day, and then described each tangible support transaction they had with any individual listed (i.e., who provided what service or good, and for how long). Individuals' scores on Support Received and Support Provided were obtained by (a) converting each material support transaction into dollar amounts, using current market rates (interrater reliability = .87); (b) summing providing and receiving transactions separately over the nine activity logs; and (c) transforming the resulting scores by log 10 (due to extreme skewness and kurtosis).

Factor analysis of the bimonthly research questionnaire yielded the Economic Stress, Congregational Involvement, and Life Satisfaction measures

---

[1]The plan to recruit a proportionally larger sample in the Fellowship congregation was integral to the continuing research program in the setting (Maton, 1986).

used in the current study (see Maton, 1987).[2] The Economic Stress measure contained seven items designed by the investigator. An example of an item is "It is a struggle to stretch my (or my family's) monthly income to meet my (our) expenses and bills." The Congregational Involvement scale contained four items designed by the investigator, assessing levels of involvement, influence, and belonging. A representative item is "I am very involved in (name of congregation)." The Life Satisfaction scale contained five of the six items used by Withey and Andrews (1976) in their national survey. A representative item from the scale is "How satisfied are you with your life as a whole these days?" The mean Cronbach alpha reliabilities for the three scales were 0.87, 0.86, and 0.84, respectively, and the average test–retest reliabilities were 0.82, 0.88, and 0.63, respectively. Some evidence for the construct validity of these measures is present in the meaningful patterns of relationships obtained in the previous research (Maton, 1986, 1987).

Demographic information on sex, age, number of years in congregation, occupation, and children living in home were obtained at the time of the initial sample recruitment.

Results

High- versus Low-Support Congregations

One-way analyses of variance indicated significant differences across congregations on Support Received, $F(2, 159) = 15.97, p < .001$, and Support Provided, $F(2, 159) = 11.97$, $p < .001$. Post-hoc analyses revealed that for both support variables members of two of the congregations (Fellowship and Assembly of God) reported significantly higher levels than members of the third congregation (Church of Christ) (Scheffé test, $p < .05$). Given these significant differences across settings, the Fellowship and Assembly of God congregations were designated as High Support congregations, and the Church of Christ congregation was designated as a Low Support congregation. Additional one-way analyses of variance, with one prespecified contrast, did not reveal significant differences between the two high-support and one low-support congregation on Sex, Years in Congregation, Occupational Status, Children in Home, Economic Stress, Involvement, or Life Satisfaction. However, members of the two high-support congregations (combined $M = 31.3$) were younger than members of the low-support congregation ($M = 37.2$), contrast $t(159) = -3.69, p < .001$.

---

[2]For the current study, and the two studies reported below, copies of the measures, and additional information about measurement development, can be obtained from the author.

Zero-Order Correlations

Life satisfaction was inversely and significantly related to Economic Stress, $r(160) = -.31$, $p < .001$, and positively and significantly related to Involvement, $r(160) = .27$, $p < .001$. The zero-order correlations among variables are displayed in Table 1.

Primary Analyses

Hierarchical multiple regression analysis, with contrast coding of Setting type, was the primary data analytic method. Life satisfaction was the criterion variable. The first regression step included entrance of the five demographic variables. On the next step, the Economic Stress measure was entered. Then, the two Setting contrast variables were entered. The contrast of interest—Setting Support—compared the two high support congregations with the low support congregation.[3] Contrast coding of Setting Support allows a direct comparison of the two high-support settings versus the low-support congregation based on an equivalent contribution of the two high-support congregations (i.e., independent of sample size; an unweighted means analysis, Cohen & Cohen, 1975). Next, the Economic Stress × Setting interaction terms were entered, with the contrast of interest comparing the two high-support settings with the one low-support setting. Then, to assess the independent contribution of the Individual Experience predictor variables beyond setting variables, Support Received, Support Provided, and Involvement were entered if they explained additional, significant variance. Finally, to assess the independent contribution of potential stress-buffering interactions at the individual level, the Economic Stress × Individual Experience interaction terms were entered if they explained additional significant variance.

Table 2 presents the step R^2 and standardized regression weights (βs) for the regression analysis. Economic Stress was inversely and significantly related to life satisfaction, $\beta = -0.41$, $p < .001$. The Setting Support contrast did not explain significant variance in life satisfaction. However, the Economic Stress by Setting Support interaction was significant and in the predicted direction, $\beta = 0.81$, $p < .05$. Figure 1 reveals the differing slopes of the regression lines for the high- and low-support congregations (following

---

[3]For the current study (and the other two studies reported below), the exact nature of the coding of the remaining orthogonal contrast (or contrasts) is not important, since the research hypothesis focused only on comparisons between settings high and low on setting support. However, all contrasts must be simultaneously entered into the equation, so that the unweighted means analysis would be operative, and so that all variance between settings would be accounted for (prior to entrance of the individual experience variables) (Cohen & Cohen, 1975).

Table 1. Correlation Matrix of Variables for Congregational Members ($N = 162$)

Variable	1	2	3	4	5	6	7	8	9	10	11
1. Sex[a]	—										
2. Age	-.04	—									
3. Years in congregation	-.11	.15[d]	—								
4. Occupational status	-.26[f]	.13[d]	.07	—							
5. Children in home[b]	.06	-.38[f]	-.15[d]	-.14[d]	—						
6. Economic stress	-.07	-.10	.10	-.10	.06	—					
7. Setting support[c]	-.09	-.34[f]	.09	.06	.13[d]	-.02	—				
8. Involvement	-.03	-.10	.35[f]	.08	.21[e]	-.13[d]	.12	—			
9. Support received	.04	-.29[f]	.21[e]	-.07	.15[d]	.15[d]	.37[f]	.41[f]	—		
10. Support provided	-.07	-.07	.17[d]	.03	.15[d]	-.19[e]	.33[f]	.36[f]	.38[f]	—	
11. Life satisfaction	.06	.00	-.01	.02	.11	-.31[f]	.12	.27[f]	.07	.12	—

[a]1 = male, 2 = female.
[b]1 = no children living at home, 2 = children living at home.
[c]1 = member of low-support congregation, 2 = member of high-support congregation.
[d]$p < .05$.
[e]$p < .01$.
[f]$p < .001$.

Table 2. Step R^2 and β from Hierarchical Multiple Regression
Analysis of Life Satisfaction for Members of High- and Low-
Support Congregations ($N = 162$)[a]

Variable sets	Step R^2	β
Demographics	.020	
Economic stress	.095[c]	−.41[c]
Setting	.013	
Economic stress × setting	.037[b]	
Economic stress × setting support contrast		.81[b]
Individual experience	.037[c]	
Involvement		.22[c]

[a] Occupational Status, Years in Congregation, Age, Sex, and Children Living at Home were the demographic variables entered simultaneously in Step 1. Setting main effect and interaction components were represented through two contrast coded variables entered simultaneously in Steps 3 and 4, respectively. Economic Stress by individual experience interaction components did not explain a significant amount of variance, when entered after the setting variables. Only significant betas from the final equation (with variables from all five steps entered) are listed.
[b] $p < .05$.
[c] $p < .001$.

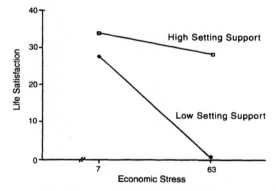

Figure 1. Regression of life satisfaction on economic stress for members of High Setting Support and Low Setting Support congregations.

Cohen & Cohen, 1975). High-stress individuals in the high-support churches reported greater life satisfaction than their counterparts in the low-support church. On the other hand, low-stress participants in the two types of settings were relatively similar on life satisfaction.

Independent of the influence of setting support, Involvement was significantly and positively related to life satisfaction, $\beta = 0.22, p < .001$. None of the Economic Stress × Individual Experience interactions explained additional significant variance in life satisfaction.

Secondary Analysis

To further examine the contributions of individual-level and setting-level variables to variance in life satisfaction, a second regression analysis was performed. For this analysis, the Individual Experience variables were made available for entrance first, with significant or near significant main or interactive effects entered. Next, the Setting Support interaction contrast was entered. Finally, all remaining main effect and interaction variables were forced to enter. A comparison of betas at different steps in the equation was used to identify Individual Experience variables whose variance overlapped with that of the Stress × Setting Support interaction, which was significant in the primary analysis.

The results indicate that, when entered prior to setting variables, the Stress × Support Received interaction, $\beta = 0.49, p < .09$, approached significance, and in the expected direction. When the Stress × Setting Support contrast was next entered, the Economic Stress × Support Received interaction was reduced substantially, $\beta = 0.32, p < .30$. This indicated some overlap of variance of the Support Received interaction with the Setting Support interaction. Finally, with all individual experience terms forced into the equation, the Stress × Setting Support interaction approached significance, $\beta = 0.72, p < .08$. Thus, independent of the entire set of individual experience variables, including the Stress × Support Received interaction, the Stress × Setting Support interaction accounted for a marginally significant amount of variance in life satisfaction.

Summary

The significant Stress × Setting Support interaction partially reflected the individual-level, Stress × Support Received interaction. On the other hand, the variance in life satisfaction explained by the Stress × Setting Support interaction was not fully accounted for by the individual experience variables. Thus, other mechanisms not tapped by the three individual experience variables included in the current study also appeared to be operative.

STUDY 2

Method

As part of a larger study on social support and organizational characteristics in mutual help groups (Maton, 1988), members of eight Compassionate Friends (bereaved parents) mutual help groups completed anonymous research questionnaires. All group leaders were told that the purpose of the study was to obtain information about members' experiences in the mutual help group and about members' current sense of well-being. The anonymous nature of the research instrument was described, as was a preferred research procedure in which the investigator would come to a meeting to describe the study, and members would complete the research forms at the start of the meeting. The groups were located in urban, suburban, and rural communities in an East Coast state.

Eight of nine groups contacted agreed to take part, and five of these eight agreed to the preferred procedure. In the other three groups, the investigator was not invited to the meeting, but each leader agreed to give out the forms to members. These members were asked to complete the forms at home and to mail them back to the investigator in a stamped, preaddressed envelope.

Of the 101 members at the eight meetings, 86 agreed to take part in the research, and 80 returned usable questionnaires (79% of the initial sample). The average age was 46.3 years, 61 were female and 19 male, all but one were white, and individuals who were employed primarily had jobs in white-collar or blue-collar occupations. Analyses revealed no significant differences on primary research variables between respondents from groups in which the investigator distributed forms versus those in which the group leaders distributed the forms. Reflecting the variations in group size, the research samples across the eight groups ranged from 5 to 26 individuals.

Measures

The Support Received and Support Provided measures focused on in-group emotional support and resulted from factor analysis of items designed by the investigator (see Maton, 1988). A representative item from the four-item Support Received scale is "Members regularly provide emotional support to me." A representative item from the five-item Support Provided scale is "I regularly provide emotional support to group members." The nine-item Group Cohesion subscale of the Group Environment Scale (Moos, Insel, & Humphrey, 1974) was included to assess an additional facet of perceived setting support. In addition, a scale to assess the development of friendships with group members was generated from factor analysis. A representative item from this five-item scale is "I have developed a close friendship with another group member." Finally, since a setting-level measure of Role Differentiation, designed by the investigator, was related to well-being in the larger mutual help group study (Maton, 1988), this scale was included in the current study. A representative item from this five-item scale is "Different members are in charge of different aspects of group functioning." All items were assessed on five-point Likert-type scales.

Cronbach alphas for the five scales ranged from 0.70 to 0.75. Some evidence for the construct validity of these measures is present in the meaningful patterns of relationships obtained in the previous research (Maton, 1988).

Bereavement stress was operationalized in terms of the recency of the death of the child, assessed in months. Many parents in Compassionate Friends groups maintain involvement for extensive periods of time, often to help others, long past the first years of intense grieving. Consistent with life stress research, it was assumed that the more recent the death, the greater the level of life stress. Bereavement stress in the sample ranged from a high of 3 months to a low of 276 months, with a median of 36 months.

Depression was assessed by the 10-item depression scale of the Hopkins Symptom Checklist (Derogatis, Lipman, Rickels, Uhlenhuth, & Covi, 1974). Self-esteem was assessed with Bachman and O'Malley's (1977) adaptation of Rosenberg's (1965) 10-item self-esteem measure. Each of these criterion measures has established reliability and validity. For ease of administration during group meetings, the depression and self-esteem items were answered on the same five-point Likert-type scales as the support items.

Demographic information included sex, age, and SES.[4] Hollingshead's (1957) two-factor index was used to calculate SES.

Results

High- versus Low-Support Groups

One-way analyses of variance indicated significant differences across mutual help groups on Cohesion, $F(7, 72) = 2.52$, $p < .05$, and Role Differentiation, $F(7, 72) = 4.42$, $p < .001$, but not for Support Received, Support Provided, or Friendship. A post-hoc analysis did not indicate differences across pairs of groups on Cohesion (Scheffé test). However, a comparison on the Cohesion variable between the four groups with higher means and the four groups with lower means was highly significant, contrast $t(72) = 3.65$, $p < .0001$. Given this highly significant finding on the Cohesion support variable, the four high Cohesion groups were designated as the High Setting Support groups in the current study.[5]

---

[4]Length of time in group was not included as a covariate since its high correlation with bereavement recency, $t(78) = .80, p < .0001$, indicated an extreme redundancy with the primary life stress measure.

[5]Given the theoretical assumption that settings that differ significantly on support indices differ in stress-buffering capacity, Cohesion was chosen as the key variable on which to differentiate high- and low-support settings. Cohesion differed significantly between groups, whereas the other indices of support did not. Of note, however, at the group level of analysis ($N = 8$ groups), Cohesion and Support Received were significantly related, $r = .72, p < .05$.

One-way analyses of variance with an a priori contrast comparing the four high- with the four low-support settings did not reveal significant differences on bereavement stress, sex, social class, support provided, support received, friendship, or self-esteem (although the results for social class and bereavement were marginally significant). However, the four groups high on Setting Support did contain members who were significantly older, contrast $t(73) = 2.33$, $p < .05$, and significantly less depressed, contrast $t(73) = -2.37, p < .05$.

Of special relevance for the stress-buffering hypothesis, subsample ANOVAs including only high-stress individuals (those above the median on bereavement stress) were performed. High-stress individuals in the four high-support groups reported significantly higher levels of Support Received, contrast $t(32) = 2.2$, $p < .05$, and marginally higher levels of Friendship, contrast $t(32) = 1.93$, $p < .065$, than high-stress members in the low-support groups. Finally, a full sample ANOVA revealed that the four high-support groups had significantly higher means on Role Differentiation, contrast $t(73) = 3.60$, $p < .001$, than the four low-support groups. Thus, the high-support groups were also high role differentiation groups.

Zero-Order Correlations

The zero-order correlations among variables are displayed in Table 3. Depression was inversely and significantly related to SES, Setting Support (membership in high-support settings), and Support Provided, and positively and significantly related to Gender (female), and Bereavement Stress. Self-esteem was positively and significantly related to Age, Support Received, Support Provided, Friendship, and perceptions of Cohesion. In addition, Self-esteem was positively and marginally related to Setting Support (membership in high support settings) and inversely and significantly related to Bereavement Stress.

Primary Analyses

Hierarchical multiple regression analyses comparable to those from Study 1 were performed, for depression and self-esteem separately. Age, Sex, and SES were the demographic variables, and Bereavement Stress was the life stress variable. Setting was contrast coded (seven orthogonal contrasts, with the one of interest contrasting the four high- versus the four low-support groups). Cohesion, Support Received, Support Provided, and Friendship represented the individual experience variables.

Table 4 presents the step R^2 and standardized regression weights (βs) for the primary analyses, with the setting variables entered first. As

Table 3. Correlation Matrix of Variables for Mutual Help Group Members ($N = 80$)

Variable	1	2	3	4	5	6	7	8	9	10	11	12
1. Sex[a]	—											
2. Age	-.19[e]	—										
3. SES	-.36[g]	.17	—									
4. Bereavement stress[c]	.13	-.42[g]	-.15	—								
5. Setting[d]	-.04	.34[g]	.23[g]	-.30[f]	—							
6. Support received	.15	.05	-.11	-.04	.09	—						
7. Support provided	.05	.24[f]	-.04	.33[g]	.06	.20[e]	—					
8. Friendship	.06	.08	-.20[e]	-.32[f]	.12	.32[f]	.28[f]	—				
9. Cohesion	.08	.21[e]	-.08	-.23[e]	.37[g]	.53[g]	.29[f]	.42[g]	—			
10. Role differentation	-.07	.18	.08	-.18	.39[g]	.21[e]	.14	.23[e]	.44[g]	—		
11. Depression	.25[f]	-.18	-.23[e]	.39[g]	-.20[e]	-.13	-.25[f]	-.15	-.14	-.10	—	
12. Self-esteem	-.14	.30[f]	.11	-.30[f]	.15	.22[e]	.37[g]	.27[f]	.28[f]	.11	-.71[g]	—

[a] 1 = male, 2 = female.
[b] Higher scores indicate higher SES.
[c] Higher scores indicate higher stress (i.e., the more recent the death).
[d] 1 = member of low-support group, 2 = member of high-support group.
[e] $p < .05$.
[f] $p < .01$.
[g] $p < .001$.

Table 4. Step R^2 and β from Hierarchical Multiple Regression Analysis of Depression and Self-Esteem for Members of High- and Low-Support Mutual Help Groups $(N = 80)^a$

Variable sets	Depression		Self-esteem	
	Step R^2 change	β	Step R^2 change	β
Demographics	.103^c		.100^c	
Bereavement stress	.114^d	.86^d	.036	
Setting	.095		.070	
Bereavement stress × setting	.201^b		.114	
Bereavement stress × setting support contrast		−.97^c		.89^b

^{a} Age, Sex, and Social Class were the demographic variables entered simultaneously in Step 1. Setting main effect and interaction components were represented through seven contrast coded variables entered simultaneously in Steps 3 and 4, respectively. Individual experience main effect and interaction components did not explain a significant amount of variance, when entered after the setting variables. Only significant betas from the final equation (with variables from all five steps entered) are listed.
$^b p < .06.$
$^c p < .05.$
$^d p < .01.$

expected, Bereavement Stress was significantly and positively related to depression, $\beta = 0.86$, $p < .01$. The Bereavement Stress × Setting Support interaction was significant and in the expected direction, $\beta = -0.97$, $p < .05$. Figure 2 depicts the differing slopes of the regression lines for the Stress × Setting Support interaction (following Cohen & Cohen, 1975). High-stress individuals in the high-support settings had lower depression than their high-stress counterparts in the low-support settings. Low-stress participants, on the other hand, had relatively similar levels of depression in high- and low-support settings. None of the individual experience main effects or interactions explained additional significant variance in well-being.

The relationship between Bereavement Stress and Self-esteem approached but did not achieve significance, $\beta = -0.21$, $p < .10$. Setting Support was not significantly related to Self-esteem, while the Bereavement Stress × Setting Support interaction was marginally significant and in the expected direction, $\beta = 0.89$, $p < .06$. None of the individual experience main effects or interactions explained a significant amount of remaining variance (although Friendship and Support Provided main effects approached significance, $ps < .10$).

Secondary Analyses

Two sets of secondary analyses were performed. First, as in Study 1, to further examine the contribution of individual-level and setting-level

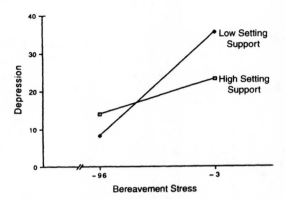

Figure 2. Regression of depression on bereavement stress for members of High Setting Support and Low Setting Support mutual help groups.

variables, the analyses were repeated with the individual experience variables entered first. For depression only, this analysis revealed a significant Bereavement Stress $\times$ Friendship interaction, $\beta = -1.23, p < .05$. When the Stress $\times$ Setting Support contrast was next entered, the Bereavement Stress $\times$ Friendship interaction was substantially reduced, $\beta = -0.55$, $p < .35$. This indicated a substantial overlap of variance of the Friendship interaction with the Setting Support interaction. Finally, with all individual experience terms forced into the equation, the Stress $\times$ Setting Support interaction continued to account for a marginally significant amount of variance in depression, $\beta = -0.82, p < .10$.

As noted above, members of the four High Setting Support groups reported higher levels of Role Differentiation along with the higher levels of Cohesion. In order to examine the combined influence of setting-level Role Differentiation and Cohesion on depression, an additional regression analysis was carried out. First, each individual was assigned their group's mean on predictor variables to yield Cohesion, Role Differentiation, Support Provided, Support Received, and Friendship group-level variables. Then, the group means on Cohesion and Role Differentiation were standardized and summed to yield a combined score for each group. This combined variable was entered along with Support Provided, Support Received, and Friendship. With all demographic variables and group-level interaction terms entered, the Life Stress by Cohesion/Role Differentiation interaction was highly significant, $\beta = -0.88, p < .005$. Further more, with all individual-level terms forced into the equation, the group-level, Life Stress $\times$ Cohesion/Role Differentiation interaction remained significant, $\beta = -0.89, p < .05$. Apparently, mutual help groups with the strongest stress-buffering potential had cumulatively higher levels of Cohesion and Role Differentiation.

Summary

The significant Stress × Setting Support interaction on depression partially reflected the individual level, Stress × Friendship interaction. On the other hand, the variance explained by the Stress × Setting Support interaction was not fully accounted for by the set of individual experience variables assessed. Other mechanisms not tapped by these four individual experience variables also appeared to be operative in the mutual help group context. At the setting level, the combination of high levels of Cohesion and Role Differentiation appeared responsible for the stress-buffering pattern of findings for depression.

STUDY 3

Method

As part of a larger study on stress and social support among the elderly (Williams & Maton, 1988), persons aged 65 or older attending senior centers were asked to participate in a structured research interview. Posters and signup tables were used to solicit participants at six senior centers. The centers were located in three metropolitan area counties adjacent to a large East Coast city.

Five trained undergraduates and one graduate student orally administered $1^{1}/_{2}$-hour to 2-hour structured interviews. Included in the interview were measures focused on life stress, social support at the center, center involvement, center cohesion, and personal well-being. Of 103 individuals interviewed, 18 were excluded because they were unable to complete all aspects of the interview (due primarily to insufficient time, or insufficient knowledge about the center due to very recent or limited involvement). The final sample comprised 85 individuals. There were no significant differences on demographic variables between those who completed and those who did not successfully complete the entire protocol. Reflecting the range in size across centers, the samples for individual centers ranged from 7 to 26.

The average age of the final sample was 73.3, 65% were female, 35% were married and living with spouses, the average SES was 41.1 (class III on Hollingshead's 5-class system), and the average length of center involvement was 4.3 years. One-way analyses of variance did not reveal significant differences across interviewers on any predictor or criterion variables.

Measures

The nine-item Cohesion subscale of the Group Environment Scale (Moos *et al.*, 1974) in slightly adapted form (the term group was changed to center) was used to assess setting-level perceptions of supportiveness. The four-item Support Received scale developed for Study 2, and the four-item Involvement scale developed for Study 1 were administered. Slight changes were made in the wording of items to make them applicable to senior centers. The Support Provided and Friendship scales used in Study 2 were also administered, with one item dropped from each scale due to lack of fit to the senior center context. All items were 5-point Likert-type scales. The alpha reliabilities of the five scales ranged from 0.72 (Friendship) to 0.87 (Cohesion).

Participants completed the 34-event Geriatric Schedule of Recent Experience (Amster & Krauss, 1974) for events during the past year. The scale is an adaptation of the Holmes and Rahe (1967) Social Readjustment Rating scale. Limitations of the scale are that it contains a number of positive events, and a large number of events that the individual may have caused (thus resulting in possible confounding with predictor and outcome variables). For primary analyses in the current study, five experienced geriatric professionals were asked to choose those negative major events on the scale unlikely to have been caused by the elderly individual. Full agreement was achieved on only three events: death of spouse, death of family member, and death of a close friend. The 57 individuals in the current study who had experienced one of these events were designated high on Bereavement Stress, and the other 28 individuals were designated low on Bereavement Stress.

Two criterion measures were included in the current study. One was the total mood disturbance score of the Profile of Mood States (POMS), a 65-adjective scale (McNair, Lorr, & Droppleman, 1981). The second was the six-item depression scale of the Brief Symptom Inventory (BSI; Derogatis & Spencer, 1982). These measures have established reliability and validity.

Demographic data included sex, age, current marital status, SES, and length of senior center involvement. SES was calculated using Hollingshead's (1957) two-factor index.

Results

High- versus Low-Support Senior Centers

One-way analyses of variance indicated marginally significant differences across senior centers on Cohesion, $F(5, 79) = 2.22, p < .06$. There were no differences on Support Received, Support Provided, Friendship, or Involvement. Although a post-hoc analysis did not indicate differences across pairs of centers on Cohesion (Scheffé test), a comparison on the Cohesion variable between the three centers with highest and lowest means was highly significant, contrast $t(79) = 2.92, p < .005$. Given this significant contrast on the Cohesion support variable, the three high Cohesion centers were designated as the High Setting Support centers in the current study. These three centers also had the three highest means on Support Received and Support Provided.

One-way analyses of variance with an a priori contrast comparing the high- versus low-support centers did not reveal significant differences on Age, Marital Status, Length of Involvement at Center, SES, Bereavement Stress, Support Provided, Support Received, Involvement, Friendship, or Depression. Marginally significant differences were found for Sex and Mood Disturbance. In contrast to Study 2, subsample ANOVAs including only high-bereavement stress individuals did not indicate any differences between high- and low-support settings on Support Received or Friendship.

Zero-Order Correlations

The zero-order correlations among variables are displayed in Table 5. Mood disturbance was inversely and significantly related to Setting Support (membership in high-support centers), Support Received, Support Provided, Friendship, Involvement, and perceptions of Cohesion. Depression was positively and significantly related to Bereavement Stress and (total) Life Event Stress, and inversely and significantly related to Support Provided, Friendship, Involvement, and perceptions of Cohesion.

Primary Analyses

Hierarchical multiple regression analyses comparable to those from Studies 1 and 2 were performed. Age, Sex, Marital Status, SES, and Length of Involvement at Center were demographic variables, and Bereavement Stress was the life stress variable. Setting was contrast coded (five orthogonal contrasts, with the one of interest contrasting the three high- versus the three low-support centers). Cohesion, Support Received, Support Provided, Friendship, and Involvement were the individual experience variables.

Table 6 presents the step R^2 and standardized regression weights (βs) for the primary regression analyses, with the Setting variables entered first. For mood disturbance, Bereavement Stress did not explain significant variance beyond the demographic variables, $\beta = 0.15$, ns. Setting Support was significantly related to the criterion variable in direct effect fashion, $\beta = -0.24$, $p < .05$. Members of the high-support centers reported significantly lower levels of mood disturbance. Independent of the setting variables, when tested individually Support Received, Support Provided, Friendship, and Involvement all had significant relationships in expected directions with mood disturbance. When these four variables were entered simultaneously as a set, a significant 14.6% of variance was explained, although none of the

Table 5. Correlation Matrix of Variables for Senior Center Members (N = 85)

Variable	1	2	3	4	5	6	7	8	9	10	11	12	13	14	15
1. Sex[a]	—														
2. Age	-.13	—													
3. SES[b]	-.10	.07	—												
4. Marital status[c]	-.23^f	-.32^h	.10	—											
5. Years in center	.24^f	.00	.01	-.06	—										
6. Bereavement stress[d]	-.08	.01	-.06	-.07	.13	—									
7. Event stress	.01	-.16	-.15	-.01	-.02	.41^h	—								
8. Setting support[e]	-.19^f	-.11	.06	.13	-.21^f	-.03	-.17	—							
9. Support received	.08	.20^f	-.00	-.22^f	.04	-.07	.02	.14	—						
10. Support provided	.22^f	.09	.04	-.15	-.04	-.19^f	-.03	.12	.65^h	—					
11. Friendship	.23^f	-.12	.01	-.00	.24^f	-.14	.05	-.12	.38^h	.48^h	—				
12. Involvement	.23^f	-.12	.00	-.21^f	.24^f	-.02	.03	-.10	.58^h	.54^h	.58^h	—			
13. Cohesion	.05	.04	-.06	-.09	-.07	-.16	-.15	.26^g	.63^h	.59^h	.32^h	.40^h	—		
14. Mood disturbance	.01	-.08	-.07	-.01	-.13	.13	.15	-.19^f	-.35^h	-.26^g	-.31^g	-.32^h	-.26^g	—	
15. Depression	-.07	.05	-.09	-.04	-.13	.21^f	.20^f	-.06	-.17	-.22^f	-.28^g	-.26^g	-.18^f	.67^h	—

[a] 1 = male, 2 = female.
[b] Higher scores indicate higher SES.
[c] 1 = not married or spouse no longer alive, 2 = married and living with spouse.
[d] 1 = no deaths during past year, 2 = death of family member or close friend.
[e] 1 = member of low-support center, 2 = member of high-support center.
[f] $p < .05$.
[g] $p < .01$.
[h] $p < .001$.

Table 6. Step R^2 and β from Hierarchical Multiple Regression Analysis of POMS-Total Mood Disturbance and BSI-Depression for Members of High- and Low-Support Senior Centers $(N = 85)^a$

Variable sets	POMS-Total mood disturbance		BSI-Depression	
	Step R^2 change	β	Step R^2 change	β
Demographics	.032		.030	
Bereavement stress	.023		$.046^b$	
Setting	.104		.058	
Setting support contrast		$-.24^b$		
Bereavement stress × setting	.068		.109	
Individual experience	$.146^c$		.062	

^{a} Age, Sex, Social Class, Marital Status, and Time in Senior Center were the demographic variables entered simultaneously in Step 1. Setting main effect and interaction components were represented through five contrast coded variables entered simultaneously in Steps 3 and 4, respectively. Involvement, Friendship, Support Received, and Support Provided each were related significantly to mood disturbance when tested individually in Step 5, and were entered simultaneously. Involvement and Friendship each were significantly related to depression when tested individually in Step 5, and were entered simultaneously. Only significant betas from the final equation (with variables from all five steps entered) are listed.
$^b p < .05.$
$^c p < .001.$

individual betas were significant. The Stress × Individual Experience interactions did not explain additional, significant variance.

For depression, neither the Setting Support main effect nor the Stress × Setting Support interaction were significant. Independent of the Setting variables, when entered individually, both Friendship, $\beta = -0.26$, $p < .05$, and Involvement, $\beta = -0.24$, $p < .05$ were significantly and inversely related to depression. When these two variables were entered simultaneously as a set, a marginally significant 6.2% of variance was explained, although neither of the individual betas were significant. None of the Stress × Individual Experience interactions, when tested individually, explained additional significant variance.

Secondary Analyses

Four sets of secondary analyses were performed. First, the relationship of individual-level Cohesion to mood disturbance was examined, since it did not explain variance independent of Setting Support in the primary analysis. When entered prior to Setting Support and the other individual experience variables, Cohesion was significantly related to mood disturbance, $\beta = -0.26, p < .025$. However, with Setting Support entered, the relationship dropped below significance, indicating an overlap of variance. Finally, with all individual experience terms forced into the equation, Setting Support continued to be significantly related to mood disturbance, $\beta = -0.25, p < .05$.

Second, to examine the relative contributions of group-level predictors to mood disturbance the regression analysis was repeated, with each individual assigned their center's mean on each predictor variable. Demographics and Life Stress were entered prior to the group-level predictor variables. Results indicated that group-level Cohesion, $\beta = -0.26, p < .05$, and group-level Support Received, $\beta = -0.24$, $p < .05$, were each significantly and inversely related to mood disturbance when tested individually. However, both betas dropped below significance when the variables were entered simultaneously, indicating that at the group level of analysis Cohesion and Support Received were highly interrelated components of setting support.

Third, the contributions of the Individual Experience interactions were further examined by making them available for entrance into the equation prior to the setting variables. For depression only, when Support Received and Support Provided interactions were entered simultaneously, a suppression effect occurred. That is, previously nonsignificant betas became significant or approached significance. Examination of the two interactions indicated that support receipt was positively related to well-being especially for recently bereaved individuals, whereas support provision was positively related to well-being especially for nonrecently bereaved individuals. When the set of setting-level main effect and interaction variables was entered, Support Provided and Support Received individual interaction betas dropped somewhat, with neither achieving significance.

Finally, the Stress × Setting Support interactions were examined using total Life Event scores (change magnitude scores across events), instead of Bereavement Stress, as the measure of life stress. Results indicated that the Life Stress × Setting Support interaction contrast again did not explain significant variance in either criterion variable.

Cross-Study Comparisons on Predictor Variables

T tests were performed to compare senior center members with mutual help group and congregational members on predictor measures, with appropriate steps taken where necessary to make the measures comparable. Senior center members reported significantly lower levels of Cohesion, $t(163) = -2.43, p < .05$, and of Support Received, $t(163) = -4.63, p < .01$, than members of mutual help groups, while there were no differences on Friendship or Support Provided. In addition, senior center members reported lower levels of Involvement than members of congregations, $t(245) = -13.52, p < .001$.

Summary

Setting Support was related to mood disturbance in main effect but not stress-buffering fashion. The Setting Support main effect may partially reflect individual perceptions of center cohesiveness. However, other mechanisms responsible not tapped by the set of individual experience variables also appeared to be operative. Finally, and unexpectedly, at the individual level of analysis, a suppression effect involving the Support Received and Support Provided interactions emerged for the depression criterion.

DISCUSSION

The results of the three studies, taken together, underscore the potential importance of highly supportive community settings for member well-being. Congregational members high on economic stress reported greater well-being in high tangible support than low tangible support congregations. Members low on economic stress, on the other hand, had comparable levels of well-being in high- and low-support congregations. Recently bereaved parents reported greater well-being in high cohesion than low cohesion mutual help groups. Nonrecently bereaved parents, on the other hand, had comparable levels of well-being in high and low cohesion groups. For senior centers, setting support was positively related to member well-being in high and low cohesion groups. For senior centers, setting support was positively related to member well-being, independent of member life stress level. The individual experience variables potentially responsible for linking setting-level support to individual well-being appeared to differ across the three types of community settings. The findings for each type of community setting are discussed below.

High-Support Congregations

The stress-buffering pattern of findings at the congregational level may reflect in part the capability of tangible aid from church members to buffer the deleterious effects of economic stress. Tangible aid receipt may enhance life satisfaction by reducing material deprivation and psychological strain for the financially stressed. In a supportive church context, tangible aid receipt may also contribute to well-being by engendering positive feelings of security in and belonging to a larger, caring community.

The higher levels of tangible support recieved by highly stressed members of the high-support congregations may have resulted from an emphasis in both settings on expressing religious commitment through reaching out to those in need, and on developing family-like relationships in the congregational context (Maton, 1986). These setting characteristics, encouraged by highly respected and influential leaders, appear to encourage high levels of formal (e.g., organized congregational tangible aid efforts) and informal (i.e., one-to-one) provision of support to those in need. In addition, these characteristics may have helped attract to each congregation members willing to provide (and perhaps receive) high levels of tangible aid.

Independent of tangible aid receipt, the results indicate that additional unmeasured factors also appear to contribute to the stress-buffering pattern of findings. One likely candidate may be the experience of higher levels of "spiritual support" among members in the high-support congregations. Spiritual support has been defined as support perceived from a personal, loving, and caring God (Maton, 1989). The Fellowship and Assembly of God congregations had as primary goals facilitating highly personal, intimate relationships between members and God, a setting characteristic not as salient in the low-support congregation (Maton, 1986). Perceived spiritual support may have provided members with hope, acceptance, and the belief that God's support was available, and thus enhanced the well-being of individuals facing high levels of economic stress.

Another possible stress-buffering mechanism may be greater levels of meaningful role responsibility in the two high-support churches. For instance, the Fellowship congregation was composed of five "house churches"—semiautonomous settings with ongoing religious and social functions requiring substantive member input and role contributions (Maton, 1986). The low-support congregation, with a more traditional, centralized organizational structure, likely had much lower levels of meaningful role opportunity. Meaningful roles may serve as moderators of economic stress by providing an alternate source of meaning, activity, and life satisfaction. Future research is necessary to directly examine these and other possible stress-buffering mechanisms, and their organizational ecologies, in samples of high- and low-support churches.

Mutual Help Groups

The stress-buffering pattern of findings for mutual help groups may reflect in part the capability of friendships developed with other group member to buffer the deleterious effects of recent death of a child. Friendship development for recently bereaved parents may contribute to well-being through the mutual sharing of experience, support, coping strategies, and companionship, all serving in part as antidotes to intense grief. Since Compassionate Friends groups meet only once per month, the extramural friendships developed may be a primary means of support in the daily lives of parents. The current findings are consistent with those of

Lieberman and Videka-Sherman (1985), who in a study of THEOS mutual help groups for widows found that higher levels of extramural "social linkage" differentiated mutual help group members who did and did not benefit from group involvement.

At the setting level of analysis, a number of characteristics of the high-support groups may have contributed to the stress-buffering pattern of findings. One potentially important setting variable is setting cohesion. The significantly higher levels of group cohesion in the high-support groups may have enhanced sharing, openness, and trust among members, factors likely to increase the potential for friendship development for recently bereaved individuals.

A second potentially important setting variable is the presence of widespread member participation in meaningful roles in the group. Participation in varied roles may enhance friendship development by facilitating collaborative interaction among members. In addition, meaningful role involvement may function directly as a stress-buffer by providing a source of meaning, activity, and esteem for highly stressed individuals. The strong, stress-buffering pattern of findings for a combined measure of role differentiation and cohesion underscores the potential importance of the combination of role differentiation and cohesion in the mutual help group context.

A third potentially important setting variable is the proportion of "veteran" to newer bereaved parents in a group. An average of 51% of the members in the high-support groups had been involved 3 years or more, versus an average of only 32% in the low-support groups. Group veterans may be better able to provide support and to directly encourage and facilitate friendship development among newer members. In addition, groups with more veterans contributing to group development may be more likely to achieve and maintain higher levels of cohesion and role differentiation.

Senior Centers

A stress-buffering relationship between setting support and well-being was not found for senior centers. Furthermore, subsample ANOVAs for highly stressed members did not reveal significant differences across centers on support received, friendship, support provided, or involvement. One possible explanation for these findings is that the organizational nature of senior centers does not provide a capability for marshalling higher levels of support resources to the highly stressed. The primary organizational goals of providing leisure activities and general service programs (Lowy, 1985) may limit the capability of centers to channel support towards members most in need. Furthermore, the cross-study findings of significantly lower levels of cohesion, support receipt, and involvement in senior centers than in mutual help groups and/or congregations may partially reflect limitations in the capability of senior centers to generate distinctly stress-buffering support resources.

Members of high-support centers reported significantly lower levels of mood disturbance than members of low-support centers. Cohen and Wills (1985) proposed that main effect rather than stress-buffering findings emerge when social integrative, rather than life stress specific, support resources are operative and assessed. Thus, it may be that high-support centers provided higher levels of social integration for members, a process reflected in the senior center context by higher levels of perceived cohesion. The higher levels of perceived cohesion may have stemmed from the nature of setting activities, the abilities and interpersonal attributes of setting staff, setting resources and attractiveness, or from other setting features.

Alternative explanations of the setting-level findings include the possibility that elderly persons with lower mood disturbance more often chose to attend high-support centers, or were more likely to perceive cohesiveness or social integration than higher mood disturbance individuals. In addition, the small sample of centers, and the small samples within settings may have unduly limited variance on key stress-buffering variables, or rendered statistical power too low to detect stress-buffering differences across centers. Finally, the support measures, initially developed for use in the mutual help group context, may not have been adequate for assessing aggregate setting support in the senior center context.

Unexpectedly, a suppression effect emerged for the support provided and support received interactions with stress at the individual level of analysis. Concerning the stress-buffering hypothesis, these findings suggest that a stress-buffering influence of support receipt may sometimes be masked by support providing. Additional research is necessary to replicate the suppression interaction finding and to examine the types of populations, life stressors, and setting conditions under which it may be manifest.

Limitations and Implications for Future Work

While the results of the current research suggest that setting-level factors may influence individual well-being, several aspects of the research limit the conclusions that can be drawn. First, the cross-sectional nature of the research leaves open the possibility of reverse causality and third-variable explanations of findings. For instance, it is possible that individuals with greater well-being, or better skills for coping with stress, were more likely to join settings high on setting support, or more likely to facilitate the development of highly supportive settings.

Second, the psychometric properties of the aggregate support measures need to be more fully established. To the extent factors such as individual

experience or personal well-being systematically biased perceptions of setting support, the validity of measures and findings may be threatened. Also,
the proportion of respondents to total setting membership was small in a
number of the settings, possibly limiting the validity of the aggregated
measures. Future research will benefit from measures of setting support
and cohesion not based on individual member perceptions, or from the use
of separate samples of individuals to complete setting-level and individual-
level measures (Rousseau, 1985).

Third, different measures of stress and support were used in the three
different studies, limiting any conclusions about differences in findings
across studies. In addition, whereas the support provided and received
measures differentiated significantly among congregations, the cohesion
measure differentiated among mutual help groups, and among senior centers. Future, comparative setting research will benefit from the development of multidimensional measures of life stress and setting-based support
relevant to diverse populations and settings.

Finally, the number of settings in each study was small, and the settings
studied were not randomly sampled from a larger universe of settings.
Future research based on longitudinal designs, using multiple sources of
individual and setting data, and including larger, representative samples of
settings and of individuals within settings is necessary to further establish
the meaning, robustness, and generalizability of findings.

The limitations notwithstanding, the findings of the three studies,
taken together, suggest important new directions for community psychology research and action. The potential of the community setting as a life
stress-buffer and the relevance of cross-level designs for stress-buffering
research have been demonstrated. At the individual level of analysis, different social support variables appear to be important in different types of settings; future research should continue to look for differences across types of
settings in the contributions of these, and other variables (e.g., meaningful
role involvement). At the setting level of analysis, examination of the
processes through which cohesion, role differentiation, and other organizational variables facilitate adaptive individual level resources and processes
is sorely needed. In this regard, organizational theorists have proposed conceptual models for understanding diverse community settings (e.g., Katz &
Kahn, 1978; Medvene, 1985; Moos & Lemke, 1984; Pargament et al., 1983;
Prestby & Wanderman, 1985; Sarason, 1982). Careful review of the available organizational literatures will help generate additional organizational
variables to be examined in future research. Based on the knowledge developed in such research, an expanded focus on programs and policies to
enhance the preventive (i.e., stress-buffering) and empowerment potential
of community settings should naturally follow.

ACKNOWLEDGMENTS

The author is very grateful to Beth Shinn, Chris Keys, Marc Zimmerman, and the three anonymous reviewers for useful feedback on this manuscript.

REFERENCES

Amster, L. E. & Krauss, H. H. (1974). The relationship between life crises and mental deterioration in old age. *International Journal of Aging and Human Development, 5*, 51–55.

Bachman, J. G. & O'Malley, P. M. (1977). Self-esteem in young men: A longitudinal analysis of the impact of educational and occupational attainment. *Journal of Personality and Social Psychology, 35*, 365–380.

Cohen, J. & Cohen, P. (1975). *Applied multiple regression/correlation analysis for the behavioral sciences*. Hillsdale, NJ: Erlbaum.

Cohen, S. & Wills, T. A. (1985). Stress, social support, and the buffering hypothesis. *Psychological Bulletin, 98*, 310–357.

Cronkite, R., Moos, R. H., & Finney, J. (1983). The context of adaptation: An integrative perspective on community and treatment environments. In W. A. O'Connor & B. Lubin (Eds.), *Ecological models: Applications to clinical and community mental health*. New York: Wiley.

Derogatis, L. R., Lipman, R. S., Rickels, K., Uhlenhuth, E. H., & Covi, L. (1974). The Hopkins Symptom Checklist (HSCL): A measure of primary symptom dimensions. In P. Pichot (Ed.), *Psychological measurements in psychopharmacology*. Basel, Switzerland: Karger.

Derogatis, L. R. & Spencer, P. M. (1982). *The brief symptom inventory (BSI): Administration, scoring and procedures*.

Fichter, J. *Religion and pain*. New York: Crossroad.

Gelfand, D. E. (1984). *The aging network: Programs and services* (3rd ed.). New York: Springer.

Giamartino, G. A. & Wandersman, A. (1983). Organizational climate correlates of viable urban block associations. *American Journal of Community Psychology, 11*, 529–541.

Holahan, C. J. & Moos, R. H. (1981). Social support and psychological distress: A longitudinal analysis. *Journal of Abnormal Psychology, 90*, 365–370.

Hollingshead, A. B. (1957). *Two-factor index of social position*. Unpublished manuscript, Yale University, New Haven, CT.

Holmes, T. H. & Rahe, R. H. (1967). The social readjustment scale. *Journal of Psychosomatic Research, 11*, 213–218.

Jacquet, C. H. (Ed.). (1984). *Yearbook of American and Canadian churches*. Nashville: Abingdon.

Katz, D. & Kahn, R. L. (1978). *The social psychology of organizations* (2nd ed.). New York: Wiley.

Keys, C. B. & Frank, S. (1987). Community psychology and the study of organizations: A reciprocal relationship. *American Journal of Community Psychology, 15*, 239–251.

Levy, L. H. (1976). Self-help groups: Types and psychological processes. *Journal of Applied Behavioral Science, 12*, 310–322.

Lieberman, M. A. & Videka-Sherman, L. (1985). The impact of self-help groups on the mental health of widows and widowers. *Archives of General Psychiatry, 42*, 658–683.

Lowy, L. (1985). Multipurpose senior centers. In A. Monk (Ed.), *Handbook of gerontological services* (pp. 274–300). New York: Van Nostrand Reinhold.

McNair, D. M., Lorr, M., & Droppleman, L. F. (1981). *Profile of mood states manual*. San Diego: Educational and Industrial Testing Service.

Maton, K. I. (1986). *Economic sharing among members of a religious fellowship: Patterns and psychological correlates.* Unpublished doctoral dissertation, University of Illinois at Urbana-Champaign.

Maton, K. I. (1987). Patterns and psychological correlates of material support within a religious setting: The bidirectional support hypothesis. *American Journal of Community Psychology, 15,* 185–207.

Maton, K. I. (1988). Social support, organizational characteristics, psychological well-being and group appraisal in three self-help group populations. *American Journal of Community Psychology, 16,* 53–77.

Maton, K. I. (1989). *The contributory, strengths, bidirectional corrective: Towards role enhancement, strengthened community settings, and cultural multiplicity.* Manuscript submitted for publication.

Maton, K. I. (1989). The stress-buffering role of spiritual support: Cross-sectional and prospective investigations. *Journal for the Scientific Study of Religion, 28,* 310–323.

Maton, K. I. & Pargament, K. I. (1987). Roles of religion in prevention and promotion. In L. A. Jason, R. D. Felner, R. Hess, & J. N. Mortisugu (Eds.), *Prevention: Toward a multidisciplinary approach* (pp. 161–206). New York: Haworth.

Maton, K. I. & Rappaport, J. (1984). Empowerment in a religious setting: A multivariate investigation. *Prevention in Human Services, 3,* 37–72.

Medvene, L. (1985). An organizational theory of self-help groups. *Social Policy, 15,* 35–37.

Moos, R. J., Insel, P. M., & Humphrey, B. (1974). *Preliminary manual for family environment scale, work environment scale, and group environment scale.* Palo Alto, CA: Consulting Psychologists Press.

Moos, R. H. & Lemke, S. (1984). Supportive residential settings for older people. In I. Altman, M. P. Lawton, & J. F. Wohlwill (Eds.), *Elderly people and the environment* (pp. 159–190). New York: Plenum Press.

Moos, R. H. & Moos, B. S. (1983). Adaptation and the quality of life in work and family settings. *Journal of Community Psychology, 11,* 158–170.

Moos, R. H., Shelton, R., & Petty, C. (1973). Perceived ward climate and treatment outcome. *Journal of Abnormal Psychology, 82,* 291–298.

Moos, R. H. & Van Dort, B. (1979). Student physical symptoms and the social climate of college living groups. *American Journal of Community Psychology, 7,* 31–43.

Nam, C. B. & Powers, M. G. (1968). Changes in the relative status level of workers in the United States, 1950–1960. *Social Forces, 47,* 158–170.

Pargament, K. I., Silverman, W., Johnson, S., Echemendia, R., & Snyder, S. (1983). The psychosocial climate of religious congregations. *American Journal of Community Psychology, 11,* 351–381.

Powell, T. J. (1987). *Self-help organizations and professional practice.* Silver Springs, MD.: National Association of Social Workers.

Prestby, J. E. & Wandersman, A. (1985). An empirical exploration of a framework of organizational viability: Maintaining block organizations. *Journal of Applied Behavioral Science, 21,* 287–305.

Rosenberg, M. (1965). *Society and the adolescent self-image.* Princeton, NJ: Princeton University Press.

Rousseau, D. M. (1985). Issues of level in organizational research: Multi-level and cross-level perspectives. *Research in Organizational Behavior, 7,* 1–37.

Sarason, S. B. (1982). *The culture of the school and the problem of change* (2nd ed.). Boston: Allyn & Bacon.

Shinn, M. (1987). Expanding community psychology's domain. *American Journal of Community Psychology, 15,* 555–573.

Shinn, M. (1990). Mixing and matching: Levels of conceptualization, measurement, and statistical analysis in community research. In P. H. Tolan, C. Keys, F. Chertok, & L. Jason (Eds.), *Researching community psychology: Integrating theories and methods* (pp. 111–126). Washington, DC: American Psychological Association.

Williams, V. G. & Maton, K. I. (1988). *Domains of life stress, directionality of social support, and well-being in the elderly.* Manuscript in preparation.

Withey, S. B. & Andrews (1976). *Social indicators of well-being: Americans' perceptions of life quality.* New York: Plenum Press.

13

The Impact of AIDS on a Gay Community: Changes in Sexual Behavior, Substance Use, and Mental Health

John L. Martin, Laura Dean, Marc Garcia, and William Hall

This report describes progress made to date on a study of the impact of the AIDS epidemic on the gay community of New York City. Using a model of the life stress process described by Barbara Dohrenwend and her colleagues, the AIDS epidemic was conceptualized as a community stressor resulting in two key stress-inducing events: death of loved ones due to AIDS and potential illness and death of oneself due to infection with human immunodeficiency virus (HIV). It was hypothesized that these stressors would be significantly related to three domains of health outcomes: sexual behavior, drug and alcohol use, and psychological distress. Descriptive trends over time are provided for both the health outcome variables and the stressor variables. Cross-sectional analyses for 3 years of data provide evidence in support of the main hypothesis. The implications of these findings are discussed from the standpoints of methodology, public health, and the psychology of stress processes in community settings.

Originally published in the *American Journal of Community Psychology, 17*(3) (1989): 269–293.

A Quarter Century of Community Psychology: Readings from the American Journal of Community Psychology, edited by Tracey A. Revenson *et al.* Kluwer Academic/Plenum Publishers, New York, 2002.

We use as a point of departure a general model of the life stress process which Barbara Dohrenwend and her collegues (B. S. Dohrenwend, 1978; B. S. Dohrenwend & Dohrenwend, 1981a) developed and articulated during the course of a decade of research. This model, shown in Figure 1, has received wide attention and was adopted as a heuristic guide by the Institute of Medicine panel on Stress and Life Events in 1981 (Elliot & Eisdorfer, 1982). Although this scheme is an oversimplification of a highly complex process of interrelationships and feedback loops, there are certain attributes of the model that were very useful in conceptualizing and organizing a study of the impact of the AIDS epidemic on the gay community of New York City.

First, the model explicitly provides for the measurement of the objective occurrence of life stressors, independent of individuals' reactions to those events (B. S. Dohrenwend, Dohrenwend, Dodson, & Shrout, 1984). Second, the model indicates that the influence of prior or extant environmental and personal factors on the occurrence of events must be considered and estimated (Brown & Harris, 1978, pp. 73–74; B. P. Dohrenwend, Link, Kern, Shrout, & Markowitz, 1988). Third, the model emphasizes the central role of mediating factors in determining the impact of life stressors (B. S. Dohrenwend & Dohrenwend, 1981b). Specifically, factors in the ongoing social situation, such as social supports or social burdens, and intrapersonal factors, such as self-esteem and mastery, play a critical role in

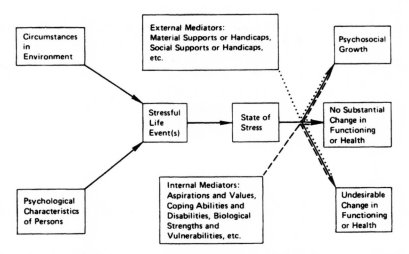

Figure 1. Model of life stress process. Adapted from B. S. Dohrenwend, 1978, *American Journal of Community Psychology, 6*, pp. 1–14.

the influence that stressors ultimately have on individual health. And fourth, the model includes not only decrements in health but also personal growth or health enhancement as possible consequences of life stressors (B. P. Dohrenwend *et al.*, 1982). Thus, the model can be fruitfully applied to adaptive as well as maladaptive human responses to environmental demands. Using this model as an organizing framework, we designed a longitudinal study of the impact of the AIDS epidemic on nonill but at-risk gay men. A major goal of the project has been to compare and evaluate specific components of the model, to determine the explanatory power of each with regard to health outcomes.

The three primary health outcomes of interest were sexual behavior, drug and alcohol use, and mental health. We expected to see an impact of the AIDS epidemic on substance-use patterns and sexual activity because these were the types of behaviors most intensively focused upon in risk-reduction literature aimed at controlling the epidemic (e.g., Bay Area Physicians for Human Rights, 1982; Berkowitz & Callen, 1983; Gay Men's Health Crisis Newsletter, 1982). Substance use and sexual activity were also behaviors that had been occurring at very high rates in particular segments of the gay community prior to the onset of the epidemic. Thus, there was room to observe a great deal of change, particularly in the direction of reductions in these behaviors.

The hypothesis that the AIDS epidemic would result in a major impact on mental health, however, was based on theoretical and empirical developments. We drew on findings derived from research on the nature and effects of stressful life events (B. S. Dohrenwend & Dohrenwend, 1974, 1978), human responses to natural and man-made disasters (B. P. Dohrenwend *et al.*, 1979; Erikson, 1976), the effects of social disorganization on mental health, (Leighton, 1955), and the central role of threat appraisal in stress responses (Lazarus, 1966). Drawing parallels between stressors studied from these perspectives and the AIDS epidemic, we reasoned that as the AIDS epidemic grew it would generate stressors capable of increasing the rate of mental disorders and psychological distress in those communities at high risk for the disease. In addition, since stressors capable of evoking mental distress might also be those same forces that influence other health-related outcomes, such as sexual behavior and substance use, findings from such a study could have both theoretical and practical implications.

It is important to note that the psychological stress of the AIDS epidemic is not, nor was it ever, equivalent for all gay men. Just as there is a definable risk gradient for AIDS illness within the gay community, which is best modeled by levels of receptive anal intercourse activity (Chmiel *et al.*, 1987; Kingsley *et al.*, 1987; Martin, García, & Beatrice, 1989; Mayer *et al.*, 1986; Moss *et al.*, 1987; Stevens *et al.*, 1986; Winkelstein, Lyman, & Padian, 1987), so is there systematic variation in the extent to which the AIDS epidemic is a stressor for the population of gay men. For some, the epidemic has destroyed their personal and social lives. For others, the epidemic has left them relatively unaffected. In order to operationalize and measure variation in the experience of AIDS-related stressors we focused on (a) bereavement of a lover and/or close friends due to AIDS (Martin, 1988a; Martin & Dean, 1989), and (b) the personal threat of developing AIDS which is brought about by knowledge of a positive HIV antibody test. (A positive HIV antibody test is generally accepted as evidence of infection with the virus that causes AIDS, and is considered by many to invariably result in morbidity and death [Institute of Medicine, 1988, pp. 35–36].)

Although the ultimate goal of this research program is to evaluate fully specified, interactive, longitudinal models of the processes leading from the experience of these stressors to various health outcomes, our first step has been more modest. That is, we have sought to establish the extent to which AIDS-related stressors impinge directly on mental health, sexual behavior, and substance-use patterns within the gay population. The purpose of this paper is to describe the progress we have made toward this end.

METHOD

Study Participant Selection

Since no sampling frame exists for enumerating gay and bisexual men we could neither draw a random sample of the community nor evaluate the sample for representativeness once it was drawn. Recognizing this limitation our goal was to generate a sample reflecting the diversity of the gay male population and avoid a narrow sample of convenience. Prespecified inclusion criteria were (a) New York City residency, (b) over 19 years of age, and (c) be a homosexual or bisexual male, defined as such by personal self-assessment. The only exclusion criterion was a diagnosis of AIDS.

The sample was recruited in early 1985 in multiple steps (Martin & Dean, 1985, 1990). First, a two-stage random probability sample was drawn of all members of gay organizations in New York City. Stratifying the 110 organizations by size (small: up to 50; medium: 51–100; and large: 100 or more), and by type (social, religious, athletic, cultural, political), half of the groups in each stratum were randomly selected to approach for assistance in subject recruitment. Due to the difficulty in recruiting black and Hispanic gay men into research programs, 100% of all groups whose membership consisted primarily of men of color were approached for assistance.

In response to this personal solicitation, 92% of the organizations we approached agreed to participate.

Having located organizations willing to participate, the head of each group was instructed to randomly select five group members to whom invitational materials would be mailed. These materials were compiled by the research team but were sent out by the group leader so that an individual's identity would not be revealed unless that person decided to enroll in the study. The response rate for this organization subsample was 76%; 131 respondents were obtained from this source.

We recruited additional respondents in less systematic ways through four other channels: (a) Face-to-face recruitment at the 1985 Gay Pride Festival ($n = 72$); (b) nurse-practitioner recruitment at a public health clinic serving young, low income, primarily heterosexual, individuals ($n = 15$); (c) enrollment of unsolicited volunteers who heard about our study and contacted us in order to participate ($n = 41$); and (d) referrals into the study through 23 pilot subjects who agreed to test the "snowball" recruitment procedures, as described below.

A total of 291 respondents were recruited directly by the research team from the above five sources. At the conclusion of the interview with each of these participants, interviewers requested respondents' cooperation in recruiting friends into the study. Each man was given recruitment materials to mail to three friends. Respondents were asked to avoid "prescreening" those friends selected for recruitment so that each individual could choose to enroll or decline enrollment on his own. This method of recruitment, through personal referrals, allowed us to penetrate gay social networks in New York City up to five generations removed from the original individuals recruited directly by us, the researchers, from the five original recruitment sources.

The final sample compiled in 1985 consisted of 746 men, 39% recruited directly though diverse community channels, and the remaining 61% recruited through snowball procedures. The data presented in this paper are based on the 624 members of the panel who have completed three annual interviews in 1985, 1986, and 1987. This represents a reinterview rate of 84% after 3 years. Adjusting for the 18 men who died during this study period, the overall response rate is 86%. A number of demographic characteristics of the panel are shown in Table 1. As of 1987, the cohort consisted primarily of well-educated men, averaging 38 years of age, with median annual incomes of $30,000 to $35,000 for 1986. Despite intensive recruitment efforts, only 10% of the cohort was black or Hispanic. Forty-two percent qualified for the operational definition of being coupled with a lover: (a) The respondent said he had a lover; (b) the lover viewed the

Table 1. Panel Sample Demographic Characteristics, 1987
(N = 624)

Demographic variable	Sample value
Age[a]	38.0 (8.7)
Years education[a]	16.5 (1.7)
Median income	$30–35K
Black or Hispanic race	10.9%
Formal religious affiliation	51.0%
Living alone	50.7%
Coupled with a lover[b]	43.1%
Father	6.2%
U.S. Veteran	13.3%

[a]Mean (*SD*).
[b]A respondent qualified as having a lover if (a) he said he had a lover, (b) his lover viewed him as his lover (reciprocity), (c) friends viewed the two as a couple (public recognition), (d) the relationship was extant for 6 months or more (duration).

respondent as his lover (reciprocity); (c) the couple's friends viewed the pair as a couple (public recognition); and (d) the relationship had been extant for 6 months or more (duration).

HIV Antibody Status

In addition to annual psychosocial data collected in face-to-face interviews, 45% (282) of the panel sample have also had blood samples assessed for HIV antibody, and a variety of hematological characteristics, on an annual basis. The fact that the blood study subsample was recruited from within the larger community sample allowed us to evaluate sample biases that may be operating in our own seroepidemiological study of HIV infection rates among gay men. To date, no significant differences on demographic variables have been found between the subsample of men enrolled in the blood study and those who declined enrollment. In addition no differences on sexual behavior variables known to increase the risk of HIV infection and AIDS (i.e., frequency of receptive anal intercourse and the number of different sexual partners) have been found between these two groups.

It should be noted that our recruitment efforts have generated a study group of gay men that is different from most other study groups (e.g., Joseph *et al.*, 1987; McKusick, Horstman, & Coates, 1985). Many findings published to date on gay men and AIDS are based on patients drawn either from sexually transmitted disease clinics (e.g., Darrow *et al.*, 1987; Mayer *et al.*, 1986) or private physician practices (e.g., Goedert *et al.*, 1984). Some of the most widely quoted epidemiologic findings are based on samples drawn from cohorts of gay men assembled in the latter half of the 1970s for the development of the Hepatitis B vaccine and subsequent efficacy trials (Stevens *et al.*, 1986). Thus, most conclusions to date have been based on samples consisting primarily of either highly visible, easily recruited, sexually active homosexuals and/or homosexuals experiencing a health problem at the time of study enrollment. Rarely are efforts made to either recruit additional subjects or adjust the sample in ways that emphasize healthy gay men or gay men who are more difficult to identify or contact.

Although these skews may not seriously affect internal comparisons (and indeed the large cohort samples have been extremely valuable in dating the introduction of HIV into the population), they may distort estimates of population characteristics on which the magnitude of the AIDS problem are based. One example of this problem is with regard to estimating HIV prevalence. While seroprevalence estimates by Jaffe and colleagues (Darrow *et al.*, 1987) indicate that about 70% of San Francisco gay men have antibody to HIV, and estimates by Stevens *et al.* (1986) put the seroprevalence rate in New York City at about 55 to 60% in 1986, our estimate of HIV seroprevalence among New York City gay men is 37% as of late 1986.[1] It is likely that this large discrepancy is due to the nature of the samples. Since the recruitment efforts in the present study were aimed at a more diverse cross-section of the gay community compared to other samples published, it may be that epidemiologic research to date has overestimated the prevalence of HIV infection within the larger homosexual population.

Data Collection Procedures

The interview schedule was developed over a 1-year period by combining extant measures where possible with newly created measures as needed. Domains of interest inquired into each year included demographic characteristics of the respondent and his lover (if he had one), relationship satisfaction, domestic and extradomestic sexual behavior, psychological distress, drug and alcohol use, AIDS-related fears, HIV antibody testing attitudes and experiences, methods of coping with the AIDS epidemic, knowledge and beliefs about AIDS, social network structure and function, availability and adequacy of social support, AIDS-related losses and illness in the social

---

[1] A total of 397 men were originally tested in early 1986, of whom 146 were HIV antibody positive. The rate of 37% remains constant when we restrict our calculation to the 282 men who were part of the panel sample as of late 1987.

network, bereavement reactions, professional service use, physical health and illness, and a number of personality characteristics (social desirability [Marlowe & Crowne, 1961], personal hardiness [Kobasa, 1979], health locus of control [Wallston *et al.*, 1978], sensation seeking [Zuckerman, 1979], and masculinity-femininity-androgyny [Bem, 1974]). Open-ended questions with tape-recorded responses were provided by respondents at prespecified points in the interview session. The majority of measures focus on the year prior to the interview as the time frame of interest.

Interviews lasted from 2 to 4 hours and were of consistent length each year. They were typically conducted in private in respondents' homes. The interviewing team consisted of both gay and nongay individuals and included 12 to 14 people per year, one third of whom were women. Written informed consent was obtained at each interview, in accordance with institutional and government guidelines.

RESULTS

Trends in Sexual Behavior, Substance Use, and Psychological Distress

The assessment of the impact of AIDS stressors on health outcomes is complicated by the fact that ongoing changes in sexual behavior, drug use, and mental health are taking place in the gay male population of New York City. Describing the extent and nature of these changes for the sample as a whole is important for both substantive and methodological reasons. The first half of this analysis provides descriptive data on trends over time in this cohort of gay men.

Sexual Behavior, 1981–1987

In the baseline interview conducted in 1985 we inquired about sexual activity not only in the year prior to the interview but also in the year prior to when the respondent first heard about AIDS. For most of the sample this date was easily recalled: July 1981. Test–retest studies conducted during the pilot work indicated that the reliability of these retrospective reports was adequate for use as a benchmark, or "pre-AIDS" reference point, against which to compare data derived from subsequent time periods (see Martin, 1986, 1987, for details of this procedure). Thus, the following descriptive trends in sexual behavior represent activity levels for yearly periods corresponding roughly to 1981, 1985, 1986, and 1987. Table 2 shows

Table 2. Percentage of Panel Sample ($N = 624$) Reporting
No Partners, One Partner, and Two or More Partners
During Four Years[a]

	Year			
Partners	1981	1985	1986	1987
None	2.7	3.0	5.0[b]	6.9[b]
One	8.1	14.0[c]	16.2	18.6
Two or more	90.2	83.0	78.8	74.5

[a]T tests for proportions comparing matched samples were used to test
differences between each yearly value and the value for the prior year:
1985 vs. 1981, 1986 vs. 1985, 1987 vs. 1986.
[b]$p < .05$.
[c]$p < .001$.

trends in sexual partner patterns from 1981 to 1987. For the pre-AIDS year
(1981) less than 3% of the cohort were celibate (i.e., no sexual contact with
another man). This proportion increased to approximately 7% in 1987, with
statistically significant increases occurring from 1985 to 1986, and 1986 to 1987.
More pronounced changes can be seen in the adoption of monogamy: in 1981
approximately 8% of the sample reported sexual contact with a single partner,
whereas in 1987 almost 19% had sex with a single partner. The statistically significant increase in monogamy occurred between 1981 and 1985, with more
gradual subsequent increases in 1986 and 1987. While the rates of celibacy and
monogamy have certainly increased, Table 2 also indicates that the majority of
gay men reported multiple partners in 1981 (90%) as well as 1987 (75%).

In order to assess sexual contact with anonymous partners, the frequency of use of extradomestic locations for sex (i.e., bathhouses, back
room bars and sex clubs, public places, and outdoors) were examined. While
the frequency of use of all types of locations declined over time, the largest
decrease occurred in the use of bathhouses: 50% of the sample attended a
bathhouse for sex at least once in 1981 whereas 8% did so in 1987
($p < .0001$).

Although sexual partner patterns are informative, the key aspect of
sexual behavior relevant to disease transmission involves specific sexual
acts. The frequency of engaging in specific sex acts as well as the percentage
of the sample abstaining from each act are informative.

The top half of Figure 2 shows the average number of episodes in
which each of 9 types of sexual activities were engaged in during each of the
four yearly periods. The reductions in mean frequency from 1981 to 1985
are all statistically significant (Martin, 1987). Using matched-pair t tests to
compare 1985 mean levels with 1987 mean levels, we found statistically

246

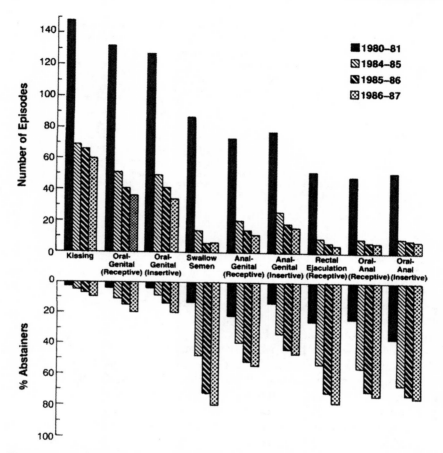

Figure 2. Mean frequency of engaging and percentage abstaining from specific sexual activities in the panel sample (*N* = 624) during 4 years.

significant declines in all nine types of sexual acts ($p < .001$). It is clear, however, that the magnitude of the declines is growing progressively smaller each year, as an asymptote in each distribution is reached. Such an asymptote is not so clearly defined in the distributions of abstainers shown in the lower half of Figure 2. The yearly increases in abstinence are statistically significant for each type of act ($p < .001$), and there does not yet appear to be a leveling off.

Two important points should be noted in Figure 2. First, as of 1987, over 50% of the sample had abstained for at least 1 year from receptive anal intercourse, whereas over 80% had abstained for at least 1 year from receiving a partner's ejaculate, either orally or rectally. Second, it is also clear that oral–genital sex is a highly preserved activity for gay men. Although abstinence from oral sex has increased over time, as of 1987 approximately 85% of the sample engaged in insertive or receptive oral sex at least once in the year. This finding demonstrates that, as a group, gay men discriminate sharply between sexual acts that carry a low risk of HIV infection (i.e., oral sex) from sexual acts that carry a high risk of HIV infection (i.e., anal intercourse). In addition, the differential changes demonstrated here indicate that investigations in this field must employ highly specific measures of sexual behavior. Global measures tapping sexual risk taking (see, for example, Martin, 1986; and Stall, McKusick, Wiley, Coates, & Ostrow, 1986) should be avoided in light of the distinct variability across types of sex acts shown in Figure 2.

Turning now to the question of risk taking during sex, we examined condom use during anal intercourse. Looking first at the percentage of the sample who engaged in receptive anal intercourse who reported "always" using a condom during this activity, we found an increase from 2% (9/490) in 1981 to 62% (176/283) in 1987 ($p < .0001$). A similar increase was also found in the frequency of consistent use of a condom during insertive anal intercourse: 2% (10/541) in 1981 compared with 58% (193/336) in 1987 ($p < .0001$).

Shifting the unit of analysis to the total number of anal intercourse episodes reported by the cohort in each yearly period, Figure 3 illustrates the percentage of condom-protected episodes (both insertive and receptive) occurring each year. It can be seen that protected episodes increased from less than 1% in 1981 to approximately 70% in 1987 ($p < .0001$).

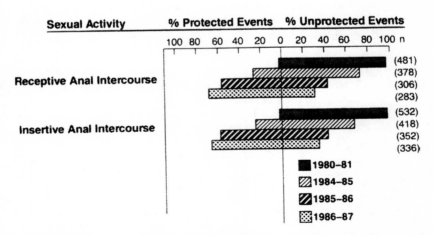

Figure 3. Proportion of condom protected and unprotected anal intercourse episodes during 4 years.

In order to determine the number of men in the sample conforming to public health risk reduction recommendations which call for either abstinence from anal intercourse or consistent condom use during intercourse we combined the data on abstainers with the data on consistent condom use. These results are shown in Table 3. It can be seen that as of 1987, 82.9% of the sample had avoided unprotected receptive anal intercourse either by abstinence or consistent condom use for at least 1 year; 77.1% had avoided unprotected insertive anal intercourse for that same time period.

These changes have clearly resulted in a public health payoff in terms of reduced rates of new HIV infections. Evidence linking behavior change with lowered incidence of infection was generated in two ways. Direct support for this conclusion comes from the observation that among the group of men who stopped engaging in receptive anal intercourse as of 1985, 22% (15/69) were HIV antibody positive. In contrast, among the group who did not stop engaging in receptive anal intercourse as of 1985, 48% (86/181) were HIV antibody positive. This represents a relative odds of 3.2, indicating that those who did not stop engaging in receptive anal intercourse were over three time more likely to be HIV positive in 1985 compared with those who did stop, $\chi^2(1) = 12.73$, $p < .001$. This protective effect of behavior change is even stronger among the 135 men who were most sexually active in the pre-AIDS year (i.e., 15 or more different sexual partners). Among those who stopped engaging in receptive anal intercourse 26% (9/34) were HIV positive. Among those who did not stop, 64% (64/101) were HIV positive (odds ratio = 5.0, $\chi^2[1] = 13.7$, $p < .001$).

The second type of evidence (which is indirect) indicating a public health payoff associated with behavior change is that in this cohort, we observed four incident seroconversions (indicative of new HIV infections among susceptible seronegative men) during a 6-month interval in 1986.

Table 3. Percentage of Panel Sample ($N = 624$) Who either Abstained from Anal Intercourse or Who Always Used a Condom with Anal Intercourse During Four Years[a]

Type of anal intercourse	Year			
	1981	1985	1986	1987
Receptive	22.9	49.0[b]	73.9[b]	82.9[b]
Insertive	14.9	43.4[b]	70.2[b]	77.1[b]

[a]T tests for proportions comparing matched samples were used to test differences between each yearly value and the value for the prior year: 1985 vs. 1981, 1986 vs. 1985, 1987 vs. 1986.
[b]$p < .001$.

This represents a half-year incidence rate of 1.6% (4/251) or 3.2% for the year. During the subsequent 12 months, we observed two incident seroconversions, representing an annual incidence rate of 0.8% (2/242), as of mid-1987. Thus, HIV infection rates have declined from over 10% per year in the early 1980s (Stevens et al., 1986), to 3% in 1986, to less than 1% in 1987.

From these figures it is quite clear that the epidemic of HIV infection in the gay community in New York City is beginning to come to a halt. Although there is not a 100% compliance with infection control guidelines in sexual behavior among gay men, the changes that have occurred have lead to a reduction in new infections to a level of 1% per year. It is crucial to note, however, that while the epidemic of new HIV infections among gay men is slowing, the incidence of new cases of AIDS illnesses continues to rise. Given a period of latency from the point of infection to significant clinical illness of 10 years or more (and the estimate continues to increase [see numerous abstracts from the IV International Conference on AIDS, Stockholm, Sweden, June 1988]), it is very likely that we will continue to see growing rates of new AIDS cases in the gay community for some time. With the continued lack of effective treatments for AIDS illnesses, the threat of this disease continues to loom for large numbers of gay men. In addition to fear of the disease itself, the social and emotional burden of helping those sick with AIDS through, what for most is, a consistent decline to death, takes a significant toll on those who survive this epidemic. Thus, it is appropriate to turn now to psychological aspects of this cohort, and examine patterns of alcohol use, drug use, and emotional distress.

Trends in Substance Use

Alcohol Abuse and Dependence, 1986–1987. Focusing on maladaptive behaviors that may be more prevalent among males, particularly when viewed as an expression of psychological distress (B. P. Dohrenwend & Dohrenwend, 1969, 1974), we attempted to measure diagnosable alcohol abuse and dependence disorders, using DSM-III (American Psychiatric Association, 1980) criteria. The Diagnostic Interview Schedule (DIS: Robins, Helzer, Croughan, & Ratcliff, 1981) section on alcoholism was included in the 1986 and 1987 versions of the interview. (See Martin & Hasin, 1990, for a detailed description of the method.) Using the standard algorithm developed by the St. Louis team, the prevalence of alcohol abuse and dependence disorders were calculated for this sample. Annual rates reported here are based on the date of the occurrence of the most recent symptom of abuse and/or dependence. The marginal values shown in Table 4 indicate that 12% of the sample met criteria for a DIS-DSM-III diagnosis of alcohol abuse or dependence in 1986. This figure dropped to less than 9% in 1987. The 2-year

Table 4. Prevalence and Incidence of DIS-DSM-III Alcohol Abuse
and Dependency among Panel Sample Members ($N = 624$) During
Two Years

Alcoholism dx. status, 1986	Alcoholism dx. Status, 1987					
	Absent		Present		Total	
	n	%	n	%	n	%
Absent	529	84.8	20	3.2	549	88.0
Present	39	6.2	36	5.8	75	12.0
Total	568	91.0	56	9.0	624	100.0

dynamics of the alcoholism diagnosis are also of interest. First, the figures in Table 4 suggest an annual incidence rate of 3.6% of new cases of DIS-DSM-III alcohol abuse or dependence among gay men. Second, approximately half of the 75 respondents who met criteria in 1986 failed to meet criteria in 1987. This finding suggests the occurrence of either (a) a remarkably high rate of remission among gay male alcoholics or (b) a problem in measurement whereby diagnostic criteria are too easily met. These data are currently under intensive study prior to conducting statistical significance tests. Although these data must be interpreted cautiously, it is clear that the types of problems associated with diagnosable alcoholism that are included in the DIS assessment instrument are not increasing in this sample. In fact, they appear to be decreasing.

Recreational Drug Use, 1981–1987. Another aspect of psychological distress may be reflected in the use of illicit drugs. Although injecting drugs is a primary risk factor for AIDS and HIV infection, only 9% of the sample had a history of injecting. More important, less than 1% reported ever sharing injection equipment. Thus, the primary interest has been in the use of noninjected drugs including marijuana, barbiturates, amphetamines, cocaine, opiates, hallucinogens, and inhaled nitrites. As with the measures of sexual behavior, the baseline interview in 1985 included a retrospective section on drug use behavior focused on the year prior to the AIDS epidemic. Thus, a benchmark, pre-AIDS year (1981), is available for comparison with 1985, 1986, and 1987. The trends in recreational drug use over these four yearly periods are shown in Figure 4. The top half of Figure 4 reflects the average number of days of drug use for each drug type, as well as for all drugs combined, for each of the 4 years. Statistically significant declines ($p < .0001$) were found for all drugs, from 1981 to 1985, except cocaine ($p < .07$) and opiates ($p < .10$). The lack of difference in cocaine use

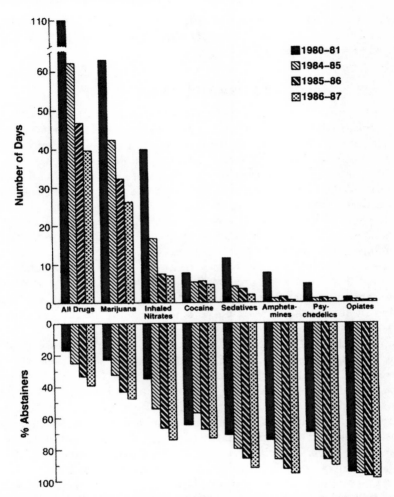

Figure 4. Mean number of days of use and percentage of abstainers in the panel sample ($N = 624$) for 4 years.

is due to the small decrease in use over time, while the lack of difference in opiate use is due to the rareness of use of opiates at all time periods in this sample. Comparing average use in 1981 with average use in 1987, Figure 4 shows a decline of over 80% in the use of inhaled nitrites, barbiturates, amphetamines, and hallucinogens. Marijuana use declined by 60% while cocaine use declined by 47% over the 6-year period. The lower half of Figure 4 indicates that many gay men abstain entirely from the use of specific drugs. Focusing on the summary measure, we found more than a doubling in the percentage of the sample that abstained from all drug use; 16% in 1981 compared with 39% in 1987.

Trends in Psychological Distress, 1985–1987

We borrowed a number of subscales from the Psychiatric Epidemiology Research Instrument (PERI: B. P. Dohrenwend, Shrout, Egri, & Mendelsohn, 1980) in order to measure various types of psychological distress symptoms. These included demoralization, sleep problems, guilt, and suicidal ideation. We also created a new measure of distress in an attempt to measure Post Traumatic Stress Response (PTSD: American Psychiatric Association, 1980) reactions to the AIDS epidemic. We modified items in the Impact of Event Scale (Horowitz, Wilner, & Alvarez, 1979), rewording them so as to be directly related to intrusive and avoidant thoughts and emotions about AIDS. Three additional items were added which contributed to the internal consistency reliability of the scale (alpha = .87). Although construct validation work remains to be done, the measure is quite sensitive to particular aspects of AIDS-related stressors and, as suggested by the findings presented here, it appears to be distinct from the measure of demoralization.

Using the PERI measures and the PTSD measure, psychological distress was assessed for 1985, 1986, and 1987. Table 5 shows mean levels of distress for the panel sample over a 3-year period. The trends shown in Table 5 for demoralization, sleep problems, guilt, and suicidal ideation indicate successive decreases in symptoms from 1985 to 1987. Statistically significant declines from 1985 to 1986, and again from 1986 to 1987, are shown for demoralization and guilt. Sleep problems declined significantly from 1986 to 1987, while suicidal ideation declined significantly from 1985 to 1986. In contrast to this pattern, stress response symptoms contained in the PTSD measure have increased on an annual basis. Although the changes from 1985 to 1986, and 1986 to 1987, are not statistically significant, the increase from 1985 to 1987 is significant ($p < .01$).

These results warrant further investigation as well as additional time points (which we are currently gathering). It is not clear at this time why depressive symptomatology of the kind tapped by the four PERI scales would be decreasing. However, the increases in PTSD-like symptoms may reflect the fact that progressively more gay men are experiencing AIDS-related stressors as the epidemic continues. We turn now to evidence that supports this proposition, and examine the relationships between AIDS-related stressors and health outcomes associated with psychological distress, drug use, and risk taking during sexual behavior.

**Table 5. Mean Levels of Psychological Distress for the Panel Sample ($N = 624$)
During Three Years[a]**

Psychological distress measure	Year					
	1985		1986		1987	
	M	SD	M	SD	M	SD
Demoralization	35.2	14.3	32.9[e]	13.6	31.8[e]	13.8
Sleep problems	4.2	2.6	4.1	2.5	3.9[c]	2.8
Guilt	4.8	3.0	4.4[e]	2.8	4.2[d]	2.8
Suicidal ideation	0.45	0.74	0.36[d]	0.66	0.37	0.67
PTSD	18.2	9.6	18.5	9.3	18.9[b]	9.5

[a]T tests for means comparing matched samples were used to test differences between each yearly
value and the value for the prior year: 1986 vs. 1985, 1987 vs. 1986.
[b]Increase from 1985 to 1987 is significant, $p < .01$.
[c]$p < .05$.
[d]$p < .01$.
[e]$p < .001$.

AIDS-Related Stressors and Health Outcomes

The following analyses represent an initial look at the longitudinal data on the associations between AIDS-related stressors (bereavement and knowledge of a positive HIV status) and sexual behavior, drug use, and psychological distress. Given the rapid changes that have characterized all aspects of the AIDS epidemic (scientific, medical, social, and political), we have approached the question cautiously and we have not attempted to model *changes* over time. Rather, using ordinary least squares regression models within each wave of data, the aim of these analyses was to determine the extent to which key associations between stressors and outcomes remained stable over time. Using results obtained from these cross-sectional analyses, we are in a better position to specify and test longitudinal models of the life stress process.

Before examining the relationships of bereavement and knowledge of being HIV positive on health outcomes, we first studied the variation in health outcomes associated with four specific demographic variables. Simultaneous regression equations were tested for 1985, 1986, and 1987, in which scores on the measures of PTSD, demoralization, drug use,[2]

[2]The summary drug use measure includes the frequency of use of illicit barbiturates, amphetamines, cocaine, and hallucinogens. We did not include marijuana or inhaled nitrites in this summary measure because each of these drugs has a distinct pattern of use and has been analyzed separately in previous research reports. See Martin (1988a).

unprotected receptive anal intercourse (RAI), and unprotected insertive anal intercourse (IAI), were each regressed on race, age, years education, and partner status. The results of these cross-sectional regression models are summarized in Table 6.

Examining the first column in Table 6 it can be seen that consistent effects associated with race were found only for PTSD symptoms. White respondents consistently reported more frequent and/or intense symptoms compared with black and Hispanic respondents. It can be seen in the second column of Table 6 that PTSD symptoms and drug use are related to age.

Table 6. Unstandardized Regression Coefficients (*SE*) Derived from Predicting Five Health Outcomes from Four Demographic Variables for Three Years (*N* = 624)[a]

Health outcome	Demographic variable			
	Race[b]	Age[c]	Education[c]	Partnered[d]
Posttraumatic stress				
1985	-3.30^g (1.24)	-0.12^g (0.04)	-0.21 (0.21)	-0.64 (0.79)
1986	-2.33^f (1.21)	-0.14^g (0.04)	-0.23 (0.21)	-1.55^f (0.76)
1987	-3.41^g (1.23)	-0.15^g (0.04)	-0.56^f (0.23)	1.60^f (0.77)
Demoralization				
1985	-1.45 (1.86)	-0.09 (0.07)	-0.86^g (0.32)	-3.17^g (1.18)
1986	-0.96 (1.76)	-0.01 (0.06)	-1.42^h (0.31)	-2.88^g (1.10)
1987	-1.75 (1.82)	-0.10 (0.06)	-1.09^g (0.33)	-1.97^e (1.14)
Unprotected RAI				
1985	0.03 (0.21)	-0.02^f (0.01)	-0.06^e (0.04)	0.76^h (0.13)
1986	0.14 (0.17)	-0.01 (0.01)	-0.03 (0.03)	0.64^h (0.11)
1987	0.13 (0.15)	-0.01 (0.01)	-0.02 (0.03)	0.52^h (0.09)
Unprotected IAI				
1985	0.22 (0.21)	0.01 (0.01)	-0.02 (0.04)	0.99^h (0.13)
1986	0.32 (0.19)	0.01 (0.01)	-0.06 (0.03)	0.85^h (0.12)
1987	0.19 (0.16)	0.01 (0.03)	-0.02 (0.03)	0.64^h (0.10)
Drug use				
1985	-0.27 (0.27)	-0.04^h (0.01)	0.02 (0.05)	-0.05 (0.17)
1986	-0.18 (0.26)	-0.03^h (0.01)	-0.01 (0.05)	-0.06 (0.16)
1987	-0.01 (0.24)	-0.02^g (0.01)	-0.04 (0.04)	-0.16 (0.15)

[a]The *F* test for each demographic variable was conducted after adjusting for the three other demographic variables (*df* = 1, 618).
[b]Black or Hispanic race = 1; white = 0.
[c]Continuous variable.
[d]Partnered with a lover = 1; single = 0.
[e]$p < .10$.
[f]$p < .05$.
[g]$p < .01$.
[h]$p < .001$.

For both of these variables the association is inverse, such that PTSD symptoms and drug use decrease as age increases.

The third column of Table 6 represents education. It can be seen that demoralization is the only variable consistently associated with years of education. This inverse association replicates prior work by the authors of the scale, showing consistently lower demoralization scores among the more highly educated (B. P. Dohrenwend et al., 1980).

The fourth column in Table 6 represents partner status in which single men are compared with partnered men. The results are complex and intriguing. Considering PTSD symptoms first, there appears to be fluctuation over time in the mean scores of partnered versus single men. However, since the effect sizes are small, it would be unwise to interpret these differences. A more consistent picture emerges with respect to demoralization. In each of the 3 years, partnered men have lower demoralization scores compared with single men. This effect, however, appears to be waning with time. It should be noted that this analysis does not take into account the incident couplings and breakups that occurred each year in the cohort (Martin, 1988b). Given the highly stressful nature of breakups, future work on the partner status–demoralization relationship over time will have to take these events into account.

The clearest and strongest associations shown in Table 6 involve the relationship between partner status and unprotected (insertive and receptive) anal intercourse or sexual risk taking. In each cross-section these results indicate that men who are in a primary relationship report significantly higher mean frequencies of unprotected intercourse compared with men who are single. This finding is important from a public health standpoint as well as a psychological standpoint: choices about risk seem to be clearly linked to the partner with whom one takes the risk.

Having established that demographic factors are important correlates of particular health outcomes, we turn now to examine the associations between AIDS-related stressors and those five health outcomes.

AIDS-Related Bereavement

The death of a lover or a close friend due to AIDS is becoming increasingly common among gay men. In 1981 the annual incidence of AIDS-related bereavement was less than 2%. By 1985 the noncumulative annual incidence had reached 18%. That figure continued to increase to 23% in 1987. These rates do not reflect the fact that of those who are bereaved, over one third have lost two or more close individuals within the same year. Some men have reported as many as six close losses in 1 year (Martin, 1988a) whereas others have been chronically bereaved of close loved ones for 3 or more consecutive years of the epidemic (Dean, Hall, & Martin, 1988). In addition, AIDS-related bereavement is not a random event in the gay population but is disproportionately concentrated among those aged 35 to 45, who are HIV antibody positive, and who have experienced one or more clinically significant signs of AIDS-related illness (Martin & Dean, 1989).

Knowledge of a Positive HIV Antibody Status

The second major AIDS-related stressor which is increasing in this cohort is knowledge of being HIV antibody positive. Such knowledge can be highly stressful because infection with HIV has serious health implications, not the least of which is a high likelihood of developing AIDS. A positive HIV antibody status is also believed to indicate infectiousness to others even in the absence of clinical symptoms of AIDS. In this cohort, 2% ($n = 13$) knew of their positive HIV status as of 1985, 6% ($n = 38$) knew as of 1986, and 9% ($n = 55$) knew as of 1987.

In order to evaluate the direct relationships between each of the AIDS-related stressors and the five health outcomes, the regression models used to test demographic effects were extended to include two additional predictors: (a) whether or not the respondent knew he was HIV antibody positive, and (b) the number of AIDS-related bereavements experienced by each respondent in the year prior to the interview. The results for each type of stressor are summarized in Table 7.

Looking first at the column summarizing bereavement results, it can be seen that there is a direct relationship between the frequency of losing someone close due to AIDS and symptoms of PTSD, demoralization, and illicit drug use. The demoralization effect disappears in 1986 but reappears in 1987 and is most likely the result of random error fluctuations. This irregularity is being studied. The link between illicit drug use and bereavement, which we reported previously (Martin, 1988a), appears to be growing weaker with time. In contrast to the indicators of psychological distress, the indicators of sexual risk taking (i.e., unprotected anal intercourse) do not appear to be consistently related to the frequency of experiencing bereavement.

The second column of Table 7 summarizes the cross-sectional associations between the five health outcomes and knowledge of a positive HIV status. These results indicate that there was no relationship between knowledge of a positive HIV status and any of the five health outcomes, for the small group who knew their status, in 1985. However, in 1986 and 1987 those who knew their positive HIV status had significantly elevated mean levels of PTSD symptoms and significantly elevated drug use scores compared with those who did not know their HIV status, positive or negative. No differences associated with knowing one's positive HIV status were

Table 7. Unstandardized Regression Coefficients *(SE)* Derived from
Predicting Five Health Outcomes from Bereavement and
Knowledge of being HIV Antibody Positive for Three Yearly
Periods $(N = 624)^a$

	Bereavement		Informed HIV antibody positive	
Health outcome	b	*SE*	b	*SE*
Posttraumatic stress				
1985	6.00^e	(0.76)	2.94	(2.54)
1986	1.83^e	(0.54)	4.78^d	(1.52)
1987	2.89^e	(0.56)	3.42^d	(1.28)
Demoralization				
1985	5.51^e	(1.18)	1.67	(3.92)
1986	0.37	(0.80)	2.11	(2.23)
1987	2.01^d	(0.84)	2.07	(1.93)
Drug use				
1985	0.53^d	(0.17)	0.94	(0.58)
1986	0.23^c	(0.11)	1.16^e	(0.33)
1987	0.20^b	(0.11)	0.93^e	(0.36)
Unprotected RAI				
1985	−0.10	(0.13)	0.49	(0.44)
1986	0.19^c	(0.08)	0.16	(0.22)
1987	0.04	(0.07)	0.23	(0.16)
Unprotected IAI				
1985	−0.13	(0.14)	0.14	(0.45)
1986	0.19^c	(0.09)	0.01	(0.24)
1987	−0.14	(0.07)	−0.02	(0.17)

^{a}The F tests for bereavement were conducted after adjusting for race, age, education,
lover status, and knowledge of being HIV antibody positive. The F tests for knowledge
of being HIV positive were conducted after adjusting for race, age, education, lover
status, and bereavement; $(df = 1, 617)$.
$^b p < .10.$
$^c p < .05.$
$^d p < .01.$
$^e p < .001.$

found for demoralization or frequency of unprotected anal intercourse
(either insertive or receptive).

SUMMARY AND DISCUSSION

The descriptive data presented in the first half of this paper indicate
that as a group gay men in this sample have undergone major changes in the
course of the AIDS epidemic. Sexual activity has decreased dramatically

while efforts aimed at reducing the risk of all types of disease transmission during sex have been incorporated into most gay men's sexual habits. Illicit drug use has become much less prevalent, and as of 1987 was largely limited to marijuana use. The rate of alcohol abuse and dependence appears to have declined, at the same time that depressive symptomatology involving demoralization, sleep problems, guilt, and suicidal ideation have also decreased. These trends suggest that, overall, the mental and physical health of the gay community of New York City may actually be improving as the AIDS epidemic progresses. Of course, such a conclusion applies only to those who are surviving the epidemic. Yet even among these survivors, there are important mental and physical health outcomes that are clearly tied to AIDS-related stressors and sociodemographic factors.

The one type of psychological distress that has increased from 1985 to 1987 for the sample as a whole has been PTSD-like symptoms associated with intrusive and avoidant thoughts and emotions about AIDS. This is also the particular type of psychological distress that appears to be most reactive to the AIDS-related stressors of bereavement and knowledge of a positive HIV antibody status. Since the occurrence of both of these stressors is increasing each year in this cohort, this may explain the differential increase in PTSD-like symptoms compared with decreases in depressive symptoms. Clearly, further work is required to disentangle these trends.

Considering the issue of either taking risk for oneself, or imposing a risk on one's partner, the lack of association between unprotected anal intercourse and knowledge of a positive HIV status was surprising. While it is premature to conclude that such knowledge has no effect on risk taking during sexual behavior, the present negative results certainly call into question the idea that HIV testing is a useful or efficacious public health intervention as a means of changing risky behavior among gay men. Indeed, more refined analyses of our own data to date indicate that knowledge of a positive HIV status may lead to increased tendency to engage in unprotected receptive anal intercourse (i.e., increased risk taking for oneself [Martin, 1988c]). In light of the extreme changes that have already occurred in sexual behavior patterns, the public health gains associated with HIV testing for the gay population as a whole may be quite small.

The one variable found to be a strong and consistent predictor of unprotected anal intercourse, in both receptive and insertive modes, was partner status. Gay men involved in a primary relationship engaged in higher risk sexual behavior more frequently than gay men who were single. Further work is needed to determine the elements of the primary relationship that may account for this differential. What is clear, however, is that unlike the early years of the epidemic, the more recent years are characterized by risk taking with known, intimate, primary partners, rather than anonymous partners contacted in extradomestic locations.

In conclusion, the results presented here indicate that AIDS-related bereavement and knowledge of a positive HIV status are directly related to increased psychological distress, particularly PTSD-like symptoms and illicit drug use. These stressors, however, do not appear to predict levels of risk-taking behavior during sex. The findings are consistent with prior work demonstrating that stressors and psychological distress are indeed significantly and directly related, but there are limitations with respect to the health outcomes we might expect to be directly influenced by stressors. Thus, it is also clear from these findings that there is a great deal more to learn about the pathways leading from the experience of stressors to various health outcomes.

The emphasis on mediating factors so central to the model of stress processes outlined by Barbara Dohrenwend, with which we began, is very well conceived. Our future work must focus on situational and personal characteristics that either sharpen or reduce the associations we have demonstrated between demographic factors, AIDS-related stressors, and deleterious health outcomes. Such a direction will not only lead us to theoretical advances in our understanding of the costs of adaptation to severe life stressors but also point the way toward effective interventions, prevention efforts, and therapeutic efforts.

ACKNOWLEDGMENTS

This research was supported by a grant from the National Institute of Mental Health (R01 MH39557) and by the New York City Department of Health. The authors thank Bruce Dohrenwend, Patrick Shrout, Mary Clare Lennon, Deborah Hasin, and Jennifer Kelsey for their consultation and advice on the collection and analyses of these data. We also acknowledge the support of Jennifer Ho for her expert administrative assistance on all aspects of the project. Most important of all, thanks to the men in the gay community for their continued involvement and support of this project.

REFERENCES

American Psychiatric Association. (1980). *Diagnostic and statistical manual of mental disorders* (3rd ed.). Washington, DC: Author.

Bay Area Physicians for Human Rights. (1982). Kaposi's sarcoma in gay men. San Francisco: Author.

Bem, S. L. (1974). The measurement of psychological androgyny. *Journal of Consulting and Clinical Psychology, 42,* 155–162.

Berkowitz, R. & Callen, M. (1983). How to have sex in an epidemic: One approach. New York: News From the Front Publications.

Brown, G. W. & Harris, T. (1978). *Social origins of depression.* New York: Free Press.

Chmiel, J. S., Detels, R., Kaslow, R. A., Van Raden, M., Kingsley, L. A., & Brookmeyer, R. (1987). Factors associated with prevalent human immunodeficiency virus (HIV) infection in the Multicenter AIDS cohort study. *American Journal of Epidemiology, 126,* 568–577.

Darrow, W. W., Echenberg, D F., Jaffe, H. W., O'Malley, P. M., Byers, R. H., Getchell, J. P., & Curran, J. W. (1987). Risk factors for human immunodeficiency virus (HIV) infections in homosexual men. *American Journal of Public Health, 77,* 479–483.

Dean, L., Hall, W., & Martin, J. L. (1988). Chronic and intermittent AIDS-related bereavement in a panel of homosexual men in New York City. *Journal of Palliative Care, 4,* 54–57.

Dohrenwend, B. P. & Dohrenwend, B. S. (1969). *Social status and psychological disorder: A causal inquiry.* New York: Wiley.

Dohrenwend, B. P. & Dohrenwend, B. S. (1974). Social and cultural influences on psychopathology. *Annual Review of Psychology, 25,* 417–452.

Dohrenwend, B. P., Dohrenwend, B. S., Kasl, S., Warheit, G. J., Bartlett, G. S., Goldsteen, R. L., Goldsteen, K., & Martin, J. L. (1979). *Report of the Public Health and Safety Task Force on behavioral effects to the President's Commission on the accident at Three Mile Island* (Stock #052-003-00732-1, pp. 257–308). Washington, DC: U.S. Government Printing Office.

Dohrenwend, B. P., Link, B. G., Kern, R., Shrout, P. E., & Markowitz, J. (1988). Measuring life events: The problem of variability within event categories. In B. Cooper (ed.), *Psychiatric epidemiology: Progress and prospects.* London: Croom Helm.

Dohrenwend, B. P., Pearlin, L., Clayton, P., Riley, M., Hamburg, B., Rose, R. M., & Dohrenwend, B. S., (1982). Report on stress and life events. In G. R. Elliot & C. Eisdorfer (Eds.), *Stress and human health: Analysis and implications of research* (pp. 55–80). New York: Springer.

Dohrenwend, B. P., Shrout, P. E., Egri, G., & Mendelsohn, F. S. (1980). Nonspecific psychological distress and other dimensions of psychopathology: Measures for use in the general population. *Archives of General Psychiatry, 37,* 1229–1236.

Dohrenwend, B. S. (1978). Social stress and community psychology. *American Journal of Community Psychology, 6,* 1–14.

Dohrenwend, B. S. & Dohrenwend, B. P. (1974). Overview and prospects for research on stressful life events. In B. S. Dohrenwend & B. P. Dohrenwend (Eds.), *Stressful life events: Their nature and effects* (pp. 313–331). New York: Wiley.

Dohrenwend, B. S. & Dohrenwend, B. P. (1978). Some issues in research on stressful life events. *Journal of Nervous and Mental Disease, 166,* 7–15.

Dohrenwend, B. S. & Dohrenwend, B. P. (1981a). Socioenvironmental factors, stress, and psychopathology. Part 2: Hypotheses about stress processes linking social class to various types of psychopathology. *American Journal of Community Psychology, 9,* 146–159.

Dohrenwend, B. S. & Dohrenwend, B. P. (1981b). Life stress and illness: Formulation of the issues. In B. S. Dohrenwend & B. P. Dohrenwend (Eds.), *Stressful life events and their contexts.* New York: Neale Watson Academic Publications.

Dohrenwend, B. S., Dohrenwend, B. P., Dodson, M., & Shrout, P. E. (1984). Symptoms, hassles, social supports and life events: The problem of confounded measures. *Journal of Abnormal Psychology, 93,* 222–230.

Elliot, G. R. & Eisdorfer, C. (Eds.). (1982). *Stress and human health: Analysis and implications of research.* New York: Springer.

Erikson, K. T., (1976). *Everything in its path: Destruction of community in the Buffalo Creek flood.* New York: Simon & Schuster.

Gay Men's Health Crisis. (1982). GMHC Newsletter, No. 1. New York: Author.

Goedert, J. J., Biggar, R. J., Winn, D. M., Greene, M. H., Mann, D. L., Gallo, R. C., Sarngadharan, M. G., Weiss, S. H., Grossman, R. J., Bodner, A. J., Strong, D. M., & Blattner, W. A. (1984).

Determinants of retrovirus (HTLV-III) antibody and immunodeficiency conditions in homosexual men. *Lancet, 1*, 711–715.

Horowitz, M. J., Wilner, N., & Alvarez, W. (1979). Impact of event scale: A study of subjective stress. *Psychosomatic Medicine, 41*, 209–218.

Institute of Medicine. (1988). *Confronting AIDS: Update 1988*. National Academy Press: Washington, DC.

Joseph, J. G., Montgomery, S. B., Emmons, C. A., Kessler, R. C., Ostrow, D. G., Wortman, C. B., O'Brien, K., Eller, M., & Eshleman, S. (1987). Magnitude and determinants of risk reduction: Longitudinal analysis of a cohort at risk for AIDS. *Psychological Health, 1*, 73–96.

Kingsley, L. A., Kaslow, R., Rinaldo, C. R. Jr., Detre, K., Odaka, N., Van Raden, M., Detels, R., Polk, B. F., Chmiel, J., Kelsey, S. F., Ostrow, D., & Visscher, B. (1987). Risk factors for seroconversion to human immunodeficiency virus among male homosexuals. *Lancet, 1*, 345–349.

Kobasa, S. C. (1979). Stressful life events, personality, and health: An inquiry into hardiness. *Journal of Personality and Social Psychology, 37*, 1–11.

Lazarus, R. S. (1966). *Psychological stress and the coping process*. New York: McGraw-Hill.

Leighton, A. H. (1955). Psychiatric disorder and the social environment: An outline for a frame of reference. *Psychiatry, 18*, 367–383.

Marlowe, D. & Crowne, D. F. (1961). Social desirability and response to perceived situational demands. *Journal of Consulting Psychology, 25*, 109–115.

Martin, J. L. (1986). AIDS risk reduction recommendations and sexual behavior patterns among gay men: A multifactorial categorical approach to assessing change. *Health Education Quarterly, 13*(4), 347–358.

Martin, J. L. (1987). The impact of AIDS on gay male sexual behavior patterns in New York City. *American Journal of Public Health, 77*, 578–581.

Martin, J. L. (1988a, August). *The role of the primary relationship in gay men's health*. Paper presented at the 96th annual conference of the American Psychological Association, Atlanta.

Martin, J. L. (1988b, June). *The influence of knowledge of HIV antibody status on subsequent sexual behavior patterns in a cohort of gay men*. Paper presented at the IV International Conference on AIDS, Stockholm, Sweden.

Martin, J. L, (1988c). Psychological consequences of AIDS-related bereavement among gay men. *Journal of Consulting and Clinical Psychology, 56*, 856–862.

Martin, J. L. & Dean, L. (1985, November). *The impact of AIDS on New York City gay men: Development of a community sample*. Paper presented at the 113th annual meeting of the American Public Health Association, Washington, DC.

Martin, J. L. & Dean, L. (1989). Risk factors for AIDS-related bereavement in a cohort of homosexul men in New York City. In B. Cooper & T. Helgason (Eds.), *Epidemiology and the prevention of mental disorders*. London: Routledge.

Martin, J. L. & Dean, L. (1990). Development of a community sample of gay men for an epidemiologic study of AIDS. *American Behavioral Scientist, 33*, 546–561.

Martin, J. L., Garcia, M. A., & Beatrice, S. (1989). Sexual behavior changes and HIV antibody in a cohort of New York City gay men. *American Journal of Public Health, 79*, 501–503.

Martin, J. L. & Hasin, D. S. (1990). Drinking, alcoholism, and sexual behavior. *Drugs and Society, 5*, 49–67.

Mayer, K. H., Ayotte, D., Groopman, J. E., Stoddard, A., Sarngadharan, M., & Gallo, R. (1986). Association of human T-lymphotropic virus type III antibodies with sexual and other behaviors in a cohort of homosexual men from Boston with and without generalized lymphadenopathy. *American Journal of Medicine, 80*, 357–363.

McKusick, L., Horstman, W., & Coates, T. J. (1985). AIDS and sexual behavior reported by gay men in San Francisco. *American Journal of Public Health*, 75, 493–496.

Moss, A. R., Osmond, D., Bacchetti, P., Chermann, J. C., Barre-Sinoussi, F., & Carlson, J. (1987). Risk factors for AIDS and HIV seropositivity in homosexual men. *American Journal of Epidemiology*, 125, 1035–1047.

Robins, L. N., Helzer, J. E., Croughan, J., & Ratcliff, K. S. (1981). National Institute of Mental Health Diagnostic Interview Schedule: Its history, characteristics and validity. *Archives of General Psychiatry*, 38, 381–389.

Stall, R., McKusick, L., Wiley, J., Coates, T. J., & Ostrow, D. G. (1986). Alcohol and drug use during sexual activity and compliance with safe sex guidelines for AIDS: The AIDS behavioral research project. *Health Education Quarterly*, 13, 359–371.

Stevens, C. E., Taylor, P. E., Zang, E. A., Morrison, J. M., Harley, E. J., de Cordoba, S. R., Bacino, C., Ting, R. C. Y., Bodner, A. J., Sarngadharan, M. G., Gallo, R. C., & Rubinstein, P. (1986). Human T-cell lymphotropic virus type III infection in a cohort of homosexual men in New York City. *Journal of the American Medical Association*, 265, 2267–2272.

Wallston, K. A., Wallston, B. S., & DeVellis, R. (1978). Development of the multidimensional health locus of control (MHCC) scales. *Health Education Monographs*, 6, 169–180.

Winkelstein, W. Jr., Lyman, D. M., & Padian, N. S. (1987). Sexual practices and risk of infection by the AIDS-associated retrovirus: The San Francisco Men's Health Study. *Journal of the American Medical Association*, 257, 321–325.

Zuckerman, M. (1979). *Sensation seeking: Beyond the optimal level of arousal*. Hillsdale NJ: Lawrence Erlbaum.

V

The 1990s

14

Sense of Community in the Urban Environment: A Catalyst for Participation and Community Development

David M. Chavis and Abraham Wandersman

Social programs need to identify catalysts for action which can be targeted in order to effectively and efficiently meet their goals. A model illustrates how a sense of community can have a catalytic effect on local action (i.e., participation in a block association) by affecting the perception of the environment, social relations, and one's perceived control and empowerment. The model is tested and confirmed through path-analytic and longitudinal techniques.

Solving problems through voluntary participation in local community institutions and organizations is an American tradition (Bellah, Madsen, Sullivan, Swidler, & Tripton; 1985), which is increasingly considered by contemporary policy analysts to be vital for effective urban service delivery (Rich, 1979), health promotion and disease prevention (Green, 1986), crime and drug abuse prevention (Curtis, 1987), welfare reform (Moynihan, 1986), and mental health service delivery (Naparstek, Beigel, & Spiro, 1982). It has been difficult to achieve precision in our empirical understanding of

Originally published in the *American Journal of Community Psychology*, *18*(1) (1990): 55–81.

A Quarter Century of Community Psychology: *Readings from the* American Journal of Community Psychology, edited by Tracey A. Revenson *et al.* Kluwer Academic/Plenum Publishers, New York, 2002.

this phenomenon and the process that occurs at the individual and community level.

Several types of communities have been identified by the social sciences: community as a place, community as relationships, and community as collective political power (Gusfield, 1975; Heller, 1989; Suttles, 1972). For all of these types of community, there exists a process for improving the quality of community life as portrayed in such terms as "community development," "community building," and "community organization." A central mechanism in this process is individuals' participation in voluntary organizations which produce collective and individual goods. These groups include neighborhood organizations, professional associations, self-help groups, churches, political parties, advocacy organizations, or unions.

Citizen participation in community organizations has been viewed as a major method for improving the quality of the physical environment, enhancing services, preventing crime, and improving social conditions (e.g., Ahlbrandt & Cunningham, 1979; Altshuler, 1970; Churchman, 1987; Florin, 1989; Hallman, 1974, 1984; Mayer, 1984; Morris & Hess, 1975; Perlman, 1976; Yates, 1973; Yin, 1977).

Sense of community is a phrase commonly used by citizens, politicians, and social scientists, to characterize the relationship between the individual and the social structure (e.g., having a sense of community or lacking a sense of community). This often-cited overarching value of community psychology (Sarason, 1974) has received relatively little theoretical or empirical attention until recently (e.g., McMillan & Chavis, 1986; Newbrough & Chavis, 1986a, 1986b).

In this article we empirically explore a model which posits that three important components influence an individual's participation in voluntary neighborhood organizations and that sense of community plays a catalytic role in mobilizing the three components. The three components are *the perception of the environment, one's social relations*, and *one's perceived control and empowerment within the community*.

The community development process is rooted within the context of the physical and social environment of the community. The community development process, as examined in this study, focuses on the development of human ecologies by empowering the community. The focus of this approach is a holistic one, concerned with the development of a community's human, economic, and environmental resources. The building of a sense of community acts as a mechanism to stimulate the healthy development of the environment and the people who inhabit it. Based on McMillan and Chavis' (1986) theoretical definition of sense of community, a community development process stimulates opportunities for membership, influence, mutual needs to be met, and shared emotional ties and support. The stronger the sense of community, the more influence the members will feel they have on their immediate environment (McMillan & Chavis, 1986). It is through this process that a sense of community can contribute to individual and community development. The relationship between a sense of community and community competence (its problem-solving ability) through collective effort is reciprocal.

Although there has been little empirical research within the community development literature relevant to these components, there is empirical support in the social sciences for the importance of each of the three components. In general, the literature on each component has been developed separately. We briefly review literature relevant to each of these three components.

PERCEPTION OF THE COMMUNITY ENVIRONMENT

Perception of the environment involves judgments about the environment (e.g., perceived qualities of the environment, satisfaction with the environment, problems in the environment). Judgments are made about the degree to which the environment or a specific aspect of the environment is positive or negative to the individual. If it is viewed negatively, it can lead to stress and/or arousal (Baum, Singer, & Baum, 1981; Wandersman, Andrews, Riddle, & Fancett, 1983). Literature reviews have concluded that, in general, there are substantive relationships between the qualities of the physical environment, the social environment (e.g., social interaction and sense of belonging), and residential satisfaction (e.g., Rohe, 1985; Taylor, 1982; Weidemann & Anderson, 1985). Negative signs in the environment (e.g., incivilities such as litter, abandoned cars, or gangs on the street) can lead to fear of crime, lower property values, and social withdrawal (Ahlbrandt & Cunningham, 1979; Lewis & Salem, 1981; Perkins, Florin, Rich, Wandersman, & Chavis, 1990; Skogan & Maxfield, 1981; Taylor, 1988). A sense of community or social cohesion has been found to moderate negative environmental factors such as crowding (Aiello & Baum, 1979; Freedman, 1975).

On the other hand, the perception of environmental problems can serve as a motivator to action. Most neighborhood organizations are formed as a response to the threat or reality of physical deterioration (Crenson, 1978; Lavrakas, 1980). Wandersman, Jakubs, and Giamartino (1981) found a curvilinear relationship between perception of environmental problems and individual participation in a block organization. The highest level of participation was among residents perceiving a moderate amount of problems on the block. Florin and Wandersman (1984) found that perception of the environment can influence an individual's participation in an organization formed to improve the community.

A sense of community is associated with the symbolic interaction that occurs through the use of the physical environment (Brower, 1980). For example, as people identify with their neighborhood, they personalize their homes which contributes to the development of common symbols (Brown, 1987; Taylor, 1988). Common symbols are a part of the membership component of a sense of community described by McMillan and Chavis (1986) (e.g., language, clothes, neighborhood name). Territorial markers and the creation of defensible space often deter neighborhood crime (Newman, 1972) which facilitates social interaction. This perception can lead to feelings of security, order, friendliness, etc. As residents feel safer and more secure in their community, they are likely to interact more with their neighbors, feel a greater sense of community, and have more incentive to participate.

SOCIAL RELATIONS

Social relations refers to the interactions among neighbors such as borrowing or lending tools, informal visiting, and asking for help in an emergency (Unger & Wandersman, 1985). Through this interaction, neighbors provide each other with emotional/personal, instrumental, and informational support.

When people feel a sense of community, they are more apt to interact with the residents in their neighborhood (Chavis, Hogge, McMillan, & Wandersman, 1986; Unger & Wandersman, 1982). At the same time, the positive face-to-face contact of neighboring continues to enhance the shared emotional connection that helps to maintain a sense of community (McMillan & Chavis, 1986).

The social network in a neighborhood develops, supports, and supplements the efforts of the neighborhood association by sharing information about the association, fostering the coproduction of services, such as sanitation and security, through informal social control (Rich, 1979). In general, residents who socially interact with their neighbors are more likely to be aware of local voluntary organizations and become members (Wandersman & Giamartino, 1980; Wandersman et al., 1981). This is particularly true for neighbors who have more friends in their neighborhood and close ties with neighbors whom they rely upon for socioemotional and instrumental support (Ahlbrandt & Cunningham, 1979; Hunter, 1974).

The presence of social networks within a neighborhood helps regulate social behavior through normative mechanisms called informal social control (cf. Merry, 1987). In an extensive review of the literature, Greenberg and Rohe (1986) concluded that while much more research needs to be done, there is evidence for a negative relationship between informal social control and crime rates. They suggested that neighborhood organizations can increase this form of social control.

PERCEIVED CONTROL AND EMPOWERMENT

The importance of the concepts of control and empowerment have been established in several areas of psychology including clinical psychology (Seligman, 1975), social psychology (Langer, 1983), environmental psychology (S. Cohen & Sherrod, 1978), and community psychology (Rappaport, 1981, 1987). Perceived control relates to the beliefs an individual has about the relationship between actions (behavior) and outcomes.

Florin applied a cognitive social learning approach to this phenomenon, whereby expectancies of individual and collective control were used to predict participation (Florin, Friedmann, Wandersman, & Meier, 1987; Florin & Wandersman, 1984). Individuals evaluate the likelihood that their own individual efforts (self-efficacy) or a group of people working together (collective efficacy) can solve a neighborhood problem (Bandura, 1986). This expectancy can influence behavior (e.g., participation in a block organization). Locus of control (generalized expectancies about outcomes being related to one's own actions or to luck, chance, or powerful others) has also been empirically related to participation (Abramowitz, 1974; Berck & Williams, 1980; Florin & Wandersman, 1984; Zimmerman & Rappaport, 1988). The results of research trying to link locus of control with participation have been inconsistent.

The areas of expectancy and control relate to both theory and research on empowerment (Rappaport, 1987; Zimmerman, 2000; Zimmerman & Rappaport, 1988). Empowerment is "a process by which individuals gain mastery or control over their own lives and democratic participation in the life of their community" (Zimmerman & Rappaport, 1988, p. 726). Zimmerman and Rappaport suggested that "participation may be an important mechanism for the development of psychological empowerment because participants can gain experience organizing people, identifying resources, and developing strategies for achieving goals" (p. 727).

A positive relationship between a sense of community and empowerment has been theoretically suggested (Chavis & Newbrough, 1986; Rappaport, 1977; 1987) but not fully established through research. Maton and Rappaport (1984) found that the development of a sense of community in a religious community was related to psychological empowerment. Bachrach and Zautra (1985) found a sense of community was positively related to "problem oriented coping" (taking action to solve the problem) when people are faced with an environmental problem.

A MODEL OF SENSE OF COMMUNITY AND PARTICIPATION IN A VOLUNTARY NEIGHBORHOOD ASSOCIATION

Our review of the literature indicates that a sense of community has been shown to be related to at least four domains of scientific investigation relevant to community development: the perception of the environment, social relations, control and empowerment, and participation in neighborhood action. We hypothesize that a sense of community acts as a catalyst for changes in these domains that promote the positive development of a community through participation in local voluntary associations. The purpose of this study was to empirically investigate a model of relations among these four domains (see Figure 1). This pattern of relations was derived from the research reviewed earlier. Local action, in this case one's level of participation in voluntary neighborhood associations (block, tenant, or civic associations) was considered the proximal variable because it is through these behaviors that actual ecological changes can occur. Perceptions of the environment, perceived and actual social relations, and a sense of individual and collective control interact to influence those

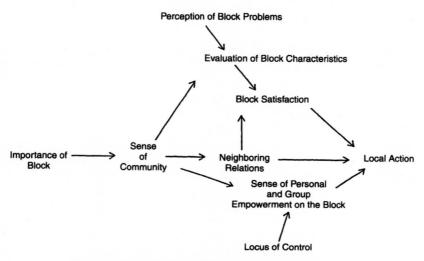

Figure 1. General path model for determinants of local action.

participatory behaviors. Over time these relationships are bidirectional and transactional.

Since we believe that these domains must be viewed in context, we have placed the importance of the block as a starting point in the model. The catalytic role of a sense of community is dependent on the importance of that environment or "community" to the individual. Durkheim (1983/1947), Gusfield (1975), Suttles (1972), and Wellman (1979) are among the social theorists that have noted the evolution or "liberation" of community from solely the traditional proxemic residential concept. Diversity of life-styles along with advances in transportation and communication allow for different types and numerous layers of community. However, the neighborhood still plays a vitally important role in the life of many people, including those limited in their mobility, their ability to integrate into the larger social systems, or their resources (Fried, 1984; Taylor, 1988; Thoits, 1982; Unger & Wandersman, 1985).

A sense of community is posited to modify these perceptions and behaviors in manners conducive to participation or other forms of local action. If an individual has a strong sense of community, the perception of environmental conditions is hypothesized to be evaluated more positively so that satisfaction with the environment is increased; one's general inclination towards the control of reinforcers (locus of control) and a sense of community are hypothesized to influence one's sense of individual and collective control over the residential environment. The character and extent of social relations and behaviors are influenced by a sense of community as well. These three domains interact to influence the level of participation in local action.

We conducted two studies in order to investigate the pattern of relations or *processes* depicted in our model. The first study of cross-sectional data attempts to validate the model. The second study identifies potential directions of influence among the key variables in the model using longitudinal data. We emphasize again that these relationships are seen as being generally bidirectional and transactional. Causal modeling was used only to further validate a relationship between the key constructs in this model.

NEIGHBORHOOD DESCRIPTION

The Waverly–Belmont neighborhood in Nashville was typical of many American transitional urban neighborhoods. Following a post-World War II exodus to the suburbs by white middle-class residents, the neighborhood experienced decreasing property values, increased crime, and a general physical deterioration. Low- and middle-income blacks, displaced by urban renewal and highway construction, moved into the area. Beginning in the 1970s there had been a reverse migration to urban areas such as this one which offered spacious older homes and the conveniences and amenities of an urban location (Clay, 1979). Houses are primarily one- and two-unit dwellings with a few multiple-unit (3 to 4 units) structures interspersed.

The neighborhood had approximately 55% nonwhite residents and 45% white residents according to the 1980 census (U.S. Census Bureau, 1980). Blacks comprised 95.6% of the nonwhite population or 53.2% of the entire neighborhood. Individual city blocks tended to have primarily either white or black residents of varying socioeconomic status. (A "block" refers to the properties on both sides of a resident's street that face each other, with cross streets serving as block boundaries.)

A Neighborhood Housing Services program (NHS) was started in this neighborhood to capitalize on the "back to the city" movement and to upgrade the conditions for existing residents. The NHS of Nashville, 1 of 195 programs then operating in 140 cities across the United States, is a locally controlled nonprofit partnership of lenders, government officials, and neighborhood residents dedicated to the revitalization of neighborhoods. The changing economic and social forces of the neighborhood, fueled in part by the NHS program, led to its revival during the later half of the 1970s. As part of its program NHS became involved in a community organizing effort that resulted in the development of 17 block associations by the summer of 1978. Members of the research team assisted in this organizing effort and provided other services to the research project (cf. Chavis & Wandersman, 1986).

PROCESS MODEL VALIDATION (STUDY 1)

Sample and Design

The sample for this study was drawn from the 1,213 respondents interviewed during the summer of 1979. The sample approximated the distribution reported by the U.S. Census Bureau with 48.3% white respondents, 51.1% black respondents, and 0.6% other racial minorities. Respondents were 56.8% female and 43.2% male. For this analysis respondents were selected from the eight blocks that had active block associations in 1979 ($N = 423$). The respondents were adult (18 years or older; range = 18–93 years) residents of the Waverly–Belmont neighborhood in Nashville.

Trained interviewers attempted to interview all adult residents on the 39 blocks selected for the study and recorded all responses to a survey. Respondents were paid $3.50 for their participation in an interview which lasted from 45 to 75 min. The model in Figure 1 was tested through path analysis using structural equations estimated by the ordinary least squares method of multiple regression to determine the antecedents of local action.

Measures

Table 1 lists measures used in this study. The independent variables were *the importance of the block* (Measure A), the respondent's *sense of community score* (Measure B3 from Table 1), *locus of control* (Levenson, 1974) and perception of the level of block problems (e.g., crime, sanitation, housing quality; Measure E). The sense of community score (Measure B3) was used because the interactive score was believed to be conceptually more appropriate (i.e., the value of a sense of community is a function of the importance to the individual of having a sense of community with that specific group). The Locus of Control Scale (Levenson, 1974) has been associated with psychological empowerment (Zimmerman & Rappaport, 1988). It consists of three subscales: internal control, chance, and powerful others.

Intervening variables were *neighboring relations, sense of personal power to influence block conditions, sense of group* (neighbors') *power over the block, evaluation of block qualities* (e.g., safe or unsafe, clean or dirty, etc.), and *satisfaction with the block* (Measures C, D1–2, F, G5). Factor

Table 1. Measures

A.	Importance of block
	Some people care a lot about the kind of block they live on. For others, the block is not important. How important is what your block is like to you? Range 1–5; not at all important–important.
B.	Sense of community
	B1. Do you feel a sense of community with others on this block? (For example, do you share interests and concerns with them?) Range 1–5; not at all a great deal.
	B2. How important is it to you to feel a sense of community with people on the block? Range 1–5; not important–very important.
	B3. Sense of community score (self-report)—interactive score was developed by multiplying B1 by B2.
C.	Neighboring relations
	Range 1–5; none–almost everyone; average of the following 10 items:
	1. How many people who live on your block would you recognize?
	2. How many of the names do you know of people who live on this block?
	3. How many people on this block would you say you have a neighborhood relationship?
	4. How many people on this block do you see socially at least three or four times a year?

Table 1. *Continued*

---

5. How many people on this block do you consider close friends?

With how many people on your block would you feel comfortable having the following contacts?

6. asking to borrow a tool
7. talking about a personal problem
8. asking to watch your house while you are away
9. asking to help you with a house repair
10. asking for a ride when your car is not working.

D. Sense of personal and group empowerment on the block
   D1. Personal: How much influence do you feel you have in getting the block the way you want it to be? Range 1–5; no influence–much influence.
   D2. Group: If there was a problem in receiving some services from the city, do you think people on the block could get the problem solved? Range 1–5; definitely–not definitely.

E. Block problems
   Sum of 18 items concerning block conditions. Range 1–4; not a problem, minor problem, moderate problem, major problem. Conditions: Street pavement, condition of houses, alley pavement, lighting of streets, water and sewage, traffic, police services, crime, noisy neighbors, condition of sidewalks, drainage, garbage collection, rats, streets signs/traffic lights, vacant lots, unkept lawns, stray dogs, fire protection.

F. Evaluation of block
   Mean of seven semantic differential items ranged 1–6; dangerous–safe, unattractive–attractive, messy–neat, noisy–quiet, houses need repair-houses in good condition, streets and walks need repair–streets and walks are in good condition, bad place to raise kids–good to raise kids.

G. Block satisfaction
   G1. All things considered how satisfied or dissatisfied are you with this block as a place to live? Range 1–5; very dissatisfied–very satisfied.
   G2. Respondents were asked to rate their block right now on a scale of 0–10 from the worst possible way this block could be to best possible way it could be.
   G3. Same as G2 except respondents were asked to rate their block as to the way they expected it to be 1 year later.
   G4. How much does this block meet your needs and values of what a block should be like? Range 1–5; not at all–to a great deal.
   G5. Block satisfaction factor score: A factor analysis was performed on items G1–G4. Factor scores were created through this procedure.

H. Local action
   Index of the level of participation in block associations: (a) nonmember; (b) member only attended and occasionally talked at meetings; (c) worker (also, encouraged neighbors to come to meetings and/or did work on a committee or outside the meetings, and/or hosted a meeting at home; (d) leader (also, acted as an officer or committee leader of organization). Unger and Wandersman (1982) reported that these groups formed a Guttman scale with a coefficient of reliability of .99 and a coefficient of scalability of .98.

analysis was used to generate a factor score from four indicators of one's satisfaction with his/her block. This analysis identified one factor that explained approximately 57% of the variance in the four items. The factor score was used to represent block satisfaction in the analysis.

Local action, the dependent variable, was represented by the level of participation in the block association (i.e., nonmember, member, worker, or leader, Measure H from Table 1).

Results

A multiple regression analysis was performed including all the variables represented in the model presented in Figure 1, using one's level of participation as the dependent variable. The predictor variables explained 23% of the variance. The zero-order correlations between the variables in the model under study are shown in Table 2. A sense of community was found to have a relatively strong direct bivariate relationship with all the predictor variables except the perception of block problems and the locus of control measures.

A path analysis for participation in block associations is shown in Table 3. Path analysis was performed based on the recursive model (Asher, 1983) in Figure 1. Ordinary least squares regression analysis was used— regressing each item on all items posited as causally prior to it. Standardized path coefficients that were significant at the .05 level or higher are reported. The residual path coefficient (X_R) (Asher, 1983) represents the correlation of that variable with unobserved variables. The residual path coefficients or latent variables (Bentler, 1980) were calculated using the R^2 adjusted for shrinkage (J. Cohen & Cohen, 1975, p. 106). The adjusted R^2 or $\bar{R}^2$ is also reported in Table 3. Figure 2 illustrates the findings of the path analysis.

While explaining only a moderate amount of variance, this model clearly demonstrates the central role played by a sense of community. The relationships hypothesized in Figure 1 were confirmed by this study, except that block satisfaction did not have the expected direct effect on local action. A sense of community was found to have a positive influence on one's perception of the environment, social relations, and the perceived control the person had over the immediate environment.

The strongest path to participation was through a sense of community, through neighboring relations, which influenced the degree to which a person became involved in the block association. A sense of community also had a moderate direct impact on participation in the block association.

An estimate of the indirect effect of sense of community, as recommended by Alwin and Hauser (1975), can be derived by multiplying the

Table 2. Zero-Order Correlation Matrix of Path Items[a]

	1	2	3	4	5	6	7	8	9	10	11	12
1. Level of participation	—	.30	.17	.20	.40	.09	.08	.31	.21	-.01	-.01	.11
2. Personal power		—	.26	.25	.31	.24	-.09	.33	.18	-.05	-.03	.09
3. Group power			—	.44	.31	.37	-.17	.40	.31	-.18	-.03	.14
4. Block satisfaction				—	.34	.59	-.29	.44	.45	-.07	.02	.20
5. Neighbor relations					—	.18	.04	.46	.33	-.15	-.16	.19
6. Evaluation of block						—	-.45	.32	.37	-.14	-.02	.11
7. Block problems							—	-.06	-.09	.06	-.02	-.10
8. Sense of community								—	.42	-.07	.05	.09
9. Importance of block									—	-.17	-.11	.24
10. Powerful others										—	.60	-.24
11. Chance											—	-.15
12. Internal control												1.00

[a]$N = 420$.

Table 3. Path Analysis of Antecedents of Participation in Block Associations

Dependent variable	R^2	$\bar{R}^{2b}$	\multicolumn{9}{c}{Equation with significant path coefficients[a]}									
			2	3	4	5	6	SOC	ImpB	P.O.	Bprob	$X_r{}^c$
1. Level of participation	.23	.20	.18	—	—	.27	—	.13	—	—	—	.89
2. Personal power	.16	.14	—	.13	—	.17	—	.18	—	—	—	.93
3. Group power	.20	.19	—	—	—	—	—	.33	.10	-.15	—	.90
4. Block satisfaction	.50	.49	—	—	—	.10	.48	.22	.09	—	—	.71
5. Neighbor relations	.25	.24	—	—	.15	—	—	.38	.11	—	.12	.87
6. Evaluation of block	.34	.33	—	—	—	—	—	.18	.26	—	-.41	.81

[a]Standardized values. SOC = Sense of community (C4), ImpB = Importance of the block, P.O. = Powerful others subscale (Locus of control), Bproh = Block problems.
[b]$\bar{R}^2$ = adjusted for shrinkage.
[c]Residual path coefficient calculated as $\sqrt{1 - R^2}$.

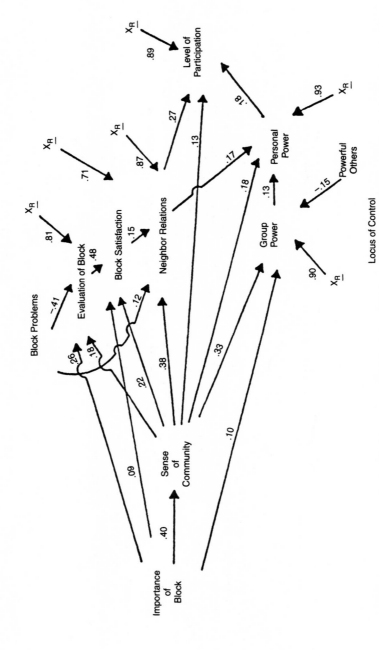

Figure 2. Path diagram with standardized path coefficients of antecedents of a person's level of participation in block associations. $N = 420$.

path coefficients. For example, in addition to the direct effect a sense of community has on one's level of participation (.13), it has an almost equal indirect effect of .10 through neighbor relations as well as smaller indirect impact through other variables. The importance of the block to the individual had its own direct effect on the evaluation of the block and sense of group power, even though it was not hypothesized to do so.

LONGITUDINAL ANALYSIS TO IDENTIFY POTENTIAL DIRECTIONALITY OF INFLUENCE (STUDY 2)

The path analysis study was limited in its ability to confirm causal relations because all measures were collected at the same time. To further test the causal inferences of our process model, we conducted a longitudinal analysis looking at the relationship between selected variables at two points in time, 1 year apart. Variables related to increased local action and perceived or subjective empowerment (perceived personal and group power) were examined.

Procedures and Instruments

The procedures and instruments were identical to those described for the previous study.

Sample and Design

The sample for this study was 349 respondents who were interviewed at both Time 1 (Summer 1978) and Time 2 (Summer 1979). This sample was demographically different from the sample used in the previous study; 64.5% were female and 62.5% blacks. The average age of these respondents (at Time 1) was 45.9 years old, while the average age for the entire Time 1 sample was 40.4 years.

A hierarchical multiple regression technique was used to improve the estimation of the causal parameters in the analysis as recommended by Cook and Campbell (1979), Heise (1975), and Kessler and Greenberg (1981). The Time 2 score for each measure was the dependent variable with the measures from the prior year acting as the independent variables. Time 1 measures were entered in a hierarchical form, whereby the dependent variable in Time 1 was entered into the equation first. The remaining variance would account for the change between Time 2 and Time 1 and will be called the "change variance" (J. Cohen, personal communication with

J. Tanaka, March 17, 1987). The standardized path (regression) coefficient illuminated the strength of each variable across time.

Results

Analyses were performed on the entire sample ($N = 349$) to confirm relations between a sense of community, social relations, subjective empowerment, and one's level of participation. A significant causal relationship across the periods chosen for this study was not found for the Chance and Powerful Others subscales of the Locus of Control Scale. Table 4 shows the models successfully inferring a causal relationship between a sense of community and the three indicators of perceived control and empowerment (perceived personal power and group power on the block and the Internal Control sub-scale of the Locus of Control Scale). For each pair of variables there are two structural equations containing the *standardized* path coefficients between the two items in Time 1 with one of the items in Time 2 as the dependent variable. Since the items have been standardized, a comparison of the relative size of the coefficients clarifies causal inferences (Cook & Campbell, 1979).

Table 4 (top) shows the close association over time between the perception of personal power and a sense of community. Perceived personal power at Time 1 has little, if any, effect on a sense of community at Time 2. However, one's sense of community and perceived personal power at Time 1

Table 4. Longitudinal Path Analysis Using Hierarchical Regression Method: Sense of Community (SOC) and Empowerment

Model[a]	R^2	Change variance[b]
SOC and personal power (PP), $n = 314$		
$SOC_2 = SOC_1 (.51)^d + PP_1 (.08)$	$.30^d$	ns
$PP_2 = PP_1 (.23)^d + SOC_1 (.23)^d$	$.15^d$	$.04^d$
		$F(2, 311) = 29.06$
SOC and group power (GP), $n = 315$		
$SOC_2 = SOC_1 (.54)^d + GP_1 (.03)$	$.29^d$	ns
$GP_2 = GP_1 (.21) + SOC_1 (.22)^d$	$.10^d$	$.04^d$
		$F(2, 312) = 18.99$
SOC and internal locus of control (ILC), $n = 303$		
$SOC_2 = SOC_1 (.55)^d + ILC_1 (-.03)$	$.29^d$	ns
$ILC_2 = ILC_1 (.21)^d + SOC_1 (.12)$	$.06^d$	$.02^c$
		$F(2, 301) = 10.15$

[a]Numbers in parentheses are the standardized regression coefficient for the variable at Time 1.
[b]Change variance is the R^2 change after the DV in Time 1 was entered into equation. $F = F$ change.
[c]$p \le .05$.
[d]$p \le .0001$.

Table 5. Longitudinal Path Analysis Using Hierarchical Regression Method: Sense of Community (SOC) Neighboring (NR)

Model[a]	R^2	Change variance[b]
SOC and neighbor relations (NR)		
$SOC_2 = SOC_1 (.48)^d + NR_1 (.13)^c$	$.31^d$	.01
		$(F = 5.7)$
$NR_2 = NR_1 (.38)^d + SOC_1 (.19)^d$	$.25^d$	.03
		$(F = 11.98)$

[a]Numbers in parentheses are the standardized regression coefficient for the variable at Time 1.
[b]Change variance is the R^2 change after the DV in Time 1 was entered into equation. $F = F$ change.
[c]$p \le .05$.
[d]$p \le .0001$.

have an equal effect on one's personal power over block conditions at Time 2. In Table 4 (middle), similar results are shown for sense of community and a sense of group power. A sense of community influences one's sense of group power the following year as much as did his/her earlier sense of group power. Table 4 (bottom) shows a weak but significant influence of a sense of community on a person's internal control. The findings of this part of the study suggest that some aspect of having a sense of community leads to an increased sense of personal and group control, and, to a lesser degree, a generalized perception of having internal control of reinforcers.

A sense of community was found to contribute to neighboring relations (Table 5). An examination of the standardized path coefficients showed that a sense of community in Time 1 was strongly linked to neighboring in Time 2. The reciprocal nature of this relationship, as stated earlier, is demonstrated by the unique variance contributed by neighboring relations in Time 1 to a person's sense of community in Time 2.

Participation, Sense of Community, and Empowerment

The effects of participation in block organizations are reported in Table 6. A subsample of the respondents who lived on a block that had an active block association during both years were selected ($n = 143$). Individuals' level of participation remained fairly constant from Time 1 to Time 2 as indicated by a path coefficient of .65. Table 6 shows the strong interdependence of participation and a sense of community. Examination of the path coefficients showed that participation at Time 1 contributed significantly to a sense of community at Time 2, and a sense of community at Time 1 contributed almost as powerfully to participation at Time 2.

A sense of personal power appeared to precede one's participation based on the analysis reported in Table 6. However, a sense of group power

Table 6. Longitudinal Path Analysis Using Hierarchical Regression Method: Participation, Sense of Community, Personal Power and Internal Locus of Control

Model[a]	R^2	Change variance[b]
Participation (PART) and sense of community (SOC), $n = 141$		
$PART_2 = PART_1\ (.65)^d + SOC_1\ (.15)^c$	$.44^d$	$.02^c$
		$(F = 4.5)$
$SOC_2 = SOC_1\ (.51)^d + PART_1\ (.19)^c$	$.28^d$	$.03^c$
		$(F = 5.69)$
Participation (PART) and internal locus of control (ILC), $n = 142$		
$PART_2 = PART_1\ (.65)^d + ILC_1\ (.04)$	$.42^d$	ns
$ILC_2 = ILC_1\ (.13)^c + PART_1\ (.20)^c$	$.24^c$	$.04^c$
		$(F = 5.4)$
Participation (PART) and personal power (PP), $n = 141$		
$PART_2 = PART_1\ (.65)^d + PP_1\ (.17)^c$	$.45^d$	$.03^c$
		$(F = 6.5)$
$PP_2 = PP_1\ (.34)^c + PART_1\ (.17)^c$	$.13^d$	$.03^c$
		$(F = 3.8)$

[a]Numbers in parentheses are the standardized regression coefficient for the variable at Time 1.
[b]Change variance is the R^2 change after the DV in Time 1 was entered into equation. $F = F$ change.
[c]$p \leq .05$.
[d]$p \leq .0001$.

did *not* show any *significant* relationship with participation in the block association. These last two results showed that individual and group power are independent of each other, though they might be tied together through a sense of community (see Table 4). A minimal sense of personal power is necessary for an individual to get involved in the association. Through the development of sense of community, a sense of group power will develop.

This analysis also revealed (Table 6, middle) that participation on the block level can have a weak yet significant positive influence on one's internal control of reinforcers. There was an insignificant relationship between participation and the other locus of control subscales.

DISCUSSION

This study attempted to determine the influence a sense of community has in stimulating participation. The results presented in Figure 2 graphically illustrate how the structure of a person's residential ecology (both physical and social) and a sense of empowerment influence their level of participation in block associations. These findings support the model in which a sense of community plays a catalytic role in stimulating satisfaction with one's residential environment, encouraging neighboring relations, and enhancing one's perception of personal and group empowerment to influence what goes on around their homes.

The contributions of other variables to participation seem to be channeled through the level of one's sense of community. Figure 2 also shows that a sense of community contributed significant unique, though sometimes low, variance in almost every direction of the path model leading to participation in the block association. The pervasiveness of the causal influence of a sense of community found in the path analysis was confirmed through the longitudinal path analysis. It is also important to note that the assumption that most of the relations are interactive rather than unidirectional was verified in the longitudinal analysis. While the causal directions for inferences among these variables should be considered representative of only these two points in time, it is reasonable to assume that the selection of other or additional time lags would continue to show the transactional nature of these constructs.

In the neighborhood environment a sense of community can be both a cause and effect of local action. People feel more secure with their neighbors when they have a sense of community. They are more likely to feel comfortable coming to their first meeting of an association and because of regular communication among neighbors, they are more likely to hear about it.

The determinants of participation in block associations were well accounted for by this model. The 23% of the variance explained by the multiple regression was considerably better than the results of earlier studies that relied on traditional demographic variables to predict participation (see Florin & Wandersman, 1984; Wandersman & Florin, 1981). The major difference between the two models was the inclusion of neighbor relations (a behavior) in the present investigation. Neighbor relations contributed significantly more than any other item to the prediction of the level of participation. Neighboring behavior plays an important role in the initial formation and maintenance of a block association (Unger & Wandersman, 1983; Wandersman et al., 1981). Neighbors communicate information specifically relevant to the block association's activities (e.g., meeting times) and provide information on outside resources (Froland, Pancoast, Chapman, & Kimboko, 1981; Granovetter, 1973). Many communities can address their problems through informal mechanisms provided by strong neighbor relations (Crenson, 1978; Unger & Wandersman, 1985) and may not resort to formal organizations.

Figure 2 shows that a sense of community can mediate the perception of block problems leading to greater satisfaction with the block and more positive impressions which can lead to neighborhood stability and growth

(Ahlbrandt & Brophy, 1975; Bradford & Marino, 1977; Goetze, 1979; Pearce, 1979; Pol, Guy, & Bush, 1982).

A sense of community is also important for neighborhood development, as our results suggest, because it contributes a sense of individual and group empowerment that helps neighbors to collectively act to meet their shared needs. When people share a strong sense of community they are motivated and empowered to change problems they face, and are better able to mediate the negative effects of things over which they have no control. A sense of community is the glue that can hold together a community development effort.

This study provides support for aspects of the theory of sense of community presented by McMillan and Chavis (1986). The influence and need meeting elements of a sense of community were demonstrated. A sense of community was positively related to changes in one's sense of group or personal power. One's level of participation was also demonstrated to be affected by a sense of community. Prestby, Wandersman, Florin, Rich, and Chavis (1990) demonstrated how participation in block associations met instrumental and social needs of members. The community development process is "activated" when citizens perceive their ability to influence events in order to obtain needs through participation in collective action.

Participation in local action is important for community development, but it is not a sufficient goal. Participation does not insure the alleviation of problems facing the community. In order for local action to be effective, participants must have or develop the skills necessary to address community needs. Leaders must be skilled at running and directing the organization. The environment (government, service agencies) should be supportive of the association's growth and domain. Finally, the association must address issues that are in the self-interest of its members. Locality-based organizations, such as block associations, must make sure that they are active in areas that address the needs and interests of their constituents. Otherwise, success will not alleviate sources of stress nor enhance the quality or quantity of participation.

Focusing on a sense of community for purposes of community development can have many benefits for the neighborhood. Social programs, in order to be effective and efficient, need to determine "triggering devices" or catalysts for their established goals to serve as targets for programmatic efforts. This type of approach requires determining mechanisms among and within people that could serve as a catalyst for change. Our research suggests that a sense of community is one such mechanism. The elements of a sense of community (McMillan & Chavis, 1986) offer a guide to activate this process; programs should be developed that foster membership, increase influence, meet needs, and develop a shared emotional connection among community members.

The use of path analysis and longitudinal analysis treated the phenomenon as a *process*, consistent with earlier definitions of empowerment (Rappaport, 1987). Unlike earlier explorations (i.e., Zimmerman & Rappaport, 1988), we explicitly examined perceived control or empowerment within a neighborhood context. Zimmerman and Rappaport (1988) used global or general measures of empowerment to differentiate groups of people from different contexts. We argue that empowerment is "context specific" so that a person may feel empowered in one setting (e.g., at home) and without control in another (e.g., at work). Correlations reported in Table 3 between the contextual empowerment variables (perceived personal and group power on the block) and the level of participation were much higher (.30 and .17, respectively) than correlations between the global Locus of Control Scales and participation (−.01, −.01, .11 for Powerful Others, Chance, and Internal control subscales, respectively).

This study also views empowerment as a collective or group experience as well as an individual process. Recent studies (e.g., Kieffer, 1984; Zimmerman & Rappaport, 1988) examined empowerment solely as an individual process. We find that perceived individual control and perceived collective control operate independently yet interact over time. Heller (1989) cautioned community psychologists that empowerment has been given individualistic connotations that can further inhibit our field's ability to foster collective strategies for achieving greater power for disenfranchised groups.

Limitations of the Current Study and Directions for Future Research

A more deliberate and elaborate attempt at studying the full effects of a sense of community is needed. The study presented in this paper was developed from data collected by a research project not originally designed for the purposes of this investigation. Some of the results presented are significant, yet explain a small percentage of the variance. This sometimes leads to findings that are suggestive at best. Future research should offer more items per concept (e.g., importance of the block, sense of group and individual empowerment), provide more measurement points, have larger samples, and incorporate objective environmental and social indicators, and include a variety of neighborhoods for comparative purposes.

This investigation was further limited because it focused entirely on the *perception* of empowerment. It did not determine whether or not the block association was actually successful in improving the quality of life or increasing the residents' capacity for self-determination. Future research needs to delineate perceived empowerment from actual empowerment in terms of their causes, effects, and the processes (Swift & Levin, 1987). Research has demonstrated the effectiveness of these organizations for improving the quality of life: reducing crime and improving housing (Florin, 1979; Wandersman, Unger, Florin, & Chavis, unpublished manuscript).

An additional limitation of this study was its analysis of only individual level variables. Complete investigation of community development should include examinations at the organizational, community (microsystem) and macrosystems level. Emerging theories must recognize the changes that occur at all these levels simultaneously as well as changes in relationships between these levels.

The strength of a sense of community as a catalyst for the community development process was apparently demonstrated even with these limitations. Given the limitations of the instruments, it should be considered important that significant relations among the longitudinal measures could be found at all. The findings are consistent with a model based on substantial earlier theory and research. Therefore, the probability that these results are a chance occurrence is greatly reduced (Nunnally, 1978), though the actual strength of these relations is still not fully known.

Future theoretical and empirical work should focus on the developmental process of community. We often tend to study community in a static manner. E. Cohen (1976) presented one of the few examples of the dynamic quality of community. Development of community is very similar to human development: Both are "living" or active systems. Therefore, we must look at development as a process. Gordon (1975) said that development "is influenced by what has gone on before. It is not, however, simply a process of adding on .... What emerges is a new organization" (p. 5). Communities are an open system influenced by their environment as well as by their internal structures. The development of community (like human development) is inseparable from its environment. We should work to identify qualities of residential environments that are conducive to community development. To extend this analogy, we anticipate that future investigation will show that there are developmental milestones in the development of community much akin to the function of milestones in human development. Recognition of these critical points is integral to community development strategies that successfully resist neighborhood decline.

Self-help through local action is a driving force within a successful community development effort. Research on community building and self-help organizations can aid in the development of new social programs and can also improve existing ones. Techniques and programs to empower people and their communities could be an area of expertise for the community psychologist (e.g., leadership training, organization development and maintenance, coalition development). An appropriate question for research on this topic is: Do the formal (organizations) or the informal mechanisms (support systems) of a community better enable people to cope with community problems (e.g., crime, unemployment, lack of resources, etc.)? Also, it is important to determine whether coping as a community enhances individuals' abilities to cope in their personal lives. If it does, how is the link between individual and collective empowerment established? When is stimulating formal mechanisms important and when are informal mechanisms appropriate for dealing with individual and community problems?

CONCLUSION

Community psychologists should consider the development of human ecologies, particularly those mediating structures such as the home, neighborhood, work, and voluntary associations, around the value and elements of a sense of community (Chavis & Newbrough, 1986). This study, and others reviewed earlier in this article, demonstrate the pervasive catalytic effects a sense of community can have for different levels and types of change. Community development should not be limited to residential environments. We must be open to where the potential for developing community may exist in other settings. The development of practical skills and techniques that can be used in the community development process will ensure a unique and valued role for the community psychologist in our society.

Our greatest challenge lies not in how to effectively research empowerment but how to participate in it and encourage it. A redistribution of actual power is inevitable in order to effectively generate a sense of empowerment. This process has tremendous potential for social conflict. As the definition of our field (Rappaport, 1987) and social reality (i.e., greater disenfranchisement) moves us to call for empowering those most at risk (the poor, ethnic minorities, victims of discrimination, the physically disabled, etc.), are we ready to do what it really takes to bring about that change? Are we willing to actively commit our personal and professional resources to struggle and take the risks necessary to really empower poor communities? How will we deal with the social conflict that will occur in the process of helping the powerless to become empowered? The answer to these questions will determine the external validity of our field's commitment to empowerment.

ACKNOWLEDGMENTS

This research was funded, in part, by a National Science Foundation grant #BNS-78-08827 to the Center for Community Studies, John F. Kennedy

Center for Research on Education and Human Development, George Peabody College, Nashville, Tennessee. The authors thank Paul Florin, Robert Innes, Barry Lee, J. R. Newbrough, and Richard Rich for their comments on earlier versions of this paper.

REFERENCES

Abramowitz, S. L. (1974). Research on internal-external control and social political activism. *Psychological Reports, 34*, 619–621.

Ahlbrandt, R. S., Jr. & Brophy, P. C. (1975). *Neighborhood revitalization: Theory and practice.* Lexington, MA: Lexington Books.

Ahlbrandt, R. S. & Cunningham, J. V. (1979). *A new public policy for neighborhood preserva-tion.* New York: Praeger.

Aiello, J. R. & Baum, A. (Eds.). (1979). *Residential crowding and design.* New York: Plenum Press.

Aldwin, D. F. & Hauser, R. M. (1975). The decompsition of effects in path analysis. *American Sociological Review, 40*, 37–47.

Altshuler, A. A. (1970). *Community control: The black demand for participation in large American cities.* New York: Pegasus.

Asher, H. B. (1983). *Causal modeling* (2nd ed.). Beverly Hills: Sage.

Bachrach, K. & Zautra, A. (1985). Coping with a community stressor: The threat of a hazardous waste facility. *Journal of Health and Social Behavior, 26*, 127–141.

Bandura, A. (1986). *Social foundations of thought and action.* Englewood Cliffs, NJ: Prentice-Hall.

Baum, A., Singer, J. E., & Baum, C. S. (1981). Stress and the environment. *Journal of Social Issues, 37*, 4–35.

Bellah, R. N., Madsen, R., Sullivan, W. M. Swidler, A., & Tipton, S. M. (1985). *Habits of the heart: Individualism and committment in American life.* Berkeley: University of California Press.

Bentler, P. M. (1980). Multivariate analysis with latent variables: Casual modeling. *Annual Review of Psychology, 31*, 419–456.

Berck, P. L. & Williams, L. J. (1980). *The neighborhood organization: An emprical examination of psychosocial support.* Unpublished manuscript, Indiana/Purdue University, Indianapolis.

Bradford, C. & Marino, D. (1977). *Redlining and disinvestment as a discriminatory practice in residential mortgage loans.* Report prepared for Office of the Assistant Secretary for Fair Housing and Equal Opportunity. Washington, DC: U.S. Department of Housing and Urban Development.

Brower, S. (1980). Territory in urban settings. In I. Altman, A. Rapaport, & J. Wohwill (Eds.), *Human behavior and environment,* New York: Plenum Press.

Brown, B. B. (1987). Territoriality. In D. Stokols & I. Altman (Eds.), *Handbook of environ-mental psychology* (Vol. 1, pp. 505–531). New York: Wiley.

Chavis, D. M., Hogge, J. H., McMillan, D. W., & Wandersman, A. (1986). Sense of community through Brunswik's lens: A first look. *Journal of Community Psychology, 14*, 24–40.

Chavis, D. M. & Newbrough, J. R. (1986). The meaning of "community" in Community Psychology. *Journal of Community Psychology, 14*, 335–340.

Chavis, D. M. & Wandersman, A. (1986). Roles for research and the researcher in neighbor-hood development. In R. B. Taylor (Ed.), *Urban neighborhoods: Research and policy* (pp. 215–249). New York: Praeger.

Churchman, A. (1987). Can resident participation in neighborhood rehabilitation programs succeed? Israel's project renewal through a comparative perspective. In I. Altman & A. Wandersman (Eds.), *Neighborhood and community environments* (pp. 113–162). New York: Plenum Press.

Clay, P. L. (1979). *Neighborhood renewal.* Lexington, MA: D.C. Health.

Cohen, E. (1976). The structural transformation of the kibbutz. In G. K. Zollchan & W. Hirsh (Eds.), *Social change* (pp. 689–732). New York: Wiley.

Cohen, J. & Cohen, P. (1975). *Applied multiple regression.* Hillsdale, NJ: Erlbaum.

Cohen, S. & Sherrod, D. R. (1978). When density matters: Environmental control as a determinant of crowding effects in laboratory and residential settings. In L. Severy (Ed.), *Crowding: Theoretical and research implications for population-environment psychology.* New York: Human Sciences.

Cook, T. D. & Campbell, D. T. (1979). *Quasi-experimentation: Design and analysis issues for field settings.* Chicago: Rand McNally.

Crenson, M. A. (1978). Social networks and political processes in urban neighborhoods. *American Journal of Political Science, 22,* 578–594.

Curtis, L. A. (Ed.). (1987). Policies to prevent crime: Neighborhood, family and employment strategies. *Annals of the American Academy of Political and Social Science, 494,* 9–168.

Durkheim, E. (1947). *The division of labor in society* (G. Simpson, Trans.). New York: Free Press of Glencoe. (original work published 1893)

Florin, P. (1989). *Nurturing the grassroots: Neighborhood volunteer organizations and America's cities.* New York: Citizens Committee for New York City.

Florin, P., Friedmann, R. R., Wandersman, A., & Meier, R. (1987). *Cognitive social learning variables and behavior: Cross-cultural similarities in person × situation interaction.* Unpublished manuscript, University of Rhode Island.

Florin, P. & Wandersman, A. (1984). Cognitive social learning and participation in community development. A comparison of standard and cognitive social learning variables. *American Journal of Community Psychology, 12,* 689–708.

Freedman, J. L. (1975). *Crowding and behavior.* New York: Viking.

Fried, M. (1984). The structure and significance of community satisfaction. *Population and Environment, 7,* 61–86.

Froland, C., Pancoast, D. C., Chapman, N. J., & Kimboko, P. J. (1981). *Helping networks and human services.* Beverly Hills: Sage.

Goetze, R. (1979). *Understanding neighborhood change.* Cambridge, MA: Ballinger.

Gordon, I. J. (1975). *Human development: A transactional perspective.* New York: Harper & Row.

Granovetter, M. S. (1973). The strength of weak ties. *American Journal of Sociology, 78,* 1360–1380.

Green, L. W. (1986). The theory of participation: A qualitative analysis of its expression in national and international health policies. *Advances in Health Education and Promotion, 1(A),* 211–236.

Greenberg, S. W. & Rohe (1986). Informal social control and crime prevention in modern urban neighborhoods. In R. B. Taylor (Ed.), *Urban neighborhoods: Research and policy.* New York: Praeger.

Gusfield, J. R. (1975). *Community: A critical response.* New York: Harper Colophon Books.

Hallman, H. (1974). *Neighborhood government in metropolitan settings.* Beverly Hills: Sage.

Hallman, H. W. (1984). *Neighborhoods: Their place in urban life.* Beverly Hills: Sage.

Heise, D. R. (1975). *Casual analysis.* New York: Wiley.

Heller, K. (1989). The return to community. *American Journal of Community Psychology, 17,* 1–15.

Hunter, A. (1974). *Symbolic communities*. Chicago: University of Chicago Press.

Kessler, R. C. & Greenberg, D. F. (1981). *Linear panel analysis: Models of quantitative change*. New York: Academic Press.

Kieffer, C. H. (1984, January). Citizen empowerment: A development perspective. In J. Rappaport & R. Hess (Eds.), *Studies in empowerment: Steps toward understanding and action* (pp. 9–36). New York: Haworth.

Langer, E. J. (1983). *The psychology of control*. Beverly Hills: Sage.

Lavrakas, P. J. (1980). *Factors related to citizen involvement in personal, household and neighborhood anti-crime measures: An executive summary*. Chicago: Northwestern University Center for Urban affairs.

Levenson, H. (1974). Activism and powerful others: Distinctions within the concept of internal-external control. *Journal of Personality Assessment, 38*, 377–383.

Lewis, D. A. & Salem, G. (1981). Community crime prevention: An analysis of a developing perspective. *Crime and Delinquency, 27*, 405–421.

Maton, K. I. & Rappaport, J. (1984). Empowerment in a religious setting: A multivariate investigation. In J. Rappaport & R. Hess (Eds.), *Studies in empowerment: Steps toward understanding action* (pp. 37–72). New York: Haworth.

Mayer, N. S. (1984). *Neighborhood organizations and community development*. Washington, DC: Urban Institute Press.

Merry, S. E. (1987). Crowding, conflict, and neighborhood regulation. In I. Altman & A. Wandersman (Eds.), *Neighborhood and community environments*. (pp. 35–68). New York: Plenum Press.

McMillan, D. W. & Chavis, D. M. (1986). Sense of community: A definition and theory. *Journal of Community Psychology, 14*, 6–23.

Morris, D. E. & Hess, K. (1975). *Neighborhood power: The new localism*. Boston: Beacon.

Moynihan, D. P. (1986). *Family and nation*. San Diego: Harcourt, Brace, Jovanovich.

Naparstek, A. J., Biegal, D. E., & Spiro, H. R. (1982). *Neighborhood networks for humane mental health care*. New York: Plenum Press.

Newbrough, J. R. & Chavis, D. M. (Eds.). (1986a). Psychological Sense of Community, I: Theory and concepts. *Journal of Community Psychology, 14*(1).

Newbrough, J. R. & Chavis, D. M. (Eds.). (1986b). Psychological Sense of community, II: Research and applications. *Journal of Community Psychology, 14*(4).

Newman, O. (1972). *Defensible space*. New York: Macmillan.

Nunnally, J. (1978). *Psychometric theory* (2nd ed.). New York: McGraw Hill.

Pearce, D. M. (1979). Gatekeepers and homeseekers: Institutional factors in racial steering. *Social Problems, 26*, 2325–2342.

Perkins, D. D., Florin, P., Rich, R. C., Wandersman, A., & Chavis, D. M. (1990). Participation and the social and physical environment of residential blocks: Crime and community context. *American Journal of Community Psychology, 18*, 83–116.

Perlman, J. E. (1976). Grassrooting the system. *Social Policy, 7*(2), 4–20.

Pol, L. G., Guy, R. F., & Bush, A. J. (1982). Discrimination in the home lending market: A macro perspective. *Social Science Quarterly, 63*, 716–728.

Prestby, J. E., Wandersman, A., Florin, P., Rich, R., & Chavis, D. M. (1990). Benefits, costs, incentive management and participation in voluntary organizations: A means to understanding and promoting empowerment. *American Journal of Community Psychology, 18*, 117–150.

Rappaport, J. (1977). *Community psychology: Values, research, and action*. New York: Holt, Rinehart, & Winston.

Rappaport, J. (1981). In praise of paradox: A social policy of empowerment over prevention. *American Journal of Community Psychology, 9*, 1–26.

Rappaport, J. (1987). Terms of empowerment/exemplars of prevention: Toward a theory for community psychology. *American Journal of Community Psychology, 15*, 1–25.

Rich, R. C. (1979). The roles of neighborhood organizations in urban service delivery. *Urban Affairs Papers, 1*, 81–93.

Rohe, W. M. (1985). Urban planning and mental health. In A. Wandersman & R. Hess (Eds.), *Beyond the individual: Environmental approaches and prevention*. New York: Haworth.

Sarason, S. B. (1974). *The psychological sense of community: Prospects for a community psychology*. San Francisco: Jossey-Bass.

Seligman, M. (1975). *Helplessness: On depression, development and death*. San Francisco: Freeman.

Skogan, W. G. & Maxfield, M. G. (1981). *Coping with crime*. Beverly Hills: Sage.

Suttles, G. D. (1972). *The social construction of community*. Chicago: University of Chicago Press.

Swift, C. & Levin, G. (1987). Empowerment: An emerging mental health technology. *Journal of Primary Prevention, 7*, 242–265.

Taylor, R. B. (1982). The neighborhood physical environment and stress. In G. W. Evans (Ed.), *Environmental stress* (pp. 286–324). New York: Cambridge University Press.

Taylor, R. B. (1988). *Human territorial functioning: An empirical evolutionary perspective on individual and small group territorial cognitions, behaviors and consequences*. Cambridge, England: Cambridge University Press.

Thoits, P. A. (1982). Life stress, social support, and psychological vulnerability: Epidemiological considerations. *Journal of Community Psychology, 10*, 341–362.

Unger, D. G. & Wandersman, A. (1982). Neighboring in an urban environment. *American Journal of Community Psychology, 10*, 493–509.

Unger, D. G. & Wandersman, A. (1983). Neighboring and its role in block organizations: An exploratory report. *American Journal of Community Psychology, 11*, 291–300.

Unger, D. G. & Wandersman, A. (1985). The importance of neighbors: The social, cognitive, and affective components of neighboring. *American Journal of Community Psychology, 13*, 139–170.

Wandersman, A., Andrews, A., Riddle, D., & Fancett, C. (1983). Environmental psychology and prevention. In R. Felner, S. Farber, L. Jason, & J. Moritsugu (Eds.), *Preventive psychology: Theory, research and practice* (pp. 104–127). New York: Pergamon.

Wandersman, A. & Florin, P. (1981). A cognitive social learning approach to the crossroads of cognition, social behavior, and the environment. In J. H. Harvey (Ed.), *Cognition, social behavior, and the environment* (pp. 393–408). Hillsdale, NJ: Erlbaum.

Wandersman, A. & Giamartino, G. (1980). Community and individual differences characteristics as influences on initial participation. *American Journal of Community Psychology, 8*, 217–228.

Wandersman, A., Jakubs, J. F., & Giamartino, G. A. (1981). Participation in block organizations. *Journal of Community Action, 1*, 40–48.

Wandersman, A., Unger, D., Florin, P., & Chavis, D. M. *Impacts of small-scale community development associations*. Unpublished manuscript.

Weidemann, S. & Anderson, J. R. (1985). A conceptual framework for residential satisfaction. In I. Altman & C. M. Werner (Eds.), *Home environments*. New York: Plenum Press.

Wellman, B. (1981). Applying network analysis to the study of support in B. H. Gottlieb (Ed.), *Social networks and social support* (pp. 156–198). Beverly Hills: Sage.

Wellman, B. (1979). The community question: The intimate networks of East Yorkers. *American Journal of Sociology, 84*, 1201–1231.

Yates, D. T. (1973). *Neighborhood democracy: The politics and impact of decentralization* Lexington, MA: Lexington Books.

Yin, R. K. (1977). Goals for citizen involvement: Some possibilities and some evidence. In
      P. Marshall (Ed.), *Citizen participation certification for community development.*
      Washington, DC: NAHRO
Zimmerman, M. A. (2000). Empowerment theory: Psychological, organizational, and commu-
      nity levels of analysis. J. Rappaport & E. Seidman (Eds.), *Handbook of community psy-
      chology* (pp. 43–63). New York: Plenum Press.
Zimmerman, M. A. & Rappaport, J. (1988). Citizen participation, perceived control, and psy-
      chological empowerment. *American Journal of Community Psychology, 16,* 725–750.

15

The Adaptation of Black Graduate Students: A Social Network Approach

Darlene C. DeFour and Barton J. Hirsch

Despite the importance of increasing the number of graduate degrees awarded to members of minority groups, there has been little research on how minority students adapt to the graduate school environment. The present study examined how social integration and social support were related to academic performance and psychological well-being among 89 black graduate and professional students. Findings indicate that black graduate students were not well integrated into their academic environment. Students in relatively more integrated departments were better adjusted, had higher grades, and perceived themselves to be making good progress in their graduate work. These students were also less likely to have considered dropping out of school. Frequency of out-of-school contact with black faculty and the number of black students in the department were important social integration and social support variables. The implications of these findings for minority student retention are discussed.

For the past two decades, increasing the participation of minorities in graduate and professional education has been a policy goal. This is an important objective for several reasons. First, graduate and professional education is a major avenue for entrance into leadership and professional

Originally published in the *American Journal of Community Psychology*, *18*(3) (1990): 487–503.

A Quarter Century of Community Psychology: *Readings from the* American Journal of Community Psychology, edited by Tracey A. Revenson *et al.* Kluwer Academic/Plenum Publishers, New York, 2002.

positions in society (National Board on Graduate Education, 1976). Second, professions in a pluralistic society could be greatly enhanced by the alternative perspective brought by minority members (Moore, 1977). Third, minority professionals can serve as role models for younger generations.

The number of minority graduate students is quite low. The National Board of Graduate Education (1978) estimated that only 6–7% of the total graduate enrollment were members of minority groups (excluding Asians). Less than 5% of doctorates awarded in 1976 to individuals born in the United States were awarded to minorities. Blackwell (1981a) presented a similar picture for first-year enrollments in medical and law school. Although minority student enrollment increased from the late 1960s to the mid-1970s, this trend is reversing. Isaac (1985) reported that total black enrollment in graduate school decreased 16% between 1976 and 1982. Hispanic enrollments also appear to have peaked and to be declining.

More attention has focused on recruiting minorities to graduate school than on what happens to them in graduate school. Recruitment is certainly important, but access is not the only issue. Retention is also critical. Enrollment in graduate school is only a necessary precondition for obtaining a degree and advancement into actual professional status (Blackwell, 1983). Once enrolled, the attrition rate for minority students is greater than that for nonminorities (Astin, 1982). Despite the importance of this issue, little empirical information exists on factors that affect the success of minority graduate students. Indeed, hardly any research has been conducted on this population at all.

In one of the few studies that has been conducted, Duncan (1976) found that minority graduate students were not socially integrated into their respective departmental communities. Students reported feeling "on the fringes" of their department. Many reported rarely or never having much dialogue with other graduate students in their department about either their field or other intellectual interests. Nor did they socialize much together. Duncan (1976) and Baird (1974) reported similar patterns for faculty–student relationships. In short, black and other minority students are isolated from peers and faculty.

Prior research has indicated that social isolation can have negative influences on academic performance, well-being, and retention (Baird, 1974; Duncan, 1976; Kjerulff & Blood, 1973). Isolation provides minority students with fewer opportunities for social comparison with peers, which is an important source of evaluative feedback. The impaired social comparison process makes it difficult for the student to develop and maintain realistic conceptions of competencies and liabilities (Duncan, 1976). Isolated students conceptions of competencies and liabilities (Duncan, 1976). Isolated students cannot take advantage of informal learning opportunities such as study groups. Blackwell (1981b) suggested tha black students' isolation and exclusion from educational networks utilized by white students negatively influence their appraisal of graduate and professional school. It would not be surprising if the high rate of first-year attrition among minority students may result in part from the failure of the departmental community to develop a social climate that readily helps these students become part of the mainsteam of departmental activities.

Although minority graduate students do not appear to be well integrated into their academic surroundings, we do not have a differentiated understanding of their social ecology. We do not know if they are isolated from all department members and in all social contexts. We do not know much about their ties to individuals outside of their department and the relationship of their academic and nonacademic social networks. Specific forms of segmentation may relate differently to academic performance, well-being, and retention.

Accordingly, the purpose of the present investigation was to provide a more detailed and systematic analysis of the social networks of black graduate students. We were particularly concerned with characteristics of their social network which reflect their support and integration into the academic environment. Within this context, we focused on three different sets of network variables. First, in contrast to previous research, special attention was given to the social role and ethnic background of network members. Second, we considered the frequency of interaction and quality of social support provided by different segments of their network. Third, we assessed the extent to which different segments of the network were integrated or segmented from each other (network "boundary density"), with a particular focus on perceived relationships between black and nonblack network members. In itself, these data should provide much needed basic information on the social and academic worlds of black graduate students. We then explore how these network variables are associated with three domains of adjustment: (a) academic performance, (b) psychological well-being, and (c) the extent to which the student has considered dropping out of graduate school. The overarching hypothesis is that higher levels of integration and social support will be related to better adjustment.

METHOD

Subjects and Procedures

This study was conducted at a large Midwestern university, located within a city of 10,000. The racial composition of this community was

85.1% white, 11% black, and 2.9% other (U.S. Bureau of Census, 1981). The student body consisted of approximately 36,000 students; 7,800 of these were graduate students. Approximately 10% of the total enrollment were minority students. The total number of black graduate and law students enrolled was approximately 174 (2.2% of the total graduate enrollment). There were 30 tenure track black faculty (1.4% of the total faculty population).

The first large group of black undergraduate students arrived at this institution in 1968. However, there are no data as to when the University began to admit black graduate and professional students. Some departments have had longer histories of having black students; some departments had never had a minority student. As a result, the ecological climate varied across departments in this respect.

Data were collected through self-administered surveys mailed to potential participants at their homes. Names and addresses of black graduate and medical students were provided by the Graduate College Office on Minority Students Affairs. Names of law students were provided by the Black Law Students Association.

The mail questionnaire method of data collection yields the lowest return rates in surveys research (Moser & Kalton, 1974). Several procedures were followed to insure the highest rate possible. First, a short article describing the study was placed in the Black Graduate Student Association's (BGSA) newsletter. Second, a brief announcement about the study was made at a banquet held by BGSA. These two events were arranged before the first mailing. After the first mailing, the first author attended a BGSA meeting to explain the study and to clear up any concerns. Follow-up telephone calls were made to remind students about the survey they had received. A second mailing was executed. A letter sent from the Dean of Minority Student Affairs Office, encouraging students to participate, corresponded with the second mailing.

The final sample ($n = 89$) consisted of 44 males and 44 females and 1 additional respondent who did not indicate gender (return rate was 51%). Ages of the respondents ranged from 22 to 59 ($M = 28.37, SD = 6.33$). The majority of the respondents were single ($n = 48$) or married ($n = 29$). Various disciplines were represented (biological sciences, physical sciences, architecture, engineering, mathematics, $n = 16$; social sciences, $n = 10$; education, $n = 19$; arts, humanities, music, $n = 11$; physical education, recreation, health education, leisure studies, $n = 3$; law, $n = 9$; medicine, $n = 2$; other, $n = 16$; missing, $n = 3$). The sample included 74 full-time and 15 part-time; 36 masters, 36 PhD, 10 JD, and 8 other (including nondegree) students, and was limited to those born and educated in the United States.

Respondents and nonrespondents did not differ on any of the above demographic variables.

Instruments

Social Networks and Social Support

A social network list questionnaire was used to identify the members of each student's social network. Respondents were asked to list people that were most important to them in the following four life domains: (a) four family members ("family"), (b) three faculty members in their department ("faculty"), (c) three students in their department ("student"), and (d) six people who are important but who fit into none of the other three domains ("social/other") (co-workers, ministers, friends, etc.). Detailed information was obtained on all network members (e.g., gender, ethnicity).

Several additional variables were assessed for each network member named on the list. The frequency of out-of-school contact with departmental network members was assessed. Students responded to the following question using a 5-point scale: "About how often do you see this person outside of school?" Responses for this item were used to create separate indices of the perceived frequency of nonschool contact with departmental network members based on role (student vs. faculty) and ethnicity (black vs. nonblack).

Satisfaction with perceived support was assessed for three areas: (a) financial, (b) academic (which included any nonfinancial concern related to their departments), and (c) personal (e.g., trouble with boy/girlfriend or family crises). Subjects were asked to indicate how helpful each network member was for each of the three areas on a 5-point scale. Based on research findings that the impact of support on outcomes is influenced by who provides the support as well as what issue the support is for (e.g., Hirsch & Rapkin, 1986; House & Wells, 1976; McFarlane, Neale, Norman, Roy, & Streiner, 1981), separate indices for satisfaction with each type of support based on role (student or faculty) and ethnicity (black vs. nonblack) were computed.

To measure network density, students listed the same names which they recorded on their Social Network List into a matrix. They put an "×" in those boxes where the relevant individuals were either friends or knew each other well. Several different density variables were computed, including the density among the black members of the network (black–black ties); the density among the nonblack members of the network (nonblack–nonblack ties); and the black–nonblack boundary density (black–nonblack ties). Precise formulae for calculating density values have been reported elsewhere (Hirsch, 1980, 1981a).

Outcome Measures

Four types of outcome measures were used. The first type of measure was an index of the students' actual academic performance (objective) derived from school records. The second set of outcome measures consisted of four indicants of perceived academic performance (subjective). The third set assessed psychological well-being. The fourth type of outcome was a potential attrition index.

Objective Academic Performance

The student's cumulative grade point average (GPA) at the end of the fall, 1982 semester (the semester before the study) and the student's cumulative GPA at the end of the spring 1983 semester (the semester that the study was conducted) were averaged together. GPA was obtained from university records.

Subjective Academic Performance

Four items were used as indicants of subjective academic performance. These items assessed the students' perception of how well he or she was performing in graduate school.

Comparative Performance. Subjects responded to the question, "How well do you think you are doing compared to other graduate students in your department?" by circling either (1) *below average*, (2) *about average*, or (3) *better than average.*

Satisfaction with Performance. Subjects rated their satisfaction with their academic performance on a 5-point scale ranging from (1) *very satisfied* to (5) *very dissatisfied.* This variable was recorded so that a higher score reflects greater satisfaction.

Grades. This item assessed the students' self-report of their grades on a 6-point scale ranging from (1) *all As* to (6) *mostly below C.* This variable was recorded so that a higher score indicates a higher grade.

Comparative Progress. Students responded to the question, "Would you say that in terms of how students normally progress through your graduate department that you are ...," by circling either (1) *way behind schedule*; (2) *a bit behind schedule*; (3) *on schedule*; or (4) *ahead of schedule.*

Psychological Well-Being

Bradburn Scale. The Bradburn (1969) scale is a 10-item instrument made up of two independent dimensions, positive and negative affect.

Variables relating to the presence or absence of positive affect have no relationship to the presence or absence of negative affect. A person is considered high on psychological well-being to the degree that he or she has an excess of positive over negative affect. An individual is low in well-being to the degree to which negative affect predominates over positive affect. The best indicator of self ratings of happiness is the discrepancy between positive affect and negative affect referred to as Affect Balance Scale (Bradburn, 1969). The scale has been validated on a cross-section of people of varying backgrounds. The measure has adequate reliability.

Center for Epidemiological Studies-Depression Scale (CES-D). The CES-D scale is a self-report depression scale (Radloff, 1977). The scale consists of 20 items and was designed to measure depressive symptomatology in the general population. The reliability and validity of the measure has been demonstrated across a wide variety of demographic characteristics (Comstock & Helsing, 1976; Frerichs, Aneshenel, & Clark, 1981; Thomas, Milburn, Brown, & Gary, 1988; Weissman, Sholomskas, Pottenger, Prusoff, & Locke, 1977). Scores of 16 and above are obtained by individuals who exhibit depressive symptomatology. The mean score of the current sample ($M = 20.60, SD = 6.974, n = 87$) was almost double the mean of a community sample of black adults ($M = 11.03$, $n = 451$; reported in Thomas *et al.*, 1988). Of our respondents who completed the instrument, 69% had scores above 16. These scores are also a great deal higher than a normative sample ($M = 9.1$, $SD = 8.6$, $n = 3,932$; reported in Weissman *et al.*, 1977). The high scores on the CES-D suggest that these students are under stress; although the findings are only suggestive without a suitable comparison group.

Potential Attrition Index

Thinking About Leaving School. Students indicated whether or not they had ever considered leaving their graduate program, using the following categories: (1) *No, I never thought about it at all*; (2) *Yes, but only briefly*; (3) *Yes, I have thought about it periodically*; (4) *Yes, I think about it all of the time*.

RESULTS

The first goal of the study was to assess the degree to which black students were integrated into their departmental communities. Social integration was assessed in terms of frequency of contact with department members, and densities based or role and ethnicity. We begin by presenting data on the demographic composition of their network.

Table 1. Mean Number of Network Members by Ethnicity and
Domain

	Black network members		Nonblack network members		
	M	SD	M	SD	t
Faculty	0.65	0.85	1.99	1.07	−6.87[a]
Students	1.10	1.10	1.23	1.25	−0.80
Social/other	4.14	2.10	1.40	1.95	6.31[a]
Total	5.89	2.76	4.67	3.13	1.97

[a]$p < .001$.

Network Composition

Table 1 shows that there were small numbers of black faculty in the students' networks. This is consistent with the small numbers of black faculty on this or most campuses (e.g., Blackwell, 1981a; Mitchell, 1982). There were more nonblack than black faculty in the students' networks, but similar numbers of black and nonblack departmental peers. Numbers of black students in the department ranged from 1 to 17 for study participants.

Frequency of Contact

When students were asked how often they were in contact with members of the department outside of school, they reported meeting with black faculty more frequently than did nonblack faculty network members (Kruskal-Wallis mean ranks 136.46 and 101.51, $X^2 = 17.87, p < .001$). They also reported interacting more frequently with black students than they did with non-black students (Kruskal-Wallis mean ranks 118.32 and 85.62, $X^2 = 16.69, p < .001$).

The difference in out-of-school contact with blacks versus nonblacks was large. Nearly 75% of the respondents reported never having out of school contact with nonblack faculty, whereas only 40% (approximately) reported that to be true of black faculty. Nearly 30% interacted with black faculty outside of school on a monthly or more frequent basis, but only 15% did so with nonblack faculty. A similar picture emerged for nonschool contact with students. For nearly one third of the sample, this never took place with nonblack students (only 13% said this was true of black students). Correspondingly, nearly 60% report interacting with fellow black students weekly or daily, but only 32% do so with nonblack students.

Ethnic Density and Boundary Densities

Interrelationships between network members were assessed by examining ethnic densities. We examined the connections among members of the same ethnic background as well as between network members of different ethnic backgrounds. Most participants used only two of seven ethnic categories; information was combined accordingly into two categories: (a) black (including black American and black not American) and (b) nonblack (including all other categories). There was a greater degree of connectedness among network members of the same ethnicity than between members of different ethnicities. The highest density existed among the nonblack members of the network ($M = 60.1\%$, $SD = 32.1$) and the least between black and nonblack network members ($M = 16.1\%$, $SD = 16.0$). Density among black network members fell between these values ($M = 45.8$, $SD = 45.8$).

Given our concern with social integration, a series of more detailed analyses were conducted to clarify the nature of black–nonblack boundary density. As can be seen in Table 2, relationships are quite sparse among black family members and nonblack, academic network members. As might be expected, boundary densities are greater when we consider only ties among members of the subject's academic department. Even here, however, the extent of black–nonblack integration is quite modest. Fewer than half of the black students and nonblack faculty in the same department are seen to be connected. When we consider ties between black students and nonblack students, the figure drops to one third. There is considerable variation in the extent of these ties. On the positive side, this

Table 2. Mean Boundary Densities Between Black and Nonblack Network Members By Role

Relationship type[a]	M	SD
Family–faculty	4.2	11.5
Family–students	9.2	19.8
Family–social/other	14.0	23.4
Faculty–faculty	72.4	41.4
Faculty–student	35.0	43.6
Student–faculty	47.9	39.7
Faculty–social/other	23.1	36.9
Social/other–faculty	6.4	17.5
Student–student	32.7	42.3
Student–social/other	15.2	35.2
Social/other–student	7.9	19.7
Social/other–social/other	24.5	35.4

[a] The first domain mentioned refers to the black member of the dyad and the second refers to the nonblack member.

indicates that some black graduate students were in situations where their black fellow students, though few in number, were seen to be substantially involved with the rest of the department. Unfortunately, there were also substantial numbers who found that black peers were not only few in number but also perceived to be totally isolated in the department.

There is only one partial exception to this trend. As might be expected, when there is a black faculty member in the department, this person is generally seen to be connected to the nonblack faculty there. Nonetheless, there is considerable variation in this figure as well.

Regression Analyses of Ethnic Variables on Outcomes

We next examined how these network variables were associated with students' academic performance, intention to drop out of school, and mental health. Stepwise multiple regression analyses were conducted to assess the joint impact of the social integration and network variables on academic performance, perception of performance, and mental health. The network and social support variables selected as predictors in the analysis were those that were hypothesized to reflect their degree of social integration into the academic network. Three sets of network/support variables were selected with this goal in mind: (a) the social role and/or ethnicity of the network member; (b) the frequency of interaction and quality of social support provided; and (c) the extent to which different segments of the network were integrated or segmented from each other. In light of the ratio of predictors to subjects, the adjusted R^2s were used (Pedhazur, 1982). Table 3 contains the results of the regression analyses.

There was a mild association between higher actual GPA and greater satisfaction with nonblack financial support. Turning to the four subjective measures of performance, perceiving performance as better than average was predicted by frequent nonschool contact with black faculty, low proportion of black students in the network, and high satisfaction with black academic support. High satisfaction with academic performance was associated with more satisfactory personal support from nonblack network members. The perception of being on or ahead of schedule (comparative progress) was related to a denser black–nonblack boundary. As indicated in Table 2, the greatest proportion of these ties were between black students and nonblack faculty. Thus, the greater the perceived integration between black students and non-black faculty, the more likely the student was to perceive that he or she is on schedule.

Some of the findings concerning perceived grades are inconsistent with the results for the objective GPA. Having more black graduate students in the department is negatively associated with perceived GPA but is not associated with actual GPA.

Table 3. Predictors of Performance and Well-Being

Criterion	Predictor	Adjusted R^2	Beta	df	F
Actual GPA	Satisfaction with nonblack financial support	.05	.22	1, 87	4.45[a]
Comparative performance	Nonschool contact with black faculty	.08	.29	1, 87	8.26[b]
	Proportion of black students in the network	.13	−.25	2, 86	7.37[c]
	Satisfaction with black academic support	.16	.21	3, 85	6.50[c]
Satisfaction with performance	Satisfaction with nonblack personal support	.04	.23	1, 87	4.72[a]
Comparative progress	Black–nonblack boundary density	.07	.26	1, 87	6.22[b]
Grades (self-report)	No. of black students in the department	.18	−.43	1, 87	20.17[c]
	Nonschool contact with black faculty	.22	.23	2, 86	13.58[c]
	Nonblack density	.25	.19	3, 85	10.69[c]
Positive affect	Satisfaction with black personal support	.10	.33	1, 87	10.47[c]
	Black–nonblack boundary density	.13	.22	2, 86	15.34[c]
Affect balance scale	Satisfaction with black personal support	.09	.32	1, 87	9.70[b]
	Average nonschool contact with black faculty	.14	.24	2, 86	7.91[b]
CES-D	Satisfaction with nonblack personal support	.12	−.37	1, 87	13.43[a]
	Satisfaction with black academic support	.16	−.22	2, 86	9.40[c]

[a] $p < .05$.
[b] $p < .01$.
[c] $p < .001$.

In terms of mental health outcomes, positive affect was predicted by higher satisfaction with black network member support for personal matters and denser connections between black and nonblack network members. Positive affect is related to a set of factors concerning the degree to which an individual is involved in the external environment and social contact (Bradburn, 1969). Overall morale (positive minus negative affect) was also predicted by greater satisfaction with black personal support and more nonschool contact with black faculty members. Finally, high satisfaction with nonblack personal support and with black academic support was related to low scores on the CES-D depression scale.

Thinking About Dropping Out

An important aspect of black graduate school experience is the high rate of dropout (Astin, 1977). It is critical to assess explicitly what aspects of the departmental climate may relate to this. If these factors are known, we may be able to intervene in the process. To this end, one step in the attrition process was examined: considering leaving graduate school. A discriminant function analysis was performed to see which of the 17 social integration and network variables best distinguished those students who had never thought about leaving school ($n = 27$) from those who had considered it no matter how briefly ($n = 60$).

Table 4. Discriminant Analysis of Those Who Thought About Dropping Out versus Those Who Had Not[a]

Variable	Standard coefficient	F
Black nonblack boundary density	0.75	7.34
Nonschool contact with black faculty	0.53	5.83
Satisfaction with nonblack academic support	0.50	3.13
Satisfaction with nonblack personal support	0.48	4.41
Nonblack nonschool contact	0.34	2.92
Proportion of black students in the network	−0.86	3.74
No. of black students in the department	−0.37	3.41
Black student nonschool contact	−0.31	2.75

[a]Canonical correlation = .47, $p < .01$.

As can be seen in Table 4, optimum discrimination was obtained by including eight variables. Black graduate students were less likely to have thought about dropping out of school if their network had a denser black–nonblack boundary and if they had more contact outside of school with black faculty. Greater satisfaction with academic and personal support from nonblack members, and more contact outside of school with nonblack network members, were also related to not thinking about dropping out of school. All these findings are consistent with the social integration and support hypothesis.

On the other hand, students were likely to have thought about dropping out of school if they had a larger number of black graduate students in their department and if those students constituted a larger proportion of their social network overall. This finding, though, is consistent with results of the regression analysis on perceived grades.

DISCUSSION

Although little research has been conducted on black graduate students, our findings and those of Duncan (1976) indicate that these individuals are isolated from much of their academic environment. Whether we consider out-of-school contact with nonblack faculty or students, or perceived ties between the black and nonblack members of their department, the findings are consistent in suggesting that black students are not well integrated into their departments.

As hypothesized, the extent of black graduate students' social integration was related to their psychological well-being and academic performance. Students in better integrated departments were better adjusted and perceived themselves to be making good progress in their graduate work. These students were also less likely to have considered dropping out of school.

Although consistent associations were found between indices of social integration and adjustment, we must be careful in the interpretation of these results. The research relied on self-report data collected at one university at one point in time. The results of the study show associations but do not demonstrate causal relationships. For example, it is possible that perceptions of academic performance influenced how frequently the student interacted with non-black department members. Those individuals who perceived themselves to be doing poorly may have separated themselves from nonblack department members. Poorer perceptions of performance could have led to social isolation.

We do not know whether nonblack graduate students are more or less isolated, as no comparable data exist for those populations. Nonetheless, if graduate study is generally more stressful for black than nonminority students, and if social support has its greatest impact on those under more stress (e.g., S. Cohen & Wills, 1985), then the extent of social integration should have a greater *effect* on black as opposed to nonminority students.

Two interesting patterns in the findings are discussed in detail. These findings concern (a) the number of black graduate students in the department, and (b) out-of-school contact with black faculty. Again, given the lack of prior research in this area, our discussion should be considered exploratory and suggestive.

We found that having more black graduate students in the department was associated with lower self-reported grades and a greater propensity to have thought of dropping out of graduate school. An interesting aspect of this finding is that an objective measure of the number of black graduate students in the department was not associated with actual GPA.

Why would the number of black graduate students in the department be unrelated to the objective measure of GPA but negatively related to these two other subjective measures? An important early investigation of networks and stress suggests one plausible explanation. In a field study of doctoral students preparing for preliminary examinations, Mechanic (1962) found that students in frequent contact with other students experienced the most stress in preparing for the examination. This frequent contact made them aware of all they did not know and heightened rather than reduced their feelings of uncertainty and inadequacy. Similar processes may unfold in departments characterized by many black graduate students. For a variety of reasons, these students tend to have considerable interaction with each other. The data indicate that these contacts were generally perceived as supportive, and supportive interactions with peers were positively related to adjustment. Nonetheless, there may be some negative side effects. A significant part of that time may be spent complaining about the stresses they are encountering. Constantly discussing negative experiences may tend to accent rather than reduce stress. The focus on negative experiences may also lead them to believe that they have done less well than is actually the case. Furthermore, the larger the number of black students, the likelier it is that one of them will talk about dropping out of school, leading others to at least entertain the idea themselves.

Further research is clearly needed to determine whether these findings can be replicated and to test these or alternative hypotheses. The nature of these results suggests that future research incorporate a triangulation of research methods (e.g., interviewing the person and members of their network to compare perceptions). Future investigators might consider alternatives to the stepwise regression procedure utilized in the present study. As pointed out by J. Cohen and Cohen (1975) the results of stepwise entry of data are sensitive to differences in interrelationships among variables, thus the findings may be unstable.

A second set of findings of considerable interest concerned out-of-school contact with black faculty. Although infrequent, this contact was consistently associated with better academic performance and psychological well-being. In social situations, casual conversations frequently turn to discussions about the field. Faculty may ask student opinions about their work and this may generate ideas for projects. The quality of the interaction may also suggest to the student that they are a valued part of the department and becoming a competent professional in their field; presumably a faculty member would not talk to them in such a manner unless the student was well regarded. Thus, such interactions can confer implicit recognition and validation of the student's academic identity (cf. Hirsch, 1981b), provide opportunities for problem solving that can lead to further academic progress, and furnish emotional sustenance at the same time. It is interesting that non-school contact with *black* faculty was important rather than contact with faculty in general. Contact with black faculty may be especially important because of their unique ability to serve as role models for black graduate students. Black faculty may serve as evidence to the student that they too can complete their graduate program and become competent professionals.

Although tentative, results of this study suggest a number of directions worth exploring in order to facilitate successful completion of graduate work by black students. The data provide empirical evidence of the importance of black faculty in any retention program. However, it is unrealistic to expect a few black faculty to be able to meet the special demands placed upon them by black graduate students, committees concerned with minority affairs, etc., while producing substantial research and meeting other requirements. The number of black faculty must be increased.

More must be done to integrate black students into their graduate department. Although in general the integration level was low, some departments do a better job of this than others. Future research could focus on the more successful departments in different fields and at different universities (especially urban and nonurban). Such research could generate useful strategic guidelines. We also need more departments to experiment with and evaluate new programs. Action and research are necessary, along with renewed commitment.

ACKNOWLEDGMENTS

This chapter is based on a dissertation submitted to the University of Illinois at Urbana-Champaign by the first author under the direction of the second author. We thank committee members Jerry Clore, Elaine Copeland, Ed Diener, and Thom Moore. The first author was supported by a National Institute of Mental Health Predoctoral trainneeship from the University of Illinois and a dissertation fellowship from the Center for Black Studies at the University of California at Santa Barbara. The second author was supported in part by The Center for Urban Affairs and Policy Research (Northwestern University).

REFERENCES

Allen, W. R. (1981). Correlates of black student adjustment, achievement, and aspirations at a predominantly white southern university. In G. E. Thomas (Ed.), *Black students in higher education* (pp. 126–141). Westport, CT: Greenwood.

Astin, A. W. (1982). *Minorities in American education.* San Francisco: Jossey-Bass.

Baird, L. I. (1974). A portrait of blacks in graduate studies. *Findings, 1,* 12–23.

Blackwell, J. E. (1981a). The access of black students to medical and law school: Trends and Bakee Implications. In G. E. Thomas (Ed.), *Black students in higher education* (pp. 185–202). Westport, CT: Greenwood.

Blackwell, J. E. (1981b). *Mainstreaming outsiders: The production of black professionals.* Bayside, NY: General Hall.

Blackwell, J. E. (1983). *Networking and mentoring: A study of cross-generational experiences of Blacks in graduate and professional school.* Atlanta: Southern Education Foundation.

Bradburn, N. M. (1969). *The structure of well-being.* Chicago: Aldine.

Cohen, J. & Cohen, P. (1975). *Applied multiple regression/correlation analysis for the behavioral sciences.* Hillsdale, NJ: Erlbaum.

Cohen, S. & Wills, T. A. (1985). Stress, social support, and the buffering hypothesis. *Psychological Bulletin, 98,* 310–357.

Comstock, G. W. & Helsing, K. J. (1976). Symptoms of depression in two communities. *Psychological Medicine, 133,* 551–563.

Duncan, B. L. (1976). Minority students. In J. Katz & R. T. Harnett (Eds.), *Scholars in the making.* Cambridge: Ballinger.

Frerichs, R., Aneshenel, C. S., & Clark, V. A. (1981). Prevalence of depression in Los Angeles County. *American Journal of Epidemiology, 113,* 691–699.

Gottlieb, B. H. (1981). Social networks and social support in community mental health. In B. H. Gottlieb (Ed.), *Social networks and social support* (pp. 11–42). Beverly Hills: Sage.

Hirsch, B. J. (1980). Natural support systems and coping with major life changes. *American Journal of Community Psychology, 8,* 159–172.

Hirsch, B. J. (1981a). Coping and adaptation in high-risk populations: Toward an integrative model. *Schizophrenia Bulletin, 7,* 164–172.

Hirsch, B. J. (1981b). Social networks and the coping process: Creating personal communities. In B. H. Gottlieb (Ed.), *Social networks and social support* (pp. 149–170). Beverly Hills: Sage.

Hirsch, B. J. & Rapkin, B. D. (1986). Multiple roles, social networks, and women's well-being. *Journal of Personality and Social Psychology, 51,* 1237–1247.

House, J. S. & Wells, J. A. (1976). Occupational stress social support, and health. In A. McLean, G. Black, & M. Collegen (Eds.), *Reducing occupational stress: Proceedings of a conference* (DHEW, NIOSH). Washington, DC: U.S. Government Printing Office.

Issac, P. D. (1985). Recruitment of minority students into graduate programs in psychology. *American Psychologist, 40*, 472–475.

Kjerulff, R. D. & Blood, M. R. (1973). A comparison of communication patterns in male and female graduate students. *Journal of Higher Education, 44*, 623–632.

McFarlane, A. H., Neale, K. A., Norman, G. R., Roy, R. G., & Streiner, D. L. (1981). Methodological issues in developing a scale to measure social support. *Schizophrenia Bulletin, 7*, 90–100.

Mechanic, D. (1962). *Students under stress.* New York: Free Press.

Mitchell, J. C. (1969). *Social networks in urban situations.* Manchester, England: Manchester University Press.

Mitchell, J. (1982). Reflections of a black social scientist: Some struggles, some doubts, some hopes. *Harvard Educational Review, 52*, 27–44.

Moore, T. (1977). Social change and community psychology. In I, Iscoe, Bloom, & C. D. Spielberger (Eds.), *Community psychology in transition.* Washington, DC: Hemisphere Press.

Moser, S. C. & Kalton, G. (1974). *Survey methods in social investigation.* New York: Basic Books.

National Board on Graduate Education. (1976). *Minority participation in graduate education,* Washington, DC: National Academy of Science.

Pedhazur, E. J. (1982). *Multiple regression in behavior research.* New York: Holt.

Radloff, L. S. (1977). The CES-D scale: A self-report depression scale for research in the general population. *Applied Psychological Measurement, 1*, 385–401.

Thomas, V. G., Milburn, N. G., Brown, D. R., & Gary, L. E. (1988). Social support and depressive symptoms among blacks. *Journal of Black Psychology, 14*, 35–45.

U.S. Bureau of the Census. (1981). *1980 census of the population,* Washington, DC: U.S. Government Printing Office.

Weissman, M. M., Sholomskas, D., Pottenger, M., Pruskoff, B. A., & Locke, B. Z. (1977). Assessing depressive symptoms in five psychiatric populations: A validation study. *American Journal of Epidemiology, 106*, 203–214.

16

Expectations and High School Change: Teacher–Researcher Collaboration to Prevent School Failure

Rhona S. Weinstein, Charles R. Soulé, Florence Collins, Joan Cone, Michelle Mehlhorn, and Karen Simontacchi

Describes the multilevel outcomes of a collaborative preventive intervention for ninth-graders at risk for school failure using qualitative and quasi-experimental methods. Teachers, administrators, and researchers implemented innovative practices communicating positive expectations for low-achieving adolescents in their transition to high school. Changes were made in the practices of curriculum, grouping, evaluation, motivation, student responsibility, and relationships (in the classroom, with parents, and in the school). Both implementation and evaluation evolved as a function of collaboration. Change was promising but not uniform. Project teachers became more positive about students and colleagues, expanded their roles, and changed school tracking policies. The 158 project students, in contrast to the 154 comparison students showed improved grades and disciplinary referrals post-intervention and increased retention in school 1 year later, but their absences rose and improved performance was not maintained. The implications of this analysis for school-based interventions and its evaluation are discussed.

Originally published in the *American Journal of Community Psychology, 19*(3) (1991): 333–363.

A Quarter Century of Community Psychology: Readings from the American Journal of Community Psychology, edited by Tracey A. Revenson *et al.* Kluwer Academic/Plenum Publishers, New York, 2002.

This paper describes the multi-level outcomes and lessons learned from a collaborative preventive intervention project aimed at systemic change in classroom and school practice. A high school and a university collaborated to prevent the school failure of "at-risk" ninth-graders, largely a minority population, during their first year of high school. Based on an expectancy communication model, teachers, administrators, and researchers developed and implemented innovative instructional practices and school policies promoting positive expectations and educational support for low-achieving adolescents at risk for school dropout. Using qualitative and quasi-experimental methods in a case study of a single school, we examine the process of collaborative change at multiple levels of the system, reflecting upon the impact of the intervention on us as researchers, the teachers, the school, and the students.

SCHOOL FAILURE AS A PROBLEM

In recent years, we have seen a flurry of national reports about the state of our schools and our persistent failure to educate large segments of our population, in particular, minorities (*A Nation at Risk*, 1983: *Children in Need*, 1987). Of enormous concern is evidence for *great inequality* in educational outcomes, *differential and higher dropout rates* for minorities as compared to majority students, and a *widening gap* in performance between groups of students over the course of schooling (*Excellence for whom*, 1984; Rumberger, 1987; Wilcox & Vincent, 1987). Although there are numerous problems in estimating the extent of the dropout problem, the available evidence, for example, in a sample of youth over 18 assessed between 1979–1982, suggests that dropout rates are higher for Blacks (23%) and Hispanics (36%) as compared to Whites (12%) (General Accounting Office, 1987).

California is among the first states to have minority children equal and now outnumber non-minority children in their schools (Guthrie & Kirst, 1988). It is also clear that early school failure predicts a continuing cycle of problems—subsequent school failure,.poor self-esteem, attendance and disciplinary problems, school dropout, unemployment, criminal activity, and mental health problems (Butler, Marsh, Sheppard, & Sheppard, 1985; Cowen, Peterson, Babigian, Izzo, & Trost, 1973; Kornberg & Caplan, 1980; Rumberger, 1987; Schorr, 1988). The cost is indeed high when schools as currently constituted might not be meeting the needs of at least half of their youngsters, given the changing demographics of our nation's schools. Urgent pleas have been made for wider efforts and early preventive programs aimed at what has come to be called "at risk" youth (Olsen, 1987).

SCHOOLING AS A RISK FACTOR: THE ROLE OF EXPECTATIONS

While certain groups of children have been identified as being at risk for school failure (the so-called educationally disadvantaged—the poor and minorities), it is increasingly clear that the school environment serves as a risk factor as well. Teacher and school effectiveness studies point to great variation between classrooms and schools in the educational outcomes achieved, despite similarity in the characteristics of the student body (Good & Weinstein, 1986; Rutter, Maughan, Mortimore & Ouston, 1979).

One important factor that places certain groups of children at risk is the operation of differential and very low academic expectations for what they can accomplish. Minorities and children from lower socio-economic classes are largely overrepresented as the target of low expectations (Alexander & Entwisle, 1987; Jones 1989). The dynamics of teacher expectations and how they can become self-fulfilling prophecies have been well illustrated within classrooms (toward individual children and between reading groups) and between classrooms (in the tracking system of high schools) (Brophy, 1983; Dusek, 1985; Oakes, 1985; Weinstein, 1989). Studies of effective schools have also pointed to the expectations of principals and teachers as powerful influences on student performance (Good & Weinstein, 1986).

Differential expectations for academic performance can often result in different opportunities to learn and different treatment in school from both teachers and peers. Our research on children's awareness of teacher expectations suggests that children (even as young as first-graders) can identify differential treatment practices that favor high over low achievers with more opportunities, choice, and positive feedback in the classroom (Weinstein & Middlestadt, 1979; Weinstein, Marshall, Brattesani, & Middlestadt, 1982; Weinstein, Marshall, Sharp, & Botkin, 1987). That children are aware of differential treatment practices and infer their relative smartness from such cues suggests a potential eroding of motivation for children at the low end of the achievement hierarchy—an erosion that might culminate in eventual school dropout. Indeed, Rumberger (1987) noted that 44% of the reasons students list for dropping out of school concern negative feelings about and experiences in school. However, motivation is far from the only issue of concern, for differential opportunity to learn, accorded on the basis of expectations, also results in different curricula and ultimately different school career paths which, once undertaken, are difficult to change.

AN EXPECTANCY COMMUNICATION MODEL FOR INTERVENTION

While the call to "raise expectations" has become a large part of recent school improvement efforts, relatively little is known about how to implement both *higher* and *more equitable* academic expectations in practice. There are surprisingly few intervention efforts targeted toward preventing the negative effects of expectancy processes in schooling. One such example is TESA, a classroom-level intervention, which trains teachers to equalize interactions with students, for example, in the distribution of praise and criticism (Kerman, 1979). Although an important effort, this project addresses only a piece of the web of low and unequal expectations that is currently institutionalized in schooling practices. Other societal legislative interventions to equalize educational opportunity, such as desegregation and mainstreaming, have remained plagued by continued segregation of groups of children at yet other levels of the system, in reading groups, tracks, and special classes (Epstein, 1985).

Our research on children's understanding of expectancy processes in the classroom suggests a theoretical model, as well as beginning empirical evidence, for the interactive characteristics of classroom and school environments which promote positive expectations for all children (Marshall & Weinstein, 1984, 1986, 1988; Weinstein, 1989). The model looks beyond patterns of differential teacher–child interaction to include the structure and organization of classroom and school life, which sets the stage for certain kinds of educational and social opportunities. Practices, such as different curriculum for different ability levels, ability-based grouping for instruction, and a single criterion for performance evaluation, heighten ability comparisons among students, with detrimental consequences for some. Alternative practices, which integrate diverse groups of students around meaningful and complex tasks, provide a variety of performance opportunities, and call for student input and control, expand definitions of ability, and increase the possibilities for motivated and successful learning of more students.

Eight features of the instructional environment are identified as critical in communicating expectations to students (see Table 1). To cre a *task environment and curriculum* (higher-order, more meaningful, more participative tasks), in *grouping for instruction* (heterogeneous, interest-based, flexible groupings), in the opportunities afforded by the *evaluation, motivation,* and *student responsibility* structures (varied performance opportunities recognizing multiple abilities, task-mastery focus, cooperative learning strategies, student-directed and student leadership opportunities), and in the *relationships in the classroom, between parents and teachers,* and

Table 1. Elements of Expectancy Communication Model

Elements	Differential practices
Curriculum	Certain tasks/curricular tracks heighten ability comparisons. Differential task allocation: highs are enriched and lows are remediated; differential curriculum lessens opportunity to learn for lows.
Grouping	Grouping by ability (reading groups, tracks) heightens ability comparisons, framing perceived competence. Ability-based inflexible grouping provides differential opportunity to learn, and limits peer contact.
Evaluation	Certain ability beliefs (that intelligence is stable, global, and distributed along a normal curve) limit the provision of varied types of performance opportunities for evaluation, creating a single set of winners/losers. Differential allocation of performance opportunities and feedback to highs and lows.
Motivation	Competitive, ego-evaluative reward systems heighten ability comparisons, limit peer interaction, decrease intrinsic motivation. Different motivators used for high (intrinsic) and low (extrinsic) achievers.
Responsibility for learning	Limited student agency restricts the uncovering of talent/competence, diminishes motivation. Differential opportunities for responsibility and choice for high and low achievers.
Class relations	Narrow academic agenda frames relationships, creating a bimodal distribution of stars and isolates, devaluing diversity and community. Differential allocation of warmth, trust, humor, and concern to high and low achievers.
Parent–class relations	Limited and narrow communication opportunities (left to problems or parent initiation) creates winner/loser families. Differential parent/class relationship for high and low achievers.
School–class relations	Limited opportunities for participation and recognition at a school-wide level leaves chances for success to just the classroom. Differential opportunities for school involvement, leadership, and reward for highs and lows.

between the classroom and the school (valuing diversity in the creation of a class community, ongoing communication and shared expectations between teachers and all parents, and access to school-wide activities and rewards).

A COLLABORATIVE PROCESS FOR SCHOOL EXPECTANCY CHANGE

How might such institutionalized and embedded expectancy practices be changed? This expectancy communication model required large-scale alterations, that is, a restructuring of instructional within-setting regularities for students (Sarason, 1971, 1982; Seidman, 1988). There have been relatively few system-oriented school change programs (e.g., Comer, 1980; Felner, Ginter, & Primavera, 1982; Solomon, Watson, Delucchi, Schaps, & Battistich, 1988) with the majority of interventions directed at improving teacher effectiveness in the classroom across a narrow range of teacher behaviors. Such studies have largely utilized a prescriptive approach, with a pre-packaged set of practices to follow. Yet organizational change theory (Beer & Walton, 1987) and longer term followup of innovations that persist in school change efforts (Berman & McLaughlin, 1978) underscore the importance of teacher/principal input and involvement, as critical factors in the successful implementation and institutionalization of innovations. This pointed to the need for a collaborative model of change, engaging researchers and school staff in a joint and creative translation of research findings into practice.

In the recent surge of school renewal efforts, there has been increased interest in school–university partnerships. Gifford (1986) has suggested that collaboration produces practice-sensitive researchers and research-sensitive practitioners, improving the potential for substantive and meaningful school change. Working within an ecological paradigm, Kelly and Kingry-Westergaard (1988) also argue that contributions to knowledge which rest on a collaborative relationship between the scientist and the research participants, enhance the validity and benefit of new knowledge. We believed that the authenticity and power of our work together would be maximized if school staff became consumers of the research literature on expectancy processes, and if we as researchers learned about the supports for and the constraints against changes in expectancy processes in the schools. Only then would we be in a position to jointly design, implement, and sustain alternative instructional practices and policies.

Multilevel Effects. With collaborative change, one might expect a fluid and multilevel process. Design and evaluation would evolve in the context of collaborative negotiation. Change would occur at multiple levels of the system. We expected that the researchers and the school staff would be touched by the process of our collaborative work together. Our successful collaboration would be the stepping stone for the creation of new practices and policies. Only when these innovations were in place in the classroom and the school, would we impact on students.

TRANSITION TO HIGH SCHOOL: OPPORTUNITY FOR PREVENTIVE INTERVENTION

Normative life transitions, such as school entry or the start of high school, represent a time of heightened sensitivity and enormous stress, with clear implications for future achievement (Felner *et al.*, 1982; Felner & Adan, 1988). As Felner and colleagues have demonstrated, straightforward systemic changes (such as having classes rather than individuals change teachers and creating homerooms) prove critical in enhancing adjustment, evidenced in project students' superior attendance rates, grade point averages, and self-concept as compared to untreated control students.

Secondary schools as currently constituted also provide severely limited contexts for adolescent development, particularly for the neediest students (Hamilton, 1984). The transition to high school can become problematic for the low-achieving adolescent (where minority and poor are overrepresented) since this is a time when expectations for academic performance are perhaps the most blatant. The widespread tracking of students into ability-based classes, with differential curricula as well as eligibility for college admission credit, immediately sends a message of difference and failure to those less academically able (Oakes, 1985). Our collaborating teachers and administrators identified the ninth grade year as the critical "make or break" year for students at risk for school failure. Preventive intervention with this group of students during their transitional year in high school became the target for our collaborative school change project.

COLLABORATIVE DEVELOPMENT OF METHODOLOGY

Entry

As Sarason and his colleagues argue in *The Preparation of Teachers* (1962, 1986), nothing about schooling will change until our teaching about "teaching" changes. Thus, our starting point became the creation of a university seminar experience which would address the expectancy literature, i.e., model it, in a way that teachers and administrators could apply it to school change efforts. We sought a diversity of perspectives in seminar membership, opening it to community teachers and administrators in addition to graduate students. We required reading of original research, systematic classroom and school observation of each of the components of the expectancy model, and a final project integrating the eight features of the model in the design of innovative lessons and policy. The seminar concept also served as a model for the school-based inservice workshops and the regularized meetings which formed the basis of the planned preventive intervention.

Our invitation to work with a school came from this seminar. A participating high school teacher asked us to join her in approaching her principal about the possibility of bringing the seminar into her school, targeting

low-achieving ninth-graders (largely a minority population) in their first
year of high school in order to prevent later school dropout. Jointly, we
planned a two-stage process: first, to hold a three-session inservice workshop with interested teachers and administrators at the high school, bringing aspects of our seminar into the school, and second, to encourage
participants of this workshop to begin collaboration on an experimental
program for at risk ninth grade students for the next academic year. Twelve
teachers (representing English, history, math, and science), the principal,
and the vice-principal participated in all three sessions of the workshops
and pledged commitment to the intervention research.

Design

Plans and Stumbling Blocks. Given our invitation into the school, we
expected smooth sailing. However, school realities, university realities, and
the often colliding expectations of individuals who differed in role as well
as personal style, slowed our progress and led to heated discussions, hard-
won compromises, and a melding of perspectives over the course of the
project. The planned intervention and its evaluation (with which we began)
was not what was, in fact, implemented. Despite the invited entry, despite
the shared concerns, there were thorny problems to address before the
intervention project was underway.

We proposed to assign participating students to at least two project
teachers in order to create a school within a school program. Project teachers would be allocated a common preparation period timed around the
lunch hour, so that teachers, administrators, and researchers could have a
regular weekly meeting of substantial length for collaborative planning.
Our work together would revolve around the implementation of the eight
factor expectancy model in classroom practices and school policies. By randomly assigning the projected entering class of approximately 120 low-
stanine (the bottom three percentiles of the achievement score distribution)
ninth-graders to project and control classes in English, history, health science,
and reading (if needed), we could evaluate the effects of the intervention
on teachers and students.

However, we encountered four problems that served to shape the
direction of the project. First, perceived scheduling constraints did not
allow for a single shared preparation period for all project teachers during
the first intervention year. Instead, some shared third period and some
shared fifth period, with all the teachers available during the lunch hour in
between. Thus, the format of our collaborative work shifted to part team
and part whole group work during the first year.

Second, enrollment realities in week three of the first intervention year (only half the expected numbers of low stanine students arrived) led to the abrupt cancellation of all the control classes. Although the project teachers volunteered to split themselves and their students into project and control classes to save the integrity of the study, we felt it to be an unwise choice. The intervention had already begun, a critical mass of participants was essential to creating systemic change, and the low N, further subdivided, would provide little statistical power for testing the effects of the program. The late date, as well as limited financial resources (hence personnel), made a search for a control school unfeasible, forcing us to think creatively about alternative designs for evaluation.

Third, given the collaborative nature of the study, our collective vision of preferred procedures to inform and protect research subjects clashed in part with the vision of the university Human Subjects Committee, necessitating a process of negotiation. Since the teachers were our collaborators in designing the study, they were not happy to be viewed as "subjects" (and hence required to sign informed consent forms). Yet given that teachers were also providing research data, the Committee wanted to apply standard procedures to protect subject rights. Some teachers refused to sign on principle as the term "subject" violated their understanding of collaboration (thus limiting the data we could collect). Regarding student involvement which required direct assessments, we were approved to solicit parental consent forms. This task proved difficult, much like the intervention program itself, in light of poor student attendance patterns, long parent work hours, and many disconnected phones. With the cancelled control group and our shift to archival student data only, we asked whether we might gain access to student records without consent, given our collaborative interest with the school staff in these records and the use of appropriate safeguards such as student ID numbers. This procedure was eventually approved enabling us to study the entire population of low achievers at the school. Just following these negotiations, human subject guidelines were rewritten to allow researchers access to student school records without informed consent as long as student identities were not revealed, as in our case. This long process of discussion proved informative about the ways in which setting and university collaborative research designs do not easily fit the language or procedures of traditional social science research.

Finally, administrators, teachers, and researchers could not agree upon the grouping assignment for students targeted for intervention. To track or to un-track unleashed lengthly emotional debates. Clearly our expectancy model pushed for heterogeneous grouping of students across ability levels. Yet school and district policy constraints as well as conflicts between teachers pulled us in other directions and forced us to compromise. Recognizing the entrenched nature of tracking, we agreed to begin within a tracked system with the goal of working towards the de-tracking of classes. For the first year of the intervention, project students were tracked into 2–3 stanine level classes in English (as always) and in history and health science (for the first time). During the second year, the band of achievement was broadened in class assignments, clearly a project outcome. More changes were to follow.

Negotiated Design. Thus, the proposed form and evaluation of our preventive intervention project underwent change as we collaborated to make it fit differing visions and unanticipated constraints. We chose a mixed qualitative and quasi-experimental empirical approach, charting both the course of the intervention over time and evidence for change at multiple levels, in the educators of teachers (us), in teachers, in school policies, and finally, as seen in the students. At the level of the student, an archival cohort design (Cook & Campbell, 1979) allowed us to evaluate the impact of the intervention by contrasting the performance of two consecutive cohorts of project students with that of a comparable group of students from two previous years' classes. Without a concurrent comparison sample of teachers and students, we were limited to data available in school records. Although enrollment was up in the second year of the intervention, we continued the same evaluation design, given the spreading effects of the intervention through the school (making a within-school control group tricky) and similar funding constraints (limiting the consideration of a control school).

Participants

School Site and Staff. The collaborative intervention project was implemented during two academic years (1986–1987 and 1987–1988) at a mid-sized urban high school with an ethnically heterogeneous student body and a minority enrollment of 68%. The school enrolled approximately 1500 students and had a certificated staff of 80. In all, 14 faculty participated in the project: ten teachers (English, reading, world history, science, computer, and special education), a counsellor, a dean, the principal, and the vice-principal. All faculty members had volunteered and had 10 or more years of experience, including several years teaching at the grade and ability level targeted for the project. Over the course of the project, three of the teachers withdrew their participation (given the heavy workload and their frustration with system constraints), one teacher left on maternity leave, and two other teachers joined in the second year. Administrative reassignment also occurred with a new principal, vice-principal, dean, and counsellor appointed.

Targeted Students. All incoming ninth-graders who were assigned to the lowest track of English classes joined in the intervention. Parents and students were informed that they were part of a special program where teachers would collaborate in their teaching of these students. Common practice at this high school, as with most high schools, placed students into four tracks of classes (honors, college preparatory, average, and low-stanine). Typically, students in the lowest track scored in the second and third stanines or percentiles in reading on the California Achievement Test (CAT). These students were placed in classes which did not earn college preparatory credit and which were generally viewed as remedial courses for the non-college bound.

Excluded from the student sample were students repeating ninth grade and students who entered ninth grade after the beginning of the school year. In all, we obtained a sample of 158 students (59 in 1986–1987 and 99 in 1987–1988) who participated in project classes. These students were contrasted to a comparison sample of 154 comparable students in their ninth grade year, drawn from cohorts in the 2 school years prior to the initiation of the intervention study (74 in 1984–1985 and 80 in 1985–1986).

Overall, this population of ninth grade students was slightly more male (54.2%) than female (45.8), with the following ethnic breakdown: 68.3% Black, 7.4% Hispanic, 4.2% Asian, 10.6% Caucasian, and 9.5% unknown. Of interest, Blacks were overrepresented and Caucasians under-represented in this population, relative to the ethnicity of the school as a whole (47.7% Black, 5.0% Hispanic, 16.3% Asian, 30.1% Caucasian, and 1.9% unknown). Academically, prior to entering ninth grade, students in the sample were performing on the low end on all measures (mean eighth grade scores were 25.42 on CAT reading percentile; 1.77 in English and 1.23 in history, on a 4-point scale). Absences were high (12.41 for English and 12.68 for history in eighth grade spring semester).

Intervention

The intervention focused on changing the classroom and school environment for at-risk ninth grade students to raise expectations for performance and motivate these adolescents to become engaged in schooling. The provision of a more positive expectancy climate was viewed as a vehicle for improving student performance and behavior in school and ultimately preventing school dropout. Rather than prescribing the innovative classroom practices and school policies, a group of teachers, administrators, and researchers collaborated in regular weekly meetings to develop, implement, and evaluate the innovations introduced. Students were programmed into one or more of the classes of participating teachers who shared a common

preparation period each day scheduled around the lunch hour. Both the
sharing of common students and of planning periods created a school
within a school program which the teachers named PACT (Promoting
Achievement through Cooperative Teaching).

The meetings served a variety of purposes, including (1) review
and discussion of research relating to the eight-component expectancy
communication model, (2) design and evaluation of innovative classroom
practices aimed at changing expectations, (3) case conferencing about students, (4) coordination of intervention efforts and policy planning with
administrators, counsellors, and deans, and (5) examination of the process
of expectancy change. These meetings created the material, programs, lesson plans, and policies that teachers then implemented in their classrooms.
Table 2 describes the types of innovative practices teachers implemented in
their classrooms.

Table 2. Innovative Positive Expectancy Practices Implemented

Elements	Innovative practices
Curriculum	Enriched curriculum materials—adapting readings from honors classes. Enriched methods of instruction—editing groups for writing, teams to create history materials.
Grouping	Regrouping strategies to help all students work with everyone. Heterogeneous grouping—moving selected students to honors classes, encouraging student involvement in school activities. Keeping opportunities open—retroactive college prep credit policy if earned.
Evaluation	Broadening performance opportunities to increase success—role plays, drama, class newsletter, peer teaching. Shared positive feedback across teachers.
Motivation	Cooperative rather than competitive teaching strategies—team learning. Focus on intrinsic motivation—encouraging student interest (community service project, choice in reading, writing).
Responsibility for learning	More active student participation—making choices, taking leadership in peer work groups, providing feedback to peers. Training in work study skills, conflict management strategies.
Class relations	Developing individual relationships with each student—individual conferences, writing assignments about being a ninth-grader and school success. Encouraging diversity of talent and views.
Parent–class relations	Reaching out to parents and bringing parents in—calls to parents with positive news, joint teacher–parent–student conferences, special evening meetings, class newsletter focused on parent writing and questions.
School–class relations	Encouraging student participation in school activities—special speakers (coaches, minority student models), creation of community service program.

Implementation Check. What can we say about the degree or fidelity of implementation of this model of high expectations? A 44-item teacher practices survey (developed as a crude implementation check) assessed the frequency with which (never, sometimes, often, always) teachers engaged in practices which instilled high expectations in students, across the eight domains of the model, e.g., "the tasks I assign are challenging and stimulate thinking," "each student has varied performance opportunities, which call for different abilities." Six teachers completed the survey early in the intervention and again at the end of the first intervention year, showing a trend for the predicted increase in positive expectancy behaviors [M(fall) = 107.8, M(spring) = 121.4; t = 2.09, df = 4, $p < .10$, one-tailed].

Analysis of our narrative records of project meetings suggested evolving but systematic attempts by each teacher to address each of the components of the model. The complexity of working toward multiple goals (learning about the negative effects of existing practices, channeling that insight into the creation of alternative practices, and supporting implementation) across diverse aspects of the school environment (the complex eight-component expectancy communication model) meant that innovative practices were put in place little by little as our collaborative team worked through cognitive and systemic constraints. Certainly, upgrading the challenge of curricular materials proved easiest to implement since materials could be adapted directly from honors level classes. Substantive changes in grouping practices (un-tracking) took longer to accomplish, with step-wise changes along the way. We also discovered that the capacity to implement innovative practices which violated long-standing norms, such as cooperative learning (in the face of competitive motivational environments), was predicated on the capacity of our team to successfully turn their own early competitive patterns into cooperative relations. What we might term full implementation of the model was never achieved. Rather, innovative practices were constantly under development and revision in the face of continual stumbling blocks. The collaboration provided the resources and the emotional support to work through the constraints. By their own report, some teachers felt more successful than others and some components of the model were easier to put in place as well.

Although we did not collect student perceptions of these changed practices, anecdotal evidence from outside evaluators of the program suggest student awareness of higher expectations. Interviewed students described their project teachers as "making sure you do your work," "our teachers care; they make you feel comfortable," and "they expect you to finish whole books, discuss them, write about them." One student wrote about the project teacher as follows:

> In Mrs. ____'s class one of my favorite teacher's she make me feel good
> about myself and she doesn't say well you ought to just stick with something

simple. She just let's you think about it and if you would like to take a
challenge and if you think that you could actually do it, then she would
encourage you to do so (Freedman, 1989).

Data Sources and Analysis

Narrative Records of Project Meetings. Detailed narrative records were
kept of the 2 years of the weekly meetings involving teachers, administrators, and researchers. These sequential records provided extensive
detail about the perceptions and attitudes of the participants, the activities
engaged in, and the conflicts aroused. An independent coder reviewed all
records to systematically identify the innovative changes introduced in
classrooms and the reported responses.

Student School Records. In addition to obtaining prior eighth grade performance, we evaluated student outcomes at two time periods, at the end of
ninth grade after 1 year of intervention (available for all students), and again
at the end of tenth grade at a 1-year post-project followup (available for the
first year project cohort and the two comparison cohorts only). Given curricular changes (the combination of English and reading classes in the second year of the intervention), the uneven number of project classes by
subject area, and several teacher withdrawals from the project, the clearest
and most consistent areas for evaluation of student academic performance
were found in English and history. Hence, the evaluation of project outcomes was limited to these two subject areas, as well as GPA, absences, disciplinary referrals, and year-end disposition, where available. Working
from school records meant that information was often limited. For example,
GPAs were not computed in eighth grade records. Disciplinary referrals
had to be constructed from counsellor records and were not available for
eighth grade and too costly to obtain at the tenth grade follow-up.

From school records we obtained the following information about
students' background, academic performance, and school behavior:
(1) gender and ethnicity, (2) prior year *pre-intervention* second semester
eighth grade CAT reading test scores, grades, and absences in English and
history, (3) *early intervention* first semester ninth grade GPA and disciplinary referrals (given unavailability of eighth grade data on these measures),
(4) *post-intervention* second semester ninth grade English and history
grades and absences, GPA, and disciplinary referrals, and (5) *1-year followup* second semester tenth grade English grades and absences (history
was not taken by all students), GPA, withdrawals, and disposition.

The four student cohorts were not found to differ significantly in
gender, ethnicity, prior year eighth grade performance in English and history,
or in prior absence rates. But the second year intervention cohort

(1987–1988) scored significantly higher than all three cohorts in entering CAT scores in reading ($F = 4.47$; $df = 3, 239$; $p < .01$), not surprisingly, given that the project was now directed toward a wider band of achievers. However, in order to maximize the N and given overall comparability of the samples at entry as well as similar patterns of results when run separately, the combined two years of project groups ($N = 158$) were contrasted to the combined comparison cohorts ($N = 154$), with students' entering CAT scores used as a covariate in all analyses.

MULTI-LEVEL PROCESSES OF CHANGE

Researchers

The process of our collaboration with school staff was planned to model the very conditions that teachers would then implement in the classroom. Early on, the narrative records of our weekly meetings revealed the teachers turning to the researchers as experts for leadership:

> I understand that you set up a program to help me discover things for myself but I guess I wanted to be fed information.

Yet our more familiar leadership stance, when unchecked, was met with resistance. The much harder and ultimately more successful route involved the sharing of leadership and the struggle for compromise. Later meetings showed increasing school staff responsibility for the project and less visible researcher presence.

We learned patience, we made trade-offs, but we also deepened our understanding. The pace of the project was slow, given the need to resolve the differing views of many participants. Committed to working with these teachers and this school, we compromised with research design and methodology. Given multiple constraints, we began working within a tracking system, seeking to improve adolescents' experiences in the lowest track whereas we had hoped that the initial intervention would dismantle the tracking system for these students. We arrived at that planned target only at the point at which all of our collaborators could support and implement these changes. In reading and writing of research (our papers were jointly authored), we learned to appreciate the teachers' perspectives and to drop our jargon. One of our collaborators became violent over the research jargon:

> If you mean a pair why the—heck—do you have to say "dyad." When every minute is precious and I wanted to know what meaning lay in this paper that could affect my teaching, I fumed at the arrogance of obfuscation.

We learned when new practices worked, when they did not, and to try again. We discovered how deeply embedded and institutionalized expectations are in the very fabric of schooling, that is, in within-district and outside-district pressures to select rather than to develop talent in students. We also saw that collaborative participant–researcher inquiry does not easily mix with the canons of social science research. Our negotiated study rocked the expectations of more formal relations between researchers and subjects, of randomized control comparisons, and of prescriptive and time-bounded interventions. Our prior theories underwent some revision as well. Having largely taken the child's point of view in the study of expectancy processes, we were perhaps less prepared for the inevitable moment when the classroom environment changed but the youngsters did not respond. Our understanding of the complexity of expectancy processes deepened and our appreciation for the person–environment transactional aspects of self-fulfilling prophecies (the students' capacities to respond) was renewed.

Teachers

The narrative records revealed the character of the changes in participating teachers over the course of the collaborative project, reflecting shifts in their attitudes and actions toward their colleagues (other teachers and administrators), their role as teachers, and their students. Change in expectations about colleagues and in role expectations occurred in the context of our weekly meetings and strengthened teachers' capacity to bring changes to their classrooms.

Attitudes Toward Colleagues. Teachers became more comfortable exposing their own teaching practices to collaborative analysis and scrutiny. In early inservice workshops, one teacher described the constraints against sharing as "an atmosphere of competition—the inference is I've done that, well, you mean you haven't done that!" This perceived competition had obviously changed into a climate of mutual respect and trust, evident in another teacher's comment, halfway into the first intervention year:

> I've become open and vulnerable to support and criticism from my colleagues in the project, seeing them as professionals who can support me and be supported by me, who are as interested as I in making the school work (Mehlhorn, 1987).

With this increased openness, came insight, new learning, and sometimes disappointment. Just as teachers were striving to go the extra mile with their students, so too, did they have to extend their patience to colleagues, each at different places regarding their perspectives on problem definition or solution. However, teachers began to learn from each other and to generate alternative strategies for problem resolution that capitalized on each other as resources as well as a more coordinated use of the school's administrative services. Teachers became more vocal and more demanding that their fellow teachers follow through on their plans, that deans and counsellors collaborate in the planning for students, and that the administrators fully support their intervention effort. Letters were sent and appointments made with the superintendent, the school board, the Parent–Teacher Association as teachers became energized to collaborate and demand accountability for student outcomes.

Role Expectations. Teachers' role definitions changed over the course of the collaborative intervention project. They began reading and sharing the research literature on teaching, subscribing to journals, and calling the university for lists of courses and readings. Project teachers also sought funding (both inside and outside the district) for their planned programs. A grant they won from a national organization funded a school-wide program for all the teachers on fostering creative writing across the curriculum. One teacher was successful in getting 16 computers from the university for her high school project class. Project teachers began to write and communicate their findings to fellow teachers, to the university community in two SUPER sponsored evening seminars, and to regional and national associations, "moving from reading and applying research to writing it" (Cone, 1989). A highlight of our collaborative writing activities was the symposium four of the teachers and the two researchers presented at the 1988 American Educational Research Association meeting in New Orleans. Part of the excitement lay in the writing itself:

> Little did we expect how much the writing would mean to us. As we wrote, we reflected on the growth that we had experienced as teachers, the effect we had had on our school, and the success our students had shown.... I can clearly remember the first day we got together to read our individual papers to each other. All of us fought back tears as we realized how much we had grown and how much we owed that growth to each other (Cone, 1989).

And part of the excitement lay in participation in and recognition by a national network of colleagues:

> [At AERA] Researchers' findings confirmed PACT philosophy and practices and offered inspiration and new techniques. Teachers were honored to attend the meeting and felt that more teachers and administrators should have the opportunity to hear presentations that offer the latest findings in educational research (Collins, 1988).

Finally, project teachers began to take a leadership and mentoring role in spreading the ideas of the PACT project to other teachers both within the school and beyond in the district, an example of their systemic impact. Lunch meetings were opened to non-project teachers around specific topics. One of the teachers applied for and won a mentor teacher award in which she implemented an adapted version of the seminar and project with faculty in a neighboring high school. In the year following the 2-year intervention project, four of the teachers delivered inservice workshops to three other schools within the district as well as at the county level to bring PACT teaching strategies to their colleagues.

Actions and Attitudes Toward Students. Teachers began to share more complex, differentiated, and positive views of student abilities. When they introduced a new lesson format, demanding different skills from students, they reported that they saw new sides of student talent. When they went the extra mile for students, for example, in responding to the student's *presence* in the classroom rather than the forgotten books and assignment, they were often rewarded with renewed enthusiasm and involvement in learning. Beginning the project with a focus on the deficits that these students bring to the classroom, over the course of our collaboration, teachers talked more and more about the capabilities these adolescents had demonstrated:

> I don't know if you collect student papers as evidence that below grade level students can think but if you do, these are to me startling examples— both boys are reading at the fifth to sixth grade level. Their papers bowled me over. I don't think my honors kids will do better.

With the more positive perceptions about these students came a renewed dedication toward making a difference and promoting positive outcomes. For example, teachers became more willing to directly confront and deal with a student–teacher conflict rather than send a student to the dean's office for disciplinary action. Quantitative evidence for change in teacher perceptions of these students can be seen in the pre- and post-intervention contrast of project and comparison students (presented in the section on students). Improvements in grades and GPA and a decrease in disciplinary referrals are in part teacher-mediated variables (not pure student qualities) and reflect the more positive teacher views of students over the course of the project.

Frustrations. Along with these very positive changes, there were also many difficult moments, and much anger and disappointment. The extent of the project students' problems was overwhelming at times. Some students did not respond at all to the changed classroom conditions. These were sad times when project teachers worked hard to maintain high expectations and hopefulness about their potential efficacy.

Teachers grew disappointed at the lack of district support for the project, at meetings which district officials cancelled because the project was not a priority, and at the ignoring of the project in district public relation efforts.

Teachers also bristled at the unevenness of administrative support for their efforts. Many meetings, many confrontations took place before the conditions for this collaborative project were ensured. There was much discouragement that this model was not adapted by administration as an organizational vehicle for the entire high school. There was anger at the administration that responsibility for these low achieving students was placed solely on the backs of project teachers ("the remedial teachers")—anger that resulted in one teacher's withdrawal from the project. Several other teachers also chose to leave because of the too heavy workload in the face of less than optimal appreciation from the administration. There was never enough time to do all that we planned and far too little support and recognition for what was accomplished. For those that continued, however, the rewards eventually outweighed these difficulties. As one project teacher shared with us at the close of the first intervention year, "This is the first year I am ending without feeling burned-out—I am enlivened and ready to go on."

The School

Policy Change. Our collaborative effort pioneered the institution of new policies regarding tracking. Although the intervention began within a heavily tracked system of teaching where the English classes for project students were not eligible for college preparatory credit at the start, project teachers gradually won support for a series of changes in class designation.

First, the school adopted a retroactive college-preparatory policy. On teacher recommendation, students who had achieved at higher levels in non-college bound English classes, would be accorded a retroactive college-prep designation on their record and moved up in the next year to a college-bound class. Second, after the second intervention year, the school integrated low-stanine students into average achievement band classes, eliminating non-college bound English classes. Third, two project teachers (and the whole department followed) offered open enrollment for their advanced placement English classes in stark contrast to the usual method of entrance exam cut-off scores. Rather than selecting students for these classes, they threw out the test results and opted for self-selection by asking interested students to sign a contract to attend daily and do the required reading and writing. One participating project student excitedly told another teacher that he was taking a class "for writers." Another project student wrote the following about the new selection procedures:

> Obviously, I'm going to like your method because I didn't pass the test the first time. There was no way I was going to pass that test—I haven't been in honors classes and I wasn't prepared to write the way you wanted me to

write. Now I'm learning. And I look around at the kids in this class and I
feel as if I am as good as they are. I'm earning As too (Cone, 1989).

Policy changes in de-tracking the system evolved from a process of negotiation between teachers and between the teachers and the administration.
Teachers grew angry at the differential treatment and status of both the
lowest achieving students and the teachers who taught these classes. Teachers
also needed to be convinced that they could effectively teach mixed-ability
classes. Over time, teachers and administrators worked through the perceived constraints of district and university mandates which kept tracking
in place and they opened the door for alternatives.

These efforts on the part of at-risk students, particularly at a time
when concern about potential school dropouts is etched on the national
agenda, brought the high school some attention as an innovator in dropout
prevention programs. The project was recognized by the Association of
California School Administrators and the National Council of Teachers on
English as a program of excellence. The project also became useful in successfully meeting the accreditation review for the Western Association of
Schools and Colleges and the State Department of Education. Particularly
as PACT teachers moved out to bring the program to other schools, the
project became part of the school's identity.

Perceptions About PACT Students. Perceptions about the abilities of
these low-achieving students underwent some change as well. A passing
teacher mistook a PACT class, deeply engaged in collaborative writing on the
computer, for an honors class. Counsellors stopped balking at teachers'
requests to move low-stanine students into honors classes. Deans perceived
that there were fewer referrals of project students for disciplinary action.
Finally, after 2 years of the PACT project, for the first time in the school's
history, two of the freshman class officers elected to the student council
were PACT students—evidence that these students were becoming identified with and integrated into the mainstream of the school's activities.

Limits of School Change. Despite changes in policies for and perceptions about these low-achieving students, the project remained somewhat
isolated as a school within a school effort, with slow generalization of the
collaborative work structure and the high expectations model to the school
as a whole. Administrative involvement was the hardest link to maintain.
Assignment changes in principal, vice-principal, deans, and counsellors
forced continual beginnings as the teachers forged working relationships
with new administrative staff each year. That these project teachers willingly
dedicated their efforts toward at-risk youngsters enabled administrators to
get off the hot seat regarding their commitment to this population. In the
press of countless other urgent educational problems, a reactive rather than
proactive stance, and shifting administrative staff, the translation of this

project firmly into every teacher's agenda within the school has yet to be made. However, the PACT teachers persist and every year more and more teachers "become involved and won over to the philosophy of research-based, teacher cooperation," as noted by an outside evaluator.

Students

Narrative records revealed that when teachers talked about student change, they reported a new enthusiasm for learning, a new responsiveness to the learning of their peers, and finally, a pride about and an identification with the school. In one class, students arrived at school half an hour early each day to work on their writing assignments on the computer. When another teacher told her class that a particular assignment was taken from an honors class, "students became motivated knowing they were using higher-level materials." Teachers told us that students pointed out the names of fellow project classmates on the school honor roll and applauded each other's work when read aloud. Several students shared lecture material with their English teacher that they had collaboratively created in a history unit on war. Attendance of project students at school athletic events was perceived to have increased and student behavior as supporters to have improved.

Using School Records to Compare Project and Comparison Students Post-Intervention. In order to assess whether the project made a difference in students' academic and behavioral performance, repeated measures ANOVAs, with group (project vs. comparison group) and time period as the independent factors, and entering CAT scores as a covariate, were conducted to measure change in these indices from end of eighth grade (pre-intervention) or first semester ninth grade (early-intervention) to end of ninth grade (post-intervention). Of most interest to us, was the Group × Time interaction, indicating a differential change over time between the intervention and comparison groups.

The ANOVA tests revealed significant interaction effects for English grades ($F = 4.80, df = 1, 310, p < .05$) and history grades ($F = 3.86, df = 1, 310, p < .05$), the two subject area classes that were evaluated in the project. That is, after 1 year of intervention, project students demonstrated greater improvement in their grades in English and history than did a comparable group of students who did not participate in the intervention (see Table 3). With regard to GPAs, the contrast was made between early-intervention, after one semester, and later-intervention, at the end of the school year. However, GPAs were obtained from school records and hence included the grades of project teachers. Although neither the Time effect nor the Group × Time interaction effect were significant, suggesting little change in GPA over time within the intervention year in either group of students, we

Table 3. Pre- and Post-Contrast of Project and Comparison Group[a]

Measures	Groups	Means End of 8th grade	Means End of 9th grade	F Group	F Time	F Group × time
Teacher-mediated change (with CAT scores as covariate)						
English	Project	1.84	2.31	8.07[d]	16.37e	4.80[d]
grades	Comparison	1.68	1.82			
History	Project	1.26	1.48	2.91[c]	3.16[c]	3.86[d]
grades	Comparison	1.19	1.18			
GPA[b]	Project	1.70	1.72	3.89[d]	0.01	0.40
	Comparison	1.53	1.51			
Referrals[b]	Project	5.38	3.64	15.51[e]	2.76[e]	12.19[e]
	Comparison	2.92	2.63			
Student-mediated change (with CAT scores as covariate)						
English	Project	12.51	15.38	0.01	16.99[e]	0.55
absences	Comparison	12.27	16.40			
History	Project	11.90	17.36	0.33	13.24[e]	7.03[e]
absences	Comparison	13.57	14.42			

[a]$N = 158$ for project students and $N = 154$ for comparison students.
[b]GPA and referrals from end of first semester to end of second semester (within ninth grade).
[c]$p < .10$.
[d]$p < .05$.
[e]$p < .01$.

did find a significant Group effect ($F = 3.89$, $df = 1, 309$, $p < .05$). This indicates that project students earned significantly higher GPAs during the intervention year (that is, both early and later) than did a comparable group of nonparticipant students. This potential project effect, appearing after one semester of intervention may, however, be due to the higher grades of project teachers.

With regard to behavioral indices, project students showed a significantly greater decrease in disciplinary referrals to the dean's office than did the comparison cohort ($F = 12.19$, $df = 1, 310$, $p < .01$) as measured from the end of the first semester to the end of the second semester of ninth grade. However, surprisingly, project students' referral rates were initially higher and remained higher than the rates of comparison students. Student absence rates were not impacted by the project. Both project and comparison students showed increased absence rates in English ($F = 16.99$, $df = 1$, 309, $p < .01$) and history ($F = 13.24$, $df = 1, 309$, $p < .01$) classes from eighth grade to the end of the ninth grade year. In fact, for history classes, given a significant Group × Time interaction finding, project students outpaced comparison students in increased absences, despite their improved grades ($F = 7.03$, $df = 1, 310$, $p < .01$).

Post-intervention, the improved grades and decreased disciplinary referrals can be seen as evidence of process change—effects that may be mediated by changes in teacher perceptions and that may precede more generalized change. However, even within project classes, the sole student-mediated variable—absence rates—was on the rise, contrary to our predictions, with history absences even greater for project than for comparison students. Possibly explaining the different patterns for English and history was the fact that the history teachers in contrast to the other departments had a more tumultuous relationship with the project (two withdrew and one joined in the second year of the project). It is also possible that something about the intervention (perhaps the increased demand and accountability) aggravated student attendance and disciplinary problems, although teachers' explanations lay in cohort differences. Teachers reported that each year this population group is tougher to reach, with greater family disintegration and poverty, variables we did not measure. Prior absence records did not differentiate the cohorts but we did not have prior disciplinary comparisons which might have distinguished the groups.

One-Year Followup. At the end of tenth grade, we were able to obtain some limited followup data on the first project cohort ($N = 59$) as compared to the combined comparison cohort of students ($N = 154$). Only English grades, GPA, English absences, and school withdrawal/disposition rates were available for analysis. All these measures reflect student-mediated changes, particularly absence and school disposition rates, but also grades from non-project teachers. We asked to what extent the intervention promoted positive outcomes and was preventive of school dropout 1 year following program completion.

At the 1-year followup, half the number of project students (18.6%) compared to comparison students (37.7%) had transferred out of the high school to other schools or unknown destinations ($x = 6.5$, $df = 1$, $p < .01$). Approximately half of these project students (6.7%) as compared to comparison students (11.7%) were referred to alternative continuation high school programs or were assumed to have dropped out. One can conclude, post-intervention, that the school had more holding power for the project students than for the comparison students and that project students were more likely to be found in regular classes than in continuation classes or out of school.

However, for those students continuing at the high school, the significant lead they demonstrated in English grades and GPA with project teachers was unfortunately not maintained with non-project teachers in the next school year. By the end of tenth grade, although projects students outperformed control students in English grades (1.74 to 1.40), they did not significantly differ from control students in English grades, nor in absences or GPA. We might note however, that given the differential attrition rates between groups, continuing project students were likely to contain more of the lowest achievers than the smaller group of continuing comparison students, possibly masking a lead in achievement. While these results are promising about the retention of these youngsters in school, the evidence is less clear regarding continued improved performance. Perhaps the intervention was not strong enough to impact student performance 1 year later.

LESSONS LEARNED

This case study represents a first step in translating our expectancy research findings into school change. In charting the multilevel effects of our collaborative intervention to raise expectations for at-risk high school students, the results show promise but they are also mixed.

Qualitative study of the collaborative process over time documents the kinds of changes that took place in researchers, teachers, and in school policy. Through compromise, the researchers learned to share the leadership of the project with school staff. In the sharing, teachers became empowered to act on behalf of students and programs to demand accountability from their colleagues and extend their professional development to encompass reading, presenting, and writing research on positive expectancy climates for at-risk students. Our collaborative efforts also changed school policy toward a liberation of these youngsters from some of the negative effects of the tracking system, enabling them to enter college-bound average achievement tracks in contrast to their previous remedial classes and opening selected advanced placement classes to student choice. However, such change was not uniform. We lost some teachers to the frustration of excessive time demands and failed administrative support. As well, we were unable to move the intervention into the mainstream of school organization as a whole, perhaps because of repeated changes in administrators. Yet the intervention still continues to *evolve* under teacher leadership, involving more and more teachers within the high school as well as other schools within the district.

But quantitative and comparative evidence for the filtered-down impact of these changes on the students as a group revealed only partial success. After 1 year of intervention, project students showed greater improvements in their grades in English and history, held higher GPAs, and reduced their disciplinary referrals more than comparable students who did not participate in the intervention. These are interactive outcomes (not pure qualities of students) and are in part the result of changed teacher perceptions, reflecting perhaps the first step in a process of change. Yet, despite more positive school performance, student absence rates (a pure student quality) continued to rise, even outpacing comparison students in history classes and disciplinary referrals (although reduced) were still higher for project students. With regard to the preventive effects of the intervention, 1 year later found more project than comparison students still enrolled at the same high school and less likely to be in a continuation program or to have dropped out. Ironically, despite the increased retention power of the program and the reduced number of students with a downward disposition (thereby heightening the difficulty of demonstrating superior performance), the achievement and attendance of project students did not exceed that of the comparison students. Was this a methodological constraint (due to differential retention rates of the two samples) or does it reflect incomplete program effects? The answer is likely both.

This intervention tackled a difficult problem (entrenched practices which communicate low expectations to students), within a hardcore population (at-risk students relatively late in their school career at the transition to high school) and with a collaborative rather than prescriptive method of inquiry. In contrast, the high school transition project of Felner and colleagues (1982, 1988) which was aimed at policy changes (in the use of homeroom teachers and class rather than student assignment to teachers) and demonstrated improvements in student adjustment, was prescriptive and in place, when the evaluation was made. Felner and colleagues also targeted all students at entry to high school. This project focused on the school's most hard-core population.

An evolving implementation may not have been strong enough to turn things around for all students in this exceedingly tough population. For example, student change may even have been greater if the overall structure of the tracking system, its messages, and learning opportunities had been changed from the start. It is also possible, given these students' needs and previous history of failure, that the intervention breadth (only two subject areas) and its length (1 academic year) may have been insufficient to have fully generalizable effects in the next academic year with other teachers. Although we improved the holding power of regular high school for these youth (reflecting perhaps a change in student attitude), we did not impact their attendance or academic performance; here, even more educational supports may be necessary. Our collaborating teachers also pointed out the important explanatory factor of individual differences among students in response to the intervention. The use of mean scores washes out the potential differential response of subgroups to the intervention. Unfortunately, our limited student data did not allow us to identify meaningful subgroups to investigate this possibility.

Given the multilevel steps of change from joint planning—to positive teacher expectations—to high expectancy classroom practices and school policies—to motivated students, perhaps it is not surprising that program effects were not uniform nor large enough to be seen at every level and with regard to all measures in a group comparison of students. Change in the underlying structural regularities of a complex real world high school is a tall order. The steps of change taken are indeed gratifying but clearly more and longer-term efforts are needed.

What does the process of collaborative intervention teach us about school-based intervention efforts and methods of evaluation? First, this case study underscores a method of intervention that is "enabling" of others and thus initiates a process. The provision of a supportive structure and a theoretical framework within which key participants created, adapted, and institutionalized innovative practice and policy, stimulated an evolving, interactive, and dynamic process of implementation and change.

Both our methods of working collaboratively and the teaching practices and policies we targeted for change were deeply constrained by layers of administrative and district edicts. The innovations we embraced proved antithetical to the ecology of the school as currently constituted (Gruber & Trickett, 1987). The empowerment of teachers to make changes in practices and policies required not only perceived agency but also the identification and construction of supportive structures that enabled that agency to be acted upon. Just the simple setting up of shared preparation periods for teachers to collaborate was a major scheduling problem during the first year, posing enormous problems for building teamwork. De-tracking the tracking system for students occurred only in stages. Each battle we faced pitted teachers against teachers or administrators or researchers as we struggled to work through differing values and systemic constraints.

We also learned that teachers, like their students, were labeled as "remedial" teachers (Finley, 1984), with lack of control over curriculum, limited performance opportunities, competitive conditions, little sense of agency, and limited relationships with colleagues. It became clear that teachers needed to change their own working conditions before they could change these conditions for students. Sarason (1990) makes this point forcefully in asking for whom do schools exist. He argues that educational reform efforts will continue to fail if they ignore the principle that "it is virtually impossible to create and sustain over time conditions for productive learning for students when they do not exist for teachers" (p. 145).

The process of school change depicted in this paper reflects newer conceptions of reform as systemic rather than narrowly-focused, as *enabling* rather than *mandating* effective practice, as engaging the natural networks of teachers rather than imposing outside delivery structures, and as requiring "steady work" rather than quick fixes (McLaughlin, 1989). Not surprisingly, Schorr (1998) concludes similarly about the qualities of successful programs which break the cycle of disadvantage for children and families. Successful programs, as need-driven, regularly engage in a process of adapting or circumventing professional and institutional constraints in order to serve the population in need.

Second, such visions of a collaborative change process and of multiple levels of outcomes within a systemic framework pose enormous challenges for the evaluation of project impact. This evolving process has implications for how and when we define or assess implementation and outcomes.

Our collaborative approach to this project, in the face of school and university realities, severely constrained the ultimate design and methodology of the evaluation, which was far too crude to fully capture the effects of the intervention. On the other hand, the collaborative model and the qualitative approach we adopted offered us tremendously rich opportunities to further our understanding of expectancy change.

Like the intervention, the evaluation evolved too. Loss of a control group meant the adoption of a descriptive and archival approach, limiting us to teacher report and student records. The natural evolution of the project resulted in shifting teacher participation and uneven membership by different subject area departments, limiting options for analysis. The collaborative inquiry with teachers ruled out the signing of subject consent forms (a university requirement) early on when trust was being developed and made an examination of teacher implementation and outcome differences a touchy subject. The use of an archival cohort design (although strengthened by the comparability of cohorts at entry, the covariate analyses, pre- and post-test comparisons, and 4 years of cohorts) could not fully control for historical or social context differences between the project and comparison groups that may explain the findings.

However, the collaborative strategy and the qualitative look at changes at the level of researcher, teacher, and school policy enhanced the quantitative, comparative look at teacher- and student-mediated program outcomes and greatly enriched our understanding of change. As this case study illustrates, the quantitative data cannot be fully understood without linking it to an understanding of the intervention process and changes in the larger school context. School-based interventions that focus only on end-point student outcomes will always miss an important part of the intervention impact. Clearly, important program effects reside at multiple levels, such as in teachers' beliefs and actions, the development of school policy, and school climate, in addition to changed student behavior.

Collaborative and systemic change projects such as these require sensitive and flexible methodologies to carefully chart the implementation of changes and outcomes at multiple levels of system and participant and most importantly, over longer periods of time. Beer and Walton (1987) suggest that intervention research is reaching a critical turning point where traditional science methodology has proven limiting—by its focus on single causes and on isolated episodes of change and by its failure to describe and to meet the needs of users. Different models of acquiring knowledge need to be developed that will expand the system context of change and continuity over time. Beer and Walton argue that "while being precise about methodology and instruments, it (traditional science) is often imprecise in depth and description of the intervention and situation" (p. 343). Newer methods have been developed to more systematically collect and test propositions in qualitative data that provide rich descriptions of process and impact (Miles & Huberman, 1984). Questions for future research include problems in implementation, teacher and student individual differences that might predict responsiveness to the intervention, and links between effective program elements and types of outcomes.

As a final note, there were clearly more ideal conditions to foster the course of this intervention. We suggest three: adequate teacher preparation time, a multilevel shared agenda, and a longer time perspective. Additional teacher preparation time would have strengthened and quickened the development of changed classroom practices and policies. More time would have reduced the frenetic pace of the project and perhaps attracted more teachers as well as prevented teacher withdrawals. The existence of conflicting agendas produced strife rather than cooperation. Although we began with the belief that we had a shared agenda between teachers, administrators, and district officials, the events of our collaboration proved us wrong. In fact, the creation of a program for at-risk students worked against us, in letting the school administration and the district off the hook, free in their eyes to attend to competing and more pressing agendas. Yet the far-reaching changes that we were negotiating (changed beliefs and opportunities for these students) required consistent and continual school level and district support. In truth, not one of us was prepared for the time it would take to systematically alter the instructional and school climate so that expectations and opportunities to learn were consistently positive and available, that is, to undo a lifelong pattern of schooling. A longer time perspective might have eased some of our disappointment and adjusted our own "too high" expectations for change.

Despite the struggles and the costs of collaboration, this way of working enabled us to perhaps go farther in our institutionalization of change, beyond classroom practices to school policies, expanding the range of innovations introduced. Collaboration helped teachers and administrators adapt the model for their own school site and their own curricular objectives. Their leadership meant that the project continues to have a life of its own, beyond the contributions of the researchers. Collaboration also oriented the researchers to the constraints inherent in changing expectancy practices in the school and the multiple layers of support for low expectations in the classroom. We were most moved when the teachers presented all of us with engraved plaques which read "Pollyanna Pedagogical Society: Charter Member," named in honor of the child of fiction who maintained an eternally hopeful attitude about the capacity of human beings. As one teacher described the hopefulness that had resulted from collaboration:

> We taught you to recognize the constraints;
> You taught us not to be stopped by them.

The next challenge is to more fully translate these effects to changed student experiences in school.

ACKNOWLEDGMENTS

This project was supported by a SUPER grant from the School of Education, University of California at Berkeley (with funds from the William and Flora Hewlett Foundation and the San Francisco Foundation) and by a University Public Health Service Biomedical Research Grant. The authors thank Drs. Bernard Gifford, Nina Gabelko, and Jon Wagner of SUPER, for their strong encouragement, Lauren Jones, for her creation of a community service program with project students, and Charles Elster, Carol Sullivan, and Robert Rosenthal, for their contribution to project development, data collection, and analysis. The comments provided by anonymous reviewers were especially helpful.

REFERENCES

Alexander, K. L. & Entwisle, D. R. (1988). Achievement in the first 2 years of school: Patterns and processes. *Monographs of the Society for Research in Child Development, 53*, 1–157.
Beer, M. & Walton, A. E. (1987). Organization change and development. *Annual Review of Psychology, 38*, 339–367.
Berman, P. & McLaughlin, M. W. (1978). *Implementing and sustaining innovations*. Santa Monica, CA: Rand.
Brophy, J. E. (1983). Research on the self-fulfilling prophecy and teacher expectations. *Journal of Educational Psychology, 75*, 631–661.
Butler, S. R., Marsh, H. W., Sheppard, M. J., & Sheppard, J. L. (1985). Seven-year longitudinal study of the early prediction of reading achievement. *Journal of Educational Psychology, 77*, 349–361.
Collins, F. A. (1988). AERA in New Orleans, *SUPER News, 4*, 3.
Comer, J. P. (1980). *School power: Implications of an intervention project*. New York: Free Press.
Committee for Economic Development (1987). *Children in need: Investment strategies for the educationally disadvantaged*. New York: CED.

Cone, J. (1989, March). *The teacher and motivation researcher relationship: Bridging the gap.* Paper presented at the Annual Meeting of the American Educational Research Association, San Francisco, CA.

Cook, T. D. & Campbell, D. T. (1979). *Quasi-experimentation: Design and analysis for field settings.* Rand McNally.

Cowen, E. L., Peterson, A., Babigian, H., Izzo, L. D., & Trost, M. A. (1973). Long-term followup of early detected vulnerable children. *Journal of Consulting and Clinical Psychology, 41,* 438–446.

Dusek, J. B. (Ed.). (1985). *Teacher expectancies.* Hillsdale, NJ: Lawrence Erlbaum.

Epstein, J. L. (1985). After the bus arrives: Resegregation in desegregated schools. *Journal of Social Issues, 41,* 23–43.

Felner, R. D. & Adan, A. M. (1988). The school transitional environment project: An ecological intervention and evaluation. In R. H. Price, E. L. Cowen, R. P. Lorion, & J. Ramos-McKay (Eds.), *14 ounces of prevention: A casebook for practitioners.* Washington, DC: American Psychological Association.

Felner, R. D., Ginter, M., & Primavera, J. (1982). Primary prevention during school transitions: Social support and environmental structure. *American Journal of Community Psychology, 10,* 277–290.

Finley, M. K. (1984). Teachers and tracking in a comprehensive high school. *Sociology of Education, 57,* 233–243.

Freedman, S. W. (1989). *The teachers, their schools, and their students.* Unpublished manuscript, University of California, National Center for the Study of Writing, Berkeley, CA.

General Accounting Office (1987). *School dropouts: Survey of local programs* (Report no. Gao/HRD-87–108). Washington, DC: GAO.

Gifford, B. R. (1986). The evolution of the school–university partnership for educational renewal. *Education and Urban Society, 19,* 77–106.

Good, T. L. & Weinstein, R. S. (1986). Schools make a difference: Evidence, criticisms, and new directions. *American Psychologist, 41,* 1090–1097.

Gruber, J. & Trickett, E. J. (1987). Can we empower others? The paradox of empowerment in the governing of an alternative public school. *American Journal of Community Psychology, 15,* 353–371.

Guthrie, J. W. & Kirst, M. W. (1988). *Conditions of education in California.* PACE (Policy Analysis for California Education), Berkeley: University of California, School of Education.

Hamilton, S. F. (1984). The secondary school in the ecology of adolescent development. *Review of Research in Education, 11,* 227–258.

Jones, L. (1989). *Teacher expectations for black and white students in contrasting classroom environments,* Masters thesis, University of California, Berkeley.

Kelly, J. G. & Kingry-Westergaard, C. (1988, September). *An epistemology for ecological research as a collaborative enterprise: Part one.* Paper presented at the Conference "Researching Community Psychology: Integrating Theories and Methodologies," sponsored by the APA Science Directorate, Chicago, IL.

Kerman, S. (1979). Teacher expectations and student achievement. *Phi Delta Kappan, 60,* 716–718.

Kornberg, M. S. & Caplan, G. (1980). Risk factors and preventive intervention in child psychopathology: A review. *Journal of Prevention, 1,* 71–133.

Marshall, H. H. & Weinstein, R. S. (1984). Classroom factors affecting students' self-evaluations: An interactional model. *Review of Educational Research, 54,* 301–325.

Marshall, H. H. & Weinstein, R. S. (1986). The classroom context of student-perceived differential teacher treatment. *Journal of Educational Psychology, 78,* 441–453.

Marshall, H. H. & Weinstein, R. S. (1988). Beyond quantitative analysis: Recontextualization of classroom factors contributing to the communication of teacher expectations. In

J. Green, J. Harker, & C. Wallet (Eds.), *Multiple analysis of classroom discourse processes.* Norwood, NJ: Ablex.

McLaughlin, M. W. (1989, April). *The Rand change agent study ten years later: Macro perspectives and micro realities.* Paper given at the Annual Meeting of the American Educational Research Association, San Francisco.

Mehlhorn, M. (1987). Teachers, researchers, administrators collaborate to aid "at risk" students. *SUPER News, 3*, 1–3.

Miles, M. B. & Huberman, A. M. (1984). *Qualitative data analysis: A sourcebook of new methods.* Beverly Hills, CA: Sage.

National Commission on Excellence in Education (1983). *A nation at risk.* Washington, DC: U.S. Department of Education.

Oakes, J. (1985). *Keeping track: How schools structure inequality.* New Haven: Yale University Press.

Olsen, L. (1987). Coalition of educators urges wider efforts for "at risk" youths. *Education Week,* June 10, 1987.

Rumberger, R. W. (1987). High school dropouts: A review of issues and evidence. *Review of Educational Research, 57,* 101–121.

Rutter, M., Maughan, B., Mortimore, P., & Ouston, J. (1979). *Fifteen thousand hours: Secondary schools and their effects on children.* Cambridge: Harvard University Press.

Sarason, S. B. (1971, 1982). *The culture of the school and the problem of change.* Boston: Allyn and Bacon.

Sarason, S. B. (1990). *The predictable failure of educational reform: Can we change course before it is too late?* San Francisco, CA: Jossey-Bass.

Sarason, S. B., Davidson, K. S., & Blatt, B. (1962, 1986). *The preparation of teachers: An unstudied problem in education.* Cambridge: Brookline (Wiley, 1st ed.).

Schorr, L. B. (1988). *Within our reach: Breaking the cycle of disadvantage.* New York: Anchor Press/Doubleday.

Seidman, E. (1988). Back to the future, community psychology: Unfolding a theory of social intervention. *American Journal of Community Psychology, 16,* 3–24.

Solomon, D., Watson, M. S., Delucchi, K. L., Schaps, E., & Battistich, V. (1988). Enhancing children's prosocial behavior in the classroom. *American Educational Research Journal, 25,* 527–554.

The Achievement Council. (1984). *Excellence for whom.* Oakland, CA.

Weinstein, R. S. (1989). Perception of classroom processes and student motivation: Children's views of self-fulfilling prophecies. In R. E. Ames & C. Ames (Eds.), *Research on motivation in education* (Vol. 3). New York: Academic Press.

Weinstein, R. S. & Middlestadt, S. E. (1979). Student perception of teacher interaction with male high and low achievers. *Journal of Educational Psychology, 71,* 421–431.

Weinstein, R. S., Marshall, H. H., Brattesani, K. A., & Middlestadt, S. E. (1982). Student perceptions of differential teacher treatment in open and traditional classrooms. *Journal of Educational Psychology, 74,* 678–692.

Weinstein, R. S., Marshall, H. H., Sharp, L., & Botkin, M. (1987). Pygmalion and the student: Age and classroom differences in children's awareness of teacher expectations. *Child Development, 58,* 1079–1093.

Wilcox, B. L. & Vincent, T. (1987). School dropout: A federal perspective. *Social Policy Report, 11,* 1–11.

17

Homelessness: What Is a Psychologist to Do?*

Marybeth Shinn

*Contrasts person-centered and structural explanations for homelessness.
Methodological problems in studies of homeless people tend to
exaggerate the role of individual deficits as causes of homelessness.
A review of data on the distribution of poverty and of inadequate and
unaffordable housing, with special emphasis on families, suggests the
importance of structural causes. Data from 700 families requesting
shelter and 524 families randomly drawn from the public assistance
case load in New York City provide more support for a structural than
for an individual deficit model. Individual demographic factors are
also important. Implications are drawn for research and action by
psychologists.*

What are the causes of homelessness? This question begs several others. First
what do we mean by homelessness? Most research on the topic is confined to
people who are sometimes called the "literal" homeless (Rossi, 1989)—those
who sleep in shelters, or on the street, in vehicles, or abandoned buildings or
other places not usually deemed fit for human habitation, although most
researchers also acknowledge the existence of a much larger group of people
who are only tenuously housed in the homes of friends or relatives.

*Presidential address presented to the Division of Community Psychology at the annual
convention of the American Psychological Association in San Francisco, August 1991.
Originally published in the *American Journal of Community Psychology*, *20*(1)
(1992): 1–24.

A Quarter Century of Community Psychology: Readings from the American Journal of
Community Psychology, edited by Tracey A. Revenson *et al.* Kluwer Academic/Plenum
Publishers, New York, 2002.

Perhaps more interesting, what do we mean by "cause?" Here the literature bifurcates into person-centered approaches and approaches that focus on structural factors. Person-centered studies typically examine a cross-section of homeless individuals and what is wrong with them. We are accumulating a large and relentlessly negative literature on rates of substance abuse and psychiatric impairment among homeless people, on their inadequate social networks or poor educational or employment histories. And too often both researchers and editorial writers slip from statements that large numbers of homeless people are _____ (substitute your favorite individual deficit here) to the assumption that the deficit of choice causes homelessness.

This focus on the individual problems of homeless people differs sharply from an analysis of structural determinants of homelessness in poverty and loss of affordable housing. McChesney (1990) has offered a useful analogy to help us understand the difference: Homelessness, she says, is like a game of musical chairs. The players are low-income households. The chairs are the housing units they can afford. If there are more low-income households than affordable housing units, some households will be left homeless when the music stops. Individual problems, even severe mental illness, do not affect the number of housing units, and they have only a marginal effect on the number of low-income households. Thus they do not *cause* homelessness. Rather they determine *vulnerability* to homelessness in a tight housing market. In the musical chairs analogy, individual problems determine only which players will be left standing (or sleeping on a heating grate) when the music stops.

This article argues that the individual-level analyses and person-centered approaches often favored by psychology are not sufficient to understand the causes of homelessness or what to do about it. I begin by discussing methodological problems in individual-level studies that have led to exaggerated estimates of the role of individual deficits in the origins of homelessness. Next, I examine more macro explanations for homelessness in increasing poverty and decreasing supplies of affordable housing, with special emphasis on homelessness among families. Third, I discuss ways of linking macro and micro explanations for homelessness, and illustrate, in part, with data from a large random study of homeless and housed poor families in New York City. Finally, I discuss implications of a multilevel approach linking situational variables and personal variables for research and action by psychologists.

METHODOLOGICAL PROBLEMS IN INDIVIDUAL-LEVEL STUDIES OF HOMELESSNESS

Homeless people are not easy to sample or to study, so that good researchers often have to settle for less than ideal designs. I do not intend to berate researchers so much as to illustrate the biases resulting from the methodological compromises they have made. The compromises include nonrandom samples; cross-sectional designs, which lead to confusion between antecedents and consequences of homelessness, biases in who is sampled, and a static picture of a dynamic process; lack of comparison groups; a focus on single adults rather than family units; and, perhaps most important, designs in which individual factors are allowed to vary but structural factors are not. Many of these compromises have led to overestimates of individual deficits as causes of homelessness.

First, most studies do not have random samples of homeless people— indeed random samples are hard to come by. So people who are most obviously homeless are most likely to be studied. A disheveled person talking loudly and gesticulating in the air will be sampled. A quiet well-dressed person in the same area late at night may be missed. Studies of nonrandom samples are often overgeneralized. One study, for example, sampled homeless individuals treated at a psychiatric emergency room and found that 97% had been previously hospitalized for psychiatric problems (Lipton, Sabatini, & Katz, 1983). The authors of this article are very clear about the specialized nature of their sample, but secondary sources sometimes report the percentage of prior hospitalization in this subgroup as an upper bound estimate of mental illness among homeless people.

Next, most studies sample a cross-section of homeless individuals at a single point in time. Mental health or substance abuse problems uncovered in these studies may be consequences as well as causes of homelessness. With a careful series of analyses, Koegel and Burnam (1988, 1992) show that symptoms indicative of antisocial personality disorder in the general population may be consequences of the homeless condition. Depression is more adequately measured but, in a significant number of cases, did not arise until after individuals became homeless; in a majority of cases it was not present 5 years earlier. A proportion of homeless alcoholics did not hit the bottle until after they had hit the street. Similarly Sosin, Colson, and Grossman (1988) found that among homeless people who had been hospitalized for psychiatric reasons, homelessness preceded the first hospitalization in almost two fifths of the cases.

Deficits in social networks may also be a consequence of homelessness rather than a cause. Several studies suggest that people receive help from families and friends before becoming literally homeless, but eventually they exhaust these interpersonal resources (Rossi, Wright, Fisher, & Willis, 1987; Shinn, Knickman, & Weitzman, 1991).

Studies conducted at a single point in time miss the dynamic processes of people's lives. Sosin, Piliavin, and Westerfelt (1990), in a longitudinal study, show that much literal homelessness is episodic, although between episodes of shelter use, sleeping in abandoned buildings, and the like, most members of their sample were only precariously housed, usually with friends, in dwellings to which they had no long-term title. Koegel, Burnam, and Farr (1990) found that only 5% of a sample of inner-city homeless adults were working at the time of the study, but a third (33%) had been employed within the last month and three fifths (59%) had been employed within the last 6 moths.

Cross-sectional studies overrepresent people who have been homeless for long and continuous periods. This is because people who became homeless in the past but had short episodes of homelessness have left the sampling frame, along with a portion of those who move in and out of homelessness. Those experiencing long, continuous episodes remain to be sampled. Several studies that have looked have found that mental health and substance-abuse problems are worse among people who have been homeless for some time or among repeat users of shelter than among new entrants to homelessness or first-time shelter requesters (Koegel & Burnam, 1988; Koegel, Burnam, & Farr, 1988; Sosin et al., 1990). Cross-sectional studies are appropriate for estimating the service needs of the mix of people who are homeless at a given time, but to the extent that the long-term homeless have more psychological or social problems than those who find housing more rapidly, cross-sectional studies again overestimate such problems among the population of all who become homeless.

Most studies of homeless individuals have no comparison groups, so that it is difficult to untangle problems associated with homelessness from those associated with poverty. Studies of families are more likely to have housed poor comparison groups, in part because a reasonable sampling frame is available in public assistance roles. Differences between groups are often smaller than might be expected on the basis of samples of homeless people alone. For example, several studies found differences between homeless and housed respondents with respect to social networks (Bassuk & Rosenberg, 1988; Fischer, Shapiro, Breakey, Anthony, & Kramer, 1986; Passero, Zax, & Zozus, 1991; Sosin et al., 1988; Wood, Valdez, Hayashi, & Shen, 1990), but others did not (Goodman, 1991; Molnar, Rath, Klein, Lowe, & Hartmann, 1991; Shinn et al., 1991), and the frequency of social contacts reported by homeless respondents in Los Angeles, Detroit, and Chicago (Farr, Koegel, & Burnam, 1986; Mowbray, Solarz, Johnson, Phillips-Smith, & Combs, 1986; Rossi et al., 1987; Sosin et al., 1988) was on a par with the frequency reported by housed-poor families in New York (Shinn et al., 1991).

Next, most studies are of single individuals, despite evidence that people in family units are an increasing proportion of the homeless population, amounting to as much as a third by some estimates. People in families, whether homeless or not, tend to have fewer mental health problems than single adults. Prior hospitalization for mental illness is hardly a perfect indicator of mental health problems, but it is reasonably objective and consistently measured across studies. Studies of single adults tend to find rates of hospitalization between 10 and 35% (in nonspecialized samples). Among adult family members the range is 4–14% (Shinn & Weitzman, 1990; Weitzman, Knickman, & Shinn, 1991).

Finally, and most important, most studies of homeless people are confined to a single city and to a single point or brief episode in historical time. Thus the poverty rate, wage rates, the characteristics of the housing market, the generosity of social benefit programs such as welfare, are all fixed. From the perspective of structural factors, these studies, no matter how large and well controlled, are essentially case studies with an n of 1 (M. A. Stegman, comments at a conference, January 31, 1991). Variance in individual connections to structural factors, such as the size of a welfare check or the amount of the rent bill, is constrained, but other individual characteristics are allowed to vary. Thus statistical models may overestimate the relative importance of individual characteristics.

Perhaps the strongest argument against a model of homelessness that begins and ends with individual deficits is historical. People with substance abuse and mental health problems, deficient social networks, and poor employment histories are nothing new. But we have not seen massive homelessness on the present scale since the Great Depression (Hopper, 1990; Hopper & Hamberg, 1984; Wright, 1989). Thus it is important to examine structural contributors to present-day homelessness in increasing poverty and decreasing supplies of affordable housing in the last dozen years.

POVERTY

To understand the relationship of poverty to homelessness, one must examine trends in both the level of poverty and how poverty is distributed. The changing distribution of poverty helps to explain why families make up an increasing share of the homeless population, and why young families, single parents, and people of color are overrepresented.

Overall, official poverty rates declined from 22% of the population in 1959 to a low of 11% in 1973, increased somewhat irregularly to a high of 15% in 1983, and declined again to 13% in 1989 (U.S. Bureau of the Census, 1991, Table 1). Patterns varied, however, among different segments of the population. Poverty among children has risen since the end of the War on Poverty, most dramatically in the years from 1979 to 1983, although it has abated somewhat since then. In 1989, 19% of children in families were poor. The situation is far worse for black and Hispanic children: 43% of

African–American children and 36% of Latino children were poor in 1989 (U.S. Bureau of the Census, 1991, Table 2). Among female-headed families with children under 18, 43% of all races, 54% of black families, and 58% of families of Hispanic origin were in poverty in 1989.

Between 1979 and 1988, there was an increase of 5.7 million poor people among families with children below 18. What accounts for this increase in poverty? The U.S. House of Representatives Committee on Ways and Means (1990) calculated that about a fifth of the increase (19.9%) or 1.1 million people was due to population growth and other demographic changes. Another fifth (19.5%, 1.1 million) was due to decreases in market income. A tenth (10%, 0.6 million) was due to changes in social insurance programs such as social security. But the lion's share of the changes, accounting for the addition of half of the total (50.6%) or 2.9 million people to the ranks of the poor, were due to erosion in welfare benefits and tightening of eligibility criteria (pp. 1053–1058).

Using a somewhat tighter definition of extreme poverty, Rossi (1989, p. 76 ff.) calculated that the number of single adults aged 22 to 59 with incomes below $4,000 per year in 1987 dollars increased from 3.1 million in 1969 to 7.2 million in 1987; among these numbers, single parents living with children made up 0.8 million in 1969 and 2.2 million in 1987. Childless adults were substantially more likely than single parents to live with parents or others. Single parents made up 59% of the 3 million living alone.

Some analysts have questioned the close linkage between poverty and homelessness because their patterns are different: The number of homeless families continued to rise throughout the 1980s, whereas the number and percentage of families in poverty decreased after 1983 (Stegman & Keys, 1991). There is no evidence that the status of the very poorest families has improved, however. Figure 1 shows how the poorest 20% of all families (including single individuals), all families with children, and single mothers with children have fared relative to the poverty line since 1973. Whereas the first two groups did recover somewhat between 1983 and 1988, the recovery never occurred for the poorest single mothers with children, from whom homeless families are disproportionately drawn. Their income remained at about a quarter of the poverty threshold. Or, to paraphrase a former president, a rising tide raises all yachts but does not do much for people who are bailing out leaky rowboats.

Since the low point in overall poverty in 1973, the distribution of income in this country has become increasingly unequal. In 1973, the poorest fifth of families (including single individuals) received 5.6% of the total amount of income, or a little over one eighth as much as the wealthiest fifth. By 1988, the poorest fifth received only 4.4% of the total, or less than one tenth as much as the wealthiest quintile (U.S. House of Representatives, 1990, p. 1073).

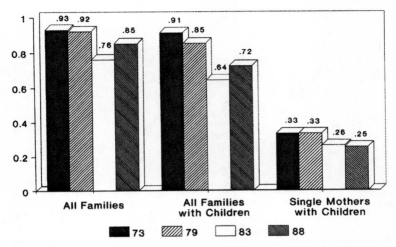

Figure 1. Trends in income as a fraction of the poverty level among the poorest 20% of each group: 1973–1988.

Note: Adjusted family income equals total pre-tax family cash income divided by the appropriate poverty threshold. Averages are weighted by persons.

Source: Committee on Ways and Means, U.S. House of Representatives 1990 Green Book, Table 39, p. 1092.

Adjustment by the poverty threshold in these and other Congressional fig-ures has the effect of adjusting for both inflation and family size. Allotments of cash income (including cash benefits) are still more lopsided.

Figure 2 shows that the distribution of income has become increasingly skewed within family types. Whereas all families and individuals, and even all families with children, experienced some growth in income between 1979 and 1987, the poorest 20% of all these family types lost ground. The decline was greatest among the poorest single mothers with children, who lost 21% of their cash income (including cash benefits such as welfare) over this period, and for the poorest young families with children, who lost 28% of their income relative to the poverty line. In absolute terms, the poorest young families were substantially better off than the poorest single mothers (51 vs. 26% of the poverty line in 1987), but their fall was more precipitous. As I note later, mothers in homeless families in New York City are substan-tially younger than mothers in housed poor families. When taxes and noncash benefits, such as food stamps and housing subsidies, are taken into account, the picture is somewhat more favorable, but still, in a period where incomes for all families were rising, incomes for the poorest families were falling. The poorest families with children lost 12% of their income relative to the poverty line from 1979 to 1987; the poorest young families lost 20% (U.S. House of Representatives, 1990, Tables 42, 43, pp. 1101–1103).

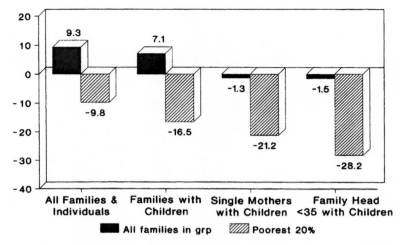

Figure 2. Percent change in family income relative to the poverty line: 1979–1987.
Note: Averages are weighted by persons.
Source: Committee on Ways and Means, U.S. House of Representatives 1990 Green Book, Tables 42 and 43.

There are three other measures by which poor people are getting poorer. One is the average dollar amount by which the incomes of poor people fall short of the official poverty thresholds. The overall deficit per family member in constant dollars was higher in the 1980s than in any prior decade and grew especially for families with female householders (Littman, 1989). In 1989, poor female-headed families with children had an average cash deficit of $5,609. The poverty thresholds in 1989 averaged $8,076 for a family of two and $12,674 for a family of four (U.S. Bureau of the Census, 1990, Table 5).

The other two measures challenge the adequacy of the poverty thresholds themselves. Poverty thresholds were originally calculated in 1955 to equal three times the cost of an economy food basket, and have been adjusted for inflation since. The original poverty threshold for a prototypical four-person family represented about half of the median income for a family of that size. Now it is more nearly a third (Watts, 1986). Thus, in terms of their standing relative to other families, poor families have lost ground. Finally, the thresholds have not been adjusted for the fact that housing is consuming an ever larger portion of poor families' budgets. By 1985, for example, the median poor family was spending 65% of its income on housing (Leonard, Dolbeare, & Lazere, 1989, p. 1). To understand the fiscal squeeze for poor people, it is important to examine changes in the housing market as well as changes in poverty.

HOUSING

McChesney (1990) suggested that the imbalance between the number of low-income households and low-income housing units was a useful way to understand the roots of homelessness. Figure 3 shows how this balance changed between 1970 and 1985. The Department of Housing and Urban Development's standard of affordability is that families should pay no more than 30% of adjusted income for housing. For a family with $10,000 in income, this works out to $250 per month. In 1970 there were 9.7 million units renting for under $250 per month (in 1985 dollars). This was approximately 2.4 million greater than the number of households with incomes below $10,000. By 1985, 1.8 million low-rent units had been lost, and the number of low-income households had increased by 4.3 million. Thus instead of a surplus of 2.4 million low-rent units, there was a 3.7 million unit deficit. Even this dramatic change understates the problem facing poor families, because, in 1985, 0.8 million of those low-rent units were vacant due to natural turnover in rental markets, structural deficiencies, or location in areas that were not considered habitable. Furthermore, occupancy of low-cost units is not restricted to low-income households. In fact, only 41% of the 11.6 million low-income renters occupied units that cost less

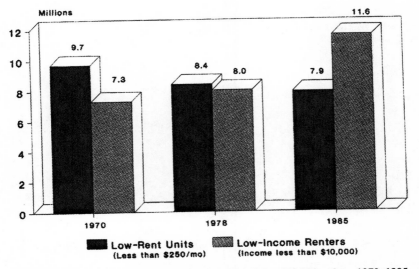

Figure 3. Rental housing shortage for households earning $10,000 or less: 1970–1985.
Note: All figures in constant 1985 dollars.
Source: Leonard, Dolbeare, and Lazere, 1989, Figure 3, based on U.S. Census Bureau, American Housing Survey, 1985.

than $250 per month (Leonard *et al.*, 1989, pp. 6–8). The poorest families faced even more severe shortages. There were 5.4 million renter households (one of six in the nation) with incomes of less than $5,000 in 1985, but only 2.1 million units they could afford by HUD's standards, a shortfall of 3.3 million units (Leonard *et al.*, 1989, pp. 8–9).

The losses in housing were due to a combination of destruction for urban renewal, abandonment, gentrification, and inadequate levels of new construction. In a development of particular relevance to homelessness among single adults, approximately 1-million single-room occupancy units—nearly half of the total supply—were lost nationwide during the 1970s (Hopper & Hamberg, 1986; Wright, 1989, p. 44).

Earlier, we saw that the distribution of incomes in this country is changing so that the rich get richer. Figure 4 tells a similar story about the distribution of housing subsidies. Budget authorizations for Federal low-income housing shrank an average of 11% per year during the Reagan years, but actual budget outlays continued to rise, in large part because of appropriations in earlier years (U.S. House of Representatives, 1990, pp. 1311–1313). The numbers of households receiving subsidies has also gone up, but this number has not kept up with increases in households in poverty (Stegman & Keyes, 1991). From 1979 to 1987, the number of poor

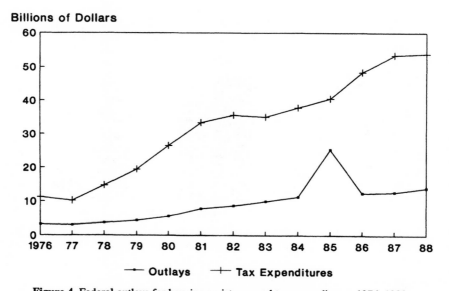

Figure 4. Federal outlays for housing assistance and tax expenditures: 1976–1988.

Source: Leonard, Dolbeare, and Lazere, 1989, Table 3; based on Low Income Housing Information Service calculations from HUD, FmHA, and Joint Tax Committee data.

renter households who received no housing assistance increased by more than a third to 5.4 million units (Leonard *et al.*, 1989, p. 31).

Over the same period there was a substantial increase in another type of federal housing assistance, namely, tax expenditures, primarily home-owner's income tax deductions for mortgage interest and property taxes. Over the past two decades, tax expenditures, which go mostly to middle-class and wealthy families, have typically been almost three and a half times as high as direct federal outlays for housing for poor families. Over two thirds of these tax expenditures, and over half of the combined total of out-lays and expenditures, goes to the top fifth of households earning $50,000 or more each year. In 1988, the average annual subsidy per household for all households with incomes below $10,000 was approximately $600; for all households with incomes above $50,000 it was about $2,000, or more than three times as much (Leonard *et al.*, pp. 31–34).

In the 13-year period from 1974 to 1987, median housing costs for all renters went up 16%. Median costs for poverty-level households rose at over twice that rate—36%. And rents for poor households living in unsub-sidized units soared 41%. In 1987, 63% of poor households paid over half of their income in rent. This included two thirds (68%) of families with heads under 65 and four fifths (80%) of families in unsubsidized rental units (Apgar, DiPasquale, Cummings, & McArdle, 1990, pp. 9, 21, 26, 34).

One response to unaffordable housing is to double up with others. The number of households with related subfamilies increased by 98% between 1980 and 1987; the number with unrelated subfamilies increased by 57%. Together, these related and unrelated subfamilies represented nearly 3 million households who were doubled up in 1987, a level that has not been seen since the years immediately after World War II (Ringheim, 1990a, p. 48).

Despite rising rents, a fifth (21%) of poor households lived in units classified as inadequate by the American Housing Survey. Renters in unsubsidized units were again at special risk (24%) as were older families (23% of those with heads over 65). Poor African–American and Latino households, who were not at special disadvantage with respect to rents, were heavily concentrated in inadequate units. One third of poor African–American families (33%) lived in inadequate housing in 1987 (Apgar *et al.*, 1990, p. 34). In fact, the proportion of *nonpoor* African–American and Latino households living in substandard conditions was greater than the proportion of *poor* white households who lived in substandard conditions (Leonard *et al.*, 1989, p. 55).

The Joint Center for Housing Studies (Apgar *et al.*, 1990) reported that only 2.5 million of 7.0 million poor households were adequately housed in units renting for less than $300/month in 1987. Among the 4.7 million unsubsidized units, fewer than a quarter (23%) were both adequate and affordable. Given these statistics, we may ask, with Rossi (1989, p. 77), not why there are so many homeless people, but why there are so few. Instead of assessing deficits among those who become homeless, we should examine the resourcefulness of the many poor individuals and families who manage to hold onto their housing.

So far we have established that, despite the small decrease in the proportion of families in poverty since the mid-1980s, the plight of the poorest families, especially young families and those headed by women, is becoming increasingly desperate. And we have seen that there has been a net loss in rental units available to poor households, skyrocketing rental burdens, and a net increase in poor households receiving no housing subsidies. We have not shown that it is those households who are poorest, those without housing subsidies, or those who are in inadequate housing who are most likely to become homeless. There are two basic strategies for doing so, one at the level of cities, and a second at the level of individuals.

Ringheim (1990b) studied a sample of eight cities and found that two factors, the proportion of renters in the total population and the proportion of low-income renters who paid more than 45% of their income in rent, accounted for 66% of the variance (adjusted R^2) in per-capita homelessness rates, as estimated by HUD. The relative contributions of income and rental rates varied from city to city (Ringheim, 1990a, 1990b). Studies at the level of cities are problematic on several grounds. The n of cities is necessarily small, so that examination of several variables is likely to yield one or two that explain a good deal of variance; changing the sample of cities might alter the results. Also, the dependent measure, rates of homelessness, is hard to assess accurately. Finally, city-level analyses are subject to the ecological fallacy from the perspective of relationships at the individual level. Nonetheless, the results are intriguing.

The second strategy is to look within a given city at the extent to which people who become homeless, as opposed to poor people who remain housed, are especially poor, or in especially high-rent or inadequate units. Such structural explanations can be contrasted with explanations at the level of individual deficits. As noted above, any study within a particular city holds constant many structural factors that one would prefer, on methodological grounds, to allow to vary. Since only variables can explain variance, these studies are biased towards finding individual correlates of homelessness.

INDIVIDUAL vs. STRUCTURAL FACTORS IN NEW YORK

My colleagues James Knickman, Beth Weitzman, and I have conducted such a study of homeless and housed but poor families in New York City.

We studied 700 families at the point when they requested shelter from the city and compared them with 524 families randomly selected from the public assistance case load. Samples of both homeless and housed families included only individuals who (a) were currently on welfare or had been on welfare within the last 6 months (90% of the shelter population in New York), (b) had not been in a shelter for at least 30 days, and (c) had children (or were pregnant). Homeless families were interviewed at Emergency Assistance Units where they had to come to request shelter. Of 969 eligible respondents screened between January and July 1988, 701 completed interviews for a response rate of 72%. One respondent met the criteria and was interviewed at two points in time; her second administration was dropped, yielding a final sample of 700.

The comparison group was randomly drawn from the public assistance roles via a multistage cluster sample. Families on public assistance in New York were required to report quarterly to Income Maintenance Centers for recertification of eligibility for welfare. We thus sampled 12 of 40 Income Maintenance Centers (with probability proportionate to size) and eligibility specialists (workers) within centers. We used these workers' appointment lists as a sampling frame, interviewing families when they showed up for appointments or, if they failed to appear, at a subsequent appointment or by phone. Of 745 families scheduled for recertification meetings who had not been in a shelter within the past month, 524 agreed to participate for a response rate of 70%. Because there were more Latino families than expected in the initial sample of 448 interviewed in March and April, we added an oversample of 76 African–American respondents in July. All interviews for both samples were conducted by Louis Harris and Associates in either English or Spanish, at the respondent's choice.

Ours is one of very few studies with large random samples of both homeless people and a housed poor comparison group. Because we interviewed families at the start of an episode of homelessness (as defined by a request for shelter) and because we confined our sample to families who had not been in shelter in the past 30 days, we avoided many of the biases in cross-sectional designs, especially the overrepresentation of the long-term homeless and confusion between antecedents and consequences of homelessness. We are now attempting to follow up the 900 families who had not already been shelter users before our first interview in both interviews and administrative records, in order to get a dynamic picture of the course of homelessness.

Our initial wave of data allows us to contrast a theory of homelessness based on individual deficits with a theory based on structural problems in poverty and lack of affordable housing. To what extent did the deficits that many studies use to explain homelessness show up in our research? Table 1 presents data on many of the individual deficits presumed to cause homelessness. The odds ratio approximates relative risk because the proportion of homeless families in the public assistance case-load is low.

Prior mental hospitalization (as a proxy for mental illness) was indeed a risk factor for homelessness, increasing relative risk fourfold, but only 4% of the homeless sample had been hospitalized. The proportion hospitalized is lower than in any previous study of homelessness. I believe there are four reasons for this: First, we sampled individuals in families, whose rates of mental hospitalization are typically in the single digits. As one service provider put it, "you have to be pretty together to hold onto your kids through an episode of homelessness." Second, we have a random sample of shelter requesters, rather than a sample of the obviously homeless, and third, we have avoided the problem inherent in cross-sectional studies of oversampling people who find it difficult to extricate themselves from homelessness. Finally, where rates of homelessness are high, as in New York, it is not only the most personally vulnerable people who lose their homes.

What about alcohol and drug problems, which are also presumed to cause homelessness? We found that 8% of homeless families, compared to 2% of housed-poor families had been in a detoxification center for drug or alcohol abuse—again a risk factor, but again one that affects only a minority of families. Because drug dealing in many shelters and welfare hotels for homeless families is rampant, more families may develop substance-abuse problems while homeless. (For more information about mental health and substance abuse, see Weitzman *et al.*, 1991.)

What about the deficient social support networks found in many studies of homeless people? We found that homeless families were actually more likely than housed families to report that they had friends and relatives, and they had been in contact with their social networks more recently. This makes a lot of sense. If you were seeking to avoid going into shelter, you too would probably be in contact with everyone you could think of who might be able to help. Great Aunt Maude would suddenly get a call from her grandniece or grandnephew.

What's more, relatives and friends *had* helped the families entering shelter. Over three quarters of the families had stayed with relatives or friends either for the longest period in the past year or for the night before entering shelter. Our data suggest that the patience or the resources of these helpers eventually ran out. For example, of 105 women who had been asked to leave by parents in the last year, only 1 said her mother or grandmother would take her in now, if asked. It is plausible that becoming homeless, moving frequently, not having an address or a phone, or simply being embarrassed about one's state would disrupt social networks of families latter on. We have no evidence that families' networks were deficient prior to becoming homeless. (For more information on social relationships, see Shinn *et al.*, 1991.)

Educational and work histories were poor among both shelter requesters and housed families. Neither played much role in predicting homelessness (see Knickman & Weitzman, 1989.)

If individual deficits were relatively unimportant in distinguishing who became homeless in our sample, were structural factors more important? All of the families in both the shelter requester and housed groups were on welfare, so their incomes were roughly comparable. Because families were interviewed at city offices, we did not feel that our promises of confidentiality would be sufficient to get accurate information about supplementary sources of income that might endanger welfare grants, so we did not ask. We do have information about families' relationships to the housing market, and this is also displayed in Table 1. Perhaps the most striking finding is that 44% of the homeless families in our study had never been able to break into the housing market in New York. That is, they had never had a place of their own for as long as a year. About one third of these families had lived with parents for the longest time in the past year; the other two thirds had doubled up with other people. Another fifth of the sample had once had a place of their own, but not in the past year. Only 37%, compared with 86% of housed families, were primary tenants in the place they

Table 1. Individual Deficits and Housing Factors as Predictors of Requesting Shelter among Poor Families in New York City

Characteristic	% Shelter requesters ($n = 700$)	% Housed families ($n = 524$)	Approximate relative risk (odds ratio)
Individual deficit model			
Mental hospitalization	4	1	4.3
Detoxification	8	2	4.6
No social ties	7	14	0.5
< 12 years of education	60	63	0.9
< 1 year full-time work	67	60	1.3
Housing model			
Never primary tenant	44	12	6.0
Primary tenant last year	37	86	0.1
Ever doubled up	81	38	6.9
3+ persons/bedroom	45	26	2.4
Subsidized housing[a]	20	33	0.5
$301 + rent[a]	36	42	0.8
2 + building problems	47	38	1.4

[a]Primary tenants only.

stayed the longest for the past year (Knickman & Weitzman, 1989; Knickman, Weitzman, Shinn, & Marcus, 1989). Each of these factors, taken singly, increased the risk of homelessness by a factor of 6 or more.

Those who were doubled up with others, and those who were not, followed distinct routes into shelter (Weitzman, Knickman, & Shinn, 1990). Two thirds of those who were doubled up left because of problems with the doubled situation. Of those who were primary tenants, almost half left because of an inability to pay the rent. Another fifth left due to building problems. Indeed 47% of the shelter requesters, compared with 38% of the housed families, had lived in a building with two or more substantial structural problems such as rats or lack of heat or running water. The relative risk was small here, because so many housed families on public assistance also lived in deplorable conditions.

Families requesting shelter were more likely than housed families to live in extremely crowded circumstances: 45% of the first group, and 26% of the second reported having three or more persons per bedroom in the place they stayed the longest during the last year. Housed families were more likely to live in public housing or housing with one or another form of subsidy. The only housing factor that did not differentiate among shelter requesters and housed families was the proportion paying over $300 per month in rent.

Although a housing model seems to differentiate homeless and poor housed families in New York City far better than a model based on individual deficits, there were a number of important individual differences between the two groups, as shown in Table 2. Many homeless families were young, and had come of age in a time when housing was very tight: 72% of the mothers in the homeless sample were 30 or under, compared to 39% of housed poor families. Being 30 or under increased the risk of homelessness by a factor of four. They were substantially more likely to be African American, despite the oversample of black respondents in the housed group, although ethnicity did not make an independent contribution to predicting homelessness after controlling for other factors (see Knickman *et al.*, 1989). They were also substantially more likely to be pregnant—34% of homeless mothers compared to 6% of housed mothers were pregnant at the time of the interview, for a relative risk of nine. Put another way, if you were on public assistance in New York in 1988 and not pregnant, you had about a 2% chance of becoming homeless in the course of a year. If you were on public assistance and pregnant, you had an 18% chance of becoming homeless. Homeless mothers were also more likely to have given birth as teenagers and within the past year. Before we resort to stereotypes about large welfare families, I point out that homeless and housed mothers of the same ages had had almost precisely the same numbers of children (although

Table 2. Other Characteristics of Shelter Requesters and Poor Housed Families

Characteristic	Shelter requesters ($n = 700$)	Housed families ($n = 524$)	Approximate relative risk (odds ratio)
Demographics			
Age ≤ 30 years	72%	39%	4.1
Ethnicity			
African American[a]	54%	32%	2.5
Hispanic	39%	60%	0.4
Other	7%	9%	0.8
Pregnant	34%	6%	9.0
Baby in past year	26%	11%	2.9
Child before 18	37%	24%	1.9
Mean number of children (ever)			
Respondent ≤ 25	1.6	1.6	
26–30	2.3	2.3	
31–40	2.8	2.7	
41+	3.2	3.9	
Public assistance history			
Parent on p.a.	52%	31%	2.4
5+ years p.a.	49%	66%	0.5
(head 30 or below)	40%	48%	0.7
(head over 30)	72%	76%	0.8
2+ "administrative" case closings	50%	26%	2.8
Victimization			
Abused or threatened	26%	16%	1.9
Childhood abuse or family separation	32%	14%	3.0
Protective services worker	9%	2%	5.6

[a]Includes oversample of African–American respondents in the housed group.

the mothers requesting shelter had fewer children with them at the time of the interview). Pregnancy seemed to destabilize whatever housing situation families were in. It may also have increased financial needs and cut into mothers' ability to earn additional income (see Weitzman, 1989).

Actions of the social service system may also have been important to homelessness: 50% of families requesting shelter, compared to 26% of housed families, had had their welfare case closed two or more times for procedural reasons while the family was still eligible for benefits. Taken alone, this variable yielded a relative risk of 2.8, but it did not hold up as a predictor of homelessness in multivariate analyses, because of its association with other variables which could have been either causes or consequences of the case closing. For example, a family who was moving from one relative to another because they had no place of their own might not receive and thus not respond to a notice to come in to recertify their eligibility for welfare, leading to loss of benefits. Alternatively, loss of benefits could lead to doubling up and frequent moves. Interestingly, although homeless families were more likely than housed families to have a parent who received public assistance, they had not been on welfare as long. This difference was diminished, but not eliminated, by controlling for respondent's age (see Knickman & Weitzman, 1989; Knickman *et al.*, 1989).

A final set of factors that differentiated homeless from housed families was a history of victimization. Homeless mothers were more likely than housed mothers to have been abused or threatened with violence by a man they were involved with. They were more likely to have been abused as children and to have been in foster care or to have run away from home. And they were more likely to have had a protective service worker assigned to their home because of child abuse or neglect (although it is not clear who the prepetrator was). Each factor, taken alone, increased risk from two to five and a half times, but they were correlated with one another. Our figures on all types of violence are likely to be underestimates, because our measures were relatively crude (see Shinn *et al.*, 1991; Weitzman *et al.*, 1991).

These findings make it clear that the effects of poverty and a tight housing market were more important than individual deficits as causes of homelessness among families in New York City, even though our study held constant features of the New York City environment that make homelessness a larger problem in New York than in many other locales. Indeed many individual problems "uncovered" in other studies could be results of homelessness rather than causes of that state. Individual factors that increased vulnerability to homelessness and affected large numbers of families included age (with those 30 and under at high risk), pregnancy (but not family size), and a history of separation from the family or victimization. Structural factors included never having been able to break into the housing market, doubling up, and overcrowding; living in subsidized housing was protective.

Other studies, particularly studies of homeless single adults, find substantially higher proportions who are mentally ill or abuse substances. I have argued that methodological problems account for some of these findings, but they do not explain them away. But to argue that substance abuse or mental illness *caused* these individuals to become homeless is to adopt a very narrow and proximal concept of causation that takes as given an ecological context of poverty and a tight housing market. Were sufficient affordable housing readily available, these individuals might still be mentally ill and they might still abuse substances, but they would not be homeless. Similarly, treating their mental health or substance-abuse problems is important and may reduce their misery, but unless such treatment is coupled with sustainable housing, it will not cure their homelessness.

This brings us to the subtitle of this article. If the root causes of homelessness lie largely in poverty and the housing market, what is the role of psychologists? We are not architects or contractors; we are not labor economists; we are not legislators. What is a psychologist to do? I believe there are roles for psychologists, especially community psychologists, in the struggle to end homelessness. Not surprisingly, they involve research and action.

ROLES FOR PSYCHOLOGISTS

Research

If we hope to understand the origins of homelessness and to do something about it, we must move beyond research paradigms that examine only what is wrong with its victims. Psychologists may not be well equipped to study changing patterns of housing construction and poverty, but we can study how these structural variables impinge on individual poor people and families. For example, we can understand vulnerability factors such as the youth of homeless families in terms of structural factors such as the steep decline in income of young families and the loss of affordable housing during the period they came of age. We can understand the overrepresentation of people of color in the ranks of the homeless in terms of their overrepresentation in the ranks of the poor and their concentration in substandard housing. These facts in turn can be understood as manifestations of enduring racism in American society. We should focus attention on variables such as these that link structural and individual levels of analysis.

Second, community psychologists and fellow travelers should study levels of analysis between the individual and macro-social policy. For example, what factors promote stability in communities and protect both the housing stock and the people who live in it? Both formal organizations such as churches and block or tenant associations and informal leadership may be important. Saegert's (1989) work on the role of older African–American women in stabilizing their buildings is an example.

Third, we should move beyond cross-sectional designs to longitudinal studies that elucidate patterns of homelessness over time. Sosin *et al.*'s (1990) study is exemplary. It showed that literal homelessness was episodic, but that very few people, once homeless, were able to obtain sustainable housing without outside assistance. Other studies, by Audrey Burnam, Pamela Fisher, Marjorie Robertson, Paul Toro, and their colleagues and by our group in New York are following their example. Even cross-sectional work can distinguish retrospectively among different patterns of homelessness (e.g., Grigsby, Baumann, Gregorich, & Roberts-Gray, 1990; Milburn, Booth, & Cerfaratti, 1991), although researchers must be wary of the sampling biases described above.

Examining the course of homelessness leads to questions about factors that help homeless people obtain and retain stable permanent housing. We should examine the coping strategies that many poor families use to maintain their housing in difficult circumstances. Again, we should not stop with individual factors, but should examine social service systems and community factors from crime or drug traffic, which may make housing unhabitable, to community organizations that act to integrate or exclude previously homeless people.

Just as different types of families follow different paths into homelessness (Weitzman et al., 1991), it seems likely that different types of families require different services and supports to extricate themselves from that state (McChesney, 1992). Factors that increase vulnerability to homelessness may be very different from those that prolong it. For example, in New York, pregnancy was a risk factor for becoming homeless but also predicted a quick exit from the shelter system, because pregnant women were given priority for permanent housing. Again, it is important to understand individual characteristics in relationship to extraindividual factors such as service systems.

Finally, we may push back the causal analysis one step beyond the structural factors I have emphasized and ask how they came to be (Blasi, 1990). How does a society of unparalleled affluence permit such destitution in its midst? How do we who are well fed, well housed, and well dressed walk by our brothers and sisters who are none of these? These are truly psychological questions. What leads a community to own and take responsibility for the homeless people in its midst rather than crying "NIMBY"— not in my backyard? How can we understand and counter the parallel phenomenon at the level of government that I call "NIMB"—not in my bailiwick? Link (1991), Toro and McDonell (1992), and others have made promising starts in this area by examining public attitudes towards homelessness. But here too we need to go beyond the level of the individual to study the organized actions of community groups and government agencies. A subsidiary concern is to understand what sorts of information and images promote change. My hunch is that qualitative work that gives voice to homeless people is important in changing public attitudes.

Action

How do we go from knowledge to action to end homelessness? If we understand homelessness as an extreme form of poverty and if structural factors such as dwindling supplies of affordable housing are critical, a key form of action is to influence the political process so as to reduce poverty and increase the construction of housing. An important role for psychologists is modesty. We should help policy makers understand the *limited* role of psychological factors such as mental illness as causes of homelessness. We should help them understand that structural factors underlie both literal homelessness and the tenuous attachment of many of our poorest citizens to their housing.

Psychologists typically want to provide services to alleviate problems, and many services from soup kitchens to substance-abuse treatment programs are needed by some homeless people. Mental health services are important to help people deal with the trauma of homelessness and with events such as violence that may have preceded or attended it. However, we must recognize that services without housing are unlikely to do more than redistribute homelessness, and we should not assume that all homeless people need any particular service other than housing.

Psychologists can also help to make systems work better for subpopulations for whom we have special expertise, for example, by virtue of knowledge of mental illness or child development. Kennedy (1989) has shown that for mentally ill individuals, it is important to match housing situations to the functional level of the person to promote well-being. Psychologists should work to create a range of supported living options for those who need them and to match persons and settings. To take just one more example, research by community psychologists and others (Felner, Primavera, & Cauce, 1981; Levine, Wesolowski, & Corbett, 1966; Peterson & Crockett, 1985) has shown that excessive numbers of school transitions are bad for children's academic performance, attendance, and self-esteem. As psychologists armed with this knowledge, we can work with shelter systems and school systems to prevent arbitrary transfers of families from place to place and to permit as much continuity for children as possible.

Finally, efforts to *prevent* homelessness include efforts to empower tenants' groups, block associations, and communities to maintain existing housing, get essential services from landlords and local governments, and maintain their communities. Work by Chavis, Florin, Perkins, Prestby, Rich, and Wandersman in a special section of the *American Journal of Community Psychology* (Wandersman & Florin, 1990) is a useful model. We can also work with developers and community groups to create housing from single-room occupancy units to single-family homes that will meet the needs of poor people for decent and affordable housing. Psychologists, even community psychologists, need to collaborate with others in this work—we do not know enough to do it alone. After all, homelessness is not simply a psychological problem.

ACKNOWLEDGMENTS

Preparation was funded by grant #RO1MH46116 from the National Institute of Mental Health. The New York City data were collected jointly with James Knickman and Beth Weitzman of the Wagner School of Public Service, New York University under a contract from the New York City Human Resources Administration to James Knickman. This paper was influenced by Hopper and Hamberg (1986) and Stegman and Keyes (1991) in ways that exceed specific citations, although the conclusions accord more with the former authors' than with the later. I thank Barbara Felton, Diane Hughes, Bruce Rapkin, and Ed Seidman for their helpful comments and Ben McDaniels, Lisa Duchon, and Beth Weitzman for checking the tables.

REFERENCES

Apgar, W. C. Jr., DiPasquale, D., Cummings, J., & McArdle, N. (1990). *The state of the nation's housing 1990*. Cambridge, MA: Joint Center for Housing Studies of Harvard University.

Bassuk, E. L. & Rosenberg, L. (1988). Why does family homelessness occur? A case-control study. *American Journal of Public Health, 78,* 783–788.

Blasi, Gary L. (1990). Social policy and social science research on homelessness. *Journal of Social Issues, 46*(4), 207–219.

Farr, R. K., Koegel, P. & Burnam, A. (1986). *A study of homelessness and mental illness in the skid row area of Los Angeles*. Los Angeles: Los Angeles County Department of Mental Health.

Felner, R. D., Primavera, J., & Cauce, A. M. (1981). The impact of school transitions: A focus for preventive efforts. *American Journal of Community Psychology, 9,* 449–459.

Fischer, P. J., Shapiro, S., Breakey, W. R., Anthony, J. C., & Kramer, M. (1986). Mental health and social characteristics of the homeless: A survey of mission users. *American Journal of Public Health, 76,* 519–524.

Goodman, L. A. (1991). The relationship between social support and family homelessness: A comparison study of homeless and housed mothers. *Journal of Community Psychology, 19,* 321–332.

Grigsby, C., Baumann, D., Gregorich, S. E., & Roberts-Gray, C. (1990). Disaffiliation to entrenchment: A model for understanding homelessness. *Journal of Social Issues, 46*(4), 141–156.

Hopper, K. (1990). Public shelter as a "hybrid institution": Homeless men in historical perspective. *Journal of Social Issues, 46*(4), 13–29.

Hopper, K. & Hamberg, J. (1986). The making of America's homeless: From skid row to new poor, 1945–1984. In R. G. Bratt, C. Hartman, & A. Meyerson (Eds.), *Critical perspectives on housing* (pp. 12–40). Philadelphia: Temple University Press.

Kennedy, C. (1989). Community integration and well-being: Toward the goals of community care. *Journal of Social Issues, 45*(3), 65–77.

Knickman, J. R. & Weitzman, B. C. (1989). *A study of homeless families in New York City: Forecasting models to target families at high risk of homelessness* (Final Report, Vol. 3). New York: Health Research Program, New York University.

Knickman, J. R., Weitzman, B. C., Shinn, M., & Marcus, E. H. (1989). *A study of homeless families in New York City: Characteristics and comparisons with other public assistance families* (Final Report, Vol. 2). New York: Health Research Program, New York University.

Koegel, P. & Burnam, M. A. (1988). Alcoholism among homeless adults in the inner city of Los Angeles. *Archives of General Psychiatry, 45*, 1011–1018.

Koegel, P. & Burnam, M. A. (1992). Problems in the assessment of mental illness among the homeless: An empirical approach. In M. J. Robertson & M. Greenblatt (Eds.), *Homelessness: A national perspective* (pp. 77–100). New York: Plenum Press.

Koegel, P., Burnam, M. A., & Farr, R. K. (1988). The prevalence of specific psychiatric disorders among homeless individuals in the inner city of Los Angeles. *Archives of General Psychiatry, 45*, 1085–1092.

Koegel, P., Burnam, M. A., & Farr, R. K. (1990). Subsistence adaptation among homeless adults in the inner city of Los Angeles. *Journal of Social Issues, 46*(4), 83–107.

Leonard, P. A., Dolbeare, C. N., & Lazere, E. B. (1989). *A place to call home: The crisis in housing for the poor.* Washington, DC: Center on Budget and Policy Priorities and Low Income Housing Information Service.

Levine, M., Wesolowski, J. C., & Corbett, F. J. (1966). Pupil turnover and academic performance in an inner city elementary school *Psychology in the Schools, 3*, 153–156.

Link, B. (1991, September). *Public attitudes toward the homeless: Compassion fatigue?* Paper presented at meeting of the American Association of Public Opinion Researchers, New York Chapter, New York.

Lipton, F. R., Sabatini, A., & Katz, S. E. (1983). Down and out in the city: The homeless mentally ill. *Hospital and Community Psychiatry, 34*, 817–821.

Littman, M. S. (1989). Poverty in the 1980's: Are the poor getting poorer? *Monthly Labor Review, 112*(6), 13–18.

McChesney, K. Y. (1990). Family homelessness: A systemic problem. *Journal of Social Issues, 46*(4), 191–205.

McChesney, K. Y. (1992). Paths to family homelessness. In M. J. Robertson & M. Greenblatt (Eds.), *Homelessness: A national perspective* (pp. 245–256). New York: Plenum Press.

Milburn, N. G., Booth, J. E., & Cerfaratti, V. (1991, August). *Discriminants of duration of homelessness among black women in shelters.* Paper presented at the meeting of the American Psychological Association, San Francisco.

Molnar, J., Rath, W. R., Klein, T. P., Lowe, C., & Hartmann, A. (1991). *Ill fares the land: The consequences of homelessness and chronic poverty for children and families in New York City.* New York: Bank Street College of Education.

Mowbray, C., Solarz, A., Johnson, S. V., Phillips-Smith, E., & Combs, C. J. (1986). *Mental health and homelessness in Detroit: A research study.* Lansing: Michigan Department of Mental Health.

Passero, J. M., Zax, M., & Zozus, R. T., Jr. (1991). Social network utilization as related to family history among the homeless. *Journal of Community Psychology, 19*, 70–78.

Peterson, A. C. & Crockett, L. (1985). Pubertal timing and grade effects on adjustment. *Journal of Youth and Adolescence, 14*, 191–206.

Ringheim, K. (1990a). *At risk of homelessness: The roles of income and rent.* New York: Praeger.

Ringheim, K. (1990b). *The structural determinants of homelessness: A study of eight cities* (Discussion paper No. 930–90). Madison, WI: Institute for Research on Poverty.

Rossi, P. H., Wright, J. D., Fisher, G. A., & Willis, G. (1987). The urban homeless: Estimating composition and size. *Science, 235*, 1336–1341.

Rossi, P. H. (1989). *Down and out in America: The origins of homelessness.* Chicago: University of Chicago Press.

Saegert, S. (1989). Unlikely leaders, extreme circumstances: Older black women building community households. *American Journal of Community Psychology, 17*, 295–316.

Shinn, M., Knickman, J. R., & Weitzman, B. C. (1991). Social relationships and vulnerability to becoming homeless among poor families. *American Psychologist, 46*, 1180–1187.

Shinn, M. & Weitzman, B. C. (1990). Research on homelessness: An introduction. *Journal of Social Issues, 46*, 1–11.

Sosin, M. R., Colson, P., & Grossman, S. (1988). *Homelessness in Chicago: Poverty and pathology, social institutions, and social change.* Chicago: University of Chicago, School of Social Service Administration.

Sosin, M., Piliavin, I., & Westerfelt, H. (1990). Toward a longitudinal analysis of homelessness. *Journal of Social Issues, 46*(4), 157–174.

Stegman, M. A. & Keyes, L. C. (1991, January). *Housing, poverty, and homelessness: A literature review and research agenda.* Paper presented at a National Institute of Mental Health/National Institute on Alcoholism and Alcohol Abuse sponsored conference, Cambridge, MA.

Toro, P. & McDonell, D. M. (1992). Beliefs, attitudes, and knowledge about homelessness: A survey of the general public. *American Journal of Community Psychology, 20*, 53–80.

U.S. Bureau of the Census (1990). *Measuring the effect of benefits and taxes on income and poverty: 1989* (Current Population Reports, Series P-60, No. 169-RD). Washington, DC: U.S. Government Printing Office.

U.S. Bureau of the Census (1991). *Poverty in the United States: 1988 and 1989* (Current Population Reports, Series P-60, No. 171). Washington, DC: U.S. Government Printing Office.

U.S. House of Representatives Committee on Ways and Means (1990). *Overview of entitlement programs: 1990 Green Book.* Washington, DC: U.S. Government Printing Office.

Wandersman, A. & Florin, P. (1990). Citizen participation, voluntary organizations, and community development: Insights for empowerment through research. Special Section, *American Journal of Community Psychology, 18*, 41–177.

Watts, H. W. (1986). Have our measures of poverty become poorer? *Focus* (University of Wisconsin-Madison Institute for Research on Poverty), *9*(2), 18–23.

Weitzman, B. C. (1989). Pregnancy and childbirth: Risk factors for homelessness? *Family Planning Perspectives, 21*(4), 175–178.

Weitzman, B. C., Knickman, J. R., & Shinn, M. (1990). Pathways to homelessness among New York City families. *Journal of Social Issues, 46*(4), 125–140.

Weitzman, B. C., Knickman, J. R., & Shinn, M., (1991). *Predictors of shelter use among low income families: Psychiatric history, substance abuse, and victimization.* Unpublished manuscript, New York University.

Wood, D., Valdez, R. B., Hayashi, T., & Shen, A. (1990). Homeless and housed families in Los Angeles: A study comparing demographic, economic and family function characteristics. *American Journal of Public Health, 80*, 1049–1052.

Wright, J. D. (1989). *Address unknown: The homeless in America.* New York: Aldine de Gruyter.

18

The Social Policy Context of Child Care: Effects on Quality

Deborah A. Phillips, Carollee Howes, and Marcy Whitebook

Examined effects on the quality of children's child care environments of (a) the stringency of state child care regulations, (b) voluntary compliance with proposed federal child care standards, and (c) the legal auspice of the center. Quality of care was assessed in 227 child care centers in five metropolitan areas. Centers in states with more stringent child care regulations tended to have better staff–child ratios, staff with more child-related training, and lower staff turnover rates. Similarly, centers that more fully complied with the ratio, group size, and training provisions of a set of proposed federal child care standards had significantly lower staff turnover rates, more age-appropriate classroom activities, less harsh and more sensitive teachers, and more teachers with specialized training. For-profit centers offered children less optimal care than did nonprofit centers. These findings are placed in the context of ecological models of research and of contemporary policy debates about child care.

Child care has been studied extensively as an environment for children's growth and development (Clarke-Stewart & Fein, 1983; Hayes, Palmer, & Zaslow, 1990). More recently, it has been conceptualized as a work environment for adult caretakers (Phillips, Howes, & Whitebook, 1991), and as

Originally published in the *American Journal of Community Psychology*, 20(1) (1992): 25–51.

A Quarter Century of Community Psychology: Readings from the American Journal of Community Psychology, edited by Tracey A. Revenson *et al.* Kluwer Academic/Plenum Publishers, New York, 2002.

a source of family support (Powell, 1987). Child care also exists within a policy context that is likely to influence how it affects children, caretakers, and families. Specifically, child care centers operate in the context of state regulations and under distinct legal and financial auspices. This level of variation, however, has received minimal attention in child care research. The research reported here was designed to examine the effects of differing child care regulations and of profit–nonprofit status on the quality of care provided by child care centers in five states.

ECOLOGICAL FRAMEWORK OF THE STUDY

The theoretical framework for the study draws upon ecological models of research (Bronfenbrenner, 1979; Seidman, 1987) that explicitly acknowledge the multiple levels of environmental influence on individual behavior and development. Individuals are placed at the core of several concentric layers of influence, ranging from their immediate environments (microsystem) to the ideologies that prevail in their culture (macrosystem). Outer layers of influence are theorized to constrain the characteristics, quality, and effects of more immediate environments. Accordingly, efforts to go beyond the environments that individuals inhabit in their daily lives to understand precisely how other levels of environmental influence affect these daily settings and, ultimately, how their influence reaches the individual are of particular interest.

Ecological models are particularly well-suited to the study of child care insofar as the child is embedded in the immediate classroom (microsystem), which is directly affected by other settings in the community—such as child care training programs—that do not contain the child (exosystem). These two systems are in turn affected by the broader economic and political structures—such as child care regulations—that influence how social institutions are organized in our society (macrosystem). The least studied of these layers in all areas of psychological research, including research on child care, is the outermost, macrosystem of influence. This is a particularly troubling oversight among community psychologists insofar as many of the factors discussed in this subfield's theoretical literature, including ideological and political influences (Price, 1989; Rappaport, 1981; Reppucci, 1985; Seidman, 1988), reside in the macrosystem. Moreover, ecological theory acknowledges that different environmental levels are more or less amenable to intervention by different mechanisms. We suggest that policy mechanisms are best suited to macrosystem interventions, namely, those interventions that focus on broad patterns of funding, organizational structure and incentives, and regulation.

The research reported here is part of a larger study of child care whose design was based on ecological frameworks for research (Whitebook, Howes, & Phillips, 1990). Specifically, we examined the differing levels of environmental influence represented by the quality of children's immediate classrooms, by the adult work environment in the participating child care centers, by the legal–financial structure of the centers, and by the stringency of the state child care regulations with which each center was required to comply. This report focuses on the relation between the macrosystem, represented by policies reflected in state child care regulations and centers' legal auspices, and the quality of the immediate microsystem of the child's classroom. As such, we hope to provide an example of community-based policy research. Before discussing the measurement of child care quality, we provide an overview of the regulatory and legal context of child care.

THE REGULATORY CONTEXT OF CHILD CARE

In every state, child care centers are required to comply with regulations that establish a threshold of quality below which children's development is presumably compromised. Safety and health precautions figure prominently in these regulations, but the majority also include provisions regarding staff training, staff–child ratios, and maximum group sizes. States vary widely, however, in the stringency of these regulations (Phillips, Lande, & Goldberg, 1990). For example, centers in Massachusetts are required to have 2 caregivers per 7 infants, whereas centers in Georgia are permitted to have 1 caregiver per 7 infants.

Given that the central purpose of these regulations is to affect the quality of care that is provided to children, a key policy issue concerns the effectiveness with which this function is served. This, of course, requires a sample of child care centers from several states. The National Child Care Staffing Study (Whitebook et al., 1990) offers this sample. Child care centers were recruited from five sites in states that include the most stringent (Massachusetts) and the most lax (Georgia) child care regulations. In the absence of samples of this nature, there has been virtually no information on the relation between regulation and quality of care.

A related question about the influence of regulations on child care quality concerns the issue of compliance. Do centers that comply with regulations that reflect prevailing definitions of high quality care actually offer higher quality care than centers that do not comply? This requires that the observed quality of care in a diverse sample of centers be compared to a uniform benchmark. We selected the Federal Interagency Day Care

Requirements (FIDCR), adopted in 1980 and almost immediately rescinded, as this benchmark. Among an array of provisions, the FIDCR reflect a professional consensus about three core ingredients of quality: the ratio of children per adult caregiver, the maximum number of children in a given classroom (group size), and the child-related training of the teaching staff. The FIDCR, therefore, offer the opportunity to examine the potential influence of federal standards on child care quality, and, more generally, provide an appropriate voluntary benchmark with which to explore the relation between regulatory compliance and child care quality.

THE LEGAL CONTEXT OF CHILD CARE

In addition to varying in compliance with standards, centers vary in their financial and legal auspice. Some centers are for-profit organizations whereas others operate on a nonprofit basis. Our interest in examining differences in quality of care based on the auspice of the center has both theoretical and empirical origins.

Traditionally, nonprofit entities have claimed to offer higher quality services than are available in the for-profit sector. The nonprofits' claims of higher quality are based on the theory of "contract failure" (Hansmann, 1980; Nelson & Krashinsky, 1973) which addresses situations in which the consumer is not able to evaluate adequately the quality of services and thus an opportunity for exploitation exists. Because nonprofit organizations cannot distribute profits to those who control the organization, the motivation for exploitation, in the form of cutting costs and reducing quality, is presumably reduced. For-profit organizations, in contrast, are viewed as having both legal sanction and motivation to make increased profits by exploiting consumers. Little is known about the applicability of notions of contract failure to child care, but an obvious first step is to assess the basic assumption that nonprofit child care centers offer higher quality care than do for-profit centers.

Available research (Coelen, Glantz, & Calore, 1979; Kagan, 1991; Kagan & Newton, 1989; 1991; Keyserling, 1972) suggests that nonprofit centers do, in fact, offer higher quality care than for-profit centers. For example, Kagan and Newton found that nonprofit centers had more "child sensitive" environments, including more sensitive and encouraging caregiver–child interactions. However, this evidence is based on single-site studies that fail to reflect the full diversity of both profit and nonprofit care, and on data that predate the recent rapid expansion in for-profit child care. We examined the implications of profit–nonprofit status for quality of care in a large sample of centers that, as noted above, reside in states that require very different levels of quality for licensing.

MEASUREMENT OF QUALITY

Empirical studies of the quality of child care are grounded in a framework that emphasizes predictive validity. Specifically, developmentalists define quality as those aspects of child care that are significantly associated with better outcomes for children, including cognitive, language, and socioemotional development (see Hayes *et al.*, 1990; Phillips & Howes, 1987). A rich research literature now supports a multimeasure approach to assessing quality of care that encompasses structural features (e.g., staff–child ratios), the developmental environment, staff–child interactions, and the stability of care. Each of these dimensions of quality captures a distinct feature of what children experience in child care. Accordingly, the field has come to adopt a strategy of convergent measurement when assessing child care quality (Zaslow, 1991). This strategy was adopted in the present study, in which each of the following aspects of quality was operationalized.

The structural characteristics of staff : child ratio and group size, and staff qualifications reflected in education and training, are often referred to as "regulatable" features of care. Although some studies fail to find significant associations between some of these features and children's development (see, e.g., Kagan & Newton, 1989, and Whitebook *et al.*, 1990, for nonsignificant group size effects), when associations are found they consistently point to higher ratios (fewer children per teacher), smaller groups, and better trained and educated staff as predictors of positive development among children in child care (Howes & Rubenstein, 1985; Howes & Stewart, 1987; Phillips, McCartney, & Scarr, 1987; Ruopp, Travers, Glantz, & Coelen, 1979; Vandell & Powers, 1983; Whitebook *et al.*, 1990).

Assessments of the developmental environment of child care that provide a comprehensive summary of the physical environment, the activities that children experience, and the quality of staff–child interactions also exist (Harms & Clifford, 1980; Sibley & Abbott-Shim, 1988). Research that relies on these assessments have consistently revealed positive associations between quality and children's development (see Hayes *et al.*, 1990, for a review of this literature).

Other measures of quality focus on the nature of staff–child interactions, such as the staff's sensitivity to children's needs. These measures are often found to mediate positive relations between the regulatable or global quality variables and child outcomes (Howes, Phillips, & Whitebook, 1992).

Finally, recent assessments of quality have pointed to the importance of stability of care (Howes & Stewart, 1987; Howes, 1988) and of stable relations between caregivers and children (Anderson, Nagle, Roberts, & Smith, 1981; Cummings, 1980) as significant predictors of children's well-being in child care. These findings have directed attention to staff turnover rates as an important quality indicator, although only one study has documented a direct link between staff turnover and children's development (Whitebook *et al.*, 1990).

HYPOTHESES

We hypothesized that policy-level variation in regulatory stringency and compliance, and in the legal–financial auspice of child care centers, influences the quality of child care that children are observed to receive. We examined three questions: (a) Does the quality of children's child care environments vary with the stringency of state child care regulations? We hypothesized that centers located in states with more stringent regulations would offer higher quality care. (b) Do centers that comply with proposed federal child care standards in the areas of staff–child ratios, group size, and staff training offer better environments for children? We hypothesized that they would. And, (c) is the legal auspice of the center associated with compliance and quality of care? We hypothesized that nonprofit centers would have higher rates of regulatory compliance and be observed to offer higher quality care to children than for-profit centers.

METHOD

Quality of care was examined in 227 child care centers in five metropolitan areas: Atlanta ($n = 46$), Boston ($n = 44$), Detroit ($n = 45$), Phoenix ($n = 45$), and Seattle ($n = 47$). These sites were selected to capture wide variation in the level of quality required by each state's child care regulations. As seen in Table 1, Massachusetts had the most stringent regulations that matched or exceeded those of each of the other sites. Michigan and Washington closely matched Massachusetts' ratio requirements (with the exception of Washington's toddler ratio), but were either silent or less stringent on group size and training. Georgia had the most lax regulations, in general, followed closely by Arizona.

Data collection took place between February and August 1988. Classroom observations and interviews with center directors and staff provided data on center characteristics and quality.

Centers

Child care centers were recruited from the five study sites using a two-part sampling strategy. First, full-year, full-day centers that had been in

Table 1. State Child Care Regulations for Ratios and Group Size, 1988[a]

State	Ratios			Group size		
	Infant	Toddler	Preschool	Infant	Toddler	Preschool
Arizona	1:5	1:6 1:8	1:15 1:20	NR	NR	NR
Georgia	1:7	1:10	1:15 1:18	NR	NR	NR
Massachusetts	2:7	1:4	1:10	7	9	20
Michigan	1:4	1:4	1:10 1:12	NR	NR	NR
Washington	1:4	1:7	1:10	8	14	20

[a]NR indicates not regulated. Infant refers to children 1 year and younger (or not walking); toddler refers to 1- and 2-year-olds; preschool refers to 3- and 4-year-olds. Where two ratios are listed for an age group, the first refers to the youngest age and the second refers to the oldest (e.g., 1:15 for 3-year-olds and 1:20 for 4-year-olds in Arizona). Only Arizona and Massachusetts require preservice training and a specified number of hours of annual, in-service training (12 hours in Arizona; 20 hours in Massachusetts).

operation for at least 9 months were identified from lists of licensed child care centers. Second, eligible centers were divided into six groups based on their location in (a) low-, middle-, or high-income U.S. Census tracts, and (b) urban or suburban neighborhoods. The final sample was then randomly selected to match the proportion of eligible centers in each of these six income and neighborhood groups. Replacement sampling was used to handle refusals.

Of all eligible centers asked to participate, 61% agreed. The participation rates in the five study sites ranged from 45–75% of all eligible centers. Refusal rates were higher among centers in middle-income (42% refused) and high-income (38% refused) census tracts than among those in low-income tracts (23% refused). Refusals were also higher among for-profit (40% refused) than nonprofit centers (21% refused). Telephone screening interviews also revealed that directors of participating centers reported higher (i.e., better) adult:child ratios than did the directors who refused to participate. This suggests that the final sample of 227 centers may be of higher-than-average quality.

Classrooms and Teachers

In each center, three classrooms were randomly selected to be observed, one each from among all available infant (4 weeks to 11 months), toddler (12 to 35 months), and preschool (36 to 59 months) classrooms. In centers that did not enroll infants, only two classrooms were observed unless a third, mixed-age classroom was available for observation. Across all participating centers, the research teams observed 643 classrooms: 85 (13%) infant, 151 (23%) toddler, 313 (49%) preschool, and 94 (15%) mixed-age classrooms. Toddler classrooms were further divided into those with young (1-year-olds) and older (2-year-olds) toddlers. The mixed-age classrooms were eliminated from all analyses reported in this article.

Two staff members from each participating classroom were interviewed and observed. Only two teachers were assigned to the majority of classrooms, but when there were more than two teachers, the participating staff were selected randomly. In classrooms with only one staff member, this individual was asked to participate. Staff participation rates were over 95% in each site. Of the final sample of 1,309 participating staff, 66% (865) were teachers and 34% (444) were assistant teachers.

Measures

Quality Assessments

Overall quality of care was assessed with the Early Childhood Environment Rating Scale (ECERS; Harms & Clifford, 1980) for each preschool classroom and the Infant-Toddler Environment Rating Scale (ITERS; Harms, Cryer, & Clifford, 1986) for each of the infant and toddler classrooms. These scales comprehensively assess the day-to-day quality of care provided to children, ranging from the safety of the equipment to the quality of teaching. Individual items (37 on the ECERS and 35 on the ITERS) are rated from a low of 1 to a high of 7. A rating of 3 on these scales indicates *minimally acceptable* quality, while a 5 indicates *good* quality. Two subscales were derived from a maximum likelihood factor analysis, with oblique rotation, of the ECERS and ITERS scale items. The first subscale, labeled Appropriate Caregiving, captured the items pertaining to child–adult interactions, supervision, and discipline. The second subscale, labeled Developmentally Appropriate Activity, captured the items pertaining to the materials, schedule, and activities. The first subscale accounted for 23% of the variance in both the preschool and infant/toddler versions of the scale (eigenvalues were 8.27 and 7.36, respectively); the second subscale accounted for 14% (eigenvalue of 5.21) and 16% (eigenvalue of 5.15) of the variance, respectively. Intercorrelations between the subscales exceeded .78 for classrooms serving all ages of children, and thus cannot be interpreted as independent, particularly if observers have adopted implicit, logical theories of quality.

The structural features of staff: child ratio and group size were assessed with classroom observations in which the numbers of adults and children were recorded at regular intervals during a 2-hour observation period. Both morning and afternoon observations were required in each classroom. The multiple observations were averaged to create a ratio and group size score for each age group of children (infants, toddlers, and preschoolers).

Staff qualifications were assessed as part of an individual interview conducted with each participating teacher. For this report, the early childhood training of the staff is used as a proxy for staff qualifications given the prominence of this variable in debates about child care regulations. This is a continuous variable, ranging from *no early childhood training* (0) to *advanced degree in early childhood education, child development, or related field* (5).

Staff–child interaction was assessed using the Arnett scale of Teacher Sensitivity. This is an observational measure, consisting of 26 items, each of which is rated from *did not occur* (1) to *occurred often* (3). Three scores accounting for 60.4% of the variance were derived from this scale using principal component analysis with varimax rotation: Harshness (9 items including critical, threatens children, and punitive; eigenvalue was 10.18), which accounted for 39.2% of the variance; Sensitivity (9 items including warm, attentive, engaged; eigenvalue was 3.92), which accounted for 15.1% of the variance; and Detachment (4 items including low levels of interaction, interest, and supervision; eigenvalue was 1.61), which accounted for 6.2% of the variance. Scores for Sensitivity and Harshness range from a low of 4 to a high of 36; scores for Detachment range from a low of 4 to a high of 16.

Staff turnover was assessed by asking each center director to indicate how many classroom staff had left the center in the past year. The annual turnover rate was calculated by dividing this number by the total number of classroom staff.

Determination of Compliance

All participating centers were classified by whether they met all, two, one, or none of three provisions—staff training, ratios, and group size—contained in the Federal Interagency Day Care Requirements (FIDCR). The FIDCR required that staff "regularly participate in specialized training." Centers whose directors indicated that they provided payment for attendance at on-site, in-service training or paid release time for off-site training and workshops were in compliance with this training provision. Ratios, based on attendance, were set at 1:3 for infants under age 2 years, 1:4 for toddlers (2 years of age), and 1:8 for preschoolers (3–6 years) in the FIDCR. Group sizes, based on attendance, were set at 6, 12, and 16 for these age groups, respectively. Centers whose infant, toddler, and preschool classrooms met or improved upon these ratio and group size limits were in compliance. For this purpose only, we combined infant (under 1 year of age) and young toddler (1-year-olds) classrooms to correspond to the FIDCR age classifications.

Determination of Auspice

Directors were asked to indicate the auspice of their center with a choice of three for-profit categories (independent, local chain, national chain) and nine nonprofit categories (independent, Head Start, parent co-operative, church sponsored, university sponsored, public or private school sponsored, corporate sponsored, government agency sponsored, and community organization sponsored). Based on the distribution of centers and policy-relevant categories, four different auspices were compared: (a) independent, for-profit centers ($n = 89$), (b) for-profit chains ($n = 18$), (c) nonprofit, nonsectarian centers ($n = 83$), and (d) sectarian centers run by churches and synagogues (also nonprofit) ($n = 37$).

Procedure

Data collection in each site was completed by a local team of research assistants. These teams were composed of individuals with dual qualifications. Each assistant had experience as a teacher, director, or support staff in the child care delivery system. Each also was an experienced, trained observer of child care and children. On average, at least two assistants spent 3 days in each center. Director interviews, taking 3 hours on average, were completed prior to any other data collection. Classroom observations were completed prior to staff interviews. Observers were unaware of the information provided by the directors, including information about the auspice of the center. However, it was not possible to assure that the observers were blind to the auspice of the center in every case. A minimum of 2 hours per classroom was required to complete the two observational measures (ECERS/ITERS and the Arnett scale), with counts of adults and children made at regular intervals during this period. Thus, the same observers assessed the structural variables such as staff:child ratios and the developmental and interactional measures of quality. However, the attentional demands of assessing these constructs simultaneously is likely to have militated against any deliberate contamination across these various types of quality measures. In most cases, each classroom was visited on more than 1 day; in all cases, both morning and afternoon activities were observed. Staff interviews required, on average, $1^{1}/_{2}$ hours.

Cross- and within-site, interrater reliabilities (percentage agreement, based on scale items) were calculated for the observational measures.

Within-site reliabilities (based on 5% of the center sample, and on agree-ment at the item level) exceeded 90% agreement in each site for the ECERS/ITERS factors, the factors from the Arnett scale, and ratio and group size counts. Cross-site reliabilities, determined at the midpoint of data collection by having one research assistant from each site travel to two other sites, were above 85% agreement for all pairs of sites for each of the observational measures. Test–retest reliabilities for the interviews were computed for 10 directors and 10 teaching staff who were not participating in the study. Test–retest reliability, averaging across all items on the director interview, was $r = .82$ (range $= .79$ to $.94$). Reliability, averaging across all items on the staff interview, was $r = .79$ (range $= .71$ to $.92$).

Plan of Analysis

The quality variables that we report were measured at different units or levels. Staff turnover was assessed at the center level. Ratio, group size, and the ITERS/ECERS subscales of Appropriate Caregiving and Developmentally Appropriate Activities were measured at the classroom level. And, staff education and the three Arnett scales (Sensitivity, Harshness, Detachment) were measured at the staff level. The analyses were, therefore, conducted on different units of analysis corresponding to these differing levels of measurement: center, classroom, and staff.

To determine whether child care centers in states with differing child care regulations differ significantly in quality of care, several MANOVAs were conducted, followed by univariate analyses in the case of significant MANOVAs. Scheffé tests were used to make post hoc comparisons of group means. Three one-way MANOVAs (with site as the independent variable) were conducted on the ratio and group size variables, respectively, for infant, toddler, and preschool classrooms. Three one-way MANOVAs were conducted to examine site effects on the two ITERS and ECERS subscales and the four staff-level variables, respectively. A one-way ANOVA was conducted on staff turnover. To determine whether centers that show differing levels of compliance with the FIDCR and that operate under differing auspices offer differing qualities of care, these same analy-ses were rerun with the four levels of compliance and, then, the four levels of auspice substituting for site as the independent variable. The com-pliance analyses did not include the dependent measures of ratio and group size given that these variables were used to determine each center's degree of FIDCR compliance. The results for the site analyses are presented first, followed by those that examine the effects of compliance with the FIDCR and center auspice, respectively.

RESULTS

Effects of State Regulation

Did the observed pattern of quality correspond to the site-specific differences in the level of quality required by state child care regulations (see Table 1)? Table 2 presents the observed ratios and group sizes by the age of children in the classroom in each of the study sites. The MANOVAs run on the observed ratios and group sizes were significant for all age groups: $F(16, 449) = 6.34$ for infants, $F(16, 531) = 4.44$ for toddlers, $F(16, 603) = 5.88$ for preschoolers, all $ps < .001$. The univariate analyses revealed that the sites differed significantly in observed ratios for each age group but did not differ in group sizes.

Centers in the three sites (Boston, Detroit, and Seattle) in which infant ratios of $1:4$ or $2:7$ were required were observed to have significantly lower (better) ratios than the centers in Atlanta where the state required only a $1:7$ ratio for infants. Differences in observed toddler and preschool ratios also mapped closely onto the relative stringency of state requirements.

Table 2. Observed Ratios and Group Sizes by Age Group of Classroom and Study Site[a]

Quality indicator	Atlanta	Detroit	Boston	Phoenix	Seattle	Comparisons	F
Ratios							
Infant							
M	5.07	2.66	2.53	4.07	2.82	B,D,S < A	14.49[b]
SD	1.66	1.05	0.79	0.78	0.77		
Toddler							
M	6.72	3.59	3.43	6.35	5.20	B,D < A	8.96[b]
SD	2.56	0.64	0.46	2.50	2.28	B < P	
Preschool							
M	10.23	5.48	7.59	10.35	7.57	B,D,S < A,P	17.73[b]
SD	4.01	1.60	3.40	4.95	3.08		
Group size							
Infant							
M	7.97	6.27	6.33	6.92	6.57		ns
SD	3.38	3.41	1.97	3.01	3.69		
Toddler							
M	10.80	8.82	9.71	8.89	8.63		ns
SD	4.20	3.19	5.38	3.12	4.18		
Preschool							
M	15.15	13.07	14.82	14.59	13.48		ns
SD	5.12	4.10	6.45	5.54	5.82		

[a]All means are least squares means. A = Atlanta, B = Boston, D = Detroit, P = Phoenix, S = Seattle.
[b]$p < .001$.

Centers in Boston and Detroit, with a 1:4 requirement, had significantly lower toddler ratios than did centers in Atlanta with its 1:10 requirement. Toddler ratios in Boston were also significantly lower than those in Phoenix. For preschoolers, centers in Boston, Detroit, and Seattle offered significantly better ratios than did centers in either Atlanta or Phoenix.

The one-way MANOVAs for site for all remaining quality variables were significant: $F(8, 436) = 6.39$ for the infant/toddler ITERS factors, $F(8, 558) = 8.83$ for the preschool ECERS factors, $F(16, 3905) = 34.66$ for the four staff-level variables, all $ps < .001$. Table 3 presents the means and standard deviations for the remaining quality variables. Staff turnover was significantly higher in the Phoenix centers than those in either Boston or Detroit.

Table 3. Turnover, Classroom Quality, Staff–Child Interaction, and Staff Qualifications by Study Site[a]

Quality indicator	Atlanta	Detroit	Boston	Phoenix	Seattle	Comparisons	F
Turnover (%)							
M	53	29	27	65	40	B,D < P	7.52[c]
SD	0.47	0.17	0.23	0.63	0.29		
Caregiving: infants and toddlers							
M	3.61	4.72	5.32	4.34	4.05	B,D,P > A	10.15[c]
SD	1.18	1.01	1.64	1.03	1.15	D > S	
Activities: infants and toddlers							
M	3.15	3.88	4.24	3.67	3.09	B,D > A,S	7.83[c]
SD	1.03	0.77	1.34	0.90	0.88		
Caregiving: preschool							
M	4.02	4.61	4.63	4.51	4.25	B,D > A	4.00[b]
SD	0.96	0.80	1.09	1.03	1.00		
Activities: preschool							
M	3.29	4.28	3.50	3.61	3.19	B > A,D,S,P	9.40[c]
SD	1.10	0.82	1.22	0.99	0.95		
Harshness							
M	16.17	14.44	14.66	14.83	14.05	B,D,S,P < A	9.15[c]
SD	4.29	4.26	4.80	3.89	4.14		
Sensitivity							
M	23.20	27.90	31.90	28.47	29.94	B,D,P,S > A	69.51[c]
SD	5.20	5.09	8.28	5.36	6.88	D > A,B,P,S, S > B	
Detachment							
M	6.64	6.83	5.75	5.69	6.41	D,P < A,B	9.74[c]
SD	2.79	2.73	2.88	1.97	2.81		
Early childhood training							
M	1.04	2.23	1.30	1.15	1.57	B > A,D,P,S	28.93[c]
SD	1.20	1.62	1.42	1.23	1.55	S > A,P	

[a]All means are least squares means, with the exception of turnover rates, which were run as an ANOVA. A = Atlanta, B = Boston, D = Detroit, P = Phoenix, S = Seattle.
[b]$p < .01$.
[c]$p < .001$.

The Atlanta centers were second only to Phoenix in the average turnover rate, but this mean was not significantly different from those in the other sites.

Classroom quality, assessed with the appropriate caregiving and developmentally appropriate activity scales, differed significantly by site. In the infant and toddler rooms, caregiving was of significantly lower quality in Atlanta than in Boston, Detroit, or Phoenix. The centers in Seattle also offered significantly poorer caregiving to infants and toddlers than did centers in Detroit. For preschoolers, the quality of caregiving was significantly higher in Boston and Detroit than in Atlanta. With respect to the activities subscale, infant and toddler classrooms in Boston and Detroit offered significantly higher quality care than did classrooms in Atlanta or Seattle. Preschool classrooms in Boston offered significantly more appropriate activities than did those in all other sites.

Variation in the staff-level quality variables did not map as closely onto the varying stringency of state regulations as did the other quality variables. Teachers in Atlanta were observed to be significantly more harsh with the children in their care than were the teachers in all other sites. However, teachers in both Atlanta and Boston were observed to be more detached than were teachers in Detroit and Phoenix. The teachers' sensitivity towards the children also varied significantly by site, such that teachers in Atlanta were significantly less sensitive than those in all other sites, and teachers in Detroit were significantly more sensitive than those in all other sites. In addition, teachers in Boston were significantly less sensitive than those in Seattle. With respect to the early childhood training of the teachers, those in Boston had significantly more training, on average, than did the teachers in all sites. Teachers in Seattle had significantly more training than those in Atlanta or Phoenix.

Effects of Compliance with the FIDCR

Table 4 presents the means and percentage of centers in each site that complied with none, some, and all of the FIDCR regulations governing ratios, group size, and staff training. A one-way ANOVA, with site as the independent variable, run on the average compliance score revealed that Boston centers were significantly more fully in compliance with the FIDCR than were the centers in Phoenix or Atlanta, $F(4, 222) = 14.05, p < .0001$. The centers in both Detroit and Seattle were also more fully in compliance than were the Atlanta centers.

Table 5, which presents the means and standard deviations for each of the compliance groups, reveals significant differences in the quality of care based on the center's degree of compliance with the FIDCR: $ps < .001$ for all MANOVAs: $F(6, 438) = 12.49$ for the infant/toddler ITERS factors, $F(6, 560) = 4.81$ for the preschool ECERS factors, $F(12, 3244) = 11.52$ for the four staff-level variables.

Table 4. Compliance of Center by Study Site

Site	No. of provisions met[a]			
	None	1	2	3
Atlanta	21.7	67.4	10.9	0
Boston	0	36.4	20.5	43.2
Detroit	6.7	35.6	35.6	22.2
Phoenix	20.0	44.4	31.1	4.4
Seattle	8.5	40.4	27.7	23.4

[a]Numbers in the table are percentages of centers.

Table 5. Turnover, Classroom Quality, Staff–Child Interaction, and Staff Qualifications by FIDCR Compliance[a]

Quality indicator	No. of FIDCR provisions met				Comparisons	F
	None	1	2	3		
Turnover (%)						
M	65	42	45	29	0>3	4.31[b]
SD	0.53	0.47	0.33	0.21		
Caregiving: infants and toddlers						
M	3.04	4.25	4.05	5.51	1,2,3>0	21.28[c]
SD	0.95	1.15	1.18	0.97	3>1,2	
Activities: infants and toddlers						
M	2.45	3.62	3.37	4.12	1,2,3>0	18.72[c]
SD	0.56	0.98	1.07	0.70	3>2	
Caregiving: preschool						
M	3.73	4.40	4.38	4.73	1,2,3>0	7.26[c]
SD	0.88	1.05	1.00	0.87	3>2	
Activities: preschool						
M	2.76	3.67	3.49	3.85	1,2,3>0	7.90[c]
SD	0.76	1.19	1.11	0.93		
Harshness						
M	15.91	14.63	15.29	14.11	1,3<0	6.90[c]
SD	4.78	4.30	4.52	3.63	3<2	
Sensitivity						
M	25.58	27.46	29.42	30.23	1,2,3>0	19.60[c]
SD	6.91	6.87	7.11	6.28	2,3>1	
Detachment						
M	6.40	6.36	6.07	6.22		ns
SD	2.38	2.83	2.67	2.59		
Early childhood training						
M	0.95	1.36	1.49	1.93	1,2,3>0	15.24[c]
SD	1.15	1.39	1.48	1.66	3>1,2	

[a]All means are least squares means, with the exception of turnover rates, which were run as an ANOVA. A = Atlanta, B = Boston, D = Detroit, P = Phoenix, S = Seattle.
[b]$p < .01$.
[c]$p < .001$.

Staff turnover rates were significantly higher in centers that met none of the FIDCR provisions than in those that met all of the provisions. The quality of caregiving and the appropriateness of the activities offered to the children also differed significantly for centers that showed varying degrees of compliance with the FIDCR. In the infant and toddler rooms, caregiving was of significantly lower quality in the centers that met none of the FIDCR provisions than in the centers that met some or all of the provisions. And, caregiving in the centers that met some (either one or two) of the provisions was of significantly lower quality than in the centers that met all of the provisions. For preschoolers, the quality of caregiving was significantly poorer in centers that met none of the provisions compared to centers that met some or all of the provisions, and in centers that met two of the provisions compared to those that met all three. With respect to the activities subscale, infant and toddler classrooms in centers that met none of the provisions were of significantly poorer quality than were classrooms in centers that met some or all of the provisions, and those that met two of the provisions were of poorer quality than those that met all three. Preschool classrooms in centers that met none of the provisions offered significantly less appropriate activities than did those that met some or all of the provisions.

Variation in the staff-level quality variables was also significantly associated with FIDCR compliance, but the univariate analyses showed effects only for staff harshness, sensitivity, and early childhood training. Teachers in centers that met none of the FIDCR provisions were observed to be significantly more harsh with the children in their care than were the teachers in centers that met one or all three, but not two, of the provisions. In addition, teachers in centers that met two of the provisions were significantly more harsh than were teachers in centers that met all three of the provisions. With respect to sensitivity, teachers in centers that met none of the FIDCR provisions were significantly less sensitive than teachers in centers that met some or all of the provisions, and teachers in centers that met only one of the provisions were significantly less sensitive than teachers in centers that met two or all three of the provisions. Teachers in centers that met none of the provisions also had significantly less early childhood training than teachers in all other centers and those in centers that met all of the provisions had significantly more early childhood training than did teachers in all other centers.

Given these differences in quality based on FIDCR compliance, it is of interest to know which of the FIDCR provisions—ratios, group size, or training—were most often violated by the noncomplying centers. Of the 227 centers, 185 were not in full compliance with these three FIDCR provisions. Of these 185 centers, only 20% failed to meet the training requirement.

However, 82.7% failed to meet the ratio requirements and 79.3% failed to meet the group size requirements.

Effects of Auspice

The auspice of the centers also significantly distinguished centers that provided varying quality of care. The MANOVAs for the structural quality measures were $F(6, 150) = 2.31, p < .05$ for infants; $F(6, 272) = 4.54, p < .001$ for toddlers, $F(6, 532) = 8.87, p < .001$ for preschoolers. The MANOVAs for the remaining quality measures were: $F(6, 438) = 10.79$ for the infant/toddler ITERS factors, $F(6, 560) = 15.99$ for the preschool ECERS factors, $F(12, 3244) = 10.64$ for the four staff-level variables, all $ps < .001$. Table 6 presents the means and standard deviations for the ratio and group size measures. Table 7 presents these data for all other quality variables.

Table 6. Observed Ratios and Group Sizes by Age Group of Classroom and Auspice[a]

Quality indicator	For-profit		Nonprofit		Comparisons	F
	Independent	Chain	Nonsectarian	Sectarian		
Ratios						
Infant						
M	4.31	4.60	3.25	3.83	N < C	2.73[b]
SD	1.93	0.59	1.41	1.25		
Toddler						
M	6.52	6.95	4.74	5.08	N < C,I	6.95[c]
SD	2.57	2.62	2.11	2.14		
Preschool						
M	9.58	11.45	6.76	7.38	N < C,I	14.95[c]
SD	4.95	3.35	2.76	2.47	S < I	
Group Size						
Infant						
M	6.94	8.13	7.26	5.44		ns
SD	3.74	3.44	2.85	2.30		
Toddler						
M	9.71	8.95	9.96	9.29		ns
SD	4.45	3.25	3.82	3.05		
Preschool						
M	14.51	16.65	14.43	12.24	C > S	3.43[b]
SD	5.76	4.13	5.67	4.23		

[a]All means are least squares means. I = independent, C = chain, N = nonsectarian, and S = sectarian.
[b]$p < .05$.
[c]$p < .001$.

Table 7. Turnover, Classroom Quality, Staff–Child Interaction, and Staff Qualifications by Auspice[a]

Quality indicator	For-profit		Nonprofit		Comparisons	F
	Independent	Chain	Nonsectarian	Sectarian		
Turnover (%)						
M	51	74	30	36	N,S < C	8.01[b]
SD	0.54	0.47	0.23	0.23	N < I	
Caregiving: infants and toddlers						
M	3.72	3.79	4.74	3.98	N > I,C	11.70[b]
SD	1.29	0.91	1.18	0.91		
Activities: infants and toddlers						
M	2.97	3.38	4.06	3.14	N > I,C	21.24[b]
SD	0.88	0.76	0.97	1.02	N > S	
Caregiving: preschool						
M	4.05	4.30	4.73	4.57	N,S > I	9.41[b]
SD	1.01	0.82	0.99	0.90		
Activities: preschool						
M	3.05	3.56	4.24	3.38	N,C > I	26.97[b]
SD	0.92	0.82	1.10	0.97	N > S	
Harshness						
M	15.40	15.18	14.35	14.54	N < I	5.26[b]
SD	4.70	4.01	4.03	4.10		
Sensitivity						
M	27.36	27.76	28.99	28.99	N > I	5.24[b]
SD	7.25	6.21	6.65	7.24		
Detachment						
M	6.22	5.95	6.43	6.15		ns
SD	2.60	2.49	2.77	2.87		
Early childhood training						
M	1.18	1.16	1.94	1.15	N > I,C,S	28.04[b]
SD	1.33	1.17	1.57	1.39		

[a] All means are least squares means, with the exception of turnover rates, which were run as an ANOVA. I = independent, C = chain, N = nonsectarian, and S = sectarian.
[b] $p < .001$.

The for-profit chains were observed to have significantly higher (poorer) ratios than were the nonsectarian nonprofit centers for all age groups. The independent for-profit centers also had significantly higher ratios for toddlers and preschoolers than did the nonsectarian nonprofit centers. For preschoolers only, the independent for-profit centers also differed significantly from the sectarian nonprofit centers.

Group size failed to differentiate centers based on their auspice, with one exception. The for-profit chains were observed to have significantly larger preschool groups than were the sectarian nonprofit centers.

Staff turnover was significantly higher in the for-profit chains than in either the religious or nonreligious nonprofit centers, and in the independent for-profit centers than in the nonreligious nonprofit centers.

The quality of caregiving and the appropriateness of the activities offered to the children also differed significantly for centers of differing auspices. In the infant and toddler rooms, the quality of the caregiving and of the activities was significantly lower in the independent for-profit centers and the chains than in the nonsectarian nonprofit centers. In addition, the quality of the activities for infants and toddlers was significantly lower in the sectarian centers than in the other nonprofit centers. For preschoolers, the quality of caregiving was significantly poorer in the independent for-profit centers than in either group of nonprofit centers. The quality of the activities in the preschool rooms was significantly poorer in the independent for-profits than in either the chains or the nonsectarian nonprofit centers and in the sectarian than the nonsectarian nonprofit centers.

Variation in the staff-level quality variables was also significantly associated with auspice, but the univariate analyses showed effects only for staff harshness, sensitivity, and early childhood training. Teachers in the independent for-profit centers were significantly more harsh and less sensitive than teachers in nonsectarian nonprofit centers. Teachers in both types of for-profit centers had significantly less early childhood training than those in nonsectarian nonprofit centers and teachers in the religious centers had significantly less training than those in nonsectarian nonprofit centers.

Our final analysis examined differences in degree of compliance with the FIDCR based on center auspice. Table 8 presents the percentages of centers of each auspice in full, partial, or no compliance with the FIDCR. The chi-square, $\chi^2(3) = 8.48$, $p < .001$, revealed that nonprofit centers were significantly more likely to be in full compliance and significantly less likely to be totally out of compliance with the FIDCR than were for-profit centers.

Table 8. Associations between Center Auspice and Degree of Compliance with the FIDCR

Auspice	No. of provisions met[a]			
	None	1	2	3
Independent, for-profit	19.1	46.1	25.8	9.0
Chain, for-profit	16.7	50.0	33.3	0
Nonsectarian, nonprofit	2.4	47.0	20.5	30.1
Sectarian, nonprofit	10.8	35.1	29.7	24.3

[a]Numbers in the table are percentages of centres.

DISCUSSION

Ecological models of research have directed attention to the potential impact of public and private policies on the quality of children's environments. Growing interest in this level of analysis has not, however, been matched by empirical efforts to document policy effects. In this context, the most important contribution of the research reported here lies in the consistency with which it documents associations between child care policy—both regulatory and financial-legal dimensions of policy—and the quality of the child care environments that children experience on a daily basis. Quality of care varied systematically and significantly with the state in which the centers resided, the centers' degree of compliance with the most recent set of proposed federal child care standards, and the financial–legal auspices under which the centers operated.

Regulatory Effects

Centers that resided in states with more stringent child care regulations tended to offer higher quality care than did centers that resided in states with relatively lax regulations. This pattern was most characteristic of those dimensions of quality—ratios and staff training—that are regulated by the states, although differences in the sites' average staff turnover rates also mapped closely onto the relative ranking of the regulations. However, the quality of caregiving, appropriateness of the activities, and the specific teacher behaviors that were observed, while significantly associated with site, corresponded less closely to the stringency of the states' regulations. These dimensions of quality are not directly regulated and are likely affected by aspects of care that are quite far removed from the purview of licensing, such as the qualifications of the center director, the amount of supervision that occurs, and the adult work environment.

This pattern of results linking state regulatory stringency to quality of care has direct implications for efforts to upgrade state child care regulations. The data suggest that such efforts will likely produce more developmentally beneficial child care environments for young children.

Compliance with the FIDCR also distinguished lower and higher quality centers on dimensions other than the ratio, group size, and training provisions by which we determined compliance. Centers in full compliance, as compared to partial or noncompliance, with the FIDCR had significantly lower staff turnover rates, higher quality of caregiving and of classroom activities, less harsh and more sensitive teachers, and more teachers with specialized training. The significant differences that emerged for centers in partial and full compliance suggest that the full complement of ratio, group size, and training provisions must be met to assure high quality care. Given that for the centers not in full compliance, the ratio and group size requirements were far more likely to be "failed" than were the training requirements, these provisions appear to be particularly important regulatory dimensions of quality.

These conclusions about regulatory effects on quality of care are based on two assumptions that require further examination. First, we have assumed that the differences found for centers in different study sites are associated with variation in the stringency of the state child care regulations that applied to each site. We did not, however, directly assess the influence of state regulations and, as a result, cannot rule out the possibility that other unmeasured factors that distinguished our sites (e.g., unemployment rates, training opportunities for child care providers) may explain the site effects. The teasing apart of state-level effects, particularly those associated with regulation, on the quality of child care is an important direction for future research.

Second, we have assumed that quality variation based on compliance with the FIDCR can provide data about the possible effects of national child care standards. However, the FIDCR have not been implemented and, as a consequence, we cannot generalize from the effects of voluntary compliance to the context of mandatory federal regulation. It has been postulated, for example, that one effect of mandatory federal regulations would be to drive poorer quality centers out of the market thus creating a supply shortage (Lehrman & Pace, 1985; Orton & Langham, 1980). Research that examines the positive and negative consequences of mandatory regulation is sorely needed. Although it is a challenge to ponder the design of such a study, pre- and posttest studies of states that toughen their child care regulations could provide a reasonable assessment of how the imposition of federal standards would affect both the supply and quality of local child care markets.

Similarly, in some states, centers that receive government funds are required to comply with more stringent standards than are nonsubsidized centers. These two classes of centers offer an obvious comparison with which to examine the effects of imposing presumably more stringent federal standards. There is some evidence to suggest, for example, that federally subsidized centers that were required to comply with federal standards in the late 1970s had better staff:child ratios and offered a broader range of supplementary services than did nonsubsidized centers that were exempt from the federal standards (Grotberg, 1980).

In addition to pointing to directions for future research, the findings reported here have important implications for our interpretations of previous research on the quality of child care. The child development literature on child care quality has been restricted to single-site studies that fail to consider the influence of the local regulatory, market, and political context within which child care operates. If the developmental effects of care are examined in a site characterized by relatively low-quality care (e.g., Atlanta), it is likely that detrimental effects will be documented, whereas the opposite portrait of child care effects would likely emerge in a high-quality site. A systematic review of the existing literature with this framework in mind would be extremely useful.

Auspice Effects

The finding that quality of care was generally poorer in for-profit than in nonprofit centers corroborates prior evidence that for-profit centers, on average, offer children less optimal care than do nonprofit centers (Coelen *et al.*, 1979; Kagan & Newton, 1989; Keyserling, 1972). What these findings add to this literature is evidence that there is variation within these two auspices and also across different measures of quality and for quality outcomes for different ages of children. The quality of care in for-profit chains sometimes differed significantly from what we observed to typify independent for-profit centers and, in general, church-affiliated nonprofit centers were of lower quality than nonsectarian nonprofit centers. With respect to age, although chains did not differ from the nonprofit centers in the quality of the activities they offered preschoolers, they did offer significantly less appropriate activities and lower quality caregiving to infants and toddlers.

These findings raise the important question of *why* auspice influences quality. In general, although there has been ample attention to the various distinctions between profit and nonprofit service delivery, particularly in the area of health and mental health care (Estes & Alford, 1990; Pattison & Katz, 1983; Simons, 1989), the relation between auspice and quality is not well understood. Assumptions about contract failure offer one framework for understanding the sources of auspice-related differences in quality, however the data we report do not provide a complete assessment of this theory.

Another influential distinction between nonprofit and for-profit child care concerns the distribution of center resources to aspects of care that are or are not associated with quality of care. For example, several studies have linked staff salaries to turnover (Hyson, 1982; Jorde-Bloom, 1988; Kontos & Stremmel, 1987; Whitebook, Howes, Friedman, & Darrah, 1982; Whitebook *et al.*, 1990) and to the observed quality of caregiving (Whitebook *et al.*, 1990). The for-profit centers that were examined in this study spent a smaller proportion of their income on staff salaries and, in fact, paid their staff significantly poorer salaries that did the nonprofit centers (Whitebook *et al.*, 1990). Other explanations are also plausible, including possible auspice-based differences in access to in-kind resources and subsidies (see Culkin, Morris, & Helburn, 1991), in the employment preferences of trained child care teachers, in governance and decision-making, and in philosophies of care.

These findings must also be placed in the broader policy context of the increasing privatization of child care, and other services, in the United States (Kahn & Kamerman, 1987; Simons, 1989). Privatization refers to the shift of power and investment from the government to the private sector, and the realignment of federal involvement from supply-side to demand-side support (Kagan, 1991). In the last decade, nonprofit services, including child care services, have absorbed large losses of government support. At the same time, for-profit services have proliferated in a wide range of health and service sectors, including child care (Kahn & Kamerman, 1987; Simons, 1989).

This trend has fueled tensions between for-profit and nonprofit providers of child care, with claims of greater cost-effectiveness and responsiveness to parent needs on the part of for-profit providers and claims of higher quality and greater equity of access to care for low-income families on the part of nonprofit providers. Of immediate concern is the combined impact of the growing share of center-based care that is provided by for-profit entities and the growing documentation in support of the nonprofits' claims that for-profit programs provide lower quality care. The implications for children are potentially quite negative. Moreover, the for-profit sector has traditionally opposed state and federal efforts to upgrade child care regulation, thereby adding to the potential negative effect of privatization on the quality of child care.

Policy Implications

This research reveals the significant association between regulation, nonprofit status, and quality of care, thereby implying an association between regulation, auspice, and positive outcomes for children in child care (see Phillips, Ricciuti, Kiernan, Howes, & Whitebook, unpublished manuscript). The policy implications of this finding are far-reaching, three of which are particularly timely. One set of implications addresses assumptions about parental choice that currently prevail in policy debates about regulation. The second set of implications focuses on the current balance of federal and state responsibility for child care regulation. The third concerns the role of parent education in an increasingly diversified child care market.

Contemporary policy debates about child care quality have been framed around a fundamental tension between enhancing regulation and enhancing parental choice. Efforts to upgrade state regulations or to impose federal regulations are portrayed as restricting parental choice insofar as they may drive some programs out of the market. Our data indicate that, in fact, these efforts to improve regulation would likely improve the quality of children's daily child care settings. Assuming that parents do not seek to place their children in low-quality care, we can conclude that efforts to polarize regulation and parental choice are unfounded.

The federal government has traditionally deferred to the states in the area of child care regulation. Yet, the data reported here concerning the uneven quality of care that is required by state regulations, the link between state regulation and the actual quality of care that children experience, and the suggested association between federal regulation and quality imply that this balance of state–federal responsibility is not optimal for assuring quality child care. We, therefore, propose an expanded federal role in child care regulation.

The accumulated data about center auspice and quality notwithstanding, a blend of profit and nonprofit child care centers is likely to be an enduring feature of the center-based child care delivery system in the United States. This feature, when placed in the context of a weak regulatory system, suggests a significant role for parent education about the key ingredients of quality care and for parental monitoring of their children's care settings. To the extent that for-profit centers are responsive to consumer demand and satisfaction, assuring that parents are educated and assertive consumers may be the only immediately promising avenue for improving the quality of care offered by this large sector of the center market.

In sum, this research illustrates the importance of adopting ecological models, and including measures of macrosystem influence, when examining the quality and effects of child care. Examining multiple levels of analysis, including consideration of policy influences, offers the opportunity to generate more creative directions for future research in child care and to inform important and timely debates about child care policy.

ACKNOWLEDGMENTS

The authors thank the Foundation for Child Development, A. L. Mailman Family Foundation, Ford Foundation, Smith-Richardson Foundation, Spunk Fund, Inc., and the Carnegie Corporation for their generous support of this research. We also acknowledge the enormous contribution of the research teams in each site without whom this study would not have been possible. Michael Kiernan and Ann Ricciuti at the University of Virginia provided expert assistance with analyses. Finally, and most important, we thank the many child care directors and teachers who spent many hours enabling us to collect the data for this study.

REFERENCES

Anderson, C. W., Nagle, R. J., Roberts, W. A., & Smith, J. W. (1981). Attachment to substitute caregivers as a function of center quality and caregiver involvement. *Child Development*, 52, 53–61.

Bronfenbrenner, U. (1979). *The ecology of human development*. Cambridge, MA: Harvard University Press.

Clarke-Stewart, K. A. & Fein, G. (1983). Early childhood programs. In M. Haith & J. Campos (Eds.), *Handbook of child psychology: Vol. II. Infancy and developmental psychobiology* (pp. 917–1000). New York: Wiley.

Coelen, C., Glantz, F., & Calore, D. (1979). *Day care centers in the U.S.: A national profile*, 1976–1977. Cambridge, MA: Abt.

Culkin, M., Morris, J. R., & Helburn, S. W. (1991). Quality and the true cost of child care. *Journal of Social Issues*, 47, 71–86.

Cummings, E. M. (1980). Caregiver stability and day care. *Developmental Psychology*, 16, 31–37.

Estes, C. L. & Alford, R. R. (1990). Systemic crisis and the nonprofit sector: Toward a political economy of the nonprofit and social services sector. *Theory and Society*, 19, 173–198.

Grotberg, E. (1980). The roles of the federal government in regulation and maintenance of quality in child care. In S. Kilmer (Ed.), *Advances in early education and day care* (Vol. 1, pp. 19–45). Greenwich, CT: JAI.

Hansmann, H. B. (1980). The role of nonprofit enterprise. *Yale Law School Journal, 189*, 835–901.

Harms, T. & Clifford, R. M. (1980). *The Early Childhood Environment Rating Scale*. New York: Teachers College Press.

Harms, T., Cryer, D., & Clifford, R. M. (1986). *Infant-Toddler Environment Rating Scale*. Unpublished document, University of North Carolina, Chapel Hill.

Hayes, C., Palmer, J., & Zaslow, M. (1990). *Who cares for America's children? Child Care policy for the 1990s*. Report of the Panel on Child Care Policy, Committee on Child Development Research and Public Policy, National Research Council. Washington, DC: National Academy Press.

Howes, C. (1988). Relations between early child care and schooling. *Developmental Psychology*, 24, 53–57.

Howes, C. Phillips, D., & Whitebook, M. (1992). Thresholds of Quality: Implications for the social development of children in child care. *Child Development*, 63, 449–460.

Howes, C. & Rubenstein, J. (1985). Determinants of toddlers' experiences in daycare: Age of entry and quality of setting. *Child Care Quarterly*, 14, 140–151.

Howes, C. & Stewart, P. (1987). Child's play with adults toys, and peers: An examination of family and child care influences. *Developmental Psychology*, 23, 423–430.

Hyson, M. (1982). *Playing with kids all day: Job stress in early childhood education*. Washington, DC: Acropol.

Jorde-Bloom, P. (1988, April). *Professional orientation and structural components of early childhood programs: A social-ecological perspective*. Paper presented at the annual meetings of the American Educational Research Association, New Orleans.

Kagan, S. L. (1991). Examining profit and nonprofit child care: An odyssey of quality and auspices. *Journal of Social Issues*, 47, 87–104.

Kagan, S. L. & Newton, J. W. (1989). For-profit and nonprofit child care: Similarities and differences. *Young Children*, 45, 4–10.

Kahn, A. J. & Kamerman, S. B. (1987). *Child care: Facing the hard choices*. Dover, MA: Auburn House.

Keyserling, M. D. (1972). *Windows on day care: A report based on findings of the National Council of Jewish Women.* New York: National Council of Jewish Women.

Kontos, S. & Stremmel, A. (1988). Caregivers' perceptions of working conditions in a child care environment. *Early Childhood Research Quarterly, 3,* 77–90.

Lehrman, K. & Pace, J. (1985). Day care regulation: Serving children or bureaucrats? *Policy Analysis, 59.*

Nelson, R. & Krashinsky, M. (1973). Two major issues of public policy: Public subsidy and organization of supply. In D. R. Young & R. Nelson (Eds.), *Public policy for day care of young children.* Lexington, MA: Heath.

Orton, R. D. & Langham, B. (1980). What is government's role in quality day care? In S. Kilmer (Ed.), *Advances in early education and day care* (Vol. 1, pp. 47–62). Greenwich, CT: JAI.

Pattison, R. V. & Katz, H. M. (1983). Investor-owned and not-for-profit hospitals: A comparison based on California data. *New England Journal of Medicine, 309,* 347–353.

Phillips, D. & Howes, C. (1987). Indicators of quality in child care: Review of the research. In D. A. Phillips (Ed.), *Quality in child care: What does research tell us?* (Research Monograph of the National Association for the Education of Young Children, Vol. 1). Washington, DC: National Association for the Education of Young Children.

Phillips, D., Howes, C., & Whitebook, M. (1991). Child care as an adult work environment. *Journal of Social Issues, 47,* 49–70.

Phillips, D., Lande, J., & Goldberg, M. (1990). The state of child care regulation: A comparative analysis. *Early Childhood Research Quarterly, 5,* 151–179.

Phillips, D., McCartney, K., & Scarr, S. (1987). Child care quality and children's social development. *Developmental Psychology, 23,* 537–543.

Phillips, D., Ricciuti, A., Kiernan, M., Howes, C., & Whitebook, M. The effects of regulatory quality and center auspice on children. Unpublished manuscript.

Powell, D. R. (1987). Day care as a family support system. In S. L. Kagan, D. R. Powell, B. Weissbourd, & E. Zigler (Eds.), *America's family support programs: Perspectives and prospects* (pp. 115–132). New Haven, CT: Yale University Press.

Price, R. (1989). Bearing witness. *American Journal of Community Psychology, 17,* 151–167.

Rappaport, J. (1981). In praise of paradox: A social policy of empowerment over prevention. *American Journal of Community Psychology, 9,* 1–26.

Reppucci, N. D. (1985). Psychology in the public interest. In A. M. Rogers & C. J. Scheirer (Eds.), *The G. Stanley Hall Lecture Series* (Vol. 5, pp. 125–156). Washington, DC: American Psychological Association.

Ruopp, R., Travers, J., Glantz, F., & Coelen, C. (1979). *Children at the center: Final results of the National Day Care Study.* Boston: Abt.

Seidman, E. (1987). Toward a framework for primary prevention research. In J. Steinberg and M. Silverman (Eds.), *Preventing mental disorders: A research perspective.* Washington, DC: U.S. Government Printing Office.

Seidman, E. (1988). Back to the future. Community Psychology: Unfolding a theory of social intervention. *American Journal of Community Psychology, 16,* 3–24.

Sibley, A. & Abbott-Shim, M. (1988). *Assessment profile for early childhood programs.* Atlanta, GA: Quality Assist, Inc.

Simons, L. S. (1989). Privatization and the mental health system. *American Psychologist, 44,* 1138–1141.

Vandell, D. & Powers C. (1983). Day care quality and children's free play activities. *American Journal of Orthopsychiatry, 53,* 293–300.

Whitebook, M., Howes, C., Friedman, J., & Darrah, R. (1982). Caring for caregivers: Burnout in child care. In L. Katz (Ed.), *Current topics in early childhood education* (Vol. 4). New York: Ablex.

Whitebook, M., Howes, C., & Phillips, D. (1990). *Who cares? Child care teachers and the quality of care in America* (Final Report of the National Child Care Staffing Study). Oakland, CA: Child Care Employee Project.

Zaslow, M. J. (1991). Variation in child care quality and its implications for children. *Journal of Social Issues, 47*, 125–138.

19

What's Wrong with Empowerment

Stephanie Riger

*Although it has stimulated useful and important research and theory in
community psychology, the concept of empowerment is problematic.
This article criticizes two assumptions and values underlying the concept
of empowerment: (a) individualism, leading potentially to unmitigated
competition and conflict among those who are empowered; and (b) a
preference for traditionally masculine concepts of mastery, power, and
control over traditionally feminine concerns of communion and
cooperation. The challenge to community psychology is to develop a
vision that incorporates both empowerment and community, despite the
paradoxical nature of these two phenomena.*

Community psychologists have long emphasized the importance of context
for understanding human behavior. Leaders in our field have persuasively
argued that human actors play out their roles in particular environments
which offer specific constraints and opportunities and serve as stimuli for
action. Yet, despite our awareness of context for those we study, we do not
always apply that understanding to ourselves. My purpose here is to point
out how our context—that is, the assumptions and values underlying the
discipline of psychology in the United States—shape, sometimes without
our awareness, how we define and study key ideas in our field.

Originally published in the *American Journal of Community Psychology*, 21(3) (1993):
279–292.

A Quarter Century of Community Psychology: *Readings from the* American Journal of
Community Psychology, edited by Tracey A. Revenson *et al.* Kluwer Academic/Plenum
Publishers, New York, 2002.

To demonstrate this, I focus on the concept of empowerment, a concept at the forefront of community psychology research today. I make two points: First, psychology's emphasis on the cognitive processes of the individual leads us to study individuals' *sense of* empowerment rather than actual increases in power, thereby making the political personal. Second, the concept of empowerment, in accord with psychology's traditional emphasis on agency, mastery, and control, emphasizes concerns that have typically been associated with masculinity and men, rather than concerns typically associated with femininity and women such as community and connections with others.

EMPOWERMENT AND POWER

History and culture shape the concepts that we use to explain human action. Perhaps most important of the values shaping psychology is the belief in individualism, a belief that lies at the heart of psychology's vision of human nature. A great deal of research in psychology rests on the assumption that the healthy individual is one who is self-contained, independent and self-reliant, capable of asserting himself and influencing his environment (and I do mean *his*) and operating according to abstract principles of justice and fairness. Yet, as Sampson (1983) pointed out, "the individual that is psychology's research subject is the creation of a given sociohistorical system" rather than an exemplar of a timeless human nature (p. 46). The supposedly autonomous individual of modern psychology is the product of Western social and economic belief systems, just as our concepts of fairness are shaped by capitalist principles of equity and exchange. Recall Fromm's observation: "The underlying structure of capitalism calls for people who believe themselves to be free agents while they are actually governed by [market] forces that press them this way and that, but behind their backs" (cited in Sampson, 1983, p. 137).

Consider how the belief in individualism affects our conception of empowerment. As Rappaport (1987) presented it, empowerment refers to "a mechanism by which people, organizations, and communities gain mastery over their affairs" (p. 122). His notion of empowerment is intended to include both a psychological sense of personal control and concern with actual social influence, political power, and legal rights. As Zimmerman (2000) summarized, "Psychological empowerment includes beliefs about one's competence and efficacy, and a willingness to become involved in activities to exert control in the social and political environment. ... Psychological empowerment is a construct that integrates perceptions of personal control with behaviors to exert control" (pp. 5, 7).

Although these definitions of empowerment include actual control and influence as part of the concept, in a great deal of research actual control is conflated with the *sense of* personal control. For example, in a study of the development of community leaders, Kieffer (1984) described "the fundamental empowering transformation ... from sense of self as helpless victim to acceptance of self as assertive and efficacious citizen," whereas Ozer and Bandura (1990) consider empowerment a manifestation of people's belief in their efficacy. Sampson (1983) has pointed out psychology's tendency to reduce complex phenomena to individual psychological dynamics:

> Effort is expended in developing precise ways to measure and assess individual psychological states and perceptions and to evaluate individual behavioral outcomes. The social context within which these individual perceptions and activities take place is put off to the side, occasionally alluded to, but rarely if ever systematically addressed. (p. 12)

Sampson here was criticizing psychological research on justice, yet his comments apply as well to the predilection in community psychology to assess empowerment through individuals' perceptions.

This proclivity stems from a deeper unresolved tension within psychology between two views of human nature, one which holds that "reality creates the person" (as reflected, e.g., in behaviorism) and the opposing view that "the person creates reality" (as reflected, e.g., in cognition) (see Buss, 1978; Sampson, 1983). Many agree that the cognitivist perspective currently dominates American psychology (Baars, 1986; Gardner, 1985; Segal & Lachman, 1972; cf. Friman, Allen, Kerwin, & Larzelere, 1993). Central to this viewpoint is the belief that structures and processes within the individual's mind are the primary determinants of behavior: "For cognitivism, it is more important to understand what is going on within the person's head as she or he confronts an objective stimulus situation than it is to understand the properties of the situation itself" (Sampson, 1983, p. 87).

The consequence of the cognitivist perspective is to ignore or downplay the influence of situational or social structural factors in favor of a focus on individual perceptions. But this view artificially disconnects human behavior from the larger sociopolitical context, resulting in a search within the self for solutions to human problems (Caplan & Nelson, 1973; Prilleltesky, 1989). In the context of empowerment, if the focus of inquiry becomes not actual power but rather the *sense of* empowerment, then the political is made personal and, ironically, the status quo may be supported.

Placing primacy on the phenomenology of the individual ignores the possibility of what Marxists deem "false consciousness." The individual's experience of power or powerlessness may be unrelated to actual ability to influence, and an increase in the sense of empowerment does not always reflect an increase in actual power. Indeed, a sense of empowerment may be an illusion when so much of life is controlled by the politics and practices at a macro level. This does not mean that individuals can have no influence or that individuals' perceptions are unimportant, but rather that to reduce power to individual psychology ignores the political and historical context in which people operate. Confusing one's actual *ability* to control resources with a *sense of* empowerment depoliticizes the latter.

Theoreticians of power distinguish *power over* ("explicit or implicit dominance") from *power to* ("the opportunity to act more freely within some realms ... through power sharing") and *power from* ("the ability to resist the power of others by effectively fending off their unwanted demands") (Hollander & Offermann, 1990, p. 179). The concept of empowerment is sometimes used in a way that confounds a sense of efficacy or esteem (part of "power to") with that of actual decision-making control over resources ("power over"). Many intervention efforts aimed at empowerment increase people's power to act, for example, by enhancing their self-esteem, but do little to affect their power over resources or policies. For example, a program designed to enhance the academic success of African American college students is described as "Empowerment of African American college students." Students in the program earn higher grade point averages than comparable students not in the program, a considerable achievement (Maton, 1993). Yet this program does not address control over decision making. Although self-esteem or achievement may be related to power and control, these concepts are not the same. To consider them the same is to depoliticize the concept of empowerment.

The question arises, then, whether attempts to enhance a sense of empowerment create the illusion of power without affecting the actual distribution of power. Many interventions attempt to achieve empowerment through increasing individuals' participation in neighborhood or self-help groups. Empowerment is sometimes equated with participation, as if changing procedures will automatically lead to changes in the context or in the distribution of resources. Lewis (1994) criticized this claim in his discussion of reforms in urban education. Some changes, such as the institution of local school councils, appear to be empowering in that they give local groups more control over schools. But viewed from a larger perspective, these changes in procedure do little to affect the distribution of resources in school systems. People who participate in community organizations often feel more empowered than nonparticipants (e.g., Zimmerman, Israel, Schulz, & Checkoway, 1992), but participation does not necessarily result in more influence or control. Chavis and Wandersman (1990) found that although people developed a greater *sense of* control through participation in a neighborhood organization, they did not perceive the group as becoming more powerful over time.

Neighborhood groups are embedded in larger forces and institutions that are nonlocal and often not susceptible to local influence (Hunter & Riger, 1986). For example, Brenner (1973) has tracked the relationship between macrolevel economic fluctuations and their microlevel impact on rates of mental hospital incarcerations. Realtors, developers, banks, mortgage institutions, and other market forces, as well as local, state, and federal governments and their agencies, often affect neighborhood dynamics in ways that are difficult if not impossible for local grass-roots groups to influence. Community organizing efforts have a long history in the United States, from those of Jane Addams to Saul Alinsky and contemporary attempts to change neighborhoods through group efforts. Molotch (1973) concluded, in a review of these efforts, that the local internal sources of change have generally been relatively unsuccessful in the light of larger, external forces of change. If interventions aimed to empower do not address these larger sociopolitical forces, they may be doomed to transitory or ineffective actions. On the other hand, attempts to address these issues may bring involvement in partisan politics which may put other constraints on psychologists' effectiveness.

A paper by Serrano-García (1984) gave a poignant description of the inextricable relationship of empowerment and politics. Her group, affiliated with the university and the community mental health center, attempted an intervention in a poor Puerto Rican community. The intervention failed to reach many of its goals in part because it did not address the central issue in Puerto Rico, its political status. Members of the intervention team held a proindependence view on this issue, yet they did not reveal their political preferences to the community. Serrano-García asked:

> 1) If we maintain our partisan anonymity will the community feel betrayed? 2) If a particular group of residents chooses to work with us, and their political partisanship is well known, should we refuse, or should we accept? Does our supposed neutrality hinder our consciousness-raising efforts by forcing us to remain outside of partisan political issues? (p. 195)

These difficult questions bring to the fore the relationship between community psychology's concept of empowerment and the larger political arena within which empowerment efforts operate.

Any serious attempt to gain power (that is, power over) by those who are disempowered will prompt those who see themselves as losing power to fight back. Increasing control over resources may be permitted only until it becomes threatening to the dominant group. In reflecting on her intervention efforts, Serrano-García concluded:

> I am convinced that our project achieved the goals it did because its goals
> and strategies were and are unknown to people in power, because we are
> working with low-status people who are not recognized as a threat, and
> because we did not choose to deal with problems which directly confront
> governmental institutions. (p. 198)

Gruber and Trickett (1987) raised this issue in the context of organizational change efforts when they asked "Can we empower others?" Empowerment requires a redistribution in power, but the institutional structure that puts one group in a position to empower others also works to subvert the process of empowerment. In their study of a school's attempt to share decision making, they found that the sense of empowerment increased among students and parents, and students had greater opportunities to affect the curriculum (that is, power to), but few changes occurred in the distribution of power over, that is, in the structural distribution of power in the school. The broader context of the empowerment effort, in which control rested with teachers, undermined attempts to equalize power.

Underlying empowerment ideology is a conflict model that assumes that a society consists of separate groups possessing different levels of power and control over resources (Gutierrez, 1990). "Empowerment is by definition concerned with many who are excluded by the majority society on the basis of their demographic characteristics or of their physical or emotional difficulties, experienced either in the past or the present" (Rappaport, 1990). The outsiders compete with the insiders—and with each other—for control of resources. Livert (n.d.) raised the problem that empowerment of all underrepresented or needy groups merely increases the competition for the same resources. Empowered individuals' rational pursuit of their own best interests may end in the destruction of neighborhoods and networks of support. His solution is to balance empowerment with a commitment to the community, thereby strengthening both individuals and the community as a whole. Bond and Keys (1993) presented a hopeful example of collaboration between two potentially conflicting groups on the board of a community agency: parents and community members. Critical to their collaboration was a culture that appreciated interdependencies and the existence of people and structures that spanned the groups' boundaries.

Empowerment of all disenfranchised groups could be dangerous. I think it is instructive that empowerment is favored not only by those who would describe themselves as politically progressive but also by those who would describe themselves as conservative such as the Republican politician Jack Kemp, former Secretary of Housing and Urban Development, whose political group is called Empower America. There are some groups of outsiders that one hopes would become less empowered, rather than more powerful. For example, neo-Nazi's might be considered outsiders, marginal to mainstream society, yet few community psychologists would advocate their empowerment.

EMPOWERMENT AND COMMUNITY

The underlying assumption of empowerment theory is that of conflict rather than cooperation among groups and individuals, control rather than communion. The image of the empowered person (or group) in research and theory reflects the belief in psychology in separation, individuation, and individual mastery (for criticisms, see Sarason, 1981). Gilligan (1982) contrasted this view of human nature with an alternate vision that emphasized relatedness and interdependence as central values of human experience. Although I disagree with Gilligan's assertion that these two modes are distributed along gender lines, I concur with her claim that psychology takes as its highest value the emphasis on autonomy and separation over relationality. The mature adult in psychological research is characterized by mastery, control, and separation, rather than interdependence or relatedness. Community psychology's emphasis on empowerment follows the pattern of placing primacy on agency, mastery, and control over connectedness.

Since Freud asserted that a mentally healthy individual was one who could work and love, psychologists have contrasted agency with communion. Bakan (1966) was one of the first contemporary psychologists to make this distinction (see also Carlson, 1971; Guttmann, 1970). In his book *The Duality of Human Existence*, Bakan defined agency as an individual acting in self-protection, self-assertion, and self-expansion while communion refers to an individual's sense of being part of a larger whole, at one with others: "Agency manifests itself in the urge to master; communion in contractual cooperation" (p. 15). He further hypothesized that agency and communion are linked to gender. In his view, men's achievement strivings are directed at agentic concerns of self-assertion, attainment of status, and mastery over the environment. In contrast, women strive to achieve communion and are motivated to work cooperatively to attain a sense of harmony with others. However, Bakan did not define the concepts of agency and communion as bipolar opposites, but as separate, independent dimensions capable of coexisting within one person.

Although Bakan's formulation of agency and communion is quite broad, the sociologist Parson's (1951; Parsons & Shils, 1952; see also Bales, 1970; Johnson, 1988) earlier distinction between instrumental and expressive activity is more specific, and thus potentially more useful. In Parson's formulation, instrumental actions are attempts to control the environment whereas expressive actions are directed toward interpersonal relationships. Parsons did not use these terms as personality descriptors. Rather, the concepts of instrumentality and expressiveness refer to the way individuals interact in social systems. Instrumental activity focuses on achievement and accomplishment outside the immediate social group. In contrast, expressive activity is directed at the interpersonal interactions that exist within the group. Hence, expressive actions manifest the principles of Bakan's concept of communion, while instrumental actions manifest those of agency. Similar to Bakan, Parsons did not view instrumental and expressive behaviors as two ends of the same continuum. Rather, he stressed the need for both expressive and instrumental roles in both individuals and in social groups.

Considerable research in psychology has adhered to the distinction between these two realms of behavior, namely, the agentic/instrumental, "doing" realm and the communal/expressive, "feeling" realm. With the advent of feminist theorizing and the growing area of research focusing on the psychology of women, it has become obvious that this simple dichotomy is inadequate. Feminists have pointed out that the two domains are not equally valued in our society. Instrumental behavior is highly valued and defines what is conventionally considered to be success. Expressiveness, associated with dependency, has traditionally had a negative connotation when used to characterize individuals. Miller (1976), in her book *Toward a New Psychology of Women*, pointed out that women are punished for making relationships and connections central in their lives, although, as Gilligan (1982) emphasized, relatedness is critical to understanding women's moral actions. Yet this emphasis on women's relationality echoes the traditional concept of "separate spheres" in which woman is defined by her ties with others (Kerber, 1986), ignoring the variability that exists among women (and men). Linking some behaviors to women and others to men obscures the fact that behavior itself has no gender and can be manifested by either sex.

The concept guiding much of community psychology's work today, that of empowerment, follows the stream of research and theory which emphasizes agency, mastery, and control. Like that previous research, it tends to deny or overlook the role of connectedness in human life. I find this particularly ironic since an early and influential *phenomenon of interest* (in Rappaport's, 1987, phrase) in community psychology was the "sense of community" (Sarason, 1974), a concept that has been overshadowed recently by the emphasis on empowerment. My point is not that the study of community and connectedness should now supersede the study of empowerment, but rather that both are integral to human well-being and happiness and to well-functioning communities, and that both ought to be the objects of our study. However, little work has been done to integrate these two ideas.

Research on rape victims demonstrates the importance of both concepts to understanding human behavior. Contrast two victims: the first, Migael Scherer (1992), a white middle-class woman raped and nearly strangled one morning in a laundromat by a stranger. Scherer's experience, documented in her book, *Still Loved by the Sun: A Rape Survivor's Journal*, included encounters with sensitive police, doctors, and judges who believed her completely, skillful rape victim advocates and therapists, supportive family and friends, and so forth. She made full use of rape counseling advocates and other social services and she did not hesitate to prosecute the rapist (who was then convicted). Scherer eloquently described the feelings of smallness and vulnerability, the inability to plan more than one day at a time, and the confusion, sleeplessness, and agitation that persist long after a rape. Scherer's account is a moving description of the process by which one woman came to feel empowered and efficacious again.

Contrast her experience with that of Altavese Thomas, a poor black mother of three, gang-raped while drinking with some women friends in a poor, high-crime neighborhood. Thomas was portrayed by Michelle Fine (1992) in her critique of the view prevalent in social psychological research that "Taking-Control-Yields-Coping" (p. 62). Thomas refused to use the criminal justice system or to rely on kin. Fine argued that:

> trusting social institutions, maximizing interpersonal supports, and engaging in self-disclosure are strategies most appropriate for middle-class and affluent individuals whose interests are served by those institutions, whose social supports can multiply available resources and contacts, and for whom self-disclosure may in fact lead not only to personal change but also to structural change. (p. 69)

Scherer was in such a position: Her life circumstances permitted control and empowerment to be her primary goals in reestablishing her sense of trust in the world after the rape. She regained a sense of control in part through prosecution of the rapist, a strategy that might be considered to reflect empowerment or agency.

Thomas refused to prosecute the rapists. Her choice stemmed, however, not from a low "sense of empowerment" but because relatedness and connections took priority for her given the likelihood of retaliation if she prosecuted. The circumstances of her life did not permit the actions usually considered essential for self-efficacy. Her behavior can best be understood in light of a need to protect her family. Such a need was not necessary in Scherer's case, since that protection existed already. Considering empowerment and control as the optimal goal for a rape victim denies the reality of Thomas's circumstances. Likewise, empowerment and control may not be the appropriate goal in all community situations.

According to Hare-Mustin and Maracek (1986), autonomy and relatedness are a function not of one's gender but rather of one's position in a social hierarchy. The highly valued attributes that our society defines as agentic are those associated with power and status because autonomy and mastery require the freedom to make choices. Those not in a position of autonomy and choice must focus on connection and communal goals to survive. Accordingly, whether individuals act in an autonomous manner or operate in a communal mode reflects their relative position in the social structure. The implication is that once those lower on the hierarchy have moved up, they may move from a relatedness mode to operate on principles of autonomy and individual agency.

The focus for community psychologists ought to be on understanding how community shapes the person, in particular, on the conditions that facilitate both efficacy or personal control and also a sense of community. Paradoxically, situations which foster community may be the opposite of those which foster empowerment. Community may exist most cohesively when people experience a shared externally generated fate such as a crisis or disaster, or a condition of poverty or oppression (Panzetta, 1973). Alienation and a sense of separateness may result from the absence of crisis or stress, or from access to sufficient resources to cope by oneself. The psychological sense of community that is advocated as a goal by Sarason (1974) and others may be a function of interdependence on a material level. Ironically, when interdependence is no longer necessary, then the psychological sense of community may disappear as well.

Stack's (1974) book, *All Our Kin*, gives a moving example of this dilemma. The poor people whom she interviewed participated in daily domestic exchanges of services, goods, and money that enabled them to survive fluctuations in welfare and the exigencies of living. At the same time, the rules both of the welfare system and of the exchange network prohibited them from acquiring any surplus that might enable them to improve their economic condition or life situation. A woman in the exchange network received an unexpected inheritance of $1,500 with which she and her husband hoped to make a down payment on a home. Within a month and a half, however, the money was gone, distributed to kin for compelling reasons such as a train ticket to visit a sick relative, payment for a burial, and new winter clothing for the children. Another couple had withdrawn from the network to preserve their resources when they had acquired steady jobs, and they had bought a house and furniture. Some years later, when their marriage was dissolving, the woman began giving some of her nice clothes and furniture away to her sisters and niece. She was reestablishing her place in the exchange network by obligating others to her, creating insurance against future need. The sense of community among these people was very great: They had a strong network which could be relied upon in time of trouble. It is important to note, however, that the network which enabled them to survive also put constraints on their survival. Finding one's voice, controlling one's resources, becoming empowered may reduce the interdependence that produces a strong sense of community.

There may, however, be circumstances in which the two phenomena are not contradictory. Chavis and Wandersman (1990) suggest that sense of community is related to participation in a neighborhood association, similar to Maton and Rappaport's (1984) finding that development of a psychological sense of community and commitment were related to empowerment for members of a religious organization. Leavitt and Saegert's (1990) research on leaders in cooperative housing projects in Harlem found that shared control was the basis for empowerment. They concluded:

> Cooperatively organized endeavors of different kinds should be explored more thoroughly as means of empowering as well as serving low-income people. The real level of control a person can have over life in this society correlates highly with disposable income. The development of a co-op sector could be an alternative to the prospect that large numbers of people will be able to exert less and less control over the services and work on which they depend. (p. 231)

There is a danger, however, that community or empowerment can be substituted as a goal when what people actually need is better jobs and more income.

Zimmerman (2000) refers to organizations such as those studied by Leavitt and Saegert as "empowered organizations (i.e., those that influence the policy process and remain viable over time)" as distinct from "empowering organizations (i.e., those that contribute to the development of psychological empowerment)." While it is theoretically possible for organizations to do both simultaneously, there are difficult choices between these two goals that need to be made as organizations grow. Elsewhere I describe the dilemmas faced by some feminist organizations, such as rape crisis centers or battered women's centers started in the 1960s as part of the Women's Liberation Movement. They began as egalitarian groups, focused not only on providing services but also on sharing leadership and developing the skills of their members. As these organizations became successful, the demand for their services increased. The need for efficiency conflicted with the time-consuming process of collective decision making, and the organizations were forced to chose between widespread participation and meeting the growing demands for services. These dilemmas, which I call the "challenges of success," highlight the contradictions between the development of community and the empowerment of individuals (Riger, 1994).

If empowerment of the disenfranchised is the primary value, then what is to hold together societies made up of different groups? Competition among groups for dominance and control without the simultaneous acknowledgment of common interests can lead to a conflict like we see today in the former Yugoslavia. One of the primary tasks for community psychology, then, is to articulate the relationship between empowerment and community. Does empowerment of disenfranchised people and groups simultaneously bring about a greater sense of community and strengthen the ties that hold our society together, or does it promote certain individuals or groups at the expense of others, increasing competitiveness and lack of cohesion?

The empowered individual in community psychology need not be the individual in isolation or even in groups, fighting with others for power and control. Rather, we should consider connection as important as empowerment. This conception of community, however, challenges the belief in individual rights and freedoms which is the cornerstone of the political philosophy on which notions of empowerment rest. Pure liberalism places primacy on individual rights, not corporate or community rights. A community psychology aimed at empowerment of the individual very much accords with our dominant political philosophy.

Group or community development inevitably will clash, at some point, with that of the individual, and the empowerment of one person or group will conflict with that of another. The challenge to community psychology is to articulate a vision that encompasses not only empowerment but also community, a vision that can address the question asked by Rodney King: "Can't we all get along?" To answer this question, we need to consider differences but also similarities; those things that separate and also those we have in common; agency and also communion; empowerment and also community.

ACKNOWLEDGMENTS

I thank Dan A. Lewis and Chris Keys for their helpful comments on earlier drafts, and Julie Nelson for research on the concepts of agency and communion. An earlier version of this article was presented as an Invited Address at the American Psychological Association convention in Toronto, Canada, August 1993.

REFERENCES

Baars, B. J. (1986). *The cognitive revolution in psychology*. New York: Guilford.
Bales, R. F. (1970). *Personality and interpersonal behavior*. New York: Holt, Rinehart & Winston.
Bakan, D. (1966). *The duality of human existence*. Chicago: Rand-McNally.

Bond, M. & Keys, C. (1993). Empowerment, diversity, and collaboration: Promoting synergy on community boards. *American Journal of Community Psychology, 21*, 37–58.

Brenner, M. H. (1973). *Mental illness and the economy.* Cambridge, MA: Harvard University Press.

Buss, A. R. (1978). The structure of psychological revolutions. *Journal of the History of the Behavioral Sciences, 14*, 57–64.

Caplan, N. & Nelson, S. D. (1973). On being useful. *American Psychologist, 28*, 199–211.

Carlson, R. (1971). Sex differences in ego functioning: Exploratory studies of agency and communion. *Journal of Consulting and Clinical Psychology, 37*, 270–271.

Chavis, D. M. & Wandersman, A. (1990). Sense of community in the urban environment: A catalyst for participation and community development. *American Journal of Community Psychology, 18*, 159–162.

Fine, M. (1992). Coping with rape: Critical perspectives on consciousness. In M. Fine, *Disruptive voices: The possibilities of feminist research* (pp. 61–76). Ann Arbor: University of Michigan Press.

Friman, P. C., Allen, K. D., Kerwin, M. L. E., & Larzelere, R. (1993). Changes in modern psychology: A citation analysis of the Kuhnian displacement thesis. *American Psychologist, 438*, 658–664.

Gardner, H. (1985). *The mind's new science: A history of the cognitive revolution.* New York: Basic Books.

Gilligan, C. (1982). *In a different voice.* Cambridge, MA: Harvard University Press.

Gruber, J. & Trickett, E. J. (1987). Can we empower others? The paradox of empowerment in the governing of an alternative public school. *American Journal of Community Psychology, 15*, 353–371.

Gutierrez, L. M. (1990). Working with women of color: An empowerment perspective. *Social Work, 35*, 149–153.

Guttmann, D. (1970). Female ego styles and generational conflict. In J. Bardwick, E. Douvan, M. Horner, and D. Guttman (Eds.), *Feminine personality and conflict.* Belmont, CA: Brooks/Cole.

Hare-Mustin, R. T. & Maracek, J. (1986). Autonomy and gender: Some questions for therapists. *Psychotherapy, 23*, 205–212.

Hollander, E. P. & Offermann, L. R. (1990). Power and leadership in organizations: Relationships in transition. *American Psychologist, 45*, 179–189.

Hunter, A. & Riger, S. (1986). The meaning of community in community mental health. *Journal of Community Psychology, 14*, 55–71.

Johnson, M. M. (1988). *Strong mothers, weak wives: The search for gender equality.* Berkeley: University of California Press.

Kerber, L. (1986). Some cautionary words for historians. *Signs: Journal of Women in Culture and Society, 11*, 304–310.

Kieffer, C. (1984). Citizen empowerment: A developmental perspective. *Prevention in Human Services, 3*, 9–36.

Leavitt, J. & Saegert, S. (1990). *From abandonment to hope: Community households in Harlem.* New York: Columbia University Press.

Lewis, D. (1994). *Race and educational reform in the American metropolis.* Albany, New York: State University of New York Press.

Livert, D. E. (n.d.) Implications of an empowerment ideology for community psychology. Unpublished manuscript, George Peabody College of Vanderbilt University, Nashville, TN.

Maton, K. (1993). *Researching the foundations of empowerment: Group-based belief systems, opportunity role structures, supportive resources, and leadership.* Paper presented at the Biennial Conference of the Society for Community Research and Action, Williamsburg, VA.

Maton, K. & Rappaport, J. (1984). Empowerment in a religious setting: A multivariate investigation. *Prevention in Human Services, 3*, 37–73.

Miller, J. B. (1976). *Toward a new psychology of women*. Boston: Beacon Press.

Molotch, H. (1973). *Social justice and the city*. Baltimore: Johns Hopkins University.

Ozer, E. M. & Bandura, A. (1990). Mechanisms governing empowerment effects: A self-efficacy analysis. *Journal of Personality and Social Psychology, 58*, 472–486.

Panzetta, A. F. (1973). The concept of community: The short-circuit of the mental health movement. In B. Denner and R. H. Price (Eds.), *Community mental health: Social action and reaction* (pp. 245–259). New York: Holt, Rinehart & Winston.

Parsons, T, (1951). *The social system*. Glencoe, IL: Free Press.

Parsons, T. & Shils, E. (1952). *Toward a general theory of action*. Cambridge, MA: Harvard University Press.

Prilleltesky, I. (1989). Psychology and the status quo. *American Psychologist, 44*, 795–802.

Rappaport, J. (1987). Terms of empowerment/exemplars of prevention: Toward a theory for community psychology. *American Journal of Community Psychology, 15*, 121–144.

Rappaport, J. (1990). Research methods and the empowerment social agenda. In P. Tolan, C. Keys, F. Chertok, and L. Jason (Eds.), *Researching community psychology* (pp. 51–63). Washington, DC: American Psychological Association.

Riger, S. (1994). Challenges of success: Stages of growth in feminist organizations. *Feminist Studies, 20*, 275–300.

Sampson, E. E. (1983). *Justice and the critique of pure psychology*. New York: Plenum Press.

Sarason, S. B. (1974). *The psychological sense of community: Prospects for a community psychology*. San Francisco: Jossey-Bass.

Sarason, S. B. (1981). *Psychology misdirected*. New York: Free Press.

Scherer, M. (1992). *Still loved by the sun: A rape survivor's journal*. New York: Simon and Schuster.

Sears, D. O. (1986). College sophomores in the laboratory: Influences of a narrow data base on social psychology's view of human nature. *Journal of Personality and Social Psychology, 51*, 515–530.

Segal, E. M. & Lachman, R. (1972). Complex behavior or higher mental process: Is there a paradigm shift? *American Psychologist, 27*, 46–55.

Serrano-Garcia, I. (1984). The illusion of empowerment: Community development within a colonial context. *Prevention in Human Services, 3*, 173–200.

Stack, C. (1974). *All our kin*. New York: Harper & Row.

Zimmerman, M. A. (2000). Empowerment theory: Psychological, organizational, and community levels of analysis. In J. Rappaport and E. Seidman (Eds.), *Handbook of community psychology* (pp. 43–63). New York: Kluwer Academic/Plenum Publishers.

Zimmerman, M. A., Israel, B. A., Schulz, A., & Checkoway, B. (1992). Further explorations in empowerment theory: An empirical analysis of psychological empowerment. *American Journal of Community Psychology, 20*, 707–727.

20

The Children of Divorce Parenting Intervention: Outcome Evaluation of an Empirically Based Program

Sharlene A. Wolchik, Stephen G. West, Susan Westover,
Irwin N. Sandler, Art Martin, Julie Lustig, Jenn-Yun Tein,
and Jennifer Fisher

*Examined efficacy of an empirically based intervention using 70
divorced mothers who participated in a 12-session program or a wait-list
condition. The program targeted five putative mediators: quality of the
mother–child relationship, discipline, negative divorce events, contact
with fathers, and support from nonparental adults. Posttest comparisons
showed higher quality mother–child relationships and discipline, fewer
negative divorce events, and better mental health outcomes for program
participants than controls. More positive program effects occurred for
mothers' than children's reports of variables and for families with
poorest initial levels of functioning. Analyses indicated that improvement
in the mother–child relationship partially mediated the effects of the
program on mental health.*

Parental divorce is one of the most prevalent stressors experienced by
children in our society. In 1985, the number of divorces was the second

Originally published in the *American Journal of Community Psychology, 21*(3) (1993):
293–331.

A Quarter Century of Community Psychology: Readings from the American Journal of
Community Psychology, edited by Tracey A. Revenson *et al.* Kluwer Academic/Plenum
Publishers, New York, 2002.

highest in our history (Vital Statistics Report, 1987) and demographers expect the rate to remain high in the future (Glick, 1988). Each year, over 1 million children experience parental divorce (U.S. National Center for Health Statistics, 1991) and it is estimated that 40% of the current generation will experience parental divorce before they are 18 years old (Glick, 1988).

Parental divorce can have negative effects on children, including elevated aggression (e.g., Felner, Stolberg, & Cowen, 1975; Hetherington, Cox, & Cox, 1978; Zill, 1983), elevated anxiety (Wyman, Cowen, Hightower, & Pedro-Carroll, 1985), poor academic performance (e.g., Guidubaldi, Cleminshaw, Perry, & Mcloughlin, 1983; Zill, 1983), poor self-concept (e.g., Parish & Wigle, 1985), and poor peer relationships (e.g., Guidubaldi *et al.*, 1983; Hetherington, Cox, & Cox, 1981). Also, children of divorce are over-represented in treatment settings (Zill, 1983). The results of a meta analysis by Amato and Keith (1991) showed that although the effect sizes were generally weak, children of divorce scored lower than children from intact families on a variety of measures of adjustment. Given the high prevalence of divorce and its potential negative effects, assisting children's postdivorce adjustment is an important focus for preventive mental health programs. In this study, the efficacy of a theory-driven, parent-focused program for children of divorce was evaluated.

Prevention programs, including those targeted for children of divorce, have traditionally been developed without a strong base in the relevant empirical literature. Only rarely have program developers in any area explicitly articulated a mechanism of operation through which the intervention is expected to produce the desired outcome (Lipsey, 1990; Sechrest, West, Phillips, Redner, & Yeaton, 1979). However, researchers have recently argued that there are several important advantages to using an empirical approach to the design and evaluation of prevention programs (Coie *et al.*, 1993; Grych & Fincham, 1992; Higginbotham, West, & Forsyth, 1988; Lorion, 1985a, 1985b; Lorion, Price, & Eaton, 1989; Price, 1982; Sandler, Gersten, Reynolds, Kallgren, & Ramirez, 1988; West, Sandler, Pillow, Baca, & Gersten, 1991). In this approach, previous empirical research is used to develop an explicit "small theory" of how children's adjustment problems can be prevented or changed. The small theory is not typically intended to provide a comprehensive understanding of the etiology of the problem. Rather, it identifies a limited number of important, potentially modifiable processes that are associated with the development of the problem.

More explicitly, the use of these small theories offers several advantages related to the design and evaluation of interventions. First, developing a small theory serves an important heuristic role by forcing the investigator to specify central processes that are expected to underlie the development of psychological symptoms. Once the processes have been specified, their plausibility can be probed through explicit tests using existing or new data sets (West *et al.*, 1991). Second, the theory offers broad guidelines for the design of the intervention. The theory identifies important variables and processes through which these variables are expected to mediate between the risk factor (divorce) and symptoms. The theory indicates only where the intervention should be directed; it is largely mute with respect to the nature of the intervention for changing the specified processes. The explicit nature of the intervention is left to the intervention designer's experience, ingenuity, and understanding of previous empirical successes and failures in the intervention literature. Third, the small theory helps in the design of field research trials.

> A theory orientation provides a framework within which the researcher can address the fundamental but vexing questions of what controls to implement, what samples to use, what measures to take, and what procedures to follow. It can help guide the research to designs that have increased probability of detecting treatment effects, permit stronger causal inference, and produce more interpretable and generalizable results (Lipsey, 1990, p. 35)

Fourth, the small theory together with a careful evaluation of the implementation of the program offer strong guidance for program redesign. This information helps distinguish between aspects of the intervention that are too weak or poorly implemented to have an impact and those aspects that were well implemented but did not have their theoretically intended effect. Fifth, the data collected from randomized trials of the intervention can provide strong tests of the underlying small theory and add to our understanding of the basic processes that affect children's adjustment in stress situations (Coie *et al.*, 1993). Finally, the detailed evidence collected on the processes through which the program is theoretically expected to operate provides information that is useful in understanding the successes and failures of attempts to replicate the program.

Felner and his colleagues (Felner, Farber, & Primavera, 1983; Felner, Rowlinson, & Terre, 1986; Felner, Terre, & Rowlinson, 1988) have provided a conceptualization of transitional events that serves as a useful general framework for developing a small theory of how children develop adjustment problems after divorce. In this framework, children's adjustments is viewed as a function of the environmental stressors, and *inter*personal and *intra*personal protective resources available to the child. This general framework organizes the results of previous research that show consistent empirical support for significant associations between children's adjustment after divorce and the following environmental and interpersonal factors: (a) the quality of the child's relationship with the custodial parent (e.g., Fogas, Wolchik, & Braver, 1987; Guidubaldi, Cleminshaw, Perry, Nastasi, & Lightel, 1986; Stolberg & Bush, 1985); (b) amount of contact between the child and the noncustodial parent (e.g., Guidubaldi *et al.*, 1986; Hetherington *et al.*, 1981; Warren *et al.*, 1984); (c) negative divorce-related events including interparental conflict (e.g., Guidubaldi *et al.*, 1986; Hetherington *et al.*, 1978; Long, Forehand, Fauber, & Brody, 1987; Sandler *et al.*, 1988; Stolberg & Anker, 1984); (d) contact with and support from nonparental adults (Guidubaldi & Cleminshaw, 1983; Hetherington *et al.*, 1981; Santrock & Warshack, 1979; Wolchik, Ruehlman, Braver, & Sandler, 1989); and, (e) discipline strategies (e.g., Baldwin & Skinner, 1989; Fogas *et al.*, 1987; Santrock & Warshack, 1979). West (1990) found support for the importance of the first three of these factors [(d) and (e) were not measured] in predicting symptoms using structural equation models in two samples of recently divorced families.

Although much less frequently investigated, researchers have also reported significant associations between children's adjustment after divorce and a number of *intra*personal processes or resources. These have included level of interpersonal reasoning (Kurdek, Blisk, & Siesky, 1981), internal locus of control (Fogas, Wolchik, Braver, Freedom, & Bay, 1992; Kurdek & Berg, 1983; Kurdek *et al.*, 1981), beliefs about divorce (Kurdek & Berg, 1987; Kurdek *et al.*, 1981; Mazur, Wolchik, & Sandler, 1992; Wolchik *et al.*, 1992) and coping abilities (Armistead *et al.*, 1990; Kurdek & Sinclair, 1988; Sandler, Tein, & West, 1994).

Most prevention programs for children of divorce aim to enhance adjustment by working directly with children. In their review of child-focused programs, Grych and Fincham (1992) concluded that although these programs are widespread, evaluations of only one program, the Children of Divorce Intervention Project (Alpert-Gillis, Pedro-Carroll, & Cowen, 1989; Pedro-Carroll, & Cowen, 1985; Pedro-Carroll, Cowen, Hightower, & Guare, 1986), have shown consistently positive effects. Grych and Fincham raised other concerns about the evaluations of child-focused programs such as the limited overlap between basic research on children's adjustment to divorce and program design, and the lack of attention to examining the processes by which change occurs. Further, Grych and Fincham noted that these programs may be limited in their ability to affect meaningful levels of change because of the significant influence of familial and environmental factors on children's postdivorce adjustment.

Because most of the environmental stressors and protective factors for which there is consistent empirical support in the basic psychosocial literature are within the *parent's* rather than the *child's* control, parents seem to be ideal change agents. To date, there have been only two at least quasi-experimental evaluations of parent-based programs (Stolberg & Garrison, 1985; Warren *et al.*, 1984) and neither achieved its intended effect. In both studies *parents'* mental health *improved* as a function of participation in the interventions, whereas *children's* mental health did *not* change. Stolberg and Garrison's program emphasized adult divorce adjustment issues rather than parenting concerns and skills (A. L. Stolberg, 1988, personal communication), possibly accounting for their lack of effects on the children's mental health. Warren *et al.*, taught parenting skills, but there were likely ceiling effects on the measures of children's symptoms due to self-selection of healthy families into the intervention. In addition, since process evaluation data were not collected, the possibility that the interventions may have been too weak or poorly implemented to have their intended effects cannot be ruled out (see Sechrest *et al.*, 1979).

The current study examined the efficacy of a theory-driven, parent-based intervention for children of divorce. Our small theory focused on five putative mediators which can be influenced by parents and for which there is consistent empirical support for their associations with children's post-divorce adjustment: (a) quality of the custodial parent–child relationship, (b) contact with the noncustodial parent, (c) negative divorce-related events including interparental conflict, (d) contact with/support from non-parental adults, and (e) discipline strategies. A parent-based intervention was designed to affect these five putative mediators, with changes in these putative mediating variables, in turn, expected to lead to positive changes in children's psychological adjustment.

Because the program was designed to change specified putative mediating variables, it can be expected that those who are most deficient on these mediators will have the greatest opportunity to benefit. Furthermore, we argued that there is a considerable increase in the statistical power to detect true effects if those who are functioning well on these mediating processes are screened out of the experimental trial (Pillow, Sandler, Braver, Wolchik, & Gersten, 1991). Because the gain in statistical power is particularly important in a relatively small-scale experimental trial such as this one, we excluded families who were functioning well on these variables.

Extensive process evaluation and outcome data were collected to assess if change occurred on the putative mediating and outcome variables, to assess whether the program was implemented as intended, and to probe various hypotheses if particular putative mediators failed to change in the expected direction. The perspectives of multiple informants were obtained on both process evaluation and outcome measures. The use of multiple measures allows us to differentiate between the effects that are consistent across informants and those that are associated only with a specific reporter (T. D. Cook, 1985). Interpretation of the latter effects is more problematic since they may reflect artifacts such as demand characteristics (Orne, 1962) or they may represent "true" effects that are not reflected in the other measures because of differential access or sensitivity to information on the part of different informants (Funder & West, 1993).

METHOD

Overview

Mothers who were divorced within the past 2 years and who had at least one child between 8 and 15 years of age were recruited to participate in an intervention consisting of 10 group and 2 individual sessions. Participants were assigned randomly to either an immediate intervention group or a wait-list control group that received the intervention following the posttest assessment. Both the mother and one randomly selected child in the target age range were assessed within 2 weeks prior to the intervention and 10 to 12 weeks later on measures of the putative mediators and children's symptoms.

Participants

Participants were recruited through random sampling of court records of filings for divorce, media articles, and school presentations. Families were sent a letter about the program and, when possible, were contacted by telephone.

Participants were screened using a two-step process. In the first step, the following seven eligibility criteria were assessed in a telephone interview to verify that the family was appropriate for both the intervention and assessment. The criteria were (a) the divorce decree was granted during the last two years; (b) there was at least one child between 8 and 15 years of age; (c) the custodial/primary residential parent was female; (d) neither the custodial parent nor any child was currently in treatment for psychological problems; (e) the custodial parent had not remarried and did not have plans to remarry during the study period; (f) the custody arrangement was expected to remain stable during the study period; and (g) English was the primary language of the mother and children.

Families meeting these first-step criteria then participated in the full pretest interview described in the Measures section. Pretest interview data were used for the second stage of screening.

First, families were eliminated in which the target child did not appear to be at risk because he or she had very favorable scores on composite measure of two of the putative mediating variables, quality of the mother–child relationship and divorce-related events. Pillow *et al*. (1991) have shown that this composite measure predicts child symptoms and have established a stable cutoff score using a large normative sample ($N = 396$) of children of divorce. Given our assumption that "healthy" families would receive little benefit from exposure to the full 10-week program, children with scores at or above the top 30% of the normative sample were excluded. Of the 177 families interviewed, 46 (26%) were excluded. Mothers of these children were told that the interview indicated that they were already doing the things addressed by the program. They were then invited to participate in a 2-hour workshop on children's adjustment to divorce.

Second, because the intervention was designed to be preventive, families were identified in which either the mother or the target child had test scores indicating clinical levels of depression may be present. These individuals were excluded and referred for immediate treatment. Twenty-one (12%) children who scored 18 or more (Burbach, Farha, & Thorpe, 1986) on the Child's Depression Inventory (Kovacs, 1981) or were suicidal, as assessed with a revised version of the Child Assessment Schedule (Gersten, Beals, & Kallgren, 1991; Hodges, Kline, Stern, Cytryn, & McKnew, 1982), were excluded. One mother whose score on the Psychiatric Epidemiology Research Interview (PERI; Dohrenwend, Shrout, Egri, & Mendelsohn, 1980) Demoralization Scale exceeded 3 standard deviations above the mean of a previous sample of divorced parents ($n = 92$) was also excluded.

Ninety-four families that completed Stage 1 and Stage 2 screening were selected to be assigned randomly to the intervention or wait-list control conditions. Of these families, 15 withdrew after participating in the interview *and* before being assigned to condition. Ten families in the control condition and 14 families in the intervention condition dropped out of the study prior to the posttest. Approximately 40% of the participant loss in the intervention condition occurred prior to the first session.

Seventy families completed pretest and posttest interviews. Ninety percent of these mothers were Caucasian. The mean age of the mothers was 36.8 years ($SD = 4.9$, range = 27–50). Seventy-four percent of the mothers had attended college. The average yearly income was between $20,001 to $25,000 (range = less than $5,000 to $50,000). These families had been divorced an average of 11.0 months ($SD = 5.9$, range = 2–24) and had been physically separated an average of 23.1 months ($SD = 12.10$, range 7–69). Seventy-four percent of the families had sole maternal custody; the remainder had joint legal custody. All the interviewed children resided primarily with their mothers. In 67% of the families, the fathers lived within the Phoenix metropolitan area. The mean number of children in the family was 2.4 ($SD = 0.80$, range = 1–4). The average age of the child who was interviewed was 10.6 (SD = 2.1, range = 8–15). Of the children interviewed, 61% were male.

Procedure

Interviews lasting approximately 2 hours were conducted by trained interviewers with the mother and child separately in the family's home. Informed consent was obtained from the mother, and the child completed an assent form prior to participation.

Measures

Modifiable Risk and Protective Factors: Children's Reports of Quality of the Custodial Parent–Child Relationship

Parent–Adolescent Communication Scale—Open Family Communication Subscale (Barnes & Olson, 1982). This 10-item scale assesses the quality of communication between the mother and child. Barnes and Olson reported internal consistency and test–retest reliabilities of .87 and .78, respectively. At pretest in the current sample, coefficient α (Cronbach, 1951) = .86.

Family Routines Inventory (Jensen, James, Boyce, & Harnett, 1983). Seven items which assessed positive routines involving the mother and child were selected from this 23-item inventory. The occurrence of these items was rated using a 3-point scale (never, sometimes, a lot). For the pretest, α = .76.

Child Report of Parenting Behavior Inventory (Schaefer, 1965). The Acceptance (16 items) and Rejection (16 items) subscales were used. Scores on this inventory have been shown to discriminate normal boys from delinquents (Schaefer, 1965). The acceptance and rejection (reverse scored) subscales were combined. For the pretest, α = .88.

Discipline

Child Report of Parenting Behavior Inventory (Schaefer, 1965). The Inconsistency of Discipline (8 item) subscale was used. Scores have been shown to discriminate normal boys from delinquents (Schaefer, 1965). For the pretest, α = .68.

Negative Divorce Events

The Divorce Events Schedule for Children (Sandler, Wolchik, Braver, & Fogas, 1991). This life-events inventory is used to assess the occurrence of divorce-related events during the past month. Of the 35 events, 17 are negative, as judged by consensual ratings of children experiencing these events. Sandler *et al.* have reported a test–retest reliability of the negative events score of .85 and have shown that the occurrence of negative divorce events is significantly related to children's adjustment problems. Internal consistency is not appropriate for life events scales, where the items are not assumed to represent the same underlying construct but to be reports of the occurrence of relatively independent events (Sandler & Guenther, 1985; Finch & West, 1997).

Children's Perception Questionnaire (Emery & O'Leary, 1982). This measure of perceptions of overt interparental conflict was modified to include 4 items that were applicable to divorced families. For the pretest, $\alpha = .80$.

Contact with Father

Calendar of Time with Father. Children were asked when visits with Dad had occurred during the past 2 weeks and the time they began and ended. Interviewers recorded this information on a calendar and then, using the calendar, reviewed the information with the child and made corrections, if appropriate. The number of hours of contact during the last 2 weeks was computed.

Support from Nonparental Adults

Children's Inventory of Social Support (Wolchik *et al.*, 1989). Children were asked to list adults who provided the support, functions of recreation/play, goods and services, advice, emotional support, and positive feedback. Wolchik *et al.*, reported that support from family adults and support from nonfamily adults interacted with negative changes in divorce-related events in predicting adjustment problems. Test–retest reliability for the number of support functions received from nonparental adults was .59.

Modifiable Risk and Protective Factors: Mothers' Reports

Parent report versions of several measures were administered with items that exactly paralleled the child report versions. These included the Open Family Communication subscale ($\alpha = .82$), Family Routines Inventory ($\alpha = .66$), the acceptance and rejection (reversed scored) combined subscale ($\alpha = .91$), and consistency of discipline ($\alpha = .86$) of the Child Report of Parenting Behavior Inventory, and Divorce Events Schedule for Children.

Family Environment Scale (Moos, 1974; Moos & Moos, 1981). The 9-item control subscale was used as a measure of discipline. Moos and Moos

(1981) have reported acceptable test–retest reliabilities for this subscale. Roosa and Beals (1990) reported an internal consistency reliability of .59 for a sample of divorced families. For the pretest, Cronbach's α = .50.

O'Leary–Porter Scale (Porter & O'Leary, 1980). This measure of overt interparental conflict was modified by deleting 2 items that were not applicable to divorced families. For the pretest, Cronbach's α = .92.

Child's Contact with Father Scale. Mothers responded to the following questions about contact during the last month: hours of face to face contact; number of visits; number of different days on which contact occurred; and number of overnights. Responses to each question were transformed into z scores and these scores were summed into a composite score.

Attitude Toward Child's Relationship with Father. Mothers answered three 7-point items about their child having a close relationship with the father and four 5-point items about the father's parenting abilities (e.g., caring parent, incompetent parent). Alphas for the pretest were .79 and .90 for these two scales, respectively. In addition, mothers reported on their willingness to change visitation, if their ex-husband requested it, using a 7-point scale.

Children's Psychological Adjustment: Children's Reports

Child Depression Inventory (Kovacs, 1981). Scores on this 27-item inventory have been shown to discriminate clinically depressed and nondepressed psychiatric patients (Kovacs, 1985; Lobovits & Handal, 1985; Saylor, Finch, Spirito, & Bennett, 1984). Finch, Saylor, Edwards, and McIntosh (1987) report a test–retest reliability of .82. At pretest, α was .84.

Children's Manifest Anxiety Scale—Revised (Reynolds & Richmond, 1978). Reynolds (1982) reported support for the convergent and divergent validity of this 28-item scale. Reynolds and Richmond reported a test–retest reliability of .68. Pretest α was .87.

Youth Report of Hostility Scale (C. Cook, 1985). Aggression was measured using 30 items from the Child Behavior Checklist (Achenbach, 1978; Achenbach & Edelbrock, 1979, 1983) which were adapted into a self-report format. Items from the aggressiveness, delinquency, and hyperactivity subscales were selected if their item–factor correlations were .40 or better in the factor analyses reported by Achenbach and Edelbrock for their four age and sex groups (Achenbach, 1978; Achenbach & Edelbrock, 1979). Alpha (pretest) was .88.

Child Assessment Schedule—Revised (Gersten *et al.*, 1991; West *et al.*, 1991). The Child Assessment Schedule (CAS; Hodges *et al.*, 1982) was adapted into a structured interview format and shortened by deleting items not used for DSM-III-R (American Psychiatric Association, 1987) classification and items with low reliability coefficients. Scores on the CAS discriminate psychiatric inpatients, outpatients, and normal controls (Hodges *et al.*, 1982). Only questions pertaining to depression or conduct problems were included in the present battery. For the depression and conduct problems subscales, pretest α = .77 and .81, respectively.

Children's Psychological Adjustment: Mothers' Reports

Child Behavior Checklist (Achenbach, 1978; Achenbach & Edelbrock, 1978, 1979). Scores on this 118-item inventory discriminate clinic referred from non-referred children (Achenbach & Edelbrock). Because the sample consisted of both boys and girls and spanned a broad age range, the total behavior problem score was used, as recommended by Achenbach and Edelbrock. Achenbach and Edelbrock report a test–retest reliability of .89. Alpha (pretest) was .92.

Mother's Psychological Adjustment

PERI—Demoralization Scale (Dohrenwend *et al.*, 1980). This 27-item scale was used to exclude mothers with extreme levels of psychological distress. Scores on the PERI have been shown to be moderately related to psychiatric diagnosis (Vernon & Roberts, 1981). Alpha (pretest) was .93.

Demographic Information

Mothers provided basic demographic information including age and gender of children, household composition, length of marriage, ethnicity, occupation, educational level, income, custody arrangement, and the father's place of residence.

Design

Experimental Conditions

Recruitment and assignment were done for seven cohorts of participants. Families who remained eligible following the two-step screening process were randomly assigned to the intervention or wait-list control condition. Groups ranged in size from 6 to 8.

Wait-List Control Condition. These families were informed that their program would begin in 6 months. Families in this condition had no contact with the project staff from pretest to posttest except for scheduling of posttest interviews.

Intervention Program. Mothers attended 10 weekly group sessions and 2 individual sessions. The individual sessions occurred after the third and sixth group sessions. The program had a strong emphasis on skill acquisition and/or enhancement. Each session included a short lecture, skill demonstration, and skill practice. Participants were assigned homework after each session and in each session, difficulties and successes in implementing the skills at home were discussed. The intervention techniques used to change each mediator are shown in Table 1. Wherever possible, techniques that have previously been shown to be effective in changing the mediating processes were employed. Discipline strategies were developed using Patterson's (1975) and Forehand and McMahon's (1981) research with families. Guerney's (1977) work with parents and children was used to develop methods to enhance listening skills and Novaco's (1975) anger management techniques were modified slightly. As shown, 5 of the sessions focused primarily on changing the quality of the mother–child relationship. The last 2 sessions focused on ways to facilitate maintenance of the program skills.

Leaders. Each group was co-led by a male-female team. Four females and 4 males served as coleaders. Seven of the leaders were graduate students in clinical psychology; one was a postdoctoral candidate. Clinical

Table 1. Techniques Used to Change Putative Mediators

Putative mediator (Session)	Intervention techniques
Quality of mother–child relationship (2, 3, 3_a [individual], 4, 5)	Positive family activities Quality Time Positive attention for desirable behaviors Listening skills
Negative divorce-related events including interparental conflict (3, 4, 5, 6_a [individual])	Anger management skills Listening skills
Contact with noncustodial parent (6)	Awareness of importance of father–child relationship Reduction of obstacles to father maintaining contact with child
Contact with nonparental adults (6_a [individual])	Social network assessment Identification of potential resources Problem solving of difficulties with attempts to augment child's network
Discipline strategies (7, 8)	Clarification of rules and expectations Monitoring of misbehaviors and consequences Use of consistent discipline

experience ranged from 1.5 to 5 years. The supervisor was a clinical psychologist with more than 10 years experience working with children and parents. Leaders received intensive training which included readings and didactic information about children's postdivorce adjustment and about the theoretical and empirical bases for the program, videotapes of sessions from a pilot of this program, and role play of session material. In addition, weekly supervision (1.5 hours) was provided. Supervision focused on problems participants had in using the program skills and ways to enhance compliance with homework assignments.

Integrity of the Intervention

Several steps were taken to ensure that the intervention was delivered as planned. First, the content and format of all sessions (group and individual) were described in detailed outlines, which leaders used as they delivered the sessions. Second, extensive training and ongoing supervision were provided. Third, a careful process evaluation was undertaken to ensure that the intervention was delivered as planned (Sechrest et al., 1979).

The process evaluation had five major components.

1. The time spent on each component of the session was recorded during the session. For example, in group Session 3, time spent on the following components was recorded: review of previous week's homework, positive recognition and communication, listening skills, active listening, and presentation of new homework activities.
2. Leaders recorded the attendance of each participant at group, individual, and makeup sessions immediately after each session.
3. Leaders independently rated their own and their coleader's knowledge/mastery of the material and efforts to facilitate group members' processing of the material immediately after each session. These ratings were made on 5-point scales anchored by extensive behavioral descriptions in which 1 represented low quality and 5 high quality performance.
4. Each participant evaluated the two coleaders of her group on 10 dimensions of performance at the middle and at the completion of the program. Example dimensions were "The leader relates session material to concerns I have about my children," and "The leader helps me find solutions when I have problems doing the exercises of the program." Each rating was made on a 5-point scale ranging from does not describe [leader] at all (1) to describes very well (5).
5. At the end of the program, participants reported on their usage of 22 skills taught in the program. Example skills included family pleasure breaks, anger management skills, and making consequences for

good and bad behavior clear. Participants reported on a 3-point scale (3 = an increase, 2 = no change, and 1 = a decrease). Scales involving negative behaviors (e.g., badmouthing the father) were recoded so that a score of 3 uniformly represented positive change.

RESULTS

Analyses of Subject Attrition

Of the 46 subjects assigned to the control group, 10 (22%) dropped out prior to the posttest, whereas 14 of the 48 (29%) subjects dropped out from the intervention group. Chi-square analysis did not indicate a significant difference in the attrition rates, $\chi^2(1, N = 94) = 0.68$, ns. Following the procedure of Jurs and Glass (1971), a series of two-way (Intervention Condition × Attrition Status) analyses of variance (ANOVAs) were conducted on all variables collected at *pretest*. This exploratory analysis sought to identify variables on which either of two attrition-related concerns may have occurred.

Of most importance, significant Intervention Condition × Attrition Status interactions identify variables on which differential attrition may have occurred. For mothers' reports, no significant Intervention Condition × Attrition interaction effects were found. For children's reports, 2 of the 12 ANOVAs showed significant interaction effects: one of the measures of aggression (C. Cook, 1985), $F(1, 90) = 6.94, p < .01$, and one of the measures of depression (Kovacs, 1981), $F(1, 89) = 8.05, p < .01$. Post hoc t tests (Winer, 1971) showed significant interactions indicating that completers in the control group were less aggressive ($M_C = 11.28$, $M_A = 17.80$), $t = 2.67, p < .01$, and tended to be less depressed ($M_C = 7.75$, $M_A = 10.80$), $t = 1.74, p < .10$, than attriters. In contrast, in the intervention group, completers and attriters did not differ in their reports of aggression ($M_C = 13.94$, $M_A = 11.86$), $t = 0.95$, ns, but completers reported higher levels of depression than attriters ($M_C = 9.82$, $M_A = 6.21$), $t = 2.31, p < .05$. Given that the control group completers tended to be healthier, any effects of attrition would be expected to be biased against showing positive effects of the treatment.

Of secondary importance, significant main effects of Attrition Status identify variables on which general attrition has occurred that may represent possible limits on the generalization of the findings. For mothers's reports, 1 of the 12 ANOVAs showed a significant effect. Mothers who attrited from the program reported higher levels of interparental conflict ($M = 15.5$) than those who completed the program ($M = 12.22$), $F(1, 89) = 4.36, p < .05$. For the children's reports, only 1 of the 13 ANOVAs was significant. Children who attrited from the program reported higher levels of contact with nonparental adults ($M = 20.6$) than children who completed the program ($M = 11.4$), $F(1, 90) = 13.28, p < .001$.

Process Evaluation

Attendance. Participants attended a mean of 9.6 of the 10 scheduled group sessions and both of the individual sessions. All missed group sessions were made up, hence, all participants received the full program.

Time Usage. Based on the detailed outlines, each session was broken down into four to seven major components and the time allotted to each was recorded. Comparisons of the planned time and the mean time actually allotted across the seven groups showed relatively good agreement. The presentation of 29 components (53%) deviated by less than 5 minutes, 18 (33%) deviated by 5–10 minutes, and 8 (15%) deviated by more than 10 minutes from the time planned. These data suggest that the sessions were carried out as intended and that all major program components were addressed.

Group Leaders' Ratings. Group leaders rated their own and their coleader's knowledge of session material and efforts to facilitate processing of the session material by group members. Self and coleader ratings of the same target leader showed high levels of agreement: 93 and 98% of the ratings for knowledge of session material and efforts to facilitate processing of the session material, respectively, agreed within 1 point on a 5-point scale. Aggregating across all group leaders and sessions, the mean ratings were 4.22 for knowledge and 4.49 for group facilitation.

Participants' Evaluation of Group Leaders. Aggregating across the mid-intervention and final assessment for all leaders, participants' evaluations of the performance of the group leaders were very positive. The overall mean rating across the 10 questions was 4.75 on the 5-point scale. The highest ratings were obtained for the items, "The leader explains the material in ways that make it easy for me to use with my children" ($M = 4.83$) and "The leader is easy to talk to and is willing to listen to any questions I have" ($M = 4.83$). The lowest (though still very positive) ratings were obtained for the items, "The leader's role play demonstrations make it easier for me to learn the skills of the program" ($M = 4.59$) and "The leader helps me find solutions when I have problems doing the exercises of the program" ($M = 4.65$).

Skill Usage. Participants reported favorable changes in their usage of 22 skills taught in the program ($M = 2.76$ on 3-point scale). The greatest positive changes occurred in measures of quality time spent with the child, listening skills, setting clear and consistent rules and consequences, and using positive recognition. The least amount of change occurred for seeking help with tasks from adults and badmouthing the father.

Evaluation of Program Effects on Mediating and Outcome Variables

A series of Analyses of Covariance (ANCOVA), comparing the intervention with the control group, were conducted in which the participant's pretest score was used as the covariate and participant's posttest score on the same measure was used as the dependent variable. Following Huitema (1980), in cases in which the assumption of homogeneity of regression lines was not met, an Intervention Condition × Pretest Level of Covariate interaction was added to the equation and the results were probed and interpreted following the guidelines of Huitema (1980) and Aiken and West (1991). In particular, the Johnson-Neyman (1936) procedure was used with the data from the entire sample ($N = 70$) to identify the point(s) at which the two nonparallel regression lines became significantly different. These points are then used to define regions of significance and non- significance for the treatment effect (see Aiken & West).

Graphical and statistical diagnostic procedures (see Fox, 1991) were used to detect outliers in these data.[1] In cases in which an outlier was detected, the results are reported both with and without the outlier included in the data set.

Putative Mediators

Child Report Measures

Table 2 presents pretest, posttest, and adjusted posttest means, and F values for children's reports of the mediating variables. As shown, an Intervention Condition × Pretest Level interaction was obtained on the measure of Acceptance/Rejection (Schaefer, 1965), $F(1, 66) = 4.96, p < .05$. Application of the Johnson-Neyman (1936) procedure indicated that, within the actual range of values on the Acceptance/Rejection measure observed in the present study, the regression lines for the program and control groups did not differ significantly for low pretest values (< 86.25) of parent–child relationships. However, for high pretest values, program

---

[1]Least squares estimates of interactions involving continuous variables are particularly sensitive to outliers.

Table 2. Children's Reports of Mediating Variables

Scale	n	Pretest	Posttest	Adjusted posttest	Intervention condition F	Interaction F
Communication[b]						
Control	36	42.81	43.58	42.52	0.00	
Program	34	39.85	41.18	42.54		
Positive routines[b]						
Control	36	7.69	7.89	7.53	0.91	
Program	34	6.26	7.68	8.22		
Acceptance/rejection[c]						
Control	36	85.33	85.83	—		4.96[f]
Program	34	79.89	82.91	—		
Consistency of discipline[b]						
Control	36	16.83	17.68	17.92	0.48	
Program	34	17.79	17.66	17.40		
Interparental conflict[c]						
Control	36	5.69	5.17	—		3.97[e]
Program	33	5.70	5.21	—		
Negative divorce events[c]						
Control	35	4.31	3.46	—		3.91[e]
Program	33	4.79	3.09	—		
Hours with father in last month[b,d]						
Control	25	33.36	27.85	26.25	0.32	
Program	25	29.06	30.51	31.49		
Support from non-parental adults[a]						
Control	36	12.39	16.28	15.56	5.78[f]	
Program	34	10.35	8.65	9.12		

[a] Except for interparental conflict and negative divorce-events, higher scores are more favorable.
[b] Slopes of regression lines for the two intervention conditions were parallel. Traditional ANCOVA results are reported.
[c] Slopes of regression lines were not parallel. ANCOVA includes Intervention Condition × Pretest Level interaction.
[d] Only includes families in which the father resides in the Phoenix metropolitan area.
[e] $p < .10$.
[f] $p < .05$.

participants had higher predicted values, indicating better quality relationships, than participants in the control group.

There was a marginal effect for the Intervention Condition × Pretest Score interaction for both negative divorce events, $F(1, 64) = 3.91$, $p < .10$, and interparental conflict, $F(1, 65) = 3.97$, $p < .10$. For negative divorce events, the Johnson-Neyman procedure showed that the best fitting regression line for the program group predicted lower levels of negative events on the posttest than the corresponding regression line for the control group for high (>9.44) values of negative divorce events on the pretest. The regression lines did not significantly differ in the region in which low pretest values of negative divorce events were reported. For interparental conflict, the regression lines for the two groups did not differ within the observed range of pretest scores.

The participants in the program group and control group did not differ in the reported amount of contact with the father or the consistency of discipline (Schaefer, 1965). Contrary to prediction, children in the program group (adjusted $M = 9.12$) reported receiving fewer support functions from nonparental adults than children in the control group (adjusted $M = 15.56$), $F(1, 67) = 5.78, p < 0.5$.

Parent Report Measures

The three measures of the quality of the custodial parent–child relationship showed evidence of positive effects of the program. As shown in Table 3, measures of quality of communication (Barnes & Olson, 1982), positive routines (Jensen *et al.*, 1983), and Acceptance/Rejection (Schaefer, 1965)

Table 3. Mothers' Reports of Mediating Variables

		Mean[a]		Adjusted posttest	Intervention condition F	Interaction F
Scale	n	Pretest	Posttest			
Communication[b]						
Control	36	44.53	45.09	44.90	6.56[g]	
Program	34	43.99	46.50	46.69		
Positive routines[b]						
Control	36	9.06	9.08	9.00	22.60[g]	
Program	34	8.79	10.68	10.77		
Acceptance/rejection[b]						
Control	36	86.42	89.17	88.94	3.29[e]	
Program	34	85.62	90.58	90.78		
Control[b]						
Control	36	11.88	11.65	11.84	8.69[g]	
Program	34	12.53	12.97	12.84		
Consistency of discipline[c]						
Control	36	20.64	21.42	—		6.46[f]
Program	34	19.64	22.09	—		

Table 3. *Continued*

Scale	n	Pretest	Posttest	Adjusted posttest	Intervention condition F	Interaction F
			Mean[a]			
Interparental conflict[c]						
Control	36	12.89	10.67	—		3.03[e]
Program	33	11.48	10.24	—		
Negative divorce events[c]						
Control	29	3.28	2.93	—		5.37[f]
Program	31	3.10	2.26	—		
Attitudes towards father's parenting abilities[b]						
Control	36	12.02	11.72	12.08	3.40[e]	
Program	33	13.00	13.85	13.43		
Mother's willingness to change visitation[b]						
Control	32	5.59	5.09	5.07	4.61[f]	
Program	32	5.47	5.91	5.92		
Attitudes about father–child relationship[b]						
Control	36	14.24	13.86	13.88	1.05	
Program	34	14.29	14.62	14.59		
Amount of father–child contact[h,d]						
Control	24	0.63	0.70	0.39	0.63	
program	25	−0.39	0.11	−0.24		

[a] Except for interparental conflict and negative divorce-events, higher scores are more favorable.
[b] Slopes of regression lines for the two intervention conditions were parallel. Traditional ANCOVA results are reported.
[c] Slopes of regression lines were not parallel. ANCOVA includes Intervention Condition × Pretest Level interaction.
[d] Only includes families in which the father resides in the Phoenix metropolitan area.
[e] $p < .10$.
[f] $p < .05$.
[g] $p < .01$.

had higher adjusted means in the program than the control condition, $F(1, 67) = 6.56, p < .01; 22.60, p < .01;$ and $3.29, p < .10$, respectively.

Mothers in the program condition (adjusted $M = 12.84$) reported higher scores on the measure of control (Moos & Moos, 1981) than mothers in the control condition (adjusted $M = 11.84$), $F(1, 67) = 8.69, p < .01$. The analysis of the consistency of discipline scale (Schaefer, 1965) showed a significant Intervention Condition × Pretest Score interaction, $F(1, 66) = 6.46, p < .01$. The pattern of this interaction is shown in Figure 1.

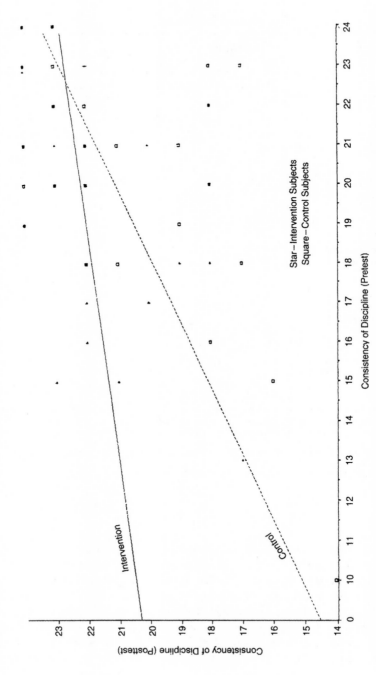

Figure 1. Interaction of pretest scores on consistency of discipline and intervention condition in predicting posttest scores on consistency of discipline.

As shown, follow-up analyses using the Johnson-Neyman (1936) procedure indicated that when pretest scores were low (< 20.2), indicating less consistent discipline, the best fitting regression line for program participants predicted significantly higher scores on the posttest than did the regression line for control group participants. However, when pretest scores were high, the difference between the regression lines for the program and control groups did not reach statistical significance.

There was a significant Intervention Condition $\times$ Pretest Score interaction for negative divorce events (Sandler, Wolchik, et al., 1991), $F(1, 56) = 5.37$, $p < .05$, and a marginal Intervention Condition $\times$ Pretest Score interaction for interparental conflict (Porter & O'Leary, 1980), $F(1, 65) = 3.03$, $p < .10$. Follow-up analysis using the Johnson-Neyman (1936) procedure showed that when a low number (< 3.7) of negative events were reported at pretest, the regression lines for the program and the control conditions did not differ. However, when a high number of negative events were reported at pretest, the regression line for the program subjects predicted significantly fewer negative events at posttest than did the regression line for the control subjects. For the measure of interparental conflict, the regression lines for the two groups did not differ within the observed range of pretest scores.

Finally, mothers in the program group (adjusted $M = 13.43$), relative to the control group (adjusted $M = 12.08$), tended to have more positive attitudes toward the father's parenting abilities, $F(1, 66) = 3.40$, $p < .10$. Also, mothers in the program reported greater willingness to change visitation if their ex-spouse requested it (adjusted $M = 5.92$) than mothers in the control group (adjusted $M = 5.07$), $F(1, 62) = 4.61$, $p < .05$. However, no differences occurred between the control and program groups in their attitudes about the father–child relationship. Comparison of the amount of contact between fathers and children, which was restricted to families in which the father lived within the Phoenix metropolitan area ($n[\text{program}] = 25$; $n[\text{control}] = 24$), showed no significant differences between the program and control groups.

Evaluation of Program Effects On Outcome Variables

Child Report Measures

The child report measures of symptoms showed mixed evidence of positive program effects. The program group (adjusted $M = 8.92$) reported a lower level of aggression (C. Cook, 1985) than the control group (adjusted $M = 12.07$), $F(1, 67) = 6.45$, $p < .01$. The program and control groups did not differ in their scores on anxiety (Reynolds & Richmond, 1978) (adjusted $Ms = 37.29$ and 38.06, respectively) or CAS conduct disorder (Gersten *et al.*, 1991) (adjusted *M*s = 15.25 and 15.21, respectively). Although the program and control groups did not differ on depression scores on the Child Depression Inventory (Kovacs, 1981) (adjusted *M*s = 6.06 and 6.77, respectively), an Intervention Condition × Pretest Level interaction was obtained on the CAS measure of depression (Gersten *et al.*, 1991), $F(1, 64) = 4.22, p < .05$. Contrary to expectation, the Johnson-Neyman procedure indicated that the program group had higher predicted scores on the posttest than the control group for high (> 21.94) levels of pretest scores. This last finding must be treated cautiously because of the presence of an extreme outlier. If this one outlier is deleted, the Intervention Condition × Pretest Score interaction is not significant, $F(1, 63) = 2.43$, ns.

Finally, a series of analyses were performed which controlled for possible differential attrition. All analyses of covariance described above were respecified to control for both pretest depression (Kovacs, 1981) and aggression (C. Cook, 1985) scores. The observed main effect of the intervention on aggression at posttest remained significant, $F(1, 65) = 6.21, p < .05$. The Pretest Level × Intervention Condition interaction for the measure of depression (Gersten *et al.*, 1991) was significant, $F(1, 61) = 4.41, p < .05$, when the same extreme outlier was included.

Parent Report Measures

Analysis of mother reports of total behavior problem score (Achenbach & Edelbrock, 1983) showed an Intervention Condition × Pretest Level interaction, $F(1, 66) = 5.64, p < .05$. This interaction is depicted in Figure 2. As can be seen, the best fitting regression line for the program group predicts significantly lower scores on the posttest than the corresponding regression line for the control group for high (> 29.93) scores on the pretest. The regression lines for the program and control groups do not differ in the region where scores on the pretest were low.

In light of the evidence reported above of differential attrition on the child report measures of depression (Kovacs, 1981) and aggression (C. Cook, 1985), this analysis was repeated controlling for the child's pretest levels on these variables. The Intervention Condition × Pretest Score interaction remained significant, $F(1, 63) = 5.35, p < .05$.

Mediational Analyses

Kenny and his associates (Baron & Kenny, 1986; Judd & Kenny, 1981) have proposed a series of criteria that must be met before claims of mediation

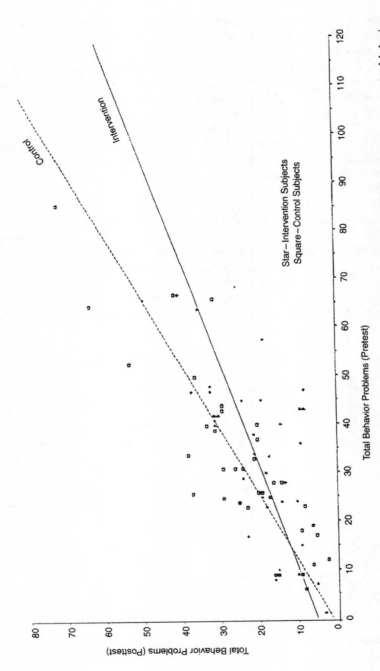

Figure 2. Interaction of pretest scores on total behavior problems and intervention condition in predicting posttest scores on total behavior problems.

can be made. The first two criteria: (a) The intervention must produce significant effects in the outcome variable, and (b) the intervention must produce significant effects in the putative mediator, have already been examined. For the parent report measures, these analyses suggested that the measures of the quality of the custodial parent–child relationship, control, consistency of discipline, negative events, and interparental conflict were candidates for a mediational analysis.

Given the relatively small sample, the effect of each potential mediating variable was assessed separately. For the analysis of the quality of the mother–child relationship, the scores for each subject on measures of acceptance/rejection, communication, and positive routines were initially standardized at pretest and posttest using the pretest mean and standard deviation for each respective measure. Composite scores were formed for each subject by taking the mean of the three standardized pretest and three standardized posttest scores, respectively. Given the Pretest Level × Intervention interactions that were obtained for several mediating and outcome variables, this effect was also included in the mediational analyses (see Baron & Kenny, 1986; James & Brett, 1984).

Figure 3 depicts a structural equation model that explicitly probes the mediational effect of the quality of the parent–child relationship composite

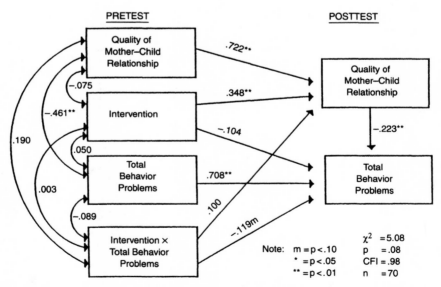

Figure 3. Structural model estimating mediation and moderated mediation of the effect of the intervention on total behavior problems.

variable.[2] The pretest measurements allow us to control for the pretest levels of the putative mediator (parent–child relationship) and outcome variable (symptoms) on their respective posttest levels. As depicted in Figure 3, the total effect of intervention on symptoms can be partitioned into a direct effect, $\beta = .10$, ns, and an indirect (mediated) effect comprised of a significant intervention to posttest mother–child relationship, $\beta = .35, p < .01$, and a significant posttest mother–child relationship to symptoms relation, $\beta = -.22$, $p < .01$. A test of the indirect effect using the multivariate delta method (Sobel, 1982, 1986) shows that it was significant, $t = 2.55, p < .01$. Based on the present data, we estimate that 43% of the main effect of the intervention on posttest mother reports of symptoms was mediated by the improved parent–child relationship. In contrast, we estimate that only 16% of the smaller intervention × pretest symptoms effect on posttest symptoms effect was mediated by the improved posttest mother reports of symptoms; this indirect effect did not attain statistical significance. We also performed a series of parallel structural equation analyses to probe the indirect effect of the intervention and the Pretest Symptoms × Intervention interaction on posttest symptoms through each of the other potential mediators (control, consistency of discipline, negative events, and interparental conflict). None of the other indirect effects met the criteria of (a) being comprised of two significant component paths and (b) having a significant overall indirect effect.

DISCUSSION

This trial represents an important step in the iterative process of developing effective prevention programs (Price, 1982; Sandler, Braver, Wolchik, Pillow, & Gersten, 1991; West et al., 1991) for children of divorce. Using a "small theory" (Lipsey, 1990) based on existing literature, an intervention was developed and implemented. The trial tested the efficacy of the program in changing the putative mediators, tested the program's efficacy in changing more distal mental health outcomes, and tested whether change on the putative mediating processes accounted for change in mental health outcomes. The pattern of results has implications for service delivery and also for understanding children's adjustment problems following divorce (see Coie et al., 1993).

According to extensive process evaluation data, the program was implemented as planned and participants felt positively about the competence of

---

[2]The loadings of these measures on a single factor at Time 1 were acceptance/rejection (.81), communication (.66), and positive routines (.40).

their group leaders. Further, participants reported using the program skills. Posttest comparisons between the experimental and control conditions, which controlled for preintervention levels, showed several positive program effects. However, the magnitude of the effects differed for mothers' and children's reports. Significant differences in the expected direction occurred for three of the four mediators measured from mothers' perspectives. Children's reports showed significant expected differences on measures of one mediator, a marginal effect on another mediator, and an unexpected difference on a third mediator. Mothers' reports also showed positive program effects for children's symptoms. Children's reports presented a more mixed picture of the effect of the program on adjustment. For several of the mediating and outcome variables, the effect of the intervention interacted with pretest levels, such that benefits were greater for those with poorest initial functioning.

The positive results of this trial contrast with those of the two previous evaluations of parent-focused interventions for children of divorce. Neither Warren *et al.* (1984) nor Stolberg and Garrison (1985) reported program effects on the proximal family environment mediating variables targeted by the program or on children's mental health outcomes. However, both studies reported positive program effects on *mother's* mental health. Differences between the current and past programs in content and delivery might help to explain the discrepant findings. First, unlike Stolberg and Garrison's program, the current program focused on changing parenting skills rather than on facilitating mother's mental health. Although Warren *et al.* also targeted parenting skills, the length of their intervention might have been insufficient to affect meaningful change. The current program involved 10 group and 2 individual sessions, providing multiple opportunities for practice and feedback. In addition, in each session, mothers discussed their use of the program skills during the previous week. Another plausible explanation for the difference involves the selection of subjects. In the current study, those potential participants who were functioning well on a subset of the targeted mediators were excluded from participation. Exclusion of this subgroup, who were unlikely to benefit from the intervention, most likely resulted in enhanced power to detect program effects (Pillow *et al.*, 1991). Support for this explanation is provided by the interactive effects that occurred for several of the mediating and outcome variables in the current trial. Finally, program fidelity might have differed across the programs. In the absence of careful process evaluation data documenting that the interventions were delivered as planned, it is not possible to rule out implementation problems as an explanation of the lack of effectiveness of the previous field trials (see Moncher & Prinz, 1991; Yeaton & Sechrest, 1981).

The program was not equally effective in changing all five of the putative mediators. Expected posttest differences occurred for both mothers' and children's reports of two of the four mediating variables on which both mothers' and children's reports were obtained: quality of the custodial parent–child relationship and negative divorce-related events. Program participants were more accepting and warm in their interactions with their children and reported fewer negative divorce-related events than did control subjects. It should be noted that the program effect for children's reports of negative divorce-related events was marginal. Expected differences occurred for mothers' but not children's reports of discipline, with program participants reporting that they were less inconsistent and less authoritarian in discipline than control subjects. Although mothers in the program reported a greater willingness to change visitation and tended to report more positive perceptions about their ex-husbands' parenting abilities, group differences in father–child contact did not occur. An unexpected effect occurred for support from nonparental adults: At posttest, children in the control group reported more support than did children in the program.

Because the process evaluation data revealed that all program components were implemented as planned, weak implementation is implausible as an explanation for the differential effectiveness of the program in changing these mediators. A more plausible explanation involves the strength of the intervention with respect to each of the mediators (Sechrest et al., 1979), as reflected in the differences in the amount of time allocated to each of the mediators. The quality of the mother–child relationship and negative divorce-related events were addressed in several sessions; the other mediators were addressed in only one or two sessions. With additional attention, positive change in other mediators might have occurred. This explanation is consistent with the results of the mediational analysis. A second explanation involves the amount of actual control mothers have over each of the putative mediators. It is reasonable to argue that mothers have greater control over the quality of the mother–child relationship, negative events, and consistency of discipline than they do over contact with fathers and support from nonparental adults. For these latter mediators, mothers may primarily serve a gatekeeping function. Programs that directly involve fathers and nonparental adults may be needed for change to occur in these mediators.

The relative intense focus on the mother–child relationship provides a possible explanation of the finding that children in the control group had more contact with nonparental adults than children in the program condition. Because of the strong focus on enhancing the mother–child relationship, children may have had less time to spend with other adults. Reflecting the success of the program in changing this component, they may have also had less need to seek support from other adults.

    The interactions of the pretest level of the variable with intervention condition that occurred for several putative mediating variables and outcome measures have both interventive and theoretical implications. These interactive effects are consistent with an emerging consensus that not all children of divorce are at risk for developing adjustment problems (Felner *et al.*, 1983, 1988; Sandler *et al.*, 1988). The success of the present program in benefiting those at highest risk speaks well for its potential to help those families in most need. The interactive findings in the context of the exclusion of 30% of the potential participants suggest that the cost effectiveness of programs for divorced families could be increased by screening out those unlikely to benefit (Pillow *et al.*, 1991). However, screening measures with adequate sensitivity and specificity need to be developed to identify families who will benefit most from the intervention (Braver, 1989; Sandler, Braver *et al.*, 1991).

    The difference in findings across reporters raises several interesting issues (see also Funder & West, 1993). One of these involves conclusions about the effectiveness of the program. Because mothers participated in the intervention and their reports of program effects were both more consistent and positive, demand characteristics might be advanced as an explanation of the findings. However, attributing the intervention effects solely to demand characteristics does not seem warranted for several reasons. First, the two other evaluations of parent programs for children of divorce (Stolberg & Garrison, 1985; Warren *et al.*, 1984) have not shown positive effects on parental reports of children's mental health. Second, children also reported positive change on some of the mediators and one of the measures of aggression. Given the relatively low correlation (.25) typically reported in the literature between parent and child reports of children's adjustment (Achenbach, McConaughy, & Howell, 1987; West *et al.*, 1991), even this partial convergence in the results can be considered to be encouraging. Third, the interviewers were kept blind to the respondent's program condition and no connection was made between the interviewer and the program leaders. The mother was also aware that her child was independently and simultaneously interviewed on similar topics, a measurement condition that minimizes bias in responding (Aiken & West, 1990). Fourth, a simple demand characteristics interpretation is inconsistent with the observed interactive effects of pretest level with program condition. A more plausible explanation of the reporter differences is that children may either be less sensitive observers of their environments than mothers or they may need longer exposure to changed conditions before reporting that changes have occurred. Preventive trials that include longitudinal assessment of program effects, ratings of the child by other knowledgeable informants such as teachers and peers, and behavioral observations of change are needed to examine these hypotheses.

   The current findings provide confirmation of one part of our small theory of processes affecting children's adjustment to divorce. As noted above, the primary focus of the intervention was on the quality of the mother–child relationship. The mediational analyses showed that the intervention positively affected the mother–child relationship, which, in turn, led to decreases in child symptoms, accounting for about 43% of the effect of the intervention on posttest child symptoms. The remaining direct effect of treatment on posttest child symptoms may reflect the sum of the non-significant, weak effects of the other four components of the intervention. Mediational analyses are very sensitive to the reliability and validity of measurement of the mediator (Baron & Kenny, 1986; Higginbotham *et al.*, 1988). Although the reliability issue can be addressed by structural equation models with latent variables, the results of such analyses can become unstable as N decreases and the number of parameters to be estimated increases (Bentler & Chou, 1988; Curran, West, & Finch, 1993). Given our relatively modest sample of 70 families in the present trial, we chose to use only manifest variable (path) models, which are far less sensitive to the problems of sample size but do not correct for unreliability in our analyses. The mother–child relationship was measured by multiple, highly reliable measures, whereas each of the other mediators was represented only by a single scale, perhaps accounting for the positive results of the former variable in the mediational analysis. Alternatively, other effects of the intervention (e.g., nonspecific treatment effects) may have contributed to the effectiveness of the intervention in reducing parent reports of child symptoms.

   There are several limitations of the current trial that need to be recognized. First, it is important to view these results as promising rather than as conclusive for several reasons including the large number of analyses that were conducted and the exclusive reliance on self-report measures. Another limitation of this trial stems from the sample size ($N = 70$). Although exact power calculations depend on the correlational structure of the data, the present design has power = .80 to detect a moderate effect ($d = .55$) in the analyses of covariance assuming the pretest–posttest correlation is .6. The power to detect the Pretest Level × Intervention interactions of the magnitude observed in this study (3–7% of the variance over and above variance accounted for by the pretest and the intervention) ranged from .50 to .70. The power of Sobel's test of indirect effects in mediational analysis is also quite low; the maximum power for the tests reported was .70. A substantially larger sample needs to be used in future trials of this parenting program to detect theoretically important smaller effects. This issue is not unique to the present trial if researchers are to be able to reliably detect small to moderate size effects: Todd and West (1993) reviewed all intervention trials published in the *Journal of Consulting and Clinical*

Psychology and the *American Journal of Community Psychology* during 1987–1991 and found that the median sample size was 60 and the semi-interval quartile range was 31. Thus, the majority of studies published in these journals included too few subjects to permit strong tests of the hypothesized effects.

The present study examined short-term effects. Follow-up data are clearly important to examine whether the program effects are maintained over time and to examine whether, with additional time, children report changes in their environments and mental health that can be attributed to intervention. Also, although the attrition rate is comparable to that in other parent-based programs for children of divorce, it is important to note that a moderate percentage of participants in both the intervention and control groups terminated involvement prior to the posttest. A careful attrition analysis did not reveal any evidence that differential attrition accounted for the observed results. However, as in any interventive trial in which attrition occurs, the possibility that differential attrition may have occurred on other unmeasured variables cannot be definitively ruled out.

Another limitation concerns the multiple foci of the current program. In this trial, we followed the strategy proposed by Sechrest *et al.* (1979) of initially testing the strongest possible multicomponent intervention. This strategy provided useful information on the overall effectiveness of the present intervention. The cost of this strategy is that we have only a limited ability to probe the contribution of each of the five components of the intervention to the outcome through mediational analyses, particularly in the present relatively small *N* design. But note that a complete examination of the additive and interactive contributions of each of the five components in a full factorial design (2^5) would require 32 conditions! Such a design is not only premature, given our current level of understanding of parent-based programs for children of divorce, but also inefficient and impractical. Further investigations are needed that include additional conditions in which one or more components have been removed from the full program package. Such dismantling (subtraction) designs in combination with mediational analyses will allow efficient further probing of the contribution of each of the components to changes in mental health outcomes (see Higginbotham *et al.*, 1988; West, Aiken, & Todd, 1993).

The promising effects of the current parent-focused study complement prior studies on child-focused interventions (Albert-Gillis *et al.*, 1989; Pedro-Carroll & Cowen, 1985; Stolberg & Garrison, 1985) to show that there are several effective approaches for improving the postdivorce adjustment of children. Important directions for future research involve replicating this parent-focused program and examining the additive effects of parent- and child-focused interventions.

ACKNOWLEDGMENTS

Support for this research was provided by the National Institute of Mental Health grant P50MH39246. The authors thank Tim Ayers, Pamela Balls-Organista, Jan Beals, Bruce Fogas, Sandra L. Harris, Paul Miller, Lisa Plaza, and Philip Poirier for their contributions to the project. We also thank the mothers and the children who participated.

REFERENCES

Achenbach, T. M. (1978). The child behavior profile: I. Boys aged 6–11. *Journal of Consulting and Clinical Psychology, 46,* 478–489.

Achenbach, T. M. & Edelbrock, C. S. (1979). The child behavior profile: II. Boys aged 12–16 and girls aged 6–11 and 12–16. *Journal of Consulting and Clinical Psychology, 47,* 223–233.

Achenbach, T. M. & Edelbrock, C. S. (1983). *Manual for the child behavior checklist and revised child behavior profile.* Burlington: University of Vermont, Department of Psychiatry.

Achenbach, T. M., McConaughy, S. H., & Howell, C. T. (1987). Child/adolescent behavioral and emotional problems: Implications of cross-informant correlations for situational specificity. *Psychological Bulletin, 101,* 213–232.

Aiken, L. S. & West, S. G. (1990). Invalidity of true experiments: Self-report pretest biases. *Evaluation Review, 14,* 374–390.

Aiken, L. S. & West, S. G. (1991). *Multiple regression: Testing and interpreting interactions.* Newbury Park, CA: Sage.

Albert-Gillis, L. J., Pedro-Carroll, J. L., & Cowen, E. L. (1989). The children of divorce intervention program: Development, implementation, and evaluation of a program for young urban children. *Journal of Consulting and Clinical Psychology, 57,* 583–589.

Amato, P. R. & Keith, B. (1991). Parental divorce and the well-being of children: A meta-analysis. *Psychological Bulletin, 110,* 26–46.

American Psychiatric Association. (1987). *Diagnostic and statistical manual of mental disorders* (3rd ed., rev.). Washington, DC: Author.

Armistead, L., McCombs, A., Forehand, R., Wierson, M., Long, N., & Fauber, R. (1990). Coping with divorce: A study of young adolescents. *Journal of Clinical Child Psychology, 19,* 79–84.

Baldwin, D. V. & Skinner, M. L. (1989). Structural model for anti-social behavior: Generalization to single-mother families. *Developmental Psychology, 25,* 45–50.

Barnes, H. & Olson, D. H. (1982). Parent–Adolescent Communication Scale. In D. H. Olson, H. I. McCubbin, H. Barnes, A. Larsen, M. Muxen, & M. Wilson (Eds.), *Family Inventories, Inventories used in a National Survey of Family Life Cycle* (pp. 33–48). St. Paul: Family Social Science, University of Minnesota.

Baron, R. M. & Kenny, D. A. (1986). The moderator–mediator distinction in social psychological research: Conceptual, strategic, and statistical considerations. *Journal of Personality and Social Psychology, 51,* 1173–1182.

Bentler, P. M. & Chou, C. P. (1988). Practical issues in structural modeling. In J. S. Long (Ed.), *Common problems/proper solutions: Avoiding error in quantitative research* (pp. 161–192). Newbury Park, CA: Sage.

Braver, S. L. (1989). *Selection issues in children of divorce preventive intervention.* Section of NIMH Grant MH39246 to establish The Center for the Prevention of Child and Family Stress at Arizona State University, Tempe.

Burbach, D. J., Farha, J. G., & Thorpe, J. S. (1986). Assessing depression in community samples of children using self-report inventories: Ethical considerations. *Journal of Abnormal Child Psychology, 14*, 579–589.

Coie, J. D., Watt, N., West, S. G., Hawkins, D., Asarnow, J., Markman, H., Ramey, S., Shure, M., & Long, B. (1993). The science of prevention: A conceptual framework and some directions for a national research program. *American Psychologist, 48,* 1013–1022.

Cook, C. (1985). *The Youth Self Report Hostility Scale.* Unpublished manuscript, Arizona State University, Program for Prevention Research, Tempe.

Cook, T. D. (1985). Post-positivist critical multiplism. In L. Shetland & M. M. Mark (Eds.), *Social science and social policy* (pp. 21–62). Beverly Hills, CA: Sage.

Cronbach, L. J. (1951). Coefficient alpha and the internal structure of tests. *Psychometrika, 16*, 297–334.

Curran, P. J., West, S. G., & Finch, J. F. (1993). *The robustness of test statistics and goodness-of-fit indices in confirmatory factor analysis.* Manuscript submitted for publication, Department of Psychology, Arizona State University, Tempe.

Dohrenwend, B. P., Shrout, P. E., Egri, G., & Mendelsohn, F. (1980). Nonspecific psychological distress and other dimensions of psychopathology. *Archives of General Psychiatry, 37*, 1229–1236.

Emery, R. E. & O'Leary, K. D. (1982). Children's perceptions of marital discord and behavior problems of boys and girls. *Journal of Abnormal Child Psychology, 10*, 11–24.

Felner, R. D., Farber, S. S., & Primavera, J. (1983). Transitions and stressful life events: A model for primary prevention. In R. D. Felner, L. A. Jason, J. N. Moritsugu, & S. S. Farber (Eds.), *Preventive psychology: Theory, research, and practice.* New York: Pergamon.

Felner, R. D., Rowlinson, R., & Terre, L. (1986). Unraveling the Gordian knot in life change events: A critical examination of crisis, stress, and transitional frameworks for prevention. In S. M. Auerbach & A. L. Stolberg (Eds.), *Children's life crisis events: Preventive intervention strategies* (pp. 39–63). New York: Hemisphere/McGraw-Hill.

Felner, R. D., Stolberg, A., & Cowen, E. L. (1975). Crisis events and school mental health referral patterns of young children. *Journal of Consulting and Clinical Psychology, 43*, 305–310.

Felner, R. D., Terre, L., & Rowlinson, R. T. (1988). A life transition framework for understanding marital dissolution and family reorganization. In S. A. Wolchik & P. Karoly (Eds.), *Children of divorce: Empirical perspectives on adjustment* (pp. 35–65). New York: Gardner.

Finch, J. F. & West, S. G. (1997). The investigation of personality structure: Statistical models. *Journal of Research in Personality, 31*, 439–485.

Finch, A. J., Saylor, C. F., Edwards, G. L., & McIntosh, J. A. (1987). Children's Depression Inventory: Reliability over repeated administrations. *Journal of Consulting and Clinical Psychology, 55*, 339–341.

Fogas, B. S., Wolchik, S. A., & Braver, S. L. (1987, August) *Parenting behavior and Psychopathology in children of divorce: Buffering effects.* Paper presented at the meeting of the American Psychological Association, New York.

Fogas, B. S., Wolchik, S. A., Braver, S. L., Freedom, D. S., & Bay, R. C. (1992). Beliefs about locus of control as a mediator of negative divorce-related events. *American Journal of Orthopsychiatry, 62*, 589–598.

Forehand, R. & McMahon, R. J. (1981). *Helping the noncompliant child: A clinician's guide to parent teaching.* New York: Guilford.

Fox, J. (1991). *Regression diagnostics.* Newbury Park, CA: Sage.

Funder, D. C. & West, S. G. (Eds.). (1993). Viewpoints on personality: Consensus, self-other agreement, and accuracy in judgments of personality [Special issue]. *Journal of Personality, 61*(4).

Gersten, J., Beats, J., & Kallgren, K. (1991). Epidemiological and preventive interventions: Parental death in childhood as a case example. *American Journal of Community Psychology, 19*, 481–500.

Glick, P. C. (1988). The role of divorce in the changing family structure: Trends and variations. In S. A. Wolchik & P. Karoly (Eds.), *Children of Divorce: Empirical Perspectives on Adjustment.* New York: Gardner.

Grych, J. H. & Finchman, F. F. (1992). Interventions for children of divorce: Toward greater integration of research and action. *Psychological Bulletin, 111*, 434–454.

Guerney, B. G. (1977). *Relationship enhancement: Skill-training programs for therapy, problem prevention, and enrichment.* San Francisco: Jossey-Bass.

Guidubaldi, J. & Cleminshaw, H. (1983, August). *Impact of family support system on children's academic and social functioning after parental divorce.* Paper presented at the meeting of the American Psychological Association, Anaheim, CA.

Guidubaldi, J., Cleminshaw, H. K., Perry, J. D., & Mcloughlin, C. S. (1983). The impact of parental divorce on children: Report of the nationwide NASP study. *School Psychology Review, 12*, 300–323.

Guidubaldi, J., Cleminshaw, H. K., Perry, J. D., Nastas, B. K., & Lightel, J. (1986). The role of selected family environment factors in children's post-divorce adjustment. *Family Relations, 35*, 141–151.

Hetherington, E. M., Cox, M., & Cox, R. (1978). The aftermath of divorce. In J. H. Stevens, Jr. & M. Matthews (Eds.), *Mother–child, father–child relations* (pp. 149–176). Washington, DC: NAEYC.

Hetherington, E. M., Cox, M., & Cox, R. (1981). Effects of divorce on parents and children. In M. Lamb (Ed.), *Nontraditional families* (pp. 233–288). Hillsdale, NJ: Erlbaum.

Higginbotham, H. N., West, S. G., & Forsyth, D. R. (1988). *Psychotherapy and behavior change: Social, cultural and methodological perspectives.* New York: Pergamon.

Hodges, K., Kline, J., Stern, L., Cytryn, L., & McKnew, D. (1982). The development of a child assessment interview for research and clinical use. *Journal of Abnormal Child Psychology, 10*, 173–189.

Huitema, B. (1980). *The analysis of covariance and alternatives.* New York: Wiley.

James, L. R. & Brett, J. M. (1984). Mediators, moderators, and tests for mediation. *Journal of Applied Psychology, 69*, 307–321.

Jensen, E. W., James, S. A., Boyce, T., & Hartnett, S. A. (1983). The Family Routines Inventory: Development and validation. *Social Science Medicine, 17*, 201–211.

Johnson, P. O. & Neyman, J. (1936). Test of certain linear hypotheses and their applications to some educational problems. *Statistical Research Memoirs, 1*, 57–93.

Judd, C. M. & Kenny, D. A. (1981). *Estimating the effects of social interventions.* New York: Cambridge University Press.

Jurs, S. G. & Glass, G. V. (1971). The effect of experimental mortality on the internal and external validity of the randomized comparative experiment. *Journal of Experimental Education, 40*, 62–66.

Kovacs, M. (1981). Rating scales to assess depression in school-aged children. *Acta Paedopsychiatrica, 46*, 305–315.

Kovacs, M. (1985). The Children's Depression Inventory (CDI). *Psychopharmacology Bulletin, 21*, 995–999.

Kurdek, L. A. & Berg, B. (1987). Children's beliefs about parental divorce scale: Psychometric characteristics and concurrent validity. *Journal of Consulting and Clinical Psychology, 55*, 712–718.

Kurdek, L. A. & Berg, B. (1983). Correlates of children's adjustment to their parents' divorce. In L. A. Kurdek (Ed.), *New directions in child development: Children and divorce* (pp. 47–60). San Francisco: Jossey-Bass.

Kurdek, L. A., Blisk, D., & Siesky, A. E. Jr. (1981). Correlates of children's long-term adjustment to their parents' divorce. *Developmental Psychology, 17,* 565–579.

Kurdek, L. A. & Sinclair, R. J. (1988). Relation of eighth graders' family structure, gender, and family environment with academic performance and school behavior. *Journal of Educational Psychology, 80,* 90–94.

Lipsey, M. W. (1990). Theory as method: Small theories of treatments. In L. Sechrest, E. Perrin, & J. Bunker (Eds.), *Research methodology: Strengthening causal interpretations of nonexperimental data* (pp. 33–51) (DHHS Publication No. 90-3454). Washington, DC: U.S. Government Printing Office.

Lobovits, D. A. & Handal, P. J. (1985). Childhood depression: Prevalence using DSM-III criteria and validity of parent and child depression scales. *Journal of Pediatric Psychology, 10,* 45–54.

Long, N., Forehand, R., Fauber, R., & Brody, G. (1987). Self-perceived and independently observed competence of young adolescents as a function of parental marital conflict and recent divorce. *Journal of Abnormal Child Psychology, 15,* 15–27.

Lorion, R. P. (1985a). Environmental approaches to prevention: The dangers of imprecision. *Prevention in Human Services, 4,* 193–205.

Lorion, R. P. (1985b). Evaluating preventive interventions: Guidelines for the serious social change agent. In R. D. Felner, L. Jason, J. Moritsugu, & S. S. Farber (Eds.), *Preventive Psychology: Theory, research, and practice in community intervention* (pp. 252–272). New York: Pergamon.

Lorion, R. P., Price, R. H., & Eaton, W. W. (1989). The prevention of child and adolescent disorders: From theory to research. In D. Shaffer & I. Phillips (Eds.), *Project prevention.* Washington, DC: American Academy of Child and Adolescent Psychiatry.

Mazur, E., Wolchik, S. A., & Sandler, I. N. (1992). Negative cognitive errors and positive illusions for negative events: Predictors of children's psychological adjustment. *Journal of Abnormal Child Psychology, 20,* 523–541.

Moncher, F. J. & Prinz, R. J. (1991). Treatment fidelity in outcome studies. *Clinical Psychology Review, 11,* 247–266.

Moos, R. H. (1974). *The social climate scales: An overview.* Palo Alto, CA: Consulting Psychologists Press.

Moos, R. & Moos, B. (1981). *Family Environment Scale Manual.* Palo Alto, CA: Consulting Psychologists Press.

Novaco, R. A. (1975). *Anger control: The development and evaluation of an experimental treatment.* Lexington, MA: D.C. Heath.

Orne, M. (1962). On the social psychology of the psychological experiment. *American Psychologist, 17,* 776–783.

Parish, T. & Wigle, S. (1985). A longitudinal study of the impact of divorce on adolescents' evaluation of self and parents. *Adolescence, 20,* 239–244.

Patterson, G. R. (1975). *Families: Applications of social learning to family life.* Champaign, IL: Research Press.

Pedro-Carroll, J. L. & Cowen, E. L. (1985). The children of divorce intervention project: An investigation of the efficacy of a school-based prevention program. *Journal of Consulting and Clinical Psychology, 53,* 603–611.

Pedro-Carroll, J. L., Cowen, E. L., Hightower, A. D., & Guare, J. C. (1986). Preventive intervention with latency-aged children of divorce: A replication study. *American Journal of Community Psychology, 14,* 277–290.

Pillow, D. R., Sandler, I., Braver, S., Wolchik, S., & Gersten, J. C. (1991). Theory-based screening for prevention: Focusing on mediating processes in children of divorce. *American Journal of Community Psychology, 19,* 809–836.

Porter, B. & O'Leary, K. D. (1980). Marital discord and childhood behavior problems. *Journal of Abnormal Child Psychology, 8,* 287–295.

Price, R. H. (1982, February). *Four domains of prevention research.* Paper presented to the National Institute of Mental Health Conference on Prevention Research, Austin, TX.

Reynolds, C. R. (1982). Convergent and divergent validity of the Revised Children's Manifest Anxiety Scale. *Educational and psychological Measurement, 42,* 1205–1212.

Reynolds, C. R. & Richmond, B. O. (1978). What I think and feel: A revised measure of children's manifest anxiety. *Journal of Abnormal Child Psychology, 6,* 271–280.

Roosa, M. W. & Beats, J. (1990). Measurement issues in family assessment: The case of the Family Environment Scale. *Family Process, 29,* 191–198.

Sandler, I. N., Braver, S. L., Wolchik, S. A., Pillow, D. R., & Gersten, J. C. (1991). Small theory and the strategic choices of prevention research. *American Journal of Community Psychology, 19,* 873–880.

Sandler, I. N., Gersten, J. C., Reynolds, K., Kallgren, C., & Ramirez, R. (1988). Using theory and data to plan support interventions: Design of a program for bereaved children. In B. Gottleib (Ed.), *Marshalling social support: Formats, processes, and effects* (pp. 53–83). Beverly Hills, CA: Sage.

Sandler, I. N. & Guenther, R. R. (1985). Assessment of life stress events. In P. Karoly (Ed.), *Measurement strategies in health psychology* (pp. 555–600). New York: Wiley.

Sandler, I. N., Tein, J., & West, S. G. (1994). Coping, stress and the psychological symptoms of children of divorce: A cross-sectional and longitudinal study. *Child Development, 65,* 1744–1763.

Sandler, I. N., Wolchik, S. A., Braver S. L., & Fogas, B. S. (1991). Stability and quality of life events and psychological symptomatology in children of divorce. *American Journal of Community Psychology, 19,* 501–520.

Santrock, J. W. & Warshak, R. (1979). Father custody and social development in boys and girls. *Journal of Social Issues, 35,* 112–125.

Saylor, C. F., Finch, A. J., Spirito, A., & Bennett, B. (1984). The Children's Depression Inventory: Systematic evaluation of psychometric properties. *Journal of Consulting and Clinical Psychology, 52,* 955–967.

Schaefer, E. S. (1965). Children's report of parental behavior: An inventory. *Child Development, 36,* 413–424.

Sechrest, L., West, S. G., Phillips, M. A., Redner, R., & Yeaton, W. (1979). Some neglected problems in evaluation research: Strength and integrity of treatments. In L. Sechrest and Associates (Eds.), *Evaluation studies review annual* (Vol. 4, pp. 15–35). Beverly Hills, CA: Sage.

Sobel, M. E. (1982). Asymptotatic confidence intervals for indirect effects in structural equation models. In S. Leinhardt (Ed.), *Sociological methodology 1982* (pp. 290–293). Washington, DC: American Sociological Association.

Sobel, M. E. (1986). Some new results on indirect effects and their standard errors in covariance structure models. In N. Tuma (Ed.), *Sociological methodology 1986* (pp. 159–186). Washington, DC: American Sociological Association.

Stolberg, A. L. & Anker, J. M. (1984). Cognitive and behavioral changes in children resulting from parental divorce and consequent environmental changes. *Journal of Divorce, 7,* 23–41.

Stolberg, A. L. & Bush, J. P. (1985). A path analysis of factors predicting children's divorce adjustment. *Journal of Clinical Child Psychology, 14,* 49–54.

Stolberg, A. L. & Garrison, K. M. (1985). Evaluating a primary prevention program for children of divorce. *American Journal of Community Psychology, 13,* 111–124.

Todd, M. & West. S. G. (1993). Methodological review of intervention evaluations published in *Journal of Consulting and Clinical Psychology* and the *American Journal of*

Community Psychology, 1987–1991. Unpublished manuscript, Arizona State University, Tempe.

U.S. National Center for Health Statistics. (1991). Monthly vital statistics report, *39* (No. 12), Advance report of final divorce statistics 1988. Washington, DC: U.S. Government Printing Office.

Vernon, S. W. & Roberts, R. E. (1991). Measuring nonspecific psychological distress and other dimensions of psychopathology. *Archives of General Psychiatry, 38,* 1239–1247.

Vital Statistics Report. (1987, December). National Center for Health Statistics, U.S. Department of Health and Human Services, *36* (No. 8, Suppl.).

Warren, N. J., Grew, R. S., Ilgen, E. L., Konanc, J. T., Bourgoondien, M. E., & Amara, I. A. (1984). *Parenting after divorce: Preventive programs for divorcing families.* Paper presented at the meeting of the National Institute of Mental Health, Washington, DC.

West, S. G. (1990, August). Structural modeling of variables mediating symptomatology for children of divorce. In I. N. Sandler (Chair), *Prevention research with children of divorce: Both theory and action.* Symposium presented at the meeting of the American Psychological Association, Boston, MA.

West, S. G., Aiken, L. S., & Todd, M. (1993). Probing the effects of individual components in multiple component prevention programs. *American Journal of Community Psychology, 21,* 571–605.

West, S. G., Sandler, I., Pillow, D. R., Baca, L., & Gersten, J. C. (1991). The use of structural equation modeling in generative research: Toward the design of a preventive intervention for bereaved children. *American Journal of Community Psychology, 19,* 459–480.

Winer, B. J. (1971). *Statistical principles in experimental design.* New York: McGraw-Hill.

Wolchik, S. A., Ramirez, R., Sandler, I. N., Fisher, J., Balls, P., & Brown, C. (1992). Inner-city poor children of divorce: Negative divorce-related events, problematic beliefs and adjustment problems. *Journal of Divorce, 19,* 1–20.

Wolchik, S. A, Ruehlman, L. S., Braver, S. L., & Sandler, I. N. (1989). Social support of children of divorce: Direct and stress buffer effects. *American Journal of Community Psychology, 17,* 485–501.

Wyman, P. A., Cowen, E. L., Hightower, A. D., & Pedro-Carroll, J. L. (1985). Perceived competence, self-esteem, and anxiety in latency aged children of divorce. *Journal of Clinical Child Psychology, 14,* 20–26.

Yeaton, W. H. & Sechrest, L. (1981). Critical dimensions in the choice and maintenance of successful treatments: Strength, integrity, and effectiveness. *Journal of Consulting and Clinical Psychology, 49,* 156–167.

Zill, N. (1983). *Happy, healthy, & insecure: A portrait of middle childhood in America.* Garden City, NY: Doubleday.

21

The Enhancement of Psychological Wellness: Challenges and Opportunities

Emory L. Cowen

Developed the concept of psychological wellness and made the case that proportionally more resources should be directed to the pursuit of this goal. Five pathways to wellness are considered, implicating aspects of individual development and the impact of contexts, settings, and policies. The five pathways are: forming wholesome early attachments; acquiring age- and ability-appropriate competencies; engineering settings that promote adaptive outcomes; fostering empowerment; and acquiring skills needed to cope effectively with life stressors. Although these noncompeting pathways have differential salience at different ages and for different groups and life conditions, each is an essential element in any comprehensive social plan to advance wellness. Examples of effective programs are cited in all five areas, including recent comprehensive, long-term programs embodying multiple pathways to wellness.

Since its very beginnings, mental health's focus and efforts have centered fixedly around (a) things that go wrong psychologically (i.e., psychopathology); (b) attempts to understand the processes by which they go wrong (pathogenesis); and (c) seeking better ways to repair things that have

Originally published in the *American Journal of Community Psychology*, 22(2) (1994): 149–179.

A Quarter Century of Community Psychology: Readings from the American Journal of Community Psychology, edited by Tracey A. Revenson *et al.* Kluwer Academic/Plenum Publishers, New York, 2002.

already gone wrong (e.g., psychotherapy). Historically, such efforts have overshadowed by far the fleeting glimpses the field has accorded to an intriguing, but directionally opposite, set of issues: What goes *right* in psychological development and adjustment, and what forces subserve such outcomes?

Mental health's focus on the pathological is reflected in its vocabulary as well as its orientation and activities. Illustratively, Hollister (1967) reported Margaret Mead's observation that although the English language had the word trauma to describe "an unfortunate blow that injures the personality," it had no word to describe an experience that strengthened personality. He proposed the word "stren" to fill that void. And, for a short while at least, that concept provided an impetus for fruitful research (Finkel, 1974; 1975). A related example: Antonovsky (1979), whose work in medical sociology focused on relationships between stressors and disease outcomes, noted that although our language had a word to describe the processes by which diseases unfold (i.e., pathogenesis), there was no parallel word to describe processes that favor healthy outcomes. He coined the word *salutogenesis* to spotlight the existence of such health-promoting processes and to direct attention to new, proactive challenges for medical sociology built around the question: "What makes for *health*, not disease?"

It is somewhat ironic that society holds much clearer views of failings in wellness than it does of wellness. Those views have long shaped mental health's de facto mandate (i.e., to repair) and derivative activities (Zax & Cowen, 1976). Efforts to repair established psychological dysfunction however, are difficult, costly, and often end in failure. The source of such failure may reside more in the refractory nature of presenting problems (i.e., the "point of address") than laxity in the field's search for effective ways to undo rooted psychological problems. To the contrary, the tenacity of that search over many decades has spawned complex multilevel "industries" (e.g., medications, psychotherapy, clinics, intensive-care facilities) dedicated to containing or minimizing psychological dysfunction. Indeed, the rising costs of such efforts (Kiesler, 1992; Kiesler, Simpkins, & Morton, 1989) and, at another level, the misery and waste of potential that human dysfunction entails, are among the pressing realities that fuel consideration of wellness-oriented prevention alternatives.

The orienting concept of psychological wellness directs attention to new conceptual formulations and derivative phenomena of interest (Jessor, 1993; Rappaport, 1987) that differ sharply from those that now guide the mental health fields. Historically, mental health professionals have been type-cast as "guardians" of wellness, with the term guardian defined narrowly as society's sanctioned repair agents for deficits in wellness. That role is an understandable outgrowth of the field's long-standing, dominant, "fight-pathology"-orientation. And, if professional involvements are to begin only after evident dysfunction presents itself, then the main options available are to repair wounds and forestall further erosion. That, at least, is how most mental health professionals have been trained and socialized, and that is the main arena in which their efforts and expertise have focused.

In a wellness framework, however, that classic role is limited to one small segment of a much more complex and temporally extended scenario. Although proactive and repair approaches may share a common view of ideal wellness outcomes, working to promote such outcomes from the start involves different concepts, target groups, and activities than restorative, or balming, efforts that begin only after clear signs of wellness erosion have appeared.

Mental health's historic emphasis on seeking to understand and undo crystallized pathology has left a residue of unresolved problems. The inability of a field to deal satisfactorily with major problems within its purview stimulates efforts to identify qualitatively different solutions to those problems. When the latter process reaches a certain point of cohesive evolution, it is called paradigm shift (Kuhn, 1970). Baldly put, the current mental health system is reactive, not proactive! Its time, efforts, and resources are allocated to visible, deeply rooted, change-resistant problems. Known limitations of this system raise the salience of a conceptually appealing alternative, that is, systematic effort to promote wellness from the start may prove to be a more humane, cost-effective, and successful strategy than struggling, however valiantly and compassionately, to undo established deficits in wellness.

The main goal of this article is to develop the preceding thesis. We first consider the nature of the terms wellness and wellness enhancement, how they differ from existing concepts and what can be gained from their usage. Next, basic pathways to wellness are described and examples of effective programs reflecting these strategies are cited. A final section summarizes the argument and suggests directions for future work within a wellness enhancement framework.

THE CONCEPT OF PSYCHOLOGICAL WELLNESS AND ITS UTILITY

Although the concept of psychological wellness has kindred predecessors (e.g., Antonovsky, 1979; Jahoda, 1958; Shoben, 1957), it has, for reasons noted above, recently come into clearer focus and more active usage (Cowen, 1991). It is not, however, a term that defines itself automatically or easily. For one thing, built into any definition of wellness (or, for that matter, sickness) are overt and covert expressions of values. Because values differ across cultures as well as among subgroups (and indeed individuals) within a culture, the ideal of a uniformly acceptable definition of the construct is illusory. Yet, because the concept is important both in its own right and as an orienting counterpoint to the yoke imposed by past dominant notions of pathology in mental health, it may be useful to underscore some of its definitional features that many people would value positively. These elements include (a) *behavioral* markers, such as eating, sleeping, and working well (mindful of Freud's simple notion of adaptation: "*Leben und Arbeiten*"), having effective interpersonal relationships, and mastering age- and ability-appropriate tasks; and (b) *psychological* markers, such as having a sense of belongingness and purpose, control over one's fate, and satisfaction with oneself and one's existence. It has also been suggested that there are *physiological* markers of wellness (Shedler, Mayman, & Manis, 1993).

I make no case for the sanctity of the specific outcome terms used to frame this contour definition of psychological wellness. Others with interest in wellness outcomes have used different, albeit conceptually kindred, designators such as gratification in living (Rappaport, 1981), life-satisfaction (Rappaport, 1987), sense of efficacy (Bandura, 1977; Crick & Dodge, 1994), and sense of coherence (Antonovsky, 1979). I also recognize that the literal operations that define these outcomes may vary some for different age groups and subcultures. Finally, my use of the term psychological wellness is not intended to convey the image of an etched in granite, immutable state. To the contrary, I believe it much more realistic to see wellness in more-or-less terms and as susceptible to buffeting and (some) change with changing circumstances.

Even so, I would argue that the "ideal" (value?) of wellness as depicted above pervades major segments of our culture including its mental health system and, thus, importantly shapes outcome objectives for diverse natural and interventive processess (e.g., child development, psychotherapy, primary prevention). So put, the mere use of the term wellness should not be seen as "boat-rocking." On the other hand, it is fair to ask how the proposed usage of the terms wellness and wellness enhancement is intended to differ from existing concepts and, importantly, what can be gained from such usage. Answering these questions requires consideration of two more specific issues: (a) continuity versus discontinuity in adjustment; and (b) usage distinctions between wellness enhancement and a currently better known (related) concept, that is, primary prevention in mental health.

The term wellness, as used here, is intended to anchor one end of a hypothetical continuum, anchored at the other end by an opposing term such as pathology (sickness). The preceding sentence seeks to highlight two points: (a) wellness should indeed be seen as an extreme point on a continuum, *not* as a category in a binary classification system; and (b) wellness is something more than/other than the absence of disease, that is, it is defined by the "extent of presence" of positive marker characteristics such as those cited above. And, for that reason, many people who fall well short of being glaring psychological casualties also fail to approach a predominant state of wellness. The two preceding points suggest that the ideal of wellness, and the goal of wellness enhancement, pertain to *all* people, not just to a limited or select portion of the population.

The preceding argument provides a base on which to consider similarities and differences between wellness enhancement and primary prevention. One key commonality is that both strategies share the abstract goal of maximizing positive (adaptive) outcomes. But for whom, and how? The latter question is to suggest that, depending on one's definitional druthers, the two strategies may differ in targeting, timing, and methodology. The Rosetta Stone in this case pivots around one's definition of primary prevention—a concept to which I have long been warmly cathected (e.g., Cowen, 1973, 1977, 1980, 1983, 1985, 1986). My initial mind's eye notion of this concept (which, I confess, remains today) featured *two* key components: (a) forestalling dysfunction (maladaptation), including in situations of known risk; and (b) promoting psychological health and well-being (Cowen, 1973). I have always seen this second element as very important.

Although these two strands continue to be acknowledged intellectually, they have not followed parallel courses. Indeed there has been a strong trend in influential quarters to define primary prevention, de facto, as disease prevention and for such a definition to guide the allocation of program and research monies. Illustratively, Dinges (1994) noted that less than 2% of the items in a new primary prevention bibliography (Trickett, Dahiyat, & Selby, 1994) focused on promotion (wellness enhancement) as opposed to disease prevention. More specifically, Koretz (1991), in a special number describing the activities of NIMH-sponsored Preventive Intervention Research Centers (PIRCs), identified as a prime objective for their work: "the prevention of specific disorders and dysfunctions." Similarly, Coie *et al.* (1993) proposed a "science of prevention" built around the overarching goal of forestalling specific "serious problems of human adaptation," for example, major mental illness, substance abuse, delinquency. In stating explicitly that "the goal of prevention science is to prevent or moderate major human dysfunctions," (p. 1013). Coie *et al.* imply that prevention efforts should be directed to those at known risk for specific maladaptive outcomes that one hopes to avert. A similar definitional emphasis shaped the focus of Mrazek and Haggerty's (1994) important compendium summarizing a spectrum of interventions designed to prevent specific mental disorders.

Because definitions are definitions, there is no basis for challenging the legitimacy of a pathology-reduction definition of primary prevention. Such a definition has, in fact, already (a) achieved considerable ascendancy in the field; and (b) spawned major national initiatives designed to prevent specific dysfunctions (e.g., depression, substance abuse, and conduct disorders in children). Hence, it is more fruitful to ask what such a definition *ex*cludes, and what might be gained by addressing those exclusions. The case made here is that a disease prevention definition of primary prevention, based on binary views of risk versus non-risk on the antecedent side, and health versus pathology on the outcome side, excludes most people. Moreover, by not centrally featuring proactive, health-building initiatives it may deflect attention from a potentially more utilitarian population-oriented outcome, that is, wellness in the many.

The wellness concept proposed here is thus broader in scope and farther reaching than current, widely espoused disease prevention concepts of primary prevention. This broader usage reflects the assumptions that (a) sound early wellness formation may, itself, be among the best possible inoculants against a range of adverse later outcomes—a view consistent with findings reported in several recent reviews (Yoshikawa, 1994; Zigler, Taussig, & Black, 1992); and (b) all people, not just those at risk, stand to profit from wellness enhancement steps. This second point, which flows naturally from a more continuous view of adaptation than is conveyed by dichotomies such as healthy–sick or risk–not at risk, suggests that wellness enhancement goals can be gainfully pursued all along a risk continuum.

Thus, the relationship between the term wellness enhancement and current risk-anchored definitions of primary prevention is *not* transitive. The former term includes, but is not limited to, primary prevention approaches (Cowen, 1994). Otherwise put, although most primary prevention goals and activities fit neatly within a wellness enhancement framework, they do not exhaust that framework. Within the latter matrix, psychological wellness is the overarching goal and the term wellness enhancement is used to describe a family of strategies for advancing that goal. Those strategies are considered in the next section.

RELEVANT PATHWAYS TO WELLNESS

At least five major input strands can act alone or in combination to enhance, or pose threats to, psychological wellness. These five strands reflecting individual, environmental, and stress-related sources differ with respect to (a) when, temporally, they are most relevant; (b) their modifiability; and (c) the specific steps needed for constructive modification to occur. We shall consider these five strands in a roughly developmental sequence, starting with two that are especially important in infancy and childhood (i.e., wholesome attachment formation, and the development of age- and ability-appropriate competencies).

The human infant develops slowly through a long dependency period that unfolds within a family microstructure. Key wellness-relevant outcomes in this period are shaped by the nature of the attachment relationship that forms between the infant and its primary caregiver (Ainsworth, 1989; Bowlby, 1982). This relationship is defined by the love and nurturance the caregiver communicates to the child, her sensitivity and responsiveness to the child's needs, and her availabity as a predictable source of comfort and support. A warm, secure early attachment is a vital early force that favors wellness. It promotes a view of self in the infant as loved and worthwhile, and as living in a safe, protected world. The absence of a secure attachment poses a direct threat to wellness both proximally and by restricting the formation of a solid base on which later wellness enhancing steps can rest. Although recent extensions of attachment theory (Ainsworth, 1989) highlight the importance of attachment relationships throughout childhood and adolescence, the form of this relationship must change to reflect ongoing processes of growth and development in the child. The caregiver's early essential role as "protector," for example, must gradually yield place to fostering the child's autonomous development and age-appropriate independence. Moreover, love and caring, which remain central to the construct throughout, must take on different forms of expression and involvement as the child matures.

Although there is a tendency to see the early attachment relationship as a relatively pure source of influence on psychological wellness, both physically and psychologically harsh living conditions can restrict opportunities for wholesome attachments to form (McLoyd, 1990). On the other hand, because the attachment relationship is bounded by caregiver–child interactions, and much is known about its attributes, it is in principle more amenable to constructive change than other more complexly rooted, less "controllable" input strands to wellness.

Beyond the crucial attachment pathway, another wellness-related task of childhood is to acquire age-appropriate cognitive and interpersonal skills. Some of these develop directly from the base of a sound attachment relationship; others grow out of learning experiences that take place in the two main contexts of a child's formative years (i.e., home and school). Several taxonomies of key early competencies have been proposed (Anderson & Messick, 1974; Strayhorn, 1988). Strayhorn's comprehensive list of 62 such skills reflects nine clusters (e.g., relationship building, handling frustration, cognitive processing) most of which are formed in the preschool years. Although Strayhorn developed this taxonomy and an associated assessment system in the context of therapy (i.e., repairing *deficits* in competence development), his framework offers a rich matrix within which to view proactively the essentials of early childhood competence development.

Thus, forming and maintaining wholesome attachment relationships and acquiring age-appropriate competencies are central pathways toward psychological wellness in the early years—important both in their own right and in terms of "setting the table" for what follows (Rutter, 1990). Successful early negotiation of these steps roots in the child a sense of efficacy, that is the belief that they can handle life's pressures and demands and, with that, a phenomenological sense of empowerment. Conversely, it is difficult to imagine how wholesome early growth toward wellness can occur without essential nutrients from the home and school soils in which the children form and the ongoing processes of child-rearing and education that are indigenous to those soils. The latter crucial shaping forces can be strengthened as generative knowledge cumulates about relationships between their defining features and wellness outcomes in children. Recognizing this point, Sarason (1993a, 1993b) argued cogently the key proactive role that education must play in wellness enhancement. Early efforts to build wellness, such as those noted, seem more compassionate and promising as *social* alternatives than struggling later to undo established deficit known to exact heavy human and societal tolls.

Whereas the wellness routes thus far considered unfold primarily around the development of individual children in family contexts, two other key routes, closer perhaps to community psychology's turf, highlight aspects of the social milieus in which people develop: (a) creating settings and social environments that favor wellness; and (b) promoting empowering conditions that offer people justice, hope, and opportunity. Although these routes are not *un*related to wellness in early childhood (e.g., their absence may limit wholesome attachment and competence development), they become more salient later because of the greater number and complexity of the systems (e.g., employment, justice) in which people interact, and the growing relevance of these systems to psychological wellness.

Influential social environments are those in which people have major interactions over long periods. Such environments have impact at different times. Whereas family and school are crucial shaping environments in the early years (Eccles *et al.*, 1993), churches, worksites, and social and community agencies take on growing significance later. Within each setting category, specific exemplars are alike in that they share a common mandate, yet different because such broad mandates (e.g., imparting knowledge) can be discharged in many different ways. Class environments, for example, can be autonomy-supportive or controlling; they can promote or discourage affiliation (Deci & Ryan, 1985; Moos, 1979). Precisely for that reason it has been argued that the school's impact comes not just from the academic learnings it provides, but importantly from a steady, if unobtrusive, stream of "affective lessons, taught through the functional dynamics of human relationships" (Ryan & Stiller, 1991, p. 1116). Those "lessons," which shape such outcomes as appropriate behaviors, friendship formation, cooperation, and competition differ appreciably across schools (Gump, 1980; Ryan & Stiller, 1991; Weinstein, 1991). Thus, while acting intentionally to discharge their mandate, settings often operate unintentionally in ways that enhance or restrict wellness (Sarason, 1993a). This raises several wellness-relevant questions: What are the different ways, structurally, in which settings can pursue their mandates? What relationships exist between these ways and wellness outcomes for setting inhabitants? Finding that differently operating settings are equally effective in realizing mandated objectives, but yield different wellness outcomes, would point to system change steps designed to enhance wellness.

The concept of empowerment, that is, gaining control over and making critical decisions about one's life (Rappaport, 1981, 1984, 1987; Swift, 1992) has attracted growing interest in many contexts as an important pathway to wellness. This development is fueled by the undeniable presence of many disempowered groups in modern society (e.g., minorities, poor people, children, the elderly, the homeless, disabled people) and the painful awareness of striking associations between disempowerment and problems of living. Empowerment theorists (Rappaport, 1981) argue that people benefit psychologically, that is, have greater gratification in living, when they gain control over their lives. Within an overall wellness framework, empowerment issues are most salient and compelling when focusing on the devastating correlates and costly sequelae of society's most floridly disempowering conditions. Albee (1982) cited racial, ethnic, age- and gender-related biases as among the most damaging of such conditions.

Empowerment notions have applicability at many levels ranging from the functioning of groups or settings to broad macrosocial realities (Rappaport, Swift, & Hess, 1984). Some of these contexts are more amenable to change than others. Unfortunately, the most influential ones are so complex and deeply rooted that they may at best change only slowly over generations. Hence, some (societal) empowerment strategies may be more difficult to bring off, certainly in the short term, than attachment or competence promotion strategies.

The pathways to wellness thus far considered have age- and situation-specific linkages. A fifth potential route, stemming from the occurrence of major life stress, is relevant to people of all ages and life situations. The term major stress includes powerful, often unpredictable occurrences such as parent divorce or death of a loved one and, even more corrosively, the chronically stressful life situations under which many children in modern society grow up. People vary greatly in how they adapt to such events and circumstances. Whereas some are devastated by them both in the short and long term, others cope well (are "resilient") even in the face of profoundly stressful life circumstances (Cicchetti & Garmezy, 1993; Cowen, Wyman, Work, & Parker, 1990; Garmezy, Masten, & Tellegen, 1984; Werner & Smith, 1982, 1992). Although the processes underlying such resilient adaptation have, rightfully, become a central focus both for prevention and developmental psychopathology, they are not yet fully understood (Cowen et al., 1990). What is clear, is that the ability to cope effectively with major life stress facilitates wellness outcomes (Antonovsky, 1979).

Five main pathways to wellness have been identified: (a) forming wholesome early attachments; (b) acquiring age-appropriate competencies; (c) exposure to settings that favor wellness outcomes; (d) having the (empowering) sense of being in control of one's fate; and (e) coping effectively with stress. Real-life wellness scenarios, however, are more complex than this simple listing implies. For one thing these strands are not fully independent. Witness the thought-provoking conclusion reported in two recent reviews (Yoshikawa, 1994; Zigler et al., 1992) that several early, comprehensive programs (i.e., with attachment, competence, and empowerment elements) for disadvantaged urban families did more to prevent delinquency than later, specifically targeted, delinquency-prevention programs. Pathways are also interdependent in that early failures to move toward wellness restrict a person's ultimate wellness potential (McLoyd, 1990). Moreover, as noted above, these pathways are differentially important (i.e., in regression language, have different beta weights) in different situations and at different points in the life-span. Whereas beta weights for attachment are crucial in infancy, and attachment and competence strands are crucial in childhood, empowerment may be more relevant cross-sectionally to wellness for an inner-city minority youth than for a 2-year-old in the suburbs.

A key point to highlight in considering these complex wellness strands is that *they are mutually enhancing elements in an elaborate system, not elements in competition with each other*. Thus, competence without empowerment may restrict wellness just as much as empowerment without competence. By contrast, the synergistic presence of both constitutes a powerful proactive force toward wellness. Thus a comprehensive solution to the wellness challenge requires that contributions reflecting diverse input strands be identified and harnessed. An exclusive emphasis on any one pathway would work against such a solution.

The ideal of promoting these five routes to wellness, singly and in combination, offers a conceptually appealing alternative to mental health's past dominant restorative ways. To develop the whole package however, calls for ways of thinking and doing that go well beyond psychology (cf. below).

And, even within psychology many of the issues at stake and tasks at hand (e.g., competence enhancement, system modification, and empowerment) are well removed from the classically defined mental health sphere. Finally, it should be noted that although each of the five identified strands reflects a constructive, theory-guided effort to enhance wellness, their supporting empirical substrates are still porous.

PROGRAMS TO ENHANCE WELLNESS

Interventions designed to enhance wellness are on the rise. Because primary prevention programs, as suggested above, constitute *one* major element in a broader wellness enhancement framework, some of the wellness enhancement programs to be cited can also be seen as primary prevention. The varied programs to be considered include ones (a) for adults and children; (b) targeted broadly to all people versus to specific risk subgroups; and (c) featuring a single route to wellness or combining several routes. A number of exemplary programs of this type have been reported in several review articles (Cowen, 1982, 1986; Hawkins, Catalano, & Miller, 1992a; Lorion, 1990; Price, Cowen, Lorion, & Ramos-McKay, 1988; Yoshikawa, 1994). The rest of this article cites examples of such programs both to illustrate actual accomplishments and potentials of the larger wellness thrust and to identify needed areas of program development and research.

Attachment

Broussard's (1977, 1989) Infant Family Resource Program provided 3 years of wellness-oriented services to mothers of high-risk babies. Its main goal was to "foster the development of the bonds of attachment between mother and infant...at jeopardy in many of the pairs" (1989, p. 193) through biweekly meetings with mothers and home visits from child development specialists. Program evaluation after 3 years, including observations of mother–child free-play and reunion episodes, showed that program children exceeded controls in coping and communication skills, balance of affect, and confidence, and were also less aggressive. Greenspan's (1981, 1982) related intervention for high-risk urban infants ages 0–6 taught parenting skills to meet the child's attachment needs, plus stage-specific skills of infancy and early childhood. This program too reduced the anticipated negative effects of adverse early-life conditions in a high-risk sample.

Relatedly, the Yale Child Welfare Project (Provence & Naylor, 1983; Seitz, Rosenbaum, & Apfel, 1985) provided young, inner-city mothers of firstborns 2$1/2$ years of pediatric care; regular instructional home visits; and periodic developmental assessments and feedback, as well as later day care for the child. The program's main goals were to provide support and promote sound parent–child attachments. Ten years after the program ended, the children in the experimental group were found to exceed those in the control group in socialization and school adjustment (Seitz *et al.*, 1985). To test the hypothesis that those gains reflected enduring, positive changes in caregiver practices and parent–child relationships, Seitz and Apfel (1994) studied the program's "diffusion" effects for siblings, born *after* it ended. Younger siblings of program children had better school attendance, needed fewer remedial or support services, and were making better school progress than their control counterparts. Specific expenditures for special services were four times greater for the younger siblings of controls, compared to program children. These intriguing findings suggest that the initial intervention yielded important direct, and indirect (diffusion), benefits through a common mediating mechanism, that is, positive changes in parenting practices and parent–child attachments.

Many wellness-oriented programs for infants and young children that seek to strengthen parent–child attachments also include competence enhancement elements. The Perry Preschool Project (Berrueta-Clement, Schweinhart, Barnett, Epstein, & Weikart, 1984; Schweinhart, Barnes, & Weikart, 1993; Schweinhart & Weikart, 1988) is a good example. It included an enriched preschool experience for 3–4-year-old black inner-city children, plus weekly $2^{1}/_{2}$ hour home visits designed to stimulate children's learning and promote effective parent–child interactions (attachments) and child-rearing approaches. Program outcomes have been tracked through participant age 27 (Schweinhart *et al.*, 1993) with important long-term benefits shown on (a) extent of schooling, literacy rates, and intellectual performance; (b) percentage employed, average monthly earnings, and percentage homeowners; (c) lower arrest rates, including drug-related arrests; and (d) fewer welfare or social service recipients. Those bellwether wellness indicators reflect major benefits to individuals and to society. Specifically, cost–benefit analysis showed that "over the lifetimes of participants the preschool program returns to the public an estimated \$7.16" (e.g., in later costs of delinquency, unemployment) "for each \$1 invested" (Schweinhart *et al.*, 1993; p. xviii).

Price *et al.* (1988) cited other programs for young children built around the goals of strengthening attachments and enhancing competencies, that have led to important socioemotional and cognitive wellness gains (e.g., Johnson, 1988; Olds, 1988; Ramey, Bryant, Campbell, Sparling, & Wasik, 1988). Levine and Perkins (1987) noted that the success of such programs often reflects a felicitous combination of competence-building and setting-change elements.

Competence Enhancement

Although wellness-oriented programs for young children often combine attachment and competence enhancement elements, competence acquisition later takes on greater importance in its own right. Effective competence training programs include broadly oriented ones versus those targeted to specific skills, and ones that train primarily academic versus primarily social competencies.

The Home Improvement Program for Preschool Youngsters (HIPPY), which began in Israel (Lombard, 1981), exemplifies the academically oriented skill-building approach. This 2-year home-based enrichment program teaches disadvantaged parents with limited formal education to use structured curricular materials to train school readiness skills in their own children. Learning to function effectively in this way is both empowering for parents and illuminates key roles they can play in their child's future education.

Trained indigenous paraprofessionals (most themselves parents) make regular home visits to go over curriculum exercises with parents and support their role as a teacher. In that sense the program also has a community-enhancing, empowering quality. HIPPY outcomes were assessed in a controlled longitudinal study that followed children from ages 4–16. Program children exceeded controls in school adjustment and achievement and had fewer grade retentions and dropouts. Over the same period, mothers of program children evidenced more positive self-concepts, pursued further education, and participated more in community activities (Lombard, 1981).

Spivack and Shure's (1974) Interpersonal Cognitive Problem Solving program teaches children a family of skills (e.g., recognizing feelings in oneself and others, generating alternative solutions, evaluating their consequences, and implementing appropriate action steps) designed to enhance adjustment. Program children acquired these skills. As they did, their adjustment improved and linkages were shown between these cognitive and adaptive gains (Shure & Spivack, 1982, 1988; Spivack & Shure, 1974). Programs to train other families of competencies such as adaptive assertiveness (Rotheram, Armstrong, & Booraem, 1982; Rotheram-Borus, 1988), also with positive findings, grew out of the same conceptual soil.

Although findings from early competence training programs were encouraging, their cumulation over time suggested that program outcomes were less robust or enduring than initially hoped (Durlak, 1983). Eventually, thinking in this area came to reflect several key conclusions: (a) Because social competence includes many different sets of skills, no single, simplistic training program can cover all its essential elements; (b) a circumscribed time-limited program exposure may not be enough to produce meaningful, enduring skill acquisition; (c) different skills and competencies "phase in" at different developmental stages.

These emergent views fueled the development of more complex (i.e., greater breadth and depth) second generation school-based competence training programs that seek to train multiple skills and competencies including ones to promote physical, as well as psychological, wellness. Some extend over several years, with age-appropriate entry points for new program materials and "booster shots" for skills taught earlier in simpler forms. They also reflect efforts to build class or school climates that support program leanings, and follow-through after the initial program ends (Elias & Clabby, 1992).

One such program, the Improving Social Awareness–Social Problem Solving Program (Elias & Clabby, 1992), is based on a 2-year social competence training curriculum designed to build, and promote application of, skills in (a) self-control, social awareness, and group participation; and (b) problem solving and social decision making. An initial evaluation (Elias, Gara, Ubriaco, Rothbaum, Clabby, & Schuyler, 1986) showed that the program reduced the impact of typical middle-school stressors. Follow-up 6 years later (Elias, Gara, Schuyler, Branden-Muller, & Sayette, 1991) documented long-term gains in program children's sense of efficacy and prosocial behavior, and reductions in pathology (e.g., depression) and socially disordered behaviors (e.g., aggression, vandalism).

Another multipronged social competence training program, the Yale-New Haven Social Problem Solving Program, conducted by teachers in fifth- to eighth-grade inner-city classes, sought to teach three families of competencies: stress management and impulse control; social problem solving and information processing; and behavioral social skills. A recent comprehensive evaluation demonstrated gains that grew directly out of the program, for example, problem-solving skills, prosocial attitudes in conflict resolution; and those reflecting generalization beyond program precepts, for example, more positive teacher ratings of adjustment and fewer self-reported delinquent acts (Weissberg & Caplan, unpublished manuscript).

A related, 20-session school-based program called the Positive Youth Development Program included units on stress management, self-esteem, problem solving, substance use and health, appropriate assertiveness, and forming social networks (Caplan et al., 1992). Conducted with urban and suburban sixth and seventh graders, this program strengthened participants' ability to handle interpersonal problems and deal with anxiety. Teacher ratings of program children showed improved conflict resolution, impulse control, and peer popularity. Program children also evidenced less receptive attitudes than controls toward substance and alcohol use (Caplan et al., 1992).

Elias and Clabby (1992) noted a growth in comprehensive, multi-year curricula that combine social competence and social problem-solving training with proactive health education, that is, to promote physical well-being and reduce risk for accidents, substance abuse, and preventable diseases and disorders. Examples of promising programs of this type can be cited (Pentz et al., 1989; Perry, Klepp, & Shultz, 1988; Perry, Klepp, & Sillers, 1989). Weissberg, Caplan, and Harwood (1991) made a strong case for developing highly comprehensive Social Competence and Health Education (C-SCAHE) programs and cited as an example the ambitious Social Development Project (Kasprow, Weissberg, et al., 1992). This district-wide kindergarten to 12th-grade program had three main components: (a) training at all grade levels to promote core cognitive, affective, and behavioral skills (e.g., critical thinking, problem solving, decision making), prosocial values about self and others, and accurate knowledge about health and interpersonal relationships; (b) developing school- and community-based activities and contexts to support acquisition of program learnings; (c) building school structures and decision-making mechanisms that involve all members of the school community in efforts to create a wholesome climate for academic and social development.

Although Weissberg and Elias (1993) noted that truly comprehensive C-SCAHE programs are both scarce and lack careful evaluation, they argued that such programs represent the wave of the future, that is, a third generation in school-based competence-promotion programs. They also listed essential desiderata for C-SCAHE programs and advanced a 20-year plan for program development and evaluation in this area.

Other programs with competence-training elements are targeted to specific objectives such as substance-abuse prevention (Hawkins et al., 1992a). Botvin and Tortu's (1988) Life Skills Training Program (LST) for adolescents is a good example. Based on a review of factors associated with the onset of substance abuse, LST seeks to provide immunizing personal and social skills, and strengthen self-control. This carefully developed 18-session program offers information on substance use; has units on decision making, improving self-concept, and handling anxiety; and trains skills in communication, overcoming shyness, boy–girl relationships, and appropriate assertiveness. LST programs have been conducted with different ethnic groups, using both teachers and peers as trainers. The program has been shown to reduce the use of the gateway substances (i.e., tobacco, alcohol, and marijuana), to which it is targeted (Botvin & Eng, 1982; Botvin, Renick, & Baker, 1983; Botvin & Tortu, 1988). St. Pierre, Kaltreider, Mark, and Aikin, (1992) have shown that (a) substance-abuse programs of this type can also be conducted effectively in community settings (i.e., Boys and Girls clubs); and (b) annual booster sessions enhance program effects.

To sum up, earlier "one-shot" social competence training programs are yielding place to more labor-intensive and ecologically valid interventions with greater breadth and continuity and a stronger emphasis on building environmental supports for the program (Elias *et al.*, 1991). There is reason to hope that these second-generation programs can contribute to the goal of enhancing wellness (Weissberg *et al.*, 1991; Weissberg & Elias, 1993). Mass-oriented, before the fact, comprehensive programs of the type described well exemplify a proactive, health-building thrust that tends to be overlooked in risk-grounded definitions of primary prevention (Coie *et al.*, 1993; Koretz, 1991).

Social Environment Change

Demonstrations of relationships between attributes of social environments and person outcomes (Deci, Vallerand, Pelletier, & Ryan, 1991; Moos, 1974, 1975, 1979) have fueled efforts to develop environments that favor wellness outcomes. A school, for example, might seek to do this by engineering cooperation among students (Gump, 1980; Sharon, 1990; Slavin, 1977). In an early example of this approach, Aronson, Blaney, Stephan, Sykes, and Snapp's (1978) "jig-saw" model of cooperative learning in fifth-grade social studies classes was shown both to reduce racial tensions and enhance student self-concept. A similar program (Wright & Cowen, 1985) led to more favorable views of the class environment and better social studies grades. Sprinthall (1984) argued that cooperative learning formats strengthen children's ego development, self-reliance, integrity, empathy, and moral judgment, and decrease their egocentricity. He attributed these wellness gains to system changes that redistribute power from teacher to students and thus enhance students' sense of stake and empowerment. This view is consistent with the demonstration of positive academic and adjustment outcomes in autonomy supportive class environments (Ryan & Stiller, 1991).

The STEP program (Felner, Ginter, & Primavera, 1982) modified the school environment in an effort to address major attendance and dropout problems of inner-city youth. Specifically, it sought to reduce the flux associated with the tough transition from junior to senior high school by creating stable student groupings and support systems and by having homeroom teachers do the guidance and administrative functions usually done by other school personnel. These proximal changes, it was hoped, would improve later educational outcomes. Evaluation of program outcomes 5 years later showed that STEP children had significantly fewer absences, higher grades and, importantly, a nearly 50% lower dropout rate than matched comparison youth (Felner & Adan, 1988). Such findings, reflecting major wellness benefits for participants and major dollar savings to society, provided a solid base on which to expand the program to junior high and middle school students. This new work confirmed behavioral and socioemotional gains for STEP participants (Felner *et al.*, 1993).

The San Ramon Project (Battistich, Solomon, Watson, Solomon, & Schaps, 1989; Solomon, Watson, Delucchi, Schaps, & Battistich, 1988), involving major system changes, reflects the trend noted above toward developing broadly based, long-term wellness enhancement programs that go well beyond a risk-grounded notion of primary prevention. This project sought to create total school environments, that is, "caring communities," that harness teacher, parent, and child involvements. Based on motivation theory (Deci & Ryan, 1985), classes strive to maximize students' feelings of autonomy, competence, and relatedness. A school-wide developmental-discipline approach seeks to promote autonomy and responsibility by having students set and uphold classroom norms and rules (which, in turn, helps them to feel valued), and by emphasizing solutions that build students' commitment to democratic values. To foster relatedness from kindergarten to sixth grade, many academic tasks are done in cooperative learning formats in small mixed-ability groups, and a schoolwide Buddies' program is used pairing older and younger students. The latter wellness-targeted program element has been proposed for widespread adoption by schools (Gartner & Riessman, 1993). Literature-based reading instruction is also used to help pupils better understand themselves, others, and prosocial values such as fairness and responsibility. The San Ramon program rests on the rationale that children engage better in school if they have a genuine stake and involvement in what they are doing and find their educational activities rewarding and challenging.

Program teachers exceeded controls in opportunities provided for student input and autonomy, use of cooperative learning, highlighting prosocial values and social understanding, warmth and supportiveness, number of helping activities in their classes, and using discipline styles that promoted responsible behavior rather than external rewards and punishments. These findings confirms that the program had been implemented as intended. Program children did at least as well as controls academically— better in some areas (e.g., reading comprehension). They were judged to be more cooperative and considerate, felt more accepted by classmates, were better able to resolve conflicts equitably and defend their views, and more willing to have peers participate in group decision making. They were also less anxious socially and had more friends at school.

The San Ramon project has documented important wellness outcomes in several key areas. Although it is primarily a conceptually driven effort in system change, the program includes significant competence enhancement, attachment, and empowerment components. The program is not a simple one; rather it calls for the synergistic involvements of parents, children, teachers, and other school personnel, and touches on all facets of the child's school functioning in internally consistent, goal-oriented ways, over the full elementary period.

The Seattle Social Development Project (Hawkins *et al.*, 1992b) is another broad-based program that spans the full elementary period. Although its long-term goal is to prevent substance abuse and delinquency, it assumes that such behaviors can be reduced in high-risk children by strengthening home and school attachments. The program does not address substance abuse directly. A two-pronged parent component seeks to provide family management and communication skills and help parents to create a conducive home-learning environment. Teaching practices such as proactive class management, interactive teaching, and cooperative learning are intended to strengthen school bonding. Social problem-solving training is provided only for first graders. Program children and controls all come from high crime neighborhoods. A program evaluation, when children entered fifth grade (Hawkins *et al.*, 1992b) showed that the experimental group, as expected, had stronger home and school attachments than the control group and evidenced lower rates of delinquency and drug use initiation (Hawkins & Lam, 1987; Hawkins, Von Cleve, & Catalano, 1991).

Some school-based (system change) programs have quite specific wellness goals. One example is Olweus's (1978, 1979, 1993) highly focused, persistent efforts over several decades to understand and reduce school bullying problems in Norway. His early studies (a) showed substantial base rates for the occurrence of school bullying and victimization; (b) identified determinants and correlates of these behaviors; and (c) documented their negative consequences for both bullies and victims. These generative findings were used to frame a major preventive (system change) intervention designed to reduce the incidence of bullying (aggressive behaviors), implemented in 42 Norwegian elementary and junior high schools. Key program goals included (a) enhancing awareness of bully-victim problems and their consequences; (b) gaining the active involvement of parents and teachers in addressing such problems; (c) developing and enforcing clearly articulated rules against bullying; and (d) providing support and protection for victims. Steps to advance those goals were taken at three levels: *school* (e.g., questionnaire survey, close supervision at lunch and recess times, school conferencing to enhance awareness), *class* (firm, enforced class rules against bullying; class discussion meetings), and *individual* (serious talks with bullies and victims and their parents; parent–teacher collaboration to counter bullying).

Key program findings after 2 years included (a) 50% reduction in "direct" and "indirect" school bullying plus fewer out-of-school bullying incidents both for boys *and* girls and across all grade levels (fourth to ninth); (b) parallel reductions in other antisocial behaviors (vandalism, fighting, theft, drunkenness, and truancy; and (c) improved social climate (order and discipline), interpersonal relationships, and attitudes to school work and school satisfaction. These wellness-related findings are important in their own right and have implications for the growing problems of school violence in contemporary society.

The complex (i.e., reflecting multiple wellness pathways) programs reviewed in this section provide evidence that children's wellness can be enhanced by informed school-based programming.

Empowerment

The gut appeal of the concept of empowerment lies in its potential for addressing irrepressible social blights. Hence the term has come into greater use in both the professional literature (Rappaport, 1981, 1987; Swift, 1992; Swift & Levin, 1987; Trickett *et al.*, 1994) and the public domain. Sarason (1993b) raised a note of caution about this development: "Empowerment has become a fashionable word. It has the ring of virtue and unquestioned morality. Some proclaim it as a panacea. If the empowerment movement is to avoid the worst excesses of sloganeering and conceptual superficiality, it will have to come to grips with issues that are as complex conceptually as they are at the level of action" (p. 260). Although Sarason did not spell out these issues concretely, his choice of the word "sloganeering" hints at one, that is, that the concept's eminent good sense may outpace its empirical support base.

People also use the term differently (e.g., to reflect an objective or phenomenological view of change in power). In this vein, Zimmerman (1990) distinguished between psychological empowerment and individually oriented conceptions of empowerment and later showed different outcomes to be associated with these definitions (Zimmerman, Israel, Schulz, & Checkoway, 1992). Concerns about how the concept is defined are heightened when, as is often the case, empowerment is not a directly assigned "commodity," but rather is intended (or inferred) as part of an ongoing system change. This definitional fuzziness hampers evaluation of the efficacy of intended empowering actions by making interpretations of outcome findings susceptible to circular explanations. Thus, if positive outcomes follow system change, the change steps taken are assumed to have been empowering. If such outcomes are *not* found, and that sometime happens (Gruber & Trickett, 1987), an apologist can argue that the steps taken were either insufficiently empowering or not of the empowering type needed.

The preceding caution points are noted as factors that currently limit the empowerment notion. At the same time, both common sense and observation suggest it to be a concept with widespread potential applicability and heuristic value. Nor do we lack examples of its fruitful application. Illustratively, a recent journal number (Wandersman & Florin, 1990) presented a set of studies documenting a range of positive empowerment effects in diverse community organizations and settings. Another way used to show such effects is the setting or program vignette, that is, a descriptive account of positive change in people or organizations (Rappaport, Davidson, Wilson, & Mitchell, 1975) seen to result from an empowering process. Rappaport *et al.* (1984) devoted a special journal number to such accounts, reflecting diverse settings and circumstances.

Realistically, however it may be difficult to pin down empowerment effects in situations where they are potentially most important (major macrosocial contexts) because of the complexity and widespread operation of other variables under such conditions. Important way-station indicators of the concept's power may be derivable under more controlled conditions by studying outcomes associated with analogous but less global constructs such as autonomy support (Deci & Ryan, 1985). Ryan and Stiller (1991), for example, reviewed an extensive body of research linking autonomy support to positive educational and adaptive outcomes in children, and Cowen (1991) suggested that acquiring stage-salient competencies may be a natural pathway to the child's sense of feeling empowered.

Comer's (1980, 1987) work in black inner-city schools can readily be viewed in empowerment terms though, content-wise, it is fundamentally a school management (system change) program in which parents and teachers share decision making and responsibility for education policy and practice. Comer (1988) justifiably viewed this as a potentially empowering process that can radiate positively to students, service providers, and the community. Among the important program outcomes he reported are long-term improvements in students' academic achievement and parallel gains in parents' morale and interest and educators' sense of program ownership. These positive changes are seen to stem from salutary system changes, that is, the empowerment of previously disempowered people.

Gottfredson's (1986) school-based program also used shared decision making as a route to empowerment, along with curricular changes and cooperative learning formats. After 3 years, program children evidenced less drug use and delinquent behavior than controls, were more closely attached to the school, and had more positive views of school rules and practices. Findings cited in this section thus suggest that gains in empowerment (i.e., being able to make important decisions that affect one's life) can enhance psychological wellness.

Coping with Stress

The ubiquitous term *stress* is used to describe many different situations that pose threats to wellness: real and perceived; mild and intense; specific and diffuse; anticipable and nonanticipable; acute and chronic. Moreover, each category includes multiple exemplars with different "tugs and pulls" and consequences. Although much evidence suggests that stress predisposes adverse physical and psychological sequelae (Auerbach & Stolberg, 1986; Honig, 1986a, 1986b; Johnson, 1986; Kornberg & Caplan, 1980; Roberts & Peterson, 1984), that broad generalization is differentially valid for different stressors (e.g., daily hassles vs. chronic, profound life-stress). The more severe, uncontrollable, broad-ranging, and enduring the stress, the greater is its risk-enhancing quality and the more likely is it to undermine wellness. Even so, for any given type and level of intensity of stress (objectively defined), the thought-provoking reality remains that people vary greatly in the extent to which they perceive the situation as stressful and the range of adaptations that follow.

The concept of childhood resilience, that is, coping and adapting well in the face of major life stress (Cicchetti & Garmezy, 1993; Cowen et al., 1990; Garmezy et al., 1984; Werner & Smith, 1982), offers a compelling case in point. Resilient youngsters, described as "healthy children in unhealthy environments" (Garmezy, 1982) and as those who "overcome the odds" (Werner & Smith, 1992), offer intriguing clues about pathways to wellness, even under the most dire conditions. That such resilient outcomes occur with no special programming or intervention, suggests that early wellness-enhancing processes such as sound attachment and competence acquisition help to forge protective attributes such as perceived self-efficacy, empathy, social problem-solving skills, and sense of security (Cowen et al., 1990; Rutter, 1990; Werner & Smith, 1982, 1992) which, in turn, act both to minimize the perceived stressfulness of life situations and to promote effective coping when stress occurs (Fonagy, Steele, Steele, Higgit, & Target, 1994). More needs to be learned how exactly these attributes operate and the processes by which they form (Rutter, 1990; Masten, Best, & Garmezy, 1991).

Although people's reactions to stress vary greatly, and it is important to understand why, many situations predispose adaptive problems for most people who experience them. These range from mild, circumscribed, anticipable events (e.g., dental or minor surgical procedures) to more intense, enduring situations (e.g., job loss, death of a loved one, parental divorce) with radiating negative ramifications, to unanticipable, dire, indeed potentially catastrophic, stressors both short term (e.g., fire, earthquake, flood, tornado) and prolonged (war, nuclear disaster, concentration camp). Such situations have been foci for wellness-enhancing interventions for several reasons: (a) they do indeed precipitate stressful reactions in many people who experience them—even securely attached, competent people; (b) victims can readily identify with others who have experienced the same stressor; and (c) successful coping equips one to deal more effectively with future stress whereas failure to cope increases susceptibility to future stress.

Effective models for short-circuiting the predictably negative consequences of stress and strengthening people's resources and skills for dealing with future stressors have been reported in such areas as bereavement (Silverman, 1988; Vachon, Lyall, Rogers, Freedman-Letofsky, & Freeman, 1980), marital disruption (Pedro-Carroll & Cowen, 1987), illness and hospitalization, natural disaster, war, and holocaust (e.g., Auerbach & Stolberg, 1986; Roberts & Peterson, 1984). Indeed, Bloom (1979) proposed a general preventive paradigm pivoting around the two-stage process of identifying stressful events and charting their damaging effects, and developing effective preventive interventions to short-circuit these predictable negative sequelae. Cowen (1980) called these two steps prevention's "generative" and "executive" components.

In summary, because stress operates to elevate risk, being able to cope effectively with it is another key pathway to wellness. This ability can be nourished both by basic steps in the child's formation and, later, by interventions that seek to defuse the negative effects of stress and promote adaptive skills.

SUMMARY AND NEW DIRECTIONS

Psychological wellness is proposed as a potentially fruitful orienting concept that directs attention to a family of genotypically unified, if phenotypically diverse, phenomena of interest. Wellness is seen not as an absolute but rather as an anchor point at the positive end of an adjustment continuum, that is, as an ideal that we should strive concertedly to approach. To do that requires (a) greater investment in efforts to promote wellness from the start rather than repair work that begins only after major wellness deficits become apparent; and (b) following diverse pathways, including those that focus on individuals, settings, community contexts, and societal structures and policies, in efforts to promote the well-being of the many. Promoting wellness is likely to be more humane, efficient, and (ultimately) more cost-effective than struggling to undo dysfunction.

Five pathways were considered as part of a comprehensive framework for wellness enhancement: forming wholesome attachment relationships; acquiring age-appropriate skills and competencies; developing settings and environments that favor positive adaptation; fostering empowerment; and acquiring skills for coping effectively with stress. These pathways are different. Each rests on its own special knowledge base and set of technologies.

Some of the latter reflect terrains familiar to psychologists; others considerably transcend psychology's normal boundaries. Hence, systematic pursuit of a wellness enhancement grail, calls for changes not only in *what* we do (focus on) but in *how* we go about doing those things, and with whom (i.e., professional collaborations and alliances).

Even those who subscribe to a narrower, risk-driven notion of primary prevention (e.g., Coie *et al.*, 1993; Koretz, 1991) recognize that because behavior is shaped by many, and diverse, influence systems (e.g., intraindividual, familial, community), the full range of prevention programming and research "will require collaborative efforts of interdisciplinary teams to achieve the diversity of expertise and breadth of intellectual focus that is necessary" and that "explanatory models must take full account of the social and community context as well as the systems operating within individuals and families" (Coie *et al.*, 1993, p. 1016). Areas cited specifically by those authors as part of a necessary collaborative effort include sociology, epidemiology, econometrics, psychopathology, criminology, child development, education, and several subareas of psychology.

If that view is valid for a primary prevention framework built around risk for pathology, and we believe it is, the need for cross-discipline inputs to program development and research is even stronger in a wellness framework that is *all*-population oriented and *not* bound by the concept of risk. Advancing all facets of the wellness concept thus calls for major inputs from social policy makers, urban planners, political scientists, child development specialists, and educators, among others. Hence it would be professionally "precious" (Sarason, Levine, Goldenberg, Cherlin, & Bennett, 1966) to assume that any single subarea of psychology (e.g., community, clinical, developmental, social)—indeed all of psychology or mental health—had, by itself, the knowledge or technology needed to meet this complex challenge. At the same time, those fields can play several legitimate and important roles in such a thrust, that relate both to their background and know-how in conceptualizing and assessing adjustment outcomes (i.e., the ultimate dependent variables in a wellness framework) and their expertise in studying particular wellness strands (e.g., attachment, competence) and developing ways to strengthen them.

Although the nature and magnitude of current unresolved problems in mental health underscore the need for pursuing wellness alternatives actively, the preceding falls well short of saying that the pathways proposed here are yet sufficiently clearly formulated or adequately documented. To the contrary, several need greater definitional clarity and all could profit from a more solid empirical base. We mean only to suggest here that enough is now known to argue that each identified strand represents a promising *potential* pathway to wellness, for which important answerable next-questions can be posed. Existing limitations notwithstanding, examples of effective programs illustrating each major pathway to wellness have been cited. Several impressive recent examples that combine multiple pathways and extend over long periods seem more valid ecologically than earlier uni-dimensional, time-limited approaches.

Thus, even though wellness enhancement approaches are not yet ready for beatification, this theoretically appealing option is well beyond being a mere pipe dream. Indeed, detailed practitioner-ready manuals are now available for conducting some effective programs of the types described (Price *et al.*, 1988). At the same time, additional generative information about the ontogenesis of wellness is needed in several ares including (a) the *in vivo* study of conditions and processes that nourish the early, spontaneous development of wellness; (b) clarifying understandings of the self-views, skills and competencies, and familial contexts and pathways that operate to advance and maintain wellness; (c) identifying settings, community structures, and policies that further support the development of wellness. In parallel, there is need to develop interventions that promote wellness, both by honing existing technology more finely and by expanding the scope and reach of this family of approaches. We need also to explore ways of blending wellness approaches to augment their overall impact, and to understand better the applicability of various approaches at different developmental levels, in different settings, and with different sociocultural groups.

Although these complex challenges structure an agenda that could easily extend for decades into the next century, the questions raised are well worth pursuing—indeed have urgency. Clear answers to them can build bridges to richer, more productive life experiences for a next generation of children and youth. There is reason to be encouraged by recent findings from programs that seek to enhance wellness, and reason to hope that a further paradigm shift toward the promotion of wellness will attract increasing interest and allocation of resources in the years to come.

ACKNOWLEDGMENT

Some ideas in this paper were first presented in a talk at the W. T. Grant Foundation-sponsored conference on "Risk, Resiliency and Development," Kiawah Island, S. Carolina, May 30, 1992. The author gratefully acknowledges support from the Grant Foundation in writing this article.

REFERENCES

Ainsworth, M. D. S. (1989). Attachments beyond infancy. *American Psychologist, 44*, 709–716.
Albee, G. W. (1982). Preventing psychopathology and promoting human potential. *American Psychologist, 37*, 1043–1050.

Anderson, S. & Messick, S. (1974). Social competence in young children. *Developmental Psychology, 10*, 282–293.

Antonovsky, A. (1979). *Health, stress and coping.* San Francisco, Jossey-Bass.

Aronson, E., Blaney, N., Stephan, C., Sikes, J., & Snapp, M. (1978). *The jigsaw classroom.* Beverly Hills, CA: Sage.

Auerbach, S. M. & Stolberg, A. L. (Eds.) (1986). *Crisis intervention with children.* Washington, DC: Hemisphere.

Bandura, A. (1977). Self-efficacy: Toward a unifying theory of behavior change. *Psychological Review, 84*, 191–215.

Battistich, V., Solomon, D. S., Watson, M., Solomon, J., & Schaps, E. (1989). Effects of an elementary school program to enhance prosocial behavior and children's cognitive social problem solving skills and strategies. *Journal of Applied Developmental Psychology, 10*, 147–169.

Berrueta-Clement, J. R., Schweinhart, L. J., Barnett, M. W., Epstein, A. S., & Weikart, D. P. (1984). *Changed lives: The effects of the Perry Preschool Program on youths through age 19.* Ypsilanti, MI: High/Scope Educational Research Foundation.

Bloom, B. L. (1979). Prevention of mental disorders: Recent advances in theory and practice. *Community Mental Health Journal, 15*, 179–191.

Botvin, G. J. & Eng, A. (1982). The efficacy of a multicomponent approach to the prevention of cigarette smoking. *Preventive Medicine, 11*, 199–211.

Botvin, G. J., Renick, N., & Baker, E. (1983). The effects of scheduling format and booster sessions on a broad spectrum psychosocial approach to smoking prevention. *Journal of Behavioral Medicine, 6*, 359–379.

Botvin, G. J. & Tortu, S. (1988). Preventing substance abuse through life skills training. In R. H. Price, E. L. Cowen, R. P. Lorion, & J. Ramos-McKay (Eds.), *14 ounces of prevention: A casebook for practitioners* (pp. 98–110). Washington, DC, American Psychological Association.

Bowlby, J. (1982). *Attachment and loss* (Vol. 1). New York: Basic Books.

Broussard, E. R. (1977). Primary prevention program for newborn infants at high risk for emotional disorder. In D. C. Klein & S. E. Goldston (Eds.), *Primary prevention: An idea whose time has come* (pp. 63–68). Rockville, MD: U. S. Department of Health, Education, and Welfare.

Broussard, E. B. (1989). The Infant-Family Resource Program: Facilitating optimal development. In R. E. Hess & J. DeLeon (Eds.), *The National Mental Health Association: 80 Years of involvement in the field of prevention* (pp. 179–224). New York: Haworth.

Caplan, M. Z., Weissberg, R. P., Grober, J. S., Sivo, P. J., Grady, K., & Jacoby, C. (1992). Social competence promotion with inner-city and suburban young adolescents: Effects on social adjustment and alcohol use. *Journal of Consulting and Clinical Psychology, 60*, 56–63.

Cicchetti, D. & Garmezy, N. (Eds.). (1993). Milestones in the development of resilience. *Development and Psychopathology, 4*, 497–783.

Coie, J. D., Watt, N. F., West, S. G., Hawkins, J. D., Asarnow, J. R., Markman, H. J., Ramey, S. L., Shure, M. B., & Long, B. (1993). The science of prevention: A conceptual framework and some directions for a national research program. *American Psychologist, 48*, 1013–1022.

Comer, J. P. (1980). *School power.* New York: Free Press.

Comer, J. P. (1987). New Haven's school-community connection. *Educational Leadership, 44*, 13–16.

Comer, J. P. (1988). Educating poor minority children. *Scientific American, 259*, 42–48.

Cowen, E. L. (1973). Social and community interventions. In P. Mussen & M. Rosenzweig (Eds.), *Annual Review of Psychology, 24*, 423–472.

Cowen, E. L. (1977). Baby-steps toward primary prevention. *American Journal of Community Psychology, 5*, 1–22.

Cowen, E. L. (1980). The wooing of primary prevention. *American Journal of Community Psychology, 8*, 258–284.

Cowen, E. L. (Ed.). (1982). Research in primary prevention in mental health. *American Journal of Community Psychology, 10*, 239–367.

Cowen, E. L. (1983). Primary prevention in mental health: Past, present and future. In R. D. Felner, L. Jason, J. Moritsugu, & S. S. Farber (Eds.), *Preventive psychology: Theory, research and practice in community interventions* (pp. 11–25). New York: Pergamon.

Cowen, E. L. (1985). Person centered approaches to primary prevention in mental health: Situation-focused and competence enhancement. *American Journal of Community Psychology, 13*, 31–48.

Cowen, E. L. (1986). Primary prevention in mental health: Ten years of retrospect and ten years of prospect. In M. Kessler & S. E. Goldston (Eds.), *A decade of progress in primary prevention* (pp. 3–45). Hanover, NH: University Press of New England.

Cowen, E. L. (1991). In pursuit of wellness. *American Psychologist, 46*, 404–408.

Cowen, E. L. (1994). Community psychology and routes to psychological wellness. In J. R. Rappaport & E. Seidman (Eds.), *Handbook of community psychology* (2nd ed.) New York: Wiley.

Cowen, E. L., Wyman, P. A., Work, W. C., & Parker, G. R. (1990). The Rochester Child Resilience Project (RCRP): Overview and summary of first year findings. *Development and Psychopathology, 2*, 193–212.

Crick, N. R. & Dodge, K. A. (1994). A review and reformulation of social information processing mechanisms in children's social adjustment. *Psychological Bulletin, 115*, 74–101.

Deci, E. L. & Ryan, R. (1985). *Intrinsic motivation and self-determination in human behavior.* New York: Plenum Press.

Deci, E. L., Vallerand, R. J., Pelletier, L. G., & Ryan, R. M. (1991). Motivation and education: The self-determination perspective, *Educational Psychologist, 26*, 325–346.

Dinges, N. (1994). Mental health promotion. In P. J. Mrazek & R. J. Haggerty (Eds.), *Reducing risks for mental disorders: Frontiers for preventive intervention* (pp. 333–355). Washington, DC: National Academy Press.

Durlak, J. (1983). Social problem-solving as a primary prevention strategy. In R. D. Felner, L. A. Jason, J. N. Moritsugu, & S. S. Farber (Eds.), *Preventive psychology: Theory, research and practice* (pp. 31–48). New York: Pergamon.

Eccles, J. S., Midgley, C., Wigfield, A., Buchaman, C. M., Reuman, D., Flanagan, C., & McIvers, D. (1993). The impact of stage-environment fit on young adolescents' experiences in schools and families. *American Psychologist, 48*, 90–101.

Elias, M. J. & Clabby, J. F. (1992). *Building social problem-solving skills: Guidelines from a school-based program.* San Francisco: Jossey-Bass.

Elias, M. J., Gara, M. A., Schuyler, T. F., Branden-Muller, L. R., & Sayette, M. A. (1991). The promotion of social competence: Longitudinal study of a school-based program. *American Journal of Orthopsychiatry, 61*, 409–417.

Elias, M. J., Gara, M., Ubriaco, M. Rothbaum, P. A., Clabby, J. F., & Schuyler, T. (1986). Impact of a preventive social problem solving program on children's coping with middle school stressors. *American Journal of Community Psychology, 14*, 259–275.

Felner, R. D. & Adan, A. M. (1988). The School Transitional Environmental Project: An ecological intervention and evaluation. In R. H. Price, E. L. Cowen, R. P. Lorion, & J. Ramos-McKay (Eds.), *14 ounces of prevention: A casebook for practitioners* (pp. 111–122). Washington, DC: American Psychological Association.

Felner, R. A., Brand, S., Adam, A. A., Mulhall, P. F., Flowers, N., Sartain, B., & DuBois, B. L. (1993). Restructuring the ecology of the school as an approach to prevention during school transitions: Longitudinal follow-up and extensions of the School Transition Environmental Project (STEP). *Prevention and Human Services, 10*, 103–136.

Felner, R. P., Ginter, M. A., & Primavera, J. (1982). Primary prevention during school transitions: Social support and environment structure. *American Journal of Community Psychology, 10,* 227–240.

Finkel, N. J. (1974). Strens and traumas: An attempt at categorization. *American Journal of Community Psychology, 2,* 265–275.

Finkel, N. J. (1975). Strens trauma and trauma resolution. *American Journal of Community Psychology, 3,* 173–178.

Fonagy, P., Steele, M., Steele, H., Higgit, A., & Target, M. (1994). The theory and practice of resilience. *Journal of Child Psychology and Psychiatry, 35,* 231–257.

Garmezy, N. (1982). Foreword. In E. E. Werner & R. S. Smith (Eds.), *Vulnerable but invincible: A study of resilient children* (pp. xiii–xix). New York: McGraw-Hill.

Garmezy, N., Masten, A. S., & Tellegen, A. (1984). Studies of stress-resistant children: A building block for developmental psychopathology. *Child Development, 55,* 97–111.

Gartner, A. & Riessman, F. (1993). Peer tutoring: Toward a new model. ERIC Digest. Washington, DC: ERIC Clearinghouse on Teaching and Teacher Education.

Gottfredson, D. C. (1986). An empirical test of school-based environmental and individual interventions to reduce the risk of delinquent behavior. *Criminology, 24,* 705–731.

Greenspan, S. I. (1981). *Psychopathology and adaptation in infancy and early childhood: Principles of clinical diagnosis and preventive intervention* (Clinical Infant Reports No. 1). New York: International Universities Press.

Greenspan, S. I. (1982). Developmental morbidity in infants in multi-risk-factor families. *Public Health Reports, 97,* 16–23.

Gruber, J. & Trickett, E. J. (1987). Can we empower others? The paradox of empowerment in the governing of an alternative public school. *American Journal of Community Psychology, 15,* 353–371.

Gump, P. V. (1980). The school as a social situation. In M. R. Rosenzweig & L. W. Porter (Eds.), *Annual Review of Psychology, 31,* 553–582.

Hawkins, J. D., Catalano, R. F., & Miller, J. Y. (1992a). Risk and protective factors for alcohol and other drug problems: Implications for substance abuse prevention. *Psychological Bulletin, 112,* 64–105.

Hawkins, J. D., Catalano, R. F., Morrison, D. M., O'Donnell, J., Abbott, R. D., & Day, L. E. (1992b). The Seattle Social Development Project: Effects of the first four years on protective factors and problem behaviors. In J. McCord & R. E. Tremblay (Eds.), *The prevention of anti-social behavior in children* (pp. 139–161). New York: Guilford.

Hawkins, J. D. & Lam, T. (1987). Teacher practices, social development, and delinquency. In J. D. Burchard & S. N. Burchard (Eds.), *The prevention of delinquent behavior* (pp. 241–274). Newbury Park, CA: Sage.

Hawkins, J. D., Von Cleve, E., & Catalano, R. F. (1991). Reducing early childhood aggression: Results of a primary prevention program. *Journal of the American Academy of Child and Adolescent Psychiatry, 30,* 208–217.

Hollister, W. G. (1967). Concept of strens in education: A challenge to curriculum development. In E. M. Bower & W. G. Hollister (Eds.), *Behavioral science frontiers in education* (pp. 193–206). New York: Wiley.

Honig, A. S. (1986a, May). Stress and coping in children (Part 1). *Young Children,* pp. 50–63.

Honig, A. S. (1986b, July). Stress and coping in children (Part 2): Interpersonal family relationships. *Young Children,* pp. 47–50.

Jahoda, M. (1958). *Current concepts of positive mental health.* New York: Basic Books.

Jessor, R. (1993). Successful adolescent development among youth in high-risk settings. *American Psychologist, 48,* 117–126.

Johnson, D. L. (1988). Primary prevention of behavior problems in young children: The Houston Parent Child Development Center. In R. H. Price, E. L. Cowen, R. P. Lorion, &

J. Ramos-McKay (Eds.), *14 ounces of prevention: A casebook for practitioners* (pp. 44–52). Washington, DC: American Psychological Association.

Johnson, J. H. (1986). *Life events as stressors in childhood and adolescence.* Newbury Park, CA: Sage.

Kasprow, W. J., Weissberg, R. P., *et al.* (1992). *New Haven Public Schools Social Development Project.* New Haven, CT: New Haven School District.

Kiesler, C. A. (1992). Some observations about the concept of the chronically mental ill. In M. Kessler, S. E., Goldston, & J. M., Joffe (Eds.), *The present and future of prevention: In honor of George W. Albee* (pp. 55–68) Newbury Park, CA: Sage.

Kiesler, C. A., Simpkins, C., & Morton, T. (1989). The psychiatric in-patient treatment of children and youth in general hospitals. *American Journal of Community Psychology, 17,* 821–830.

Koretz, D. S. (1991). Prevention-centered science in mental health. *American Journal of Community Psychology, 19,* 453–458.

Kornberg, M. S. & Caplan, G. (1980). Risk factors and preventive intervention in child psychotherapy: A review. *Journal of Prevention, 1,* 71–133.

Kuhn, T. S. (1970). *The structure of scientific revolutions,* (2nd ed.). Chicago: University of Chicago Press.

Levine, M. & Perkins, D. V. (1987). *Principles of community psychology: Perspectives and applications.* New York: Oxford University Press.

Lombard, A. D. (1991). *Success begins at home.* Lexington, MA: Lexington Books.

Lorion, R. P. (Ed.). (1990). *Protecting the children: Strategies for optimizing emotional and behavioral development.* New York: Haworth.

Masten, A. S., Best, K. M., & Garmezy, N. (1991). Resilience and development: Contributions from the study of children who overcame adversity. *Development and Psychopathology, 2,* 425–444.

McLoyd, V. C. (1990). The impact of economic hardship on Black families and children: Psychological stress, parenting and socioemotional development. *Child Development, 61,* 311–346.

Moos, R. H. (1974). *Evaluating treatment environments: A social ecological approach.* New York: Wiley.

Moos, R. H. (1975). *Evaluating correctional and community settings.* New York: Wiley.

Moos, R. H. (1979). *Evaluating educational environments.* San Francisco, CA: Jossey-Bass.

Mrazek, P. J. & Haggerty, R. J. (Eds.). (1994). *Reducing risks for mental disorders: Frontiers for preventive intervention.* Washington, DC: National Academy Press.

Olds, D. L. (1988). The prenatal/early infancy project. In R. H. Price, E. L. Cowen, R. P. Lorion, & J. Ramos-McKay (Eds.), *14 ounces of prevention: A casebook for practitioners* (pp. 9–23). Washington, DC: American Psychological Association.

Olweus, D. (1978). *Aggression in the schools: Bullies and whipping boys.* Washington, DC: Hemisphere.

Olweus, D. (1979). Stability of aggressive reaction patterns in males: A review. *Psychological Bulletin, 86,* 852–875.

Olweus, D. (1993). *Bullying at school: What we know and what we can do about it.* Cambridge, MA: Blackwell.

Pedro-Carroll, J. L. & Cowen, E. L. (1987). Preventive interventions for children of divorce. In J. P. Vincent (Ed.), *Advances in family intervention, assessment and theory* (Vol. 4, pp. 281–307). Greenwich, CT: JAI Press

Pentz, M. A., Dwyer, J. H., MacKinnon, D. P., Flay, B. R., Hansen, W. B., Wang, E. Y. I., & Johnson, C. A. (1989). A multi-community trial for primary prevention of adolescent drug abuse: Effects on drug use prevalence. *Journal of the American Medical Association, 261,* 3259–3266.

Perry, C. L., Klepp, K. I., & Shultz, J. M. (1988). Primary prevention of cardiovascular disease: Community wide strategies for youth. *Journal of Consulting and Clinical Psychology*, *56*, 358–364.

Perry, C. L., Klepp K. I., & Sillers, C. (1989). Community wide strategies for cardiovascular health. The Minnesota Heart Health Youth Program. *Health Education Research*, *4*, 87–101.

Price, R. H., Cowen, E. L., Lorion, R. P., & Ramos-McKay, J. (Eds.). (1988). *14 ounces of prevention: A casebook for practitioners*. Washington, DC: American Psychological Association.

Provence, S. & Naylor, A. (1983). *Working with disadvantaged parents and children: Scientific issues and practice*. New Haven, CT: Yale University Press.

Ramey, C. T., Bryant, D. M., Campbell, F. A., Sparling, J. J., & Wasik, B. H. (1988). In R. H. Price, E. L. Cowen, R. P. Lorion & J. Ramos-McKay (Eds.), *14 ounces of prevention: A casebook for practitioners* (pp. 32–43). Washington, DC: American Psychological Association.

Rappaport, J. (1981). In praise of paradox: A social policy of empowerment over prevention. *American Journal of Community Psychology*, *9*, 1–25.

Rappaport, J. (1984). Studies in empowerment: Introduction to the issue. *Prevention in Human Services*, *3*, 1–7.

Rappaport, J. (1987). Terms of empowerment/exemplars of prevention: Toward a theory of community psychology. *American Journal of Community Psychology*, *15*, 121–148.

Rappaport, J., Davidson, W. S., Wilson, M. N., & Mitchell, A. (1975). Alternatives to blaming the victim or the environment: Our places to stand have not moved the earth. *American Psychologist*, *30*, 525–528.

Rappaport, J., Swift, C., & Hess, R. (Eds.). (1984). Studies in empowerment: Steps toward understanding and action. *Prevention and Human Services*, *3*, 1–230.

Roberts, M. C. & Peterson, L. (1984). *Prevention of problems in childhood: Psychological research and applications*. New York: Wiley.

Rotheram, M. J., Armstrong, M., & Booraem (1992). Assertiveness training in fourth- and fifth-grade children. *American Journal of Community Psychology*, *10*, 567–582.

Rotheram-Borus, M. J., (1988). Assertiveness training with children. In R. H. Price, E. L. Cowen, R. P. Lorion, & J. Ramos-McKay (Eds.), *14 ounces of prevention: A casebook for practitioners* (pp. 83–97). Washington, DC: American Psychological Association.

Rutter, M. (1990). Psychosocial resilience and protective mechanisms. In J. Rolf, A. Masten, D. Cicchetti, K. H. Nuechterlein, & S. Weintraub (Eds.), *Risk and protective factors in the development of psychopathology* (pp. 181–214). Cambridge, England: Cambridge University Press.

Ryan, R. M. & Stiller, J., (1991). The social contexts of internalization: Parent and teacher influences on autonomy, motivation, and learning. In R. P. Pintrich & M. L. Maehr (Eds.), *Advances in motivation and achievement, Vol. 7: Goals and self-regulatory processes* (pp. 115–149). Greenwich, CT: JAI.

Sarason, S. B. (1993a). *Letters to a SERIOUS education president*. Newbury Park, CA: Corwin.

Sarason, S. B. (1993b). *The case for change: Rethinking the preparation of educators*, San Francisco, Jossey-Bass.

Sarason, S. B., Levine, M., Goldenberg, I. I., Cherlin, D. L., & Bennett, E. M. (1966). *Psychology in community settings: Clinical, educational, vocational and social aspects*. New York: Wiley.

Schweinhart, L. J., Barnes, H. V., & Weikart, D. P. (1993). *Significant benefits: The High/Scope Perry Preschool study through age 27*. Ypsilanti, MI: High Scope Press.

Schweinhart, L. J. & Weikart, D. P. (1988). The High Scope/Perry Preschool Program. In R. H. Price, E. L. Cowen, R. P. Lorion, & J. Ramos-McKay (Eds.), *14 ounces of prevention: A casebook for practitioners* (pp. 53–65). Washington, DC: American Psychological Association.

Seitz, V. & Apfel, N. H. (1994). Parent focused intervention: Diffusion effects on siblings. *Child Development, 65,* 677–683.

Seitz, V., Rosenbaum, N. K., & Apfel, N. H. (1985). Effects of family support intervention: A ten-year follow-up. *Child Development, 56,* 376–391.

Sharon, S. (1990). *Cooperative learning: Theory and research.* New York: Praeger.

Shedler, J., Mayman, M., & Manis, M. (1993). The illusion of mental health. *American Psychologist, 48,* 1117–1131.

Shoben, E. J. (1957). Toward a concept of normal personality. *American Psychologist, 12,* 183–189.

Shure, M. B. & Spivack, G. (1982). Interpersonal problem-solving in young children: A cognitive approach to prevention. *American Journal of Community Psychology, 10,* 341–356.

Shure, M. B. & Spivack, G. (1988). Interpersonal cognitive problem solving (ICPS). In R. H. Price, E. L. Cowen, R. P. Lorion, & J. Ramos-McKay (Eds.). *14 ounces of prevention: A casebook for practitioners* (pp. 69–82). Washington, DC: American Psychological Association.

Silverman, P. R. (1988). Widow-to-widow: A mutual help program for the widowed. In R. H. Price, E. L. Cowen, R. P. Lorion, & J. Ramos-McKay (Eds.). *14 ounces of prevention: A casebook for practitioners* (pp. 175–186). Washington, DC: American Psychological Association.

Slavin, R. L. (1977). Classroom reward structure: An analytical and practical review. *Journal of Educational Research, 44,* 633–650.

Solomon, D., Watson, M. S., Delucchi, K. L., Schaps, E., & Battistich, V. (1988). Enhancing children's prosocial behavior in the classroom. *American Educational Research Journal, 25,* 527–554.

Spivack, G. & Shure, M. B. (1974). *Social adjustment of young children: A cognitive approach to solving real-life problems.* San Francisco: Jossey-Bass.

Sprinthall, N. A. (1984). Primary prevention: A road paved with a plethora of promises and procrastinations. *Personnel and Guidance Journal, 62,* 491–495.

St. Pierre, T. L., Kaltreider, D. L., Mark, N. M., & Aikin, K. J. (1992). Drug prevention in a community setting: A longitudinal study of the relative effectiveness of a three-year primary prevention program in Boys and Girls Clubs across the nation. *American Journal of Community Psychology, 20,* 673–706.

Strayhorn, J. M. (1988). *The competent child: An approach to psychotherapy and preventive mental health.* New York: Guilford.

Swift, C. F. & Levin, G. (1987). Empowerment: The greening of prevention. In M. Kessler, S. E., Goldston, & J. M. Joffe. (Eds.), *The present and future of prevention: In honor of George W. Albee* (pp. 99–111). Newbury Park, CA: Sage.

Swift, C. F. (1992). Empowerment: An emerging mental health technology. *Journal of Primary Prevention, 8,* 71–94.

Trickett, E. J., Dahiyat, C., & Selby, P. (1994). *Primary prevention in mental health: An annotated bibliography.* Rockville, MD: U.S. Department of Health and Human Services.

Vachon, J. L., Lyall, M. A., Rogers, J., Freedman-Letofsky, K., & Freeman, S. (1980). A controlled study of self-help intervention for widows. *American Journal of Psychiatry, 137,* 1380–1384.

Wandersman, A. & Florin, P. (1990). Citizen participation, voluntary organizations and community development: Insights for empowerment through research. *American Journal of Community Psychology, 18,* 41–177.

Weinstein, C. S. (1991). The classroom as a social context for learning. In M. R. Rosenzweig & L. W. Porter (Eds.), *Annual Review of Psychology, 42,* 493–525.

Weissberg, R. P. & Caplan, M. Z. Promoting social competence and preventing antisocial behavior in young urban adolescents. Unpublished manuscript.

Weissberg, R. P., Caplan, M. Z., & Harwood, R. L. (1991). Promoting competence enhancing environments: A systems-based perspective on primary prevention. *Journal of Consulting and Clinical Psychology, 59,* 830–841.

Weissberg, R. P. & Elias, M. J. (1993). Enhancing young children's social competence and health behavior: An important challenge for educators, scientists, policy makers and funders. *Applied and Preventive Psychology, 2,* 179–190.

Werner, E. E. & Smith, R. S. (1982). *Vulnerable but invincible: A study of resilient children.* New York: McGraw-Hill.

Werner, E. E. & Smith, R. S. (1992). *Overcoming the odds: High risk children from birth to adulthood.* Ithaca, NY: Cornell University Press.

Wright, S. & Cowen, E. L. (1985). The effects of peer teaching on student perceptions of class environment, adjustment and academic performance. *American Journal of Community Psychology, 13,* 413–427.

Yoshikawa, H. (1994). Prevention as cumulative protection: Effects of early family support and education on chronic delinquency and its risks. *Psychological Bulletin, 115,* 28–54.

Zax, M. & Cowen, E. L. (1976). *Abnormal psychology: Changing conceptions* (2nd ed.). New York: Holt, Rinehart, & Winston.

Zigler, E., Taussig, C., & Black, K. (1992). A promising preventative for juvenile delinquency. *American Psychologist, 47,* 997–1006.

Zimmerman, M. A. (1990). Taking aim on empowerment research: On the distinction between individual and psychological conceptions. *American Journal of Community Psychology, 18,* 169–177.

Zimmerman, M. A., Israel, B. A., Schulz, A., & Checkoway, B. (1992). Further explorations in empowerment theory: An empirical analysis of psychological empowerment. *American Journal of Community Psychology, 20,* 707–728.

22

Impact of the JOBS Intervention on Unemployed Workers Varying in Risk for Depression

Amiram D. Vinokur, Richard H. Price, and Yaacov Schul

Reports the results of the JOBS II randomized field experiment that included a sample of 1,801 recent job losers, 671 of which participated in a modified version of the JOBS I intervention for unemployed workers (Caplan, Vinokur, Price, & van Ryn, 1989). The intervention focused on enhancing the sense of mastery through the acquisition of job-search and problem-solving skills, and on inoculation against setbacks. JOBS II was intended to prevent poor mental health and to promote high quality reemployment. The study tested whether the efficacy of the intervention could be increased by screening and oversampling respondents who were at higher risk for a significant increase in depressive symptoms. Results demonstrated that the intervention primarily benefited the reemployment and mental health outcomes of the high-risk respondents. This suggests the feasibility of enhancing the efficacy of this preventive intervention by targeting it for high-risk unemployed workers who could be identified prospectively.

A great deal of research has been conducted on the impact of job loss and unemployment on workers' stress and mental health (Barling, 1990; Fryer & Payne, 1986; Warr, 1983). There is strong evidence showing the adverse

Originally published in the *American Journal of Community Psychology, 23*(1) (1995): 39–74.

A Quarter Century of Community Psychology: Readings from the American Journal of Community Psychology, edited by Tracey A. Revenson *et al.* Kluwer Academic/Plenum Publishers, New York, 2002.

effects of job loss and unemployment on social and psychological functioning (e.g., Catalano, 1991; Catalano & Dooley, 1977; Dew, Bromet, &
Schulberg, 1987; Kessler, Turner, & House, 1988, 1989; Vinokur, Caplan, &
Williams, 1987), as well as on physical health (Cobb & Kasl, 1977) and on
the family (Justice & Duncan, 1977). During the thriving economy of
the 1950s and 1960s, 4–5% of the workforce was looking for a job
(Chamberlain, Cullen, & Lewin, 1980, p. 586). These percentages suggest
that even if today's economy will once again thrive, millions of individuals
will continue to be vulnerable to the harmful effects of job loss and unemployment (Reich, 1991).

Because the fundamental causes of job loss and unemployment are
rooted in societal and economic processes, remedies for their adverse social
effects must be sought in comprehensive economic and social policies
(Blinder, 1987). Although national and state social and economic policies
need to address the problems that result from unemployment, various community-based efforts can be undertaken to reduce the social and psychological impact of unemployment at the local level. For example, special
community-based intervention programs can be implemented to provide
support and coping skills to unemployed workers in their search for employment and to moderate the adverse effects of unemployment on mental
health.

The JOBS Intervention Project developed at the University of
Michigan was designed to test a preventive intervention for unemployed
workers. The intervention goals were to prevent the deterioration in mental health of unemployed workers which often results from job loss and prolonged unemployment and to promote high quality reemployment. This
intervention was designed as a job search seminar to teach participants the
most effective strategies to find appropriate positions and to enhance their
job search skills. While the seminar was aimed specifically at enhancing job
search skills, it also incorporated several components designed to enhance
participants self-esteem and sense of control, job search self-efficacy, and
inoculation against setbacks. These components were considered essential
to maintain the motivation and the persistence in job search behavior to
regain employment (Caplan, Vinokur, Price, & van Ryn, 1989). Various
aspects of these components have been discussed in the literature in terms of
effectance motivation (White, 1959), locus of control (Rotter, 1966), personal
control (Gurin, Gurin, & Morrison, 1978), self-efficacy (Bandura, 1977), and
sense of mastery (Pearlin & Schooler, 1978; Pearlin, Menaghan, Lieberman,
& Mullen, 1981). The intervention was originally tested in a large-scale, randomized experimental field study using a large heterogeneous sample of
unemployed persons who were recruited from unemployment offices in
southeastern Michigan (Caplan *et al.*, 1989).

Several reports have already provided strong evidence that the intervention accomplished its goals. Using the 1-month and 4-month follow-up data, Caplan *et al.* (1989) showed that the intervention produced higher quality reemployment in terms of earnings and job satisfaction, and higher motivation, even among those who remained unemployed. Additional analyses on these two short-term follow-ups demonstrated that participants achieved significantly better employment outcomes and mental health than their counterparts in the control group (Vinokur, Price, & Caplan, 1991). Finally, a long-term follow-up, $2\frac{1}{2}$ years later, demonstrated continued beneficial effects of the intervention on wage rates, monthly earnings and fewer episodes of job changes (Vinokur, van Ryn, Gramlich, & Price, 1991).

In later analyses of the data, we demonstrated that the beneficial mental health effects of the intervention were primarily experienced by an identifiable subgroup of respondents who were at high risk of experiencing a clinically significant setback in mental health such as experiencing a depression episode (Price, van Ryn, & Vinokur, 1992). The high-risk respondents were those identified by higher combined scores on depressive symptoms, financial strain, and low assertiveness at pretest. Both research and theory suggest that these three variables are prominent risk factors for poor mental health and continued unemployment of persons who lose their job. Several studies demonstrated that financial strain has a significant impact on depression (Kessler, Turner, & House, 1988). Further, depression symptoms may reduce the chances of reemployment (Hamilton, Hoffman, Broman, & Rauma, 1993) because of their effect on the motivation for, and effectiveness of, job search behavior. Finally, lack of assertiveness and associated social skills hinders effective interpersonal communication with potential employers and therefore reduces the chance of landing a job.

Despite the positive results obtained in the testing of the JOBS intervention, a number of questions are yet to be answered. One question is whether the retrospective identification of this subgroup could be translated into a prospective screening mechanism to increase the effectiveness of an intervention program aimed at preventing poor mental health outcomes. Furthermore, while risk status was defined and demonstrated to be an important predictor of the intervention effect on mental health, it remains to be seen whether risk status also moderates the effect of the intervention on reemployment outcomes. Recent studies implicate the increase in depressive symptomatology that follows a job loss as contributing to continuation of unemployment status (Hamilton *et al.*, 1993). However, if the JOBS intervention is more effective in reducing depressive symptomatology among high- than low-risk respondents, it may also be more effective in improving the reemployment outcomes of the high- than the low-risk respondents by shortening their period of unemployment. That is, we hypothesize that the intervention will produce greater reemployment benefits for the high-risk individuals than the low-risk ones, as had been demonstrated with respect to mental health.

A number of prevention researchers and theorists have enumerated the advantages of maximizing the effects of interventions on mental health through the identification of mediating variables and the screening and targeting of the intervention on the mediators (Brown, 1991; Emery, 1991; Pillow, Sandler, Braver, Wolchik, & Gersten, 1991; Reid, 1991).[1] We hypothesized that advanced screening of high-risk job losers and their selection into the JOBS intervention could increase the efficacy of the intervention since it would include those job losers who could benefit most from the intervention.

The purpose of this paper is to report the results of the JOBS II study, a large-scale extension of the original randomized field experiment using the JOBS intervention. The most important extension in this JOBS II study included the testing of a screening instrument and a procedure to identify, oversample, and recruit high-risk job losers, and then to randomize the high- and low-risk respondents into the intervention and a control condition. Another extension of the original study included the collection of data from a spouse or another significant other who knew the respondent well and could report on his or her mental health and role and emotional functioning. These additional reports by significant others could provide convergent validation of the respondents' report of their own mental health and role and emotional functioning and shed additional light on the interpretation of the results.

Apart from these extensions of the original study, the present JOBS II study was intended to provide an operational replication (Lykken, 1968) of the original study. Thus, the main basic features of the earlier study and the intervention, such as the sources and procedures for recruiting respondents, and for the delivery of the intervention, including its content, remained essentially the same. However, the new study included a number of important changes as well.

First, the conceptual framework that guided the JOBS II intervention focused on increasing the sense of mastery and the enhancement of

---

[1]Risk factors may include early epidemiological risk factors such as demographics as well as mediational variables involved in the process producing the problem that is intended to be prevented. For example, Pillow *et al.* (1991) suggest that interventions to prevent poor mental health of children of divorce should use screening on the mediating variables that include parental conflict and lack of parental warmth and support for the children. Similarly, interventions to prevent poor mental health of job losers, such as the JOBS II intervention, may include financial strain, which has been demonstrated to mediate the effects of job loss on depression symptomatology (Kessler *et al.*, 1987; Pearlin *et al.*, 1981).

personal control and job search self-efficacy. The importance of increasing the focus on sense of mastery and control has been highlighted by new research on these constructs in our earlier study and in research by others. For example, research findings from the JOBS I study demonstrated that increases in job-search self-efficacy had a significant impact on the intensity of job search behavior (van Ryn & Vinokur, 1992). In a similar vein, Eden and Aviram (1993) tested a similar intervention for job losers and demonstrated that their intervention increased general self-efficacy and job search behavior. More generally, enhancing a sense of mastery appears to be an essential step in reducing the risk for depression. For example, Marshall and Lang (1990) have demonstrated that mastery—and not optimism—was the critical predictor of depression among the women in their sample.

Second, changes were introduced to increase the strength, integrity, and efficiency of the intervention. The new JOBS II study included the hiring of a new team of six cotrainers and increasing their formal training from 80 to 240 hours. To increase efficiency and attendance, the intervention was shortened from eight sessions during a 2-week period (in JOBS I) to five sessions during a 1-week period (in JOBS II) with total number of intervention hours reduced by 30% (approximately from 28 to 20 hours).

Third, perhaps the most significant change in this extension of the original study occurred in the economic environment during and immediately after the time of the intervention, when the participants were searching for a new job. Whereas data from the U.S. Bureau of Labor Statistics (1988, 1992) indicate that the conditions of the labor market for job seekers became much *better* during the year following the original JOBS I intervention, these conditions became much *worse* during the year following the replication JOBS II intervention study. Thus, if the JOBS II study also replicates the beneficial effects demonstrated by the original study, it would lend a strong support to the robustness and efficacy of the JOBS program using a new set of trainers and supervisory personnel, and most important, demonstrating results under different, more difficult, conditions of labor market trajectory. Such findings would suggest the suitability and practicality of implementing this program in various community settings undergoing expansions or contractions in their labor markets. Because of these changes, the findings of the JOBS II study provide additional implications regarding the generalizability of the intervention to other settings and the nature of the economic environment.

To summarize, the goals of this paper are to examine the following four questions: (a) Was the redesigned JOBS II intervention aimed at enhancing participants' sense of mastery successful in achieving this outcome? (b) Did the intervention replicate the positive effects on reemployment and mental health outcomes obtained in JOBS I, particularly with a procedural variation that shortened the intervention, and delivered it in a different economic environment? (c) Having used a new prospective design for screening high-risk respondents, did the intervention replicate the JOBS I findings showing that the high-risk participants benefited most in terms of reduction in depression symptoms? (d) Did the findings regarding the differential positive effects of JOBS II for high-risk participants generalize to other measures of well-being, such as distress and role and emotional functioning as reported by both participants and their significant others?

METHOD

Subjects and Overview of the Design

An overview of the design of the study including the steps involved in screening and recruitment, and in pretest, and posttest data collections is displayed in Figure 1.

Method and Procedures of Recruitment

Respondents were recruited from four offices of the Michigan Employment Security Commission (MESC) in southeastern Michigan, the state agency that provides unemployment payments. Trained interviewers approached and contacted 31,560 potential respondents while they waited in the unemployment offices and briefly inquired *whether they were unemployed and were looking for a job.* Over 23,000 of those contacted were ineligible for participation because they were new entrants to the labor market, already reemployed, or were just accompanying others in line. Thus, of those contacted, only 7,956 (Figure 1, Box 2) met basic initial criteria, which also included information from the respondents that *they were not on strike or expecting to be recalled for work in the next few months, or planning to retire in the next 2 years.* Those who met all of the above initial criteria were asked to fill out a 5-page, self-administered screening questionnaire described below to determine three additional final eligibility criteria and to provide baseline pretest measures. Only 3,402 (Figure 1, Box 3) met *all* eligibility criteria for participation in the field experiment. Of the three final exclusion criteria, the first included information that the respondent had *lost his/her job and was unemployed for over 13 weeks.* The second criterion was designed to exclude respondents who were likely to introduce selection and attrition bias due to a strong preference for the program offered to the control or the experimental group. Thus the respondents were told about two programs that were being offered by the University of Michigan on how to

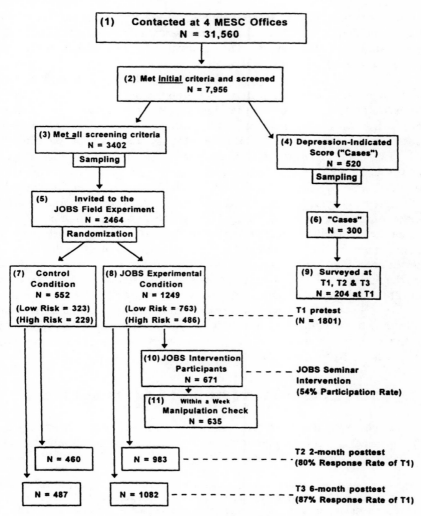

Figure 1. Research design of the JOBS II Field Study.

seek jobs. One program was described as a five half-day (Monday through Friday) seminar series (the experimental condition); the other was described as a self-guided booklet program (the control condition). To ensure equal motivation to enter one or the other condition, only persons who expressed no preference were randomly assigned to the experimental and control conditions. Of the 7,956 selected initially, those 1,159 (14.6%) who expressed a preference for one of the programs (versus having no preference) and the 108 respondents who refused both programs (1.3%) were excluded from the study but were sent the job search booklet and eliminated from the sample. The majority of those with a preference preferred the self-administered program.

The third criterion was designed to exclude those with a very high depression score indicative of a depression episode (Derogatis & Melisaratos, 1983) because the intervention was conceived of as a primary prevention program. Those 520 (6.5%) respondents who were excluded based on this criterion were not included in the design of the experiment.[2]

The screening questionnaire requested information on each respondent's name, address, telephone number, birth date, gender, and number of weeks unemployed since leaving last job. It also included an 11-item index of depression symptoms, a 3-item index of financial strain, and a 4-item index of social assertiveness. Based on the scores for the three indices, and using the regression weights reported in Price *et al.* (1992), a risk score for poor mental health was computed for each respondent. In addition, a risk status code (i.e., low = 1, high = 2) was assigned to each respondent based on the risk score. (For details on risk score and risk status see section on measures.) Of the 3,402 that met all of the criteria of eligibility (Figure 1, Box 3), 2,445 (72%) were classified as low risk but only 1,507 were invited (randomly selected) to participate in the study. Reducing the proportion of low-risk respondents was the method used to achieve oversampling of the high-risk respondents from 25 to 39%.

Randomization Procedures and Experimental Design

Each week, interviewers screened and recruited respondents at two of the four MESC offices mentioned above. Screening questionnaires were

---

[2]Although those with very high depression scores were not included in the design of the study, a random panel of 300 of the 520 with high depressive scores were selected to be followed up with our questionnaire surveys. However, all of the 520 respondents who had very high depressive symptoms were mailed our job search booklet. In addition, because they were more likely to experience a clinically significant depressive episode, we included in the material that we sent to them a community resource guide for mental health and welfare services that included addresses and phone numbers of mental health clinics and related social agencies and institutions where treatment and help can be obtained. Prior to composing the informational guide, we contacted all of the social agencies and clinics who appear on the guide to inform them about our action, and to solicit and obtain their cooperation in providing the needed help to those who would call. Having this informational guide available, we included it with the package of questionnaires that was mailed to all other respondents in the study with an accompanying letter that explained the general purpose of having this information for unemployed persons.

brought to the research office to complete the scoring of scales and determine risk status and eligibility. Subsequently, a computerized randomization procedure was used to allocate the low- and the high-risk respondents to a control condition or an experimental condition. Those randomized to the experimental condition received an invitation to participate in the JOBS intervention program in a site chosen for its proximity to the office from which they were recruited.

Experimental Condition

The JOBS seminar experimental condition consisted of five 4-hour sessions conducted during the morning hours of a 1-week period. All persons in the experimental condition were mailed an invitation to attend the seminar with a $5 bill incentive to cover transportation costs. Respondents assigned to the experimental condition were also told that they would receive a $20 check payment for completing at least 4 of the 5 sessions and a certificate of participation. The certificate was awarded at the last session.

Each training site was located in the geographical area in which recruitment to the site took place. The sites included community colleges, community centers, and rented conference rooms at local hotels. The rooms were large enough to accommodate 25 persons seated at movable chairs and tables. A semicircular seating layout was used to facilitate discussion, and small groups were formed to carry out group exercises.

The design of the five training sessions was based on the principles described in Caplan et al. (1989) and in Price and Vinokur (1995). They included the application of problem-solving and decision-making group processes, inoculation against setbacks, provision of social support and positive regard from the trainers, and learning and practicing job search skills. The intervention seminars were delivered by three pairs of male and female cotrainers to groups ranging from 12 to 22 participants ($M = 15.6$). The seminar trainers included social workers, educational counselors, and high school teachers who were themselves unemployed at the time but were looking for work. They were recruited and selected carefully to insure their suitability to follow the intervention protocol and facilitate group processes. They received approximately 240 hours of formal training by our staff which included conceptual knowledge of group processes, the theoretical bases of the intervention, and extensive rehearsal. The trainers also practiced by conducting the five session sequence twice with pilot participants. In all, the intervention was delivered to 671 participants during 22 weeks, beginning March 1, 1991 and ending August 7, 1991.

The sessions covered a wide range of substantive, skill-related topics. The topics included examples and exercises in identifying and conveying one's job-related skills, using social networks to obtain job leads, contacting potential employers, preparing job applications and resumés, and successfully going through a job interview. Each of the five sessions was standardized for the trainers in 8 to 12 pages of documentation per 4-hour session. The full details of the selection and training of the trainers' program and of the intervention are available in a comprehensive 370-page implementation manual (Curran, 1992) that can be obtained from the authors.

Intervention Quality Control. Two procedures were used to maintain a high level of trainer adherence to the protocol over the 5-month duration of the intervention. First, trainers were regularly observed by members of the research team. The observers followed a procedure worked out jointly with the trainers that allowed for constructive feedback after the end of each observed session. Second, the trainers met weekly with a staff person in charge of their training to deal with special skill-related topics that surfaced in their work as trainers.

Intervention Dropouts and Participants. Among those who were assigned to the experimental condition and became study participants by returning the Time 1 (T1) pretest questionnaire (Figure 1, Box 8; $n = 1,249$), 46% ($n = 578$) failed to show up for the intervention but continued to provide follow-up data at Time 2 (T2) and Time 3 (T3). Of those 671 who showed up (Figure 1, Box 10), 567, or 85%, showed up for at least four of the five sessions. Most of the participants who attended the beginning sessions but dropped out of the later ones indicated they had found a job during the week of the seminar.

Control Condition

The control condition consisted of a booklet briefly describing job-search methods and tips equivalent to three single-spaced pages of text. This booklet was mailed to persons after they were randomized into the control condition. The booklet contained useful information, but it was extremely brief in comparison, for example, to self-help books available on job search.

Data Collection Procedures

After completing the screening questionnaire at an MESC office, the questionnaire was processed and a risk score was calculated. Those who were eligible for participation and who were randomized into one of the experimental conditions were mailed a package including a questionnaire for themselves and a separate questionnaire for their significant other. The package included separate self-addressed stamped envelopes for returning the questionnaires, a $5 bill attached to each questionnaire, an introductory letter to the respondent and to the significant other. An enclosed cover letter described our guarantee of confidentiality, a certificate of confidentiality obtained from the federal government, and an assurance that the study was not connected with MESC.

Significant Other was defined as the spouse of the respondent if he/she was married and living with the spouse, or else someone to whom the respondent feels close to, who knows the respondent well and sees the respondent at least once a week.

T1 pretest questionnaires were mailed weekly to cohorts of respondents who were recruited to the study during the months of February through July 1991. The questionnaires were mailed about 2 weeks before the invitation for the JOBS intervention seminar to which the respondents were randomized as experimental or control respondents. Based on the respondents' reports, it took an average of 44 minutes to complete the T1 pretest questionnaire.

Program evaluation questionnaires were mailed to the respondents immediately after they completed the intervention seminar with a separate envelope to update their address so they could receive the $20 payment for participation.

On the average, two of the five sessions of each seminar group were observed by a project staff member such as the training supervisor, project directors, and assistants, and by two of the trainers who were on a rotating schedule of research assignment every third week.

T2 and T3 follow-up questionnaires were mailed to the respondents 2 and 6 months, respectively, after the week of the intervention seminar for which they were randomized as experimental or control respondents. In addition to the $5 bill that was included with these follow-up questionnaires, respondents who did not return the questionnaires within 4 weeks were sent an offer of a $12 bonus to be paid by check upon receiving their completed questionnaires. This latter incentive method, which started in the middle of Wave 2 follow-up, resulted in a substantial increase in response rate (about 14%) and accounts for the higher T3 than T2 response rate.

Measures

All of the constructs in this study were assessed with multi-item indices, and most had a coefficient alpha in the .70s and .80s. Below we present that subset of measures that were used for the analyses of this report. The full set of measures and the questionnaires are available from the authors.

Demographics were assessed using standard survey questions for reporting age, sex, education, marital status, occupation, family income, and ethnic/racial identification.

Depression was measured with a subscale of 11 items based on the Hopkins Symptom Checklist (Derogatis, Lipman, Rickles, Uhlenuth, & Covi, 1974). The 11-item scale required respondents to indicate on a 5-point scale how much (1 = *not at all* to 5 = *extremely*) they had been bothered or distressed in the last 2 weeks by various depression symptoms such as feeling blue, having thoughts of ending one's life, and crying easily. The Cronbach coefficient alpha (Nunnally, 1978) of the scale was .90.

Financial strain was measured with a 3-item index (Kessler *et al.*, 1988; Vinokur & Caplan, 1987) based on answers to three questions with 5-point rating scales. The questions asked: "How difficult is it for you to live on your total household income right now?"; "In the next two months, how much do you anticipate that you or your family will experience actual hardships such as inadequate housing, food, or medical attention?"; and "In the next two months, how much do you anticipate having to reduce your standard of living to the bare necessities of life?" The alpha coefficients for the index ranged for the three data collection waves from .84 to .90.

Assertiveness was assessed using a short 4-item index ($\alpha = .85$) based on published instruments on social reticence and shyness (Jones & Russell, 1982) and assertiveness (Galassi, Delo, Galassi, & Bastien, 1974; Rathus, 1973). The 4-item scale required respondents to indicate how strongly they agreed or disagreed (1 = *strongly agree* to 5 = *strongly disagree*) with various statements about themselves, such as "I feel inhibited in social situations," and "Most people seem to be more aggressive and assertive than I am."

Risk Score and Risk Status. A Risk score index was computed based on the screening data according to the following formula developed in Price *et al.* (1992): Risk score = (.622 * Depression score) + (.134 * Financial Strain score) − (.098 * Assertiveness score). The regression weights suggest that respondents who score higher on depression symptoms and financial strain and lower on assertiveness are at higher risk for experiencing depression in the future. Before classifying respondents into low- and high-risk status categories we excluded all 520 (6.5%) respondents (Figure 1, Box 4) who had a mean depression index *greater* than 3.00, which is considered a clinically significant indication of depression (Derogatis & Melisaratos, 1983). As already indicated, these respondents were not included in the design of the field experiment because the intervention was conceived of as a primary prevention program. Thus, to be classified in the high-risk category, respondents had to have a risk score *greater than or equal to* 1.38. Respondents who had a risk score *less* than 1.38 were classified in the low-risk status category. The 1.38 cutting point was set to obtain approximately 25% high-risk respondents before oversampling, as in Price *et al.* (1992).[3]

Distress symptoms were measured with an 18-item index assessing a variety of distress symptoms such as restlessness, anxiety, and inattentiveness. The items required the respondents to indicate on 5-point scales "how much of the time during the last two weeks have you been ..." experiencing the various symptoms. The scales range from 1 (*none of the time*) to 5 (*all of the time*). Using the same items, the spouse/significant other reported their assessment of how the focal respondent has been during the last 2 weeks. The Cronbach alpha for the focal respondent's measure was .95. For the significant other's measure assessing the focal respondent's depression symptoms the alpha coefficient was .93.

Role and emotional functioning was measured with a 15-item index developed by Caplan *et al.* (1984). The items require the respondents to indicate "how well have you been doing (in the last two weeks) with respect to ..." various role and emotional tasks such as handling responsibilities and daily demands, staying level-headed, and making the right decisions on a 5-point scale (1 = very poorly, 5 = exceptionally well). Using the same items, the respondent's spouse/significant other also reported on the role and emotional functioning of the focal respondent. The Cronbach alpha for the focal respondent and the significant other measure was .94 and .95, respectively.

The job search self-efficacy measure was developed for this study and consisted of 6 items. All respondents, regardless of reemployment status, were asked to rate how confident they felt about being able to do the following things successfully: make the best impression and get points across in an interview, contact and persuade employers to consider them for the job, complete a good job application or resumé, use friends or other contacts to

[3]In addition to the risk score that was computed based on Price *et al.*, 1992 study, we also computed a new risk score based on the data from the current study. Using the new score, we then conducted the analyses reported in the result section again. Despite some differences in the weights of the components of the old and new risk score, the results obtained using the two risk scores were the same. The two risk scores correlate .99. Furthermore, 97% of the respondents are classified into the high- or low-risk categories by either the old or the new score. Additional analyses were conducted based on two new cutting points that classify, respectively, 50 and 75% of the respondents as high risk. The results based on the currently used cutting points that classify after oversampling only 40% of the study participants as high risk were the strongest. Although not statistically significant, the results with 50% classified as high risk, were close to those based on the current cutting point. Income per month was the only outcome where the cutting point based on 50% high risk was slightly but not significantly stronger than the one based on the currently used cutting point. Thus, our cutting point for classifying high-risk respondents seems optimal for identifying a subgroup that benefits most from the intervention.

discover promising job openings, use friends and other contacts to find out about employers that need their skills, and make a good list of all the skills they have which could be used to find a job. The rating scale categories ranged from 1 (*not at all confident*) to 5 (*a great deal confident*). Ratings on these items were averaged to create a job search self-efficacy index measure with a Cronbach's alpha coefficient of .87.

The *self-esteem* measure included 8 items from Rosenberg's (1965) self-esteem scale. The items requested the respondents to rate their degree of agreement or disagreement with statements such as "On the whole I am satisfied with myself," "I am able to do things as well as most other people," "At times I think I am no good at all." The categories for the rating scales ranged from 1 (*strongly agree*) to 5 (*strongly disagree*). This 8-item measure had a Cronbach alpha coefficient of .83.

An *internal control orientation* measure was based on 10 items from the original Rotter I-E scale that were demonstrated by Gurin *et al.* (1978) to best capture a personal, rather than ideological, orientation. The items of this scale are very similar to those used in another widely used Self-Mastery scale (Pearlin & Schooler, 1978; Pearlin *et al.*, 1981). Alpha coefficients of this measure ranged from .63 to .71 across the time waves.

The *mastery* measure was constructed by computing the mean scores of the above three measures (i.e., jobs search self-efficacy, internal control orientation, and self-esteem). This combined measure was constructed following a confirmatory factor analysis that tested whether the three constructs could be accounted for by a latent factor conceived of as personal mastery. Analysis using structural equation modeling (Bentler, 1989) provided a very good fit to the model as measured by several fit indexes including Bentler and Bonnett (1980) normed, nonnormed, and comparative fit measures (NFI = .98, NNFI = .97, CFI = .98, respectively) and Hoelter's (1983) CN = 759.

Intervention Process. Assessments of the participants' immediate perception of the process within the intervention provided an indication of the intervention's integrity and strength (Yeaton & Sechrest, 1981). These assessments were based on measures that consisted of multi-item indices and covered various aspects of the intervention such as trainers' and group members' behavior, their attractiveness to the participant, social processes (e.g., freedom to participate, willingness of the group to listen to what one had to say); and practice of job-seeking skills within the sessions. It also included measures of the proximal impact of the intervention on job search self-efficacy, job search optimism, and confidence in being able to handle setbacks and self-esteem.

Reemployment. Following the definition used in our earlier JOBS I study (Caplan *et al.*, 1989), reemployment status was determined by a combination of two criteria. To be classified as "reemployed" the person had to report working *at least 20 hours* per week *and* had to characterize the number of hours being employed as "working enough." Persons working *less than 20* hours per week *and* characterizing that amount "not working enough" were classified as "not reemployed." Persons who did not clearly fall into either of these categories (28% at T2 and 22% at T3) were omitted from analyses that include the reemployment measure. This operational definition provides an unambiguous characterization since the person is coded as employed only when meeting both subjective and objective criteria. To avoid the omission of a middle subgroup that occurred in the application of the above definition, we also used another definition of reemployment status that included *all* the respondents. This definition was based solely on the reported number of work hours per week. Those working less than 20 hours per week and those working for 20 hours or more were classified, respectively, as unemployed and reemployed. In addition to reporting the number of hours working per week, respondents also provided information on their wages from which we calculated their wage rate and monthly income.

Demographic Characteristics of the Sample of Respondents Enrolled in the Study

Our study's sample, which included those who were enrolled by returning the T1 pretest questionnaire (Figure 1, Boxes 7, 8, and 9, $N = 2,005$), was composed of workers who had lost a job recently and were unemployed for no longer than 13 weeks. Nevertheless, its characteristics closely resembled the U.S. unemployed population as reported by the U.S. Bureau of Labor Statistics (1992), which also include long-term unemployed, and reentrant and new entrants to the labor market. For example, in our sample, the median age was 34.7 years ($M = 36.20, SD = 10.38$); and included 45% male, 21.5% African–American, 76% white, 41% married, and a mean of $1,881 monthly income from last job. The U.S. unemployed population during 1991 had a median age of 30.4 years; and included 58% male, 20% African–American, 76% white, 41% married and monthly earnings of $1,834.

In our sample, only 8.6% did not complete high school, 32.4% had high school education, 35.8% had some college, 13% had 4 years of college, and 10.2% had more than 4 years of college. Respondents were recruited to the study between 1 and 13 weeks following their job loss ($M = 4.11$; $SD = 3.8$). On the average, they had worked 3.85 years ($SD = 5.01$) on their last job, 43.21 hours per week ($SD = 9.52$), and earned $10.01 ($SD = 4.86$) per hour. Their mean annual income was $22,574 ($SD = $11,932$).

Response Rates, Attrition, and Effectiveness of Randomization

Attrition from T0 (Screening) to T1

Of those 2,464 who were selected, randomized and invited to participate in the field study based on their T0 (screening) data (Figure 1, Box 5), 1,801 respondents (73%) were enrolled by returning their T1 questionnaire (Figure 1, Boxes 7 and 8). Our analyses revealed that males, younger respondents, and those experiencing higher levels of financial strain were significantly more likely to drop out of the study by not returning the T1 questionnaire. However, there were no differences in attrition rates between the experimental and control condition or between low- and high-risk groups that formed our experimental design. Moreover, there were no interactions between attrition and experimental conditions on any of the variables available in the screening data including age, gender, number of weeks since job loss, depression, financial strain, and assertiveness, or the risk score (the combination of the latter 3 measures).

Attrition from T1 to T2 and T3

Of those 1,801 who enrolled in the study, 1,443 (80%) provided T2 and 1,569 (87%) provided T3 questionnaires. We also received from their significant others at T1, T2, and T3 1,483 (82%), 1,304 (90%), and 1,466 (92%) questionnaires, respectively. The higher response rate at T3 than at T2 was the result of additional follow-up contacts and higher respondent pay.

There was no significant difference in attrition between experimental and control condition nor any significant interactions between experimental conditions and risk status, consequently, the integrity of the randomization to experimental and control conditions was fully preserved (Hansen, Collins, Malotte, Johnson, & Fielding, 1985). There were no significant differences in any of the T1 variables between respondents randomized to the experimental and control conditions, nor an interaction between condition and risk status, nor between condition and any of the individual components of the risk status index, that is, depression, financial strain, and assertiveness. In addition, none of the T1 demographics or job-related variables including age, sex, education, family income, number of dependents, number of hours worked per week on last job, and wage rate on last job was associated with experimental condition.

Compared to respondents who provided data for the T2 follow-up, dropouts were significantly older (37.00 vs. 32.85 years, $p < .001$), male (vs. female) 51 vs. 44%; $p < .01$), nonwhites (33 vs. 21%; $p < .001$). They also had less education (13.16 vs. 13.60 years, $p < .001$), lower family income

($22,169 vs. $27,955; $p < .001$) and lower prior monthly income from the job they lost ($1757 vs. $1911, $p < .01$) and experienced higher financial strain (3.31 vs. 3.13, $p < .01$) than those who responded. There was also a statistically significant difference in the proportion of dropouts between the experimental and control condition at T2 (16.7% dropout in the control vs. 21.3% dropout in the experimental condition, $p < .02$). However, with more intensive follow-up at T3, the dropout difference was reduced to a nonsignificant 1.6% between the control and experimental conditions. Most important, we tested for interaction effects between dropout and experimental condition on 17 variables that included demographics and screening and pretest scores on mental health and job related variables (e.g., prior monthly income). No statistically significant interaction effect was found for either Time 2 or Time 3 dropout. Following Hansen *et al.* (1985) we conclude that differential attrition rates could not affect the internal validity of the results.

RESULTS

Manipulation Checks on the Integrity and Strength of the Intervention

Of those 1249 job seekers who were assigned to the experimental condition and were invited to the job search seminar, 671 (54%) participated in the intervention. Of these 671 participants, 85% attended at least 4 of the 5 sessions. Thus, the mean number of sessions attended was 4.27. Using a mailed self-administered questionnaire, 635 (95%) of those who attended the intervention seminar reported their evaluation and experiences within a week after the last session. Their evaluations provided uniformly strong evidence of the integrity and strength of the intervention and its immediate impact. On a series of 5-point scales ranging from 1 to 5, participants provided ratings indicating that they found the seminar relevant to their needs ($M = 4.51, SD = 0.46$), that the group process was highly positive ($M = 4.59$, $SD = 0.43$), and that their job-search optimism and their confidence in overcoming setbacks was high ($M = 4.40, 4.15; SD = .52, .68$, respectively). They also rated the trainers and their fellow group members on warmth, expertise, and helpfulness on 7-point scales ranging from 1 to 7. Again, these ratings indicated positive evaluations with mean scores of 6.77 ($SD = 0.63$) and 6.73 ($SD = 0.69$), respectively.

Finally, comparison of measures that were available at pretest T1 with the same measures collected within a week after the intervention seminar demonstrated sizable increases in self-esteem ($Ms = 4.40$ vs. 4.09), $t(631) = 12.86, p < .001$, Cohen's effect size $d = .51$, job-search self efficacy ($Ms = 4.37$ vs. 3.61), $t(631) = 22.91, p < .001, d = 1.27$, and confidence in being prepared to handle setbacks ($Ms = 4.11$ vs. 3.54), $t(631) = 17.02$, $p < .001$, $d = .86$. These findings suggest that the intervention provided the participants with the intended positive and socially supportive group process as well as raising self-esteem, job search self-efficacy, and inoculation against setbacks.

Analyses of the Experimental Effects of the Intervention

Analysis Plan

To preserve the integrity of the randomized design and avoid selection bias (Cook & Campbell, 1979), our analyses include in the experimental group all the respondents who were randomized to this group *regardless* of whether they subsequently showed up and participated in the intervention seminar. The analyses apply the General Linear Model procedure (see Cohen & Cohen, 1983) that explores the influence of three independent variables on the different outcomes. Two of the independent variables were between-subjects factors: Condition (Experimental vs. Control) and a quantitative factor, that is, the respondent's risk score. The third independent variable was a within-subject factor, namely, time of data collection (when available pretest at screening or T1, and at T2 and T3 posttests). Because respondents were randomized to the experimental conditions by site, site was also used in additional analyses as an independent factor, in addition to experimental condition, risk status, and time. However, the results of these analyses demonstrated that site had no main effect or interactive effects with the other independent variables on our outcomes. Furthermore, since the results of the analyses that excluded site as a factor were virtually the same as when site was included, and to avoid unnecessary complexity, we present the analyses that do not include the site as a factor. Similarly, the possible main and interactive effects of other factors on the dependent variables such as that of characteristics of the pair of trainers and the period of year (trainers increased experience as they trained more groups) were also tested. There were no significant main or interactive effects with risk and condition of these variables on the outcomes. These variables are therefore not included in the remaining analyses.

The pattern of differences and interactions between low- and high-risk participants and experimental conditions are displayed in figures for dependent measures that are based on indices (e.g., mastery, depression), and in tables for dependent variables that are based on interpretable natural units (e.g., reemployment status, income per month). In these figures and tables, the data are presented according to risk status in terms of low- and high-risk categories as defined prospectively and used for randomizing

Table 1. Matrix of Intercorrelations among Experimental Condition, Risk, and Dependent Variables at T2 (Lower Triangle), at T3 (Upper Triangle) and Autocorrelations (in the Diagonal)[a]

Variable	1	2	3	4	5	6	7	8	9	10	11
1. Experimental condition[b]	**1.00**	-.01	-.06	-.06	.06	.10	-.05	-.02	.02	.00	.04
2. Risk for depression	-.01	**1.00**	.38	.39	-.27	-.28	.32	.24	-.15	-.03	-.07
3. Depression	-.04	.43	**.62**	.83	-.58	-.49	.43	.45	-.27	-.16	-.19
4. Distress	NA	NA	NA	NA	-.66	-.51	.40	.48	-.30	-.13	-.15
5. Functioning	.04	-.32	-.61	NA	**.63**	.52	-.28	-.39	.40	.10	.11
6. Mastery	.07	-.33	-.52	NA	.55	**.69**	-.24	-.27	.19	.12	.20
7. Financial strain	-.04	.35	.39	NA	-.29	-.22	**.62**	.24	-.14	-.33	-.44
8. Distress SO report	-.00	.29	.45	NA	-.41	-.31	.27	**.58**	-.62	-.10	-.11
9. Functioning, SO report	-.02	-.20	-.27	NA	.43	.26	-.20	-.63	**.61**	.05	.06
10. Employment status[c]	.07	.04	-.11	NA	.02	.05	-.26	-.07	-.00	**.34**	.68
11. Monthly income	.07	-.01	-.15	NA	.06	.11	-.32	-.11	.04	.74	**.51**

[a]The number of respondents for the computed correlations ranges between 1,185 to 1,801. T2 = 2-month posttest; T3 = 6-month posttest. NA = not available; data on this variable was not collected at T2.
[b]Coded 0 = Control, 1 = Experimental.
[c]Coded 0 = Employed less than 20 hours per week, 1 = Employed 20 or more hours per week.

respondents into the experimental and control condition. The same ANOVAs were repeated using risk as a factor with low- and high-risk levels (risk status) based on our screening categorization. These analyses produced virtually the same results as those using the continuous risk score. This absence of difference provides justification for presenting the results in the figures and tables according to our prospective categorization of low- and high-risk status. The analyses of the experimental effects of the intervention are presented first on the sense of mastery, and then on the intended reemployment and mental health outcomes. Finally, we present analyses for examining the convergent validity of the intervention effects based on reports of both job seekers and their significant others. The matrix of the intercorrelations among the experimental and the dependent variables at Times 2 and 3 posttests is presented in Table 1.

Effects on Mastery as a Proximal Outcome

The JOBS II intervention was redesigned to focus on the enhancement of sense of personal mastery through addressing both the emotional and problem-solving coping tasks of the jobs seeker. We hypothesized that this intervention focus would therefore have a beneficial impact on this construct.

We then analyzed the mastery index[4] as a function of Condition (Experimental vs. Control), respondent's Risk Score, and Time of measurement (Table 2). The results of this analysis are displayed in standardized z-score units in Figure 2.

The results show that although prior to the intervention there was virtually no difference on level of mastery between the experimental and the control group, after the intervention the experimental group had higher mastery scores than the control group (for Time 2 and Time 3: Cohen's $d = .19$ and .21, respectively). The analysis produced statistically significant Condition main effect, and a Condition × Time interaction effect (respectively, $p < .05, p < .01$). As expected, the high-risk respondents had significantly lower mastery scores than the low-risk respondents $(p < .01)$. However, risk did not moderate the effect of the intervention on mastery. Thus, although we expected the JOBS intervention to result in a greater increase in sense of mastery for the high- rather than the low-risk participants, it produced the same increase for both types of participants. Next we turn to the question of whether the intent of the intervention to improve the reemployment outcomes of the participants materialized.

---

[4]The same analysis was performed separately on each component of the mastery measure and the pattern of the results was the same as that for the global mastery measure.

Table 2. Summary Table of General Linear Model Procedure of ANOVA for Mastery

Source	df	SS	MS	F
Between subjects				
Condition (C)	1	2.25	2.25	4.47[a]
Risk	1	103.4	103.4	204.86[b]
R × C	1	0.82	0.82	1.64
Error	1332	669.97	0.50	
Within subjects				
Time (T)	2	19.31	9.65	110.87[b]
T × C	2	3.56	1.78	20.43[b]
T × R	2	1.83	0.92	10.53[b]
T × R × C	2	0.03	0.02	0.19
Error (Time)	2664	231.97	0.09	

[a] $p < .05$.
[b] $p < .01$.

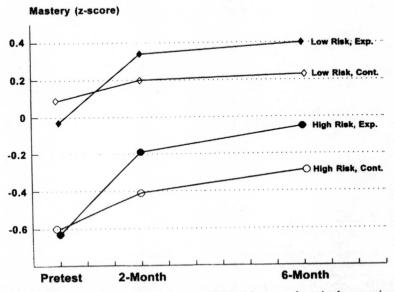

Figure 2. Mean z scores of mastery for low- and high-risk respondents in the experimental and control conditions of the JOBS field experiment.

498   Amiram D. Vinokur *et al.*

Experimental Effects on Reemployment Outcomes

Our first analysis of employment outcomes focused on rates of reemployment at T2 and T3. We performed separate analyses in which reemployment was defined either in terms of a combination of the objective and subjective criteria, or solely in terms of an objective criterion of working 20 or more hours per week.

Since both versions of the dependent variables were defined as a dichotomous variable (reemployed vs. unemployed status) logistic regression was used to analyze reemployment outcomes (Neter & Wasserman, 1974). As in the previous analyses, we examined the effects of experimental condition, the continuous risk measure, and their interaction on the dependent variable. Table 3 presents the proportion of reemployed respondents in each of the four combinations of experimental condition and risk status at the 2-month and 6-month posttests. The top and the bottom of Table 3 present the results according to the reemployment measure based first on the combined measure and second on the objective measure. At 2-month posttest, a higher proportion of both low- and high-risk respondents in the experimental group than in the control group was reemployed, Wald's $\chi^2(1) = 4.44$ and 5.79, for combined and objective criterion, respectively,

Table 3. Proportion of Reemployed Respondents According to Experimental Condition and Risk Status at 2-Month and 6-Month Follow-Up Posttest

	2-Month posttest[a]				6-Month posttest[b]			
	Experimental		Control		Experimental		Control	
	Proportion	SD	Proportion	SD	Proportion	SD	Proportion	SD
Reemployed (combined criteria)[c]								
Risk status								
Low	.34	.48	.27	.44	.59	.49	.62	.49
High	.35	.47	.29	.45	.56	.50	.46	.50
Reemployed (hours per week)[d]								
Risk status								
Low	.40	.49	.35	.48	.63	.48	.67	.47
High	.44	.50	.35	.48	.62	.49	.54	.50

[a] At T2, number of respondents in the experimental and control condition using the combined criteria was 670 and 335, respectively, and using the hours/week criteria the number was 933 and 442, respectively.
[b] At T3, number of respondents in the experimental and control condition using the combined criteria was 815 and 367, respectively, and using the hours/week criteria the number was 1,050 and 467, respectively.
[c] Reemployed respondents were those working 20 or more hours per week *and* reporting they had already been working as many hours as they need. Unemployed respondents were those working less than 20 hours per week and/or reporting not working as many hours as they need.
[d] Reemployed respondents were those working 20 or more hours per week. Unemployed respondents were those working less than 20 hours per week or not working at all.

both $p < .05$. There was no interaction between experimental condition and risk. In contrast, by the 6-month posttest, the likelihood of reemployment depended jointly on the condition and risk factors, as indicated by a significant Condition $\times$ Risk interaction, Wald's $\chi^2(1) = 4.13$ and 4.55, for combined and objective criterion, respectively, both $p < .05$. The nature of this interaction can be noted in the results showing that the likelihood of reemployment of low-risk respondents in the intervention group was not significantly different than that in the control group ($p = .44$). However, high-risk respondents in the intervention group were significantly more likely to be reemployed than high-risk controls ($p < .05$). The difference in the proportion of reemployed respondents between experimental and control conditions for the low-risk group was $-.03$ (proportions of .59 vs. 62, respectively) versus a difference of .10 for the high-risk group (.56 vs. .46, respectively, Cohen's ES $h = .20$; Cohen, 1988, pp. 180–185). The same pattern of significant results was obtained using the objective criterion for defining reemployment as presented in the bottom half of Table 3. Here, the difference in the proportion of reemployed respondents between experimental and control conditions for the low-risk group was $-.04$ (.63 vs. 67, respectively) versus a difference of .08 for the high-risk group (.62 vs. .54, respectively, Cohen's ES $h = .15$).

Next we analyzed the effects of the intervention on reported monthly income from paid work. Again, a general linear model ANOVA was performed with risk as a continuous variable and with repeated measures of monthly earnings from paid work at 2 and 6 months after the intervention. The means of monthly income are presented in Table 4 by experimental condition and risk status. Not surprisingly, the most pronounced result is the effect of time. As more respondents became reemployed, the mean monthly income significantly increased from the 2-month to the 6-month posttest, $F(1, 1208) = 163.41$, $p < .01$. In addition, experimental condition had a

Table 4. Mean Monthly Income (Dollars) of Low- and High-Risk Respondents in the JOBS Experimental and Control Condition[a]

| | 2-Month posttest | | | | 6-Month posttest | | | |
| | Experimental | | Control | | Experimental | | Control | |
Risk status	M	SD	M	SD	M	SD	M	SD
Low	733	1151	626	965	1147	1282	1192	1073
High	720	996	513	860	1098	1134	828	973

[a] Number of respondents in the low-risk and high-risk experimental condition was 511 and 313, respectively, and in the control condition the number was 231 and 157, respectively, for a total of 1,212. These numbers are the same for the 2-month and the 6-month posttest.

significant main effect on monthly income, $F(1, 1208) = 3.89, p < .05$, as well as an interaction effect of condition by risk, $F(1, 1208) = 4.50, p < .05$, with high-risk respondents benefiting more from the intervention than their counterparts in the control group in both Time 2 $(d = .22)$ and Time 3 $(d = .26)$.

Experimental Effects on Mental Health and Well-Being Outcomes

Figure 3 presents the means of depressive symptomatology at time of screening and at the two posttests. To convey information on effect size, the means are expressed in standard deviation units.

As could be expected from the way risk status was constructed (being based primarily on the depression score), with no exception the mean depression score is consistently higher for the high-risk than for the low-risk respondents (Table 5). Furthermore, whereas at the time of screening, there was no difference in mean depression between the respondents in the experimental and the control group of the respective risk groups, at both 2-month and 6-month posttests, the high-risk respondents in the experimental group had lower depression scores than their high-risk counterparts in the control group. Thus, the Condition × Time and Condition × Risk interactions were

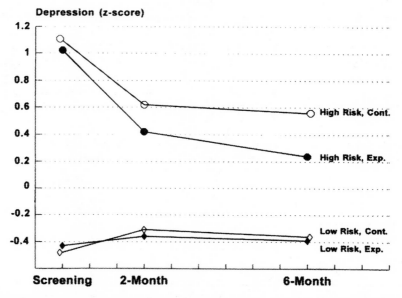

Figure 3. Mean z scores of depression symptoms for low- and high-risk respondents in the JOBS field experiment.

Table 5. Summary Table of General Linear Model Procedure
of ANOVA of Depression Symptoms

Source	df	SS	MS	F
Between subjects				
Condition (C)	1	3.12	3.12	7.63[b]
Risk	1	475.72	475.71	1161.25[b]
R × C	1	1.68	1.68	4.10[a]
Error	1331	545.25	0.41	
Within subjects				
Time (T)	2	11.20	5.60	30.25[b]
T × C	2	1.45	0.72	3.91[a]
T × R	2	50.49	25.25	136.37[b]
T × R × C	2	0.22	0.11	0.61
Error (Time)	2662	492.81	0.19	

[a] $p < .05$
[b] $p < .01$.

statistically significant (both $p < .05$). Further analyses indicated that for the low-risk respondents, none of the differences between experimentals and controls were statistically significant. In contrast, and as expected for the high-risk respondents, there was no statistical difference at screening, $t(512) = 1.38$, $p < .16$, but there was a statistically significant difference at 2-month and 6-month posttests, $t(512) = 2.02$, $d = .20$, and $t(512) = 3.08$, $d = .22$, $p < .05$ and .01, respectively. In summary, in both follow-up periods, only the high-risk respondents in the experimental group exhibited significantly lower levels of depressive symptomatology than their high-risk counterparts in the control group.

Convergent Validity of the Intervention Effects Based on the Reports of Both Job Seekers and their Significant Others

As shown in Table 1, the intercorrelations among the various measures of mental health (i.e., depression, distress) and well-being (i.e., role and emotional functioning) within each type of respondent (i.e., focal respondents and significant others) are moderate to high, mostly above .5. However, the intercorrelations between the respective measures based on the job seekers and those based on the significant others are somewhat lower, mostly about .4. These lower correlations raise the question of the extent to which the pattern of results shown with depression would replicate when the analyses are based simultaneously on the respective measures from both types of respondents.

To examine the question of the convergent validity of the effects of the intervention on mental health outcomes, we conducted multivariate analyses

(MANOVAs) of two measures that were available from both the focal respondents and their significant others only at the 6-month posttest. For each measure, the spouse/significant other provided ratings of his or her observations of the focal respondent's behaviors, reactions and symptoms, who in turn, rated his or her own experiences using the same 5-point scales. The two MANOVAs included the measure of distress symptoms and of role and emotional functioning at Time 3 posttest. Table 6 includes the results of the MANOVAs and Figure 4 presents the means (in standard deviation units) of these measures.

The analyses produced a statistically significant Condition × Risk interaction effect for both distress ($p < .05$) and functioning ($p < .01$), as well as a Risk main effect for both measures ($p < .01$), and a Condition main effect for distress ($p < .05$). As can be seen in Figure 4, the analyses produced the same consistent pattern of statistically significant results. Additional results from the MANOVA analyses revealed that, while as noted above, the Condition × Risk interactions were statistically significant, the Rater (Focal Respondent vs. Significant Other) × Condition × Risk interactions were not statistically significant ($p < .28$, and $.51$, respectively, for distress and functioning). The absence of the three-way interaction effects indicates that the pattern of Condition × Risk interaction was not different for both focal respondent and significant other data. There is virtually no difference in mean severity of distress symptoms or level of functioning between the low-risk status experimental and control group respondents ($t = 0.21$ and 0.37, respectively, for focal respondent distress and functioning, and $t = -1.09$ and 0.62, respectively, for reports of significant other). In contrast, the high-risk respondents in the experimental group displayed lower levels of distress

Table 6. Summary Table of General Linear Model Procedure of MANOVA of Distress and of Functioning

Source	df	SS	MS	F
Distress				
Condition (C)	1	2.37	2.37	4.24[a]
Risk (R)	1	127.41	127.41	228.13[b]
R × C	1	2.96	2.96	5.29[a]
Error	1418	791.96	0.56	
Functioning				
C	1	1.90	1.90	3.38
R	1	57.68	57.68	102.77[b]
R × C	1	3.95	3.95	7.04[b]
Error (Time)	1425	799.83	0.56	

[a] $p < .05$
[b] $p < .01$.

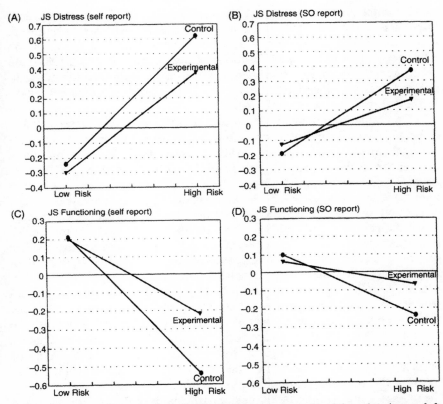

Figure 4. Mean z scores of job seeker's (JS) distress reported by job seeker (upper left-hand, Figure A), and by his/her significant other (SO) (upper right-hand, Figure B), and of job seeker's functioning reported by job seeker (lower left-hand, Figure C), and by his/her significant other (lower right-hand, Figure D) at 6-month follow-up.

symptoms and better functioning than their counterparts in the control group ($t = 2.78$, $d = .25$, and $t = -4.07$, $d = .32$, both $p < .01$, respectively, for focal respondent distress and functioning, and $t = 2.20$, $d = .20$, and $t = -2.19$, $d = .17$, both $p < .05$, respectively, for reports of significant other).

Actual Effects of Participation in the Intervention: Comparing Participants with their Control Group Counterparts

In conducting the analyses presented above, we chose to preserve the integrity of randomization in the field experiment (Cook & Campbell, 1979). Therefore, we included in the analyses all respondents who had been originally assigned to the experimental group, whether or not they were actually exposed to the JOBS Intervention Seminar. Since 46% of the experimental group respondents did not attend the JOBS intervention, the effects of the intervention and its interaction with risk status represent very conservative lower bound estimates of the true magnitude of the effects on actual participants. In terms of effect size d (Cohen, 1988), the differences between the experimental and control conditions for the high-risk respondents ranged at Time 3 from .14 (for hours working per week) to .32 (for role and emotional functioning).

Departing from the above most conservative analyses, we proceeded to estimate the JOBS intervention effects on the actual participants by comparing them with their counterparts in the control group. These counterparts are defined as the "would-be participants," that is, the subgroup of persons from the control group who would become participants were they to be invited to the intervention. For this comparison we used an analytic strategy developed by Bloom (1984) and applied to our earlier JOBS I data (Vinokur, Price, & Caplan, 1991). The estimation of the mean of the would-be participants is based on the plausible assumption, supported by the logic of randomization, that the control group consists of the same proportion of respondents who would, and others who would not, participate in the intervention as in the experimental group. Note that the known mean of the control group is composed of (equal to) the weighted contributions of the would-be participants and the would-be nonparticipants. The weights are the known proportions of participation (i.e., $p = .54$) and nonparticipation (i.e., $1 - p = .46$). Thus, to extract the desired estimated mean of the would-be participants from the mean of the total control group, we substitute the known mean of the subgroup of nonparticipants from the experimental group for the unknown mean of the would-be nonparticipants of the control group and solve the equation. (This substitution is justified on the ground that these are equivalent subgroups of persons who did not participate in the intervention.)

The application of this procedure to estimate the intervention's effects on the actual participants using all the outcomes that were examined in the full experimental analyses resulted in consistently large increases in the effect size over those produced using the full randomized groups. Without exception, we found that the estimated effects on the actual participants were nearly twice as large as those obtained using the full randomized design.[5] Specifically, compared to the results obtained using the full design,

---

[5]To compute the effect size of participation one needs to estimate the joint standard deviation of the sample of participants and the would-be participants from the control group. We estimated this standard deviation by pooling the standard variations of the participants from the experimental group with the standard deviation of the entire control group. As indicated in our earlier work (Vinokur *et al.*, 1991, see Footnote 5) and in others (Heaney, 1991), the standard deviations of the participants, the nonparticipants, and the control group are very similar, and therefore, any estimate based on these parameters is quite robust.

which ranged in effect size from .14 (for hours of work per week) to .32 (for role and emotional functioning), the estimated effect size of participation ranged from .25 to .62 (respectively, for hours of work per week and for role and emotional functioning).

DISCUSSION AND CONCLUSIONS

Like its predecessor, the JOBS II intervention was designed to provide unemployed participants with social support, job search skills, and inoculation against setbacks as necessary components for enhancing their sense of mastery. Our results show that this proximal goal of the intervention was fully accomplished. That is, the findings demonstrate that the respondents in the intervention group had significantly higher levels of mastery than their control group counterparts. However, the analyses do not provide information on which one or more of these intervention components is responsible for the results. These components were intended to reinforce each other, and it may be that all are needed to produce the desired distal outcomes, which include both reemployment in high quality jobs and mental health.

The randomized JOBS II field experiment did, indeed, produce these desired outcomes. Our analyses replicated the findings of the earlier JOBS I study regarding the beneficial effects of the intervention on reemployment and mental health. More specifically, the JOBS II study replicated the results reported by Price *et al.* (1992) regarding the differential effects of the intervention on those identified retrospectively as low- and high-risk respondents. Using *prospective* screening to identify risk for depression, our results demonstrate that the JOBS II intervention had significant effects on mental health outcomes 2 and 6 months after the intervention for the high-risk respondents. Moreover, the results extend the earlier findings in showing that the beneficial effects of the intervention for high-risk respondents apply to reemployment as well as to mental health outcomes.

Because the JOBS intervention also promotes reemployment, the issue of whether it merely promotes the reemployment of program participants at the expense of displacing other workers needs to be addressed. There is reason to believe that such displacement effects are minimal. Davidson and Woodbury (1993) have examined the issue of displacement effects of programs that are intended to promote the reemployment of workers who lost their job and qualify for unemployment compensation. They found that the displacement effects of the programs were minimal and were offset by overall improvement in the performance of the economy that results from reducing the duration of job vacancies. This acceleration of job-filling, in turn, leads to the creation of a greater number of job opportunities. Thus, if programs that promote faster reemployment succeed in reemploying people more quickly or in helping people obtain jobs more suitable for their skills, they enhance the efficiency of the labor market and ultimately, contribute to economic growth.

In summary, our analyses produced consistent findings indicating that although the intervention had practically no benefit for the low-risk participants, it benefited the high-risk participants who needed it most. Furthermore, these benefits were produced by an intervention that was significantly shorter in duration (over 1-week vs. 2-week period, and with 30% fewer meeting hours) than the original intervention. It is also worth noting that the replicated findings were produced at a time when the labor market conditions for job seekers were more difficult than those for the intervention participants in the earlier JOBS I study.

The fact that the intervention benefited only the high-risk respondents and that we have the means for screening and recruiting high-risk participants suggests that the efficacy of the intervention may be increased by providing it only to high-risk individuals. However, there is the possibility that while the low-risk participants do not benefit from the intervention, their participation in the various group processes throughout the intervention produces positive effects on the ability of the high-risk participants to benefit from the intervention. For example, by having higher self-esteem, confidence and social skills, the low-risk participants may promote effective and socially supportive interactions among group members and provide the necessary positive role models for the high-risk participants. Therefore, the exclusion of low-risk participants from the program could undermine the effectiveness of the intervention process. Accordingly, the merit of implementing the intervention exclusively for high-risk participants should not be taken for granted, but rather tested in future research.

A related caution should be exercised in designing future implementation efforts of the JOBS intervention. The caution relates to certain limitations of the external validity of our study. Two factors that limit the generalizability of the study stem from our decision to recruit respondents to the study from the state unemployment compensation offices and to restrict eligibility to those recently unemployed, that is, those who lost their job fewer than 14 weeks from time of recruitment. An additional unintended factor that limits generalizability stems from the significant dropout of younger respondents and those experiencing higher levels of financial strain. Future studies may investigate whether other demographically distinct subgroups such as the chronically unemployed and those experiencing economic hardship could benefit from the JOBS intervention, and whether modifications are needed to make the intervention effective for these particular groups.

The fact that the JOBS II intervention had significant effects on reemployment outcomes such as monthly income, as well as mental health outcomes, is of special significance. There is evidence that both outcomes have a reciprocal relationship, each one influencing the other over time. Hamilton *et al.* (1993) demonstrated that depression among auto workers experiencing layoffs contributed to prolonged unemployment. Other studies have shown that reemployment restored mental health to pre-unemployment levels through its effect on the reduction of economic hardship and financial strain (e.g., Kessler *et al.*, 1988). As our current screening data and earlier risk analyses indicate, financial strain is a significant component of high risk for mental health problems among recent job losers. Furthermore, financial strain was found to be a mediator between unemployment status and poor mental health outcomes in earlier studies (Kessler, Turner, & House, 1987, 1988) and is probably a critical mediator of negative mental health outcomes for other life events as well (Umberson, Wortman, & Kessler, 1992).

We have restricted our use of data from spouses and significant others primarily to establishing the convergent validity of measures of distress and personal functioning. Indeed, we were able to show that the JOBS II intervention had positive effects on role and emotional functioning not only as reported by focal respondents but as also observed by spouses and significant others. These findings are encouraging since they triangulate intervention effects by obtaining additional reports by natural raters in the environment of the focal respondent. Our data present additional opportunities to understand the role of spouses and significant others in supporting or undermining the coping attempts of job losers. Other research indicates that job loss may affect family processes and the well-being of both spouses (Liem & Liem, 1988; Penkower, Bromet, & Dew, 1988) and children (Justice & Duncan, 1977; Steinberg, Catalano, & Dooley, 1981). But the influence of family dynamics may also flow in the other direction; spouses or significant others may play key roles in providing social support or social undermining to job seekers, which, in turn, may affect their psychological well-being and the motivation for job search behavior. Thus, the dynamics of social support and social undermining and their role in affecting psychological well-being and the motivation for job search will be explored in subsequent analyses.

These results by themselves do not reveal the mechanisms by which the JOBS intervention has its effects. For example, the mechanisms by which JOBS II increases the likelihood of reemployment, remain unclear. As we indicated earlier, the theoretical rationale underlying the JOBS intervention aims at increasing participant motivation for job search as well as increasing job search skills. Indeed, our earlier research demonstrated that the intervention increased job search behavior (van Ryn & Vinokur, 1992). However, how such increased motivation, the intensity of job search, or skills actually lead to improved reemployment and mental health outcomes remains to be discovered. A detailed analysis of the causal mechanisms leading from exposure to the JOBS intervention to an enhanced sense of mastery may illuminate the mechanisms by which this preventive intervention has its effects and represents still another avenue for future analyses.

ACKNOWLEDGMENT

This research was supported by National Institute of Mental Health Grant No. P50MH38330 to the Michigan Prevention Research Center (Richard H. Price, Principal Investigator).

REFERENCES

Bandura, A. (1977). Self-efficacy: Toward a unifying theory of behavior change. *Psychological Review, 84*, 191–215.
Barling, J. (1990). *Employment, stress and family functioning.* New York: Wiley.
Bentler, P. M. (1989). *EOS Structural Equation Program Manual.* Los Angeles: BMDP Statistical Software.
Bentler, P. M. & Bonnett, D. G. (1980). Significance tests and goodness of fit in the analysis of covariance structures. *Psychological Bulletin, 88*, 588–606.
Blinder, A. S. (1987). *Hard heads and soft hearts: Tough minded economics for a just society.* Reading MA: Addison-Wesley.
Bloom, H. S. (1984). Accounting for no-shows in experimental evaluation designs. *Evaluation Review, 8*, 225–246.
Brown, C. H. (1991). Comparison of mediational selected strategies and sequential designs for preventive trials: Comments on a proposal by Pillow *et al. American Journal of Community Psychology, 19*, 837–846.
Caplan, R. D. Abbey, A., Abramis, D. J., Andrews, F. M., Conway, T. L., & French, J. R. P. (1984). *Tranquilizer use and well-being: A longitudinal study of social and psychological effects* (Technical Report Series). Ann Arbor: University of Michigan, Institute for Social Research.
Caplan, R. D., Vinokur, A. D., Price, R. H., & van Ryn, M. (1989). Job seeking, reemployment, and mental health: A randomized field experiment in coping with job loss. *Journal of Applied Psychology, 74*, 759–769.
Catalano, R. (1991). The health effects of economic insecurity. *American Journal of Public Health, 81*, 1148–1152.
Catalano, R. & Dooley, D. (1977). Economic predictor of depressed mood and stressful life events in a metropolitan community. *Journal of Health and Social Behavior, 18*, 292–307.
Chamberlain, N. W., Cullen, D. E., & Lewin, D. (1980). *The labor sector* (3rd ed.). New York: McGraw-Hill.
Cobb, S. & Kasl, S. V. (1977). *Termination: The consequences of job loss* (NIOSH Research Report, DHEW Publication No. 77–224). Washington, DC: U.S. Government Printing Office.
Cohen, J. (1988). *Statistical power analysis for the behavioral sciences.* (2nd ed.). Hillsdale, NJ: Erlbaum.

Cohen, J. & Cohen, P. (1983). *Applied multiple regression/correlational analysis for the behavioral sciences* (2nd ed.). Hillsdale, NJ: Erlbaum.

Cook, T. D. & Campbell, D. T. (1979). *Quasi-experimentation: Design & analysis issues for field settings.* Boston: Houghton Mifflin.

Curran, J. (1992). *JOBS: A manual for teaching people successful job search strategies.* Ann Arbor: Michigan Prevention Research Center, Institute for Social Research.

Davidson, C. & Woodbury, S. A. (1993). The displacement effect of reemployment bonus programs. *Journal of Labor Economics, 11,* 575–605.

Derogatis, L. R., Lipman, R. S., Rickles, K., Uhlenhuth, E. H., & Covi, L., (1974). The Hopkins Symptom Checklist (HSCL). In P. Pichot (Ed.), *Psychological measurements in psychopharmacology: Modem problems in pharmacopsychiatry* (Vol. 7, pp. 79–110). New York: Karger, Basel.

Derogatis, L. R. & Melisaratos, N. (1983). The brief symptom inventory: An introductory report. *Psychological Medicine, 13,* 595–605.

Dew, M. A., Bromet, E. J., & Schulberg, H. C. (1987). A comparative analysis of two community stressors' long term, mental health effects. *American Journal of Community Psychology, 15,* 167–184.

Eden, D. & Aviram, A. (1993). Self-efficacy training to speed reemployment: Helping people to help themselves. *Journal of Applied Psychology, 78,* 352–360.

Emery, R. E. (1991). Mediational screening in theory and in practice. *American Journal of Community Psychology, 19,* 853–857.

Fryer, D. & Payne, R. (1986). Being unemployed: A review of the literature on the psychological experience of unemployment. *International Review of Industrial and Organizational Psychology* (Chap. 8, pp. 235–278).

Galassi, J. P., Delo, J. S., Galassi, M. D., & Bastien, S. (1974). The college self-expression scale: A measure of assertiveness. *Behavior Therapy, 5,* 165–171.

Gurin, P., Gurin, G., & Morrison, B. M. (1978). Personal and ideological aspects of internal and external control. *Social Psychology, 41,* 275–296.

Hamilton, V. L., Hoffman, W. S., Broman, C. L., & Rauma, D. (1993). Unemployment, distress, and coping: A panel study of autoworkers. *Journal of Personality and Social Psychology, 65,* 234–247.

Heaney, C. A. (1991). Enhancing social support at the workplace: Assessing the effects of the caregiver support program. *Health Education Quarterly, 18,* 477–494.

Hansen, W. B., Collins, L. M., Malotte, C. K., Johnson, C. A., & Fielding, J. E. (1985). Attrition in prevention research. *Journal of Behavioral Medicine, 8,* 261–275.

Hoelter, J. W. (1983). The analysis of covariance structures: Goodness-of-fit indices. *Sociological Methods and Research, 11,* 325–344.

Jones, W. H. & Russell, D. (1982). The social reticence scale: An objective instrument to measure shyness. *Journal of Personality Assessment, 46,* 629–631.

Justice, B. & Duncan, D. F. (1977). Child abuse as a work-related problem. *Corrective and Social Psychiatry, and Journal of Behavior Technology. Methods and Therapy, 23,* 53–55.

Kessler, R. C., Turner, J. B., & House, J. S. (1987). Intervening processes in the relationship between unemployment and health, *Psychological Medicine, 17,* 949–961.

Kessler, R. C., Turner, J. B., & House, J. S. (1988). The effects of unemployment on health in a community survey: Main, modifying, and mediating effects. *Journal of Social Issues, 44,* 69–85.

Kessler, R. C., Turner, J. B., & House, J. S. (1989). Unemployment, reemployment, and emotional functioning in a community sample. *American Sociological Review, 54,* 648–657.

Liem, R. & Liem, J. H. (1988). The psychological effects of unemployment on workers and their families. *Journal of Social Issues, 44,* 87–105.

Lykken, D. T. (1968). Statistical significance in psychological research. *Psychological Bulletin, 70*, 151–159.

Marshall, G. N. & Lang, E. L. (1990). Optimism, self-mastery, and symptoms of depression in women professionals. *Journal of Personality and Social Psychology, 59*, 132–139.

Neter, J. & Wasserman, W. (1974). *Applied linear statistical models: Regression, analysis of variance, and experimental designs.* Homewood, IL: R. D. Irwin.

Nunnally, J. C. (1978). *Psychometric theory.* New York: McGraw-Hill.

Pearlin, L. I. & Schooler, C. (1978). The structure of coping. *Journal of Health and Social Behavior, 19*, 2–21.

Pearlin, L. I., Menaghan, E. G., Lieberman, M. A., & Mullen, J. T. (1981). The stress process. *Journal of Health and Social Behavior, 22*, 337–356.

Penkower, L., Bromet, E., & Dew, M. (1988). Husbands' layoff and wives' mental health: a prospective analysis. *Archive of General Psychiatry, 45*, 994–1000.

Pillow, D. R., Sandler, I. N., Braver, S. L., Wolchik, S. A., & Gersten, J. C. (1991). Theory-based screening for prevention: Focusing on mediating processes in children of divorce. *American Journal of Community Psychology, 19*, 809–836.

Price, R. H., van Ryn, M., & Vinokur, A. D. (1992). Impact of preventive job search intervention on the likelihood of depression among the unemployed. *Journal of Health and Social Behavior, 33*, 158–167.

Price, R. H. & Vinokur, A. D. (1995). Michigan JOBS Program: Supporting career transitions in a time of organizational downsizing. In M. London (Ed.). *Employee development and job creation: Human resource strategies for organizational growth* (pp. 191–209). Guilford.

Rathus, S. A. (1973). A 30-item schedule for assessing assertive behavior. *Behavior Therapy, 4*, 398–406.

Reich, R. B. (1991). *The work of nations: Preparing ourselves for 21st century capitalism* (1st ed.). New York: A. A. Knopf.

Reid, J. B. (1991). Mediational screening as a model for prevention research. *American Journal of Community Psychology, 19*, 867–872.

Rosenberg, M. (1965). *Society and the adolescent self-image.* Princeton, NJ: Princeton University Press.

Rotter, J. B. (1966). Generalized expectancies for internal versus external control of reinforcement. *Psychological Monographs, 80* (Whole No. 609).

Steinberg, L, Catalano, R., & Dooley, D. (1981). Economic antecedents of child abuse and neglect. *Child Development, 52*, 975–985.

Umberson, D., Wortman, C. B., & Kessler, R. C. (1992). Widowhood and depression: Explaining long-term gender difference in vulnerability. *Journal of Health and Social Behavior, 33*, 10–24.

U.S. Bureau of Labor Statistics (1988, January). *Employment and Earning* (Vol. 35). Washington, DC: U.S. Government Printing Office.

U.S. Bureau of Labor Statistics (1992, January). *Employment and Earning* (Vol. 39). Washington, DC: U.S. Government Printing Office.

van Ryn, M. & Vinokur, A. D. (1992). How did it work? An examination of the mechanisms through which a community intervention influenced job-search behavior among an unemployed sample. *American Journal of Community Psychology, 20*, 577–599.

Vinokur, A. & Caplan, R. D. (1987). Attitudes and social support: Determinants of job-seeking behavior and well-being among the unemployed. *Journal of Applied Social Psychology, 17*, 1007–1024.

Vinokur, A., Caplan, R. D., & Williams, C. C. (1987). Effects of recent and past stress on mental health: Coping with unemployment among Vietnam veterans and non-veterans. *Journal of Applied Social Psychology, 17*, 708–728.

Vinokur, A. D., Price, R. H., & Caplan, R. D. (1991). From field experiments to program implementation: Assessing the potential outcomes of an experimental intervention program for unemployed persons. *American Journal of Community Psychology, 19*, 543–562.

Vinokur, A. D., van Ryn, M., Gramlich, E. M., & Price, R. H. (1991). Long-term follow-up and benefit-cost analysis of the Jobs Project: A preventive intervention for the unemployed. *Journal of Applied Psychology, 76*, 213–219.

Warr, P. B. (1983). Job loss, unemployment and psychological well-being. In V. Allen & E. van de Vliert (Eds.), *Role transitions.* New York: Plenum Press.

White, R. W. (1959). Motivation reconsidered: The concept of competence. *Psychological Review, 66*, 297–333.

Yeaton, W. H. & Sechrest, L. (1981). Critical dimensions in the choice and maintenance of successful treatments: Strength, integrity, and effectiveness. *Journal of Consulting and Clinical Psychology, 49*, 156–157.

23

A Future for Community Psychology: The Contexts of Diversity and the Diversity of Contexts*

Edison J. Trickett

Today I revisit a premise central to community psychology since its official inception (Bennett *et al.*, 1966): the importance of developing theory, research, and intervention which locates individuals, social settings, and communities in sociocultural context. I return to this premise not because community psychology has not made significant substantive and distinctive contributions to research and practice during the last three decades but because of how much work remains to be done. We are still struggling with how to incorporate issues of culture and context into the questions we ask, the research strategies we pursue, and the ways we design and carry out interventions (Bernal & Enchautegui-de-Jesus, 1994; Leidig, 1977; Loo, Fong, & Iwamasa, 1988; Myers & Pitts, 1977; Novaco & Monahan, 1980; Trickett, Watts, & Birman, 1993; Walsh, 1987a). Incorporating culture and context more fully into the conceptual frameworks and intervention activities of the field will both further the field's originating vision and create an exciting and socially responsible agenda for the future. It represents an opportunity for community psychology to make a distinctive contribution to how we think and how we act.

In developing the argument for the importance and distinctiveness of a community psychology that integrates culture and context, I begin with the

*Society for Community Research and Action's Award for Distinguished Contribution to Theory and Research presented at the annual convention of the American Psychological Association in New York, NY, August, 1995. Originally published in the *American Journal of Community Psychology*, 24(2) (1996): 209–234.

A Quarter Century of Community Psychology: Readings from the American Journal of Community Psychology, edited by Tracey A. Revenson *et al.* Kluwer Academic/Plenum Publishers, New York, 2002.

vision of the field contained in the report of the Swampscott conference
(Bennett *et al.*, 1966). Next, three interrelated areas of scholarship are discussed which provide intellectual support for the importance of incorporating
culture and context into our future work: the development of a contextualist
philosophy of science, the emerging importance of methodological pluralism,
and the evolving paradigms in the area of human diversity. The conceptual
vehicle for this incorporation is an ecological perspective highlighted by the
title of the paper: the contexts of diversity and diversity of contexts. A contextual approach to acculturation theory and research is used to clarify some
of the many implications of the title for linking the process of acculturation to
varied social and cultural contexts. Finally, some concrete ways of attending to
culture and context in the execution and reporting of research are mentioned.

CONTEXT AND COMMUNITY PSYCHOLOGY'S ORIGINATING VISION

From the outset, both the social context in which community psychology arose and the hopes articulated at the Swampscott conference suggest
the centrality of context in the evolution of the field. The race riots, identity
politics, inequalities reflected in social institutions, and social activism in the
broader culture were reflected in the vision articulated at Swampscott.

> By the end of the conference the founders' focus was not limited to com-
> munity mental health but encompassed a broader conception of social
> interventions ... community psychologists would serve as proponents of
> the concept of community in community mental health work, advocates
> for the poor and minorities, and active participants in and contributors to
> social and political life. (Bennett *et al.*, 1966, p. 528)

The initial intent of this new field was to create a profession built on
new ways of thinking, new targets for intervention, new professional roles,
and new hopes for collaborating with citizens and communities.
Conceptually, however, such a vision firmly tied theory, research, and practice to a focus on the interdependence of people and context. Quoting
again from the Swampscott report:

> The main focus on prevention has led to a necessary concern with the
> interaction between social system structures and functions and the mental
> health of populations. Attempts at interventions in social systems, with a
> preventive emphasis, becomes a logical extension of community mental
> health services. (pp. 6–7)

Over time, much has been accomplished in the service of these broad
goals. Research traditions have developed in the assessment of important
social settings (Barker, 1968; Kelly, 1979; Moos, 1974, 1979). We have

embraced the value-driven nature of inquiry and intervention and the role of advocacy (e.g., Rappaport, 1977, 1990) and have highlighted the scholarly and social benefits of developing collaborative rather than hierarchical relationships between scholar and citizen (e.g., Kelly, 1986; Kelly & Hess, 1986; Walsh, 1987b). We now promote interventions focusing on competence, strength, and wellness rather than bumbling and pathology (Cowen, 1980, 1994; Tyler, 1978); and our contribution to preventive interventions has yielded sufficient substantive knowledge (see Trickett, Dahiyat, & Selby, 1994) to cause debate about the possible status of prevention as an area of professional certification. This last development confirms the wisdom of the warning "be careful what you wish for."

Together, these themes locate individual and group behavior in the real world with its multiple levels of influence, acknowledge that our world includes groups diverse both in resources and culture, and suggests that learning about and doing good in that real world involves creating authentic relationships that are inclusionary, negotiated, and involve the development of trust and reciprocal commitment. These strands of work do indeed provide the conceptual and empirical momentum for creating a distinctive coherent identity for community psychology.

However, the lack of widespread inclusion of multiple cultural groups as respondents (Loo *et al.*, 1988), the relative lack of multilevel research designs (see Shinn, 1996), and the lack of attention to the systemic affects of interventions illustrate the ongoing struggle for culture and context to be systematically incorporated into theory and research. Thus, we have not begun to explore the richness of such contextual questions as how empowerment is defined differently in different ethnic communities and by men and women (Gibbs & Fuery, 1994; Riger, 1993; Trickett, 1994); how to turn individually based preventive interventions into systemic resources for the settings in which they occur (Kelly & Hess, 1986; Trickett & Birman, 1989; Trickett, Kelly, & Vincent, 1985); and how to craft the research relationship between interventionist and host setting so that externally funded projects continue after the grant runs out. We are still working on the "community" of community psychology as it involves the intertwining of culture and social context.

Peeling the Contextual Onion

As Kuhn (1970) has noted, it is extraordinarily difficult to both understand the implications of one's paradigm and to change it. Part of the problem is the degree to which assumptions are implicit and hence not readily available for self-scrutiny (Sarason, 1972). Like layers of the onion, the unappreciated implications of assumptions seem to unfold gradually in a never-ending manner. And like uncovering layers of the onion, the more you uncover the more you want to cry about how little you previously understood.

Although progress is slow, the layers of the contextual onion are indeed being peeled as psychology more generally is reevaluating some of its ahistorical, acultural, and acontextual assumptions. Thus, we now understand that neither United States college students nor men necessarily represent all human beings. We now see that the laboratory is itself an ecological context with demand characteristics and experimenter influence, not a setting in which to discover context-free basic processes. We now understand that our penchant to locate problems, particularly social problems, in individuals (Caplan & Nelson, 1973; Sarason, 1981) reflects this ahistorical, acontextual, acultural mind-set, thus making classics of such books such as *Blaming the Victim* (Ryan, 1971).

But there are other, perhaps more subtle, manifestations. For example, the American Psychological Association (APA) ethical codes reflect primarily the physician's oath to do no harm to the individual without mention of the issue of community accountability, a concern explicitly mentioned in the ethical code of the American Anthropological Association (Trickett, 1998). And decontextualization of research is found in the discrepancy between the ways in which we construct our work for publication and the ways in which we actually conduct it (see Trickett, 1992). Normative publication practices suggest the unlikely proposition that descriptions of the research relationship or the settings where the research occurs are not relevant to either the replicability of the study or the validity of its findings. In these and many other ways, the imagery and influence of context has been missing, stripped from the conceptualization, investigation, and reporting of the human experience. When Sarason stated that "the implications of the obvious are not themselves obvious," I bet even he was not fully aware of all that he was implying.

Let me now turn to the three developments previously mentioned which provide contextual momentum of direct relevance to community psychology: (a) the evolution of contextualism as a philosophy of science; (b) the movement toward methodological pluralism, and (c) the evolving paradigms of human diversity and multiculturalism. Taken together, these three developments provide epistemological, methodological, and empirical support for the evolution of a community psychology that focuses on the contexts of diversity and the diversity of contexts.

PHILOSOPHY OF SCIENCE: CONTEXTUALISM AND COMMUNITY PSYCHOLOGY

In an 1985 APA symposium celebrating the 20th anniversary of the Swampscott Conference (Altman, 1987), Altman suggested that a field intent on contextualizing human behavior across different levels of analysis is well served by a world view and epistemology that provides both rationale and guidance for its intellectual journey. As community psychology has evolved, so has interest in contextualism as a philosophy of science. While the implications of a contextualist philosophy of science reach far beyond the boundaries of community psychology per se, its spirit provides both direction and energy for our field.

Its essence is nicely described by Rosnow and Georgoudi (1986).

> In short, the idea is that psychological knowledge is made concrete and is framed by relevant factors, relations, and conditions (the setting or context) within which, or among which, human acts unfold. Contextualism underscores the idea that human activity does not develop in a social vacuum, but rather it is rigorously situated within a sociohistorical and cultural context of meanings and relationships. Like a message that makes sense only in terms of the total context in which it occurs, human actions are embedded in a context of time, space, culture, and the local tacit rules of conduct.... The idea of contextualism implies that to unlock the mysteries of what makes an event meaningful we must consider, via methodological and theoretical pluralism, the wider context that "allows" or "invites" the occurrence of that event and renders it socially intelligible. (pp. 4–5)

Such a perspective serves as antidote to more positivistic assumptions. As Shweder (1990) framed it: "The ideas of a context-free environment, a meaning-free stimulus event, and a fixed meaning are probably best kept where they belong, along with placeless space, eventless time, and squared circles on that famous and fabulous list of impossible notions" (p. 8).

McGuire (1983) outlined several research implications of this epistemology in contrasting contextualism with logical empiricism. For example, he offered the assumption that from a contextualist perspective all hypotheses are true, even contradictory ones; the task is to uncover the contexts in which they hold. Some may be broadly true, some narrowly, but, quoting Blake's aphorism, he stated "Everything possible to be believed is an image of truth." The less poetic community psychologist may see this as an invitation to speculate not about any particular set of hypotheses or relationships in vacuo, such as whether or not certain kinds of competence lead to adaptive behavior in general, but about the contexts in which relationships may be expected to be confirmed and those in which they may not. It follows from this that a primary purpose of research, including research which tests theory-driven hypotheses, is to generate hypotheses about the contextual constraints of any specific piece of knowledge. In an ironic and topsy-turvy way, quantitative work may thus assume the same potential often attributed to qualitative work; that it serves, and should serve, a hypothesis generating function.

The contextualist position provides an alternative metaphor for thinking about the purposes of research. Rather than viewing research as progressing in linear effort fashion toward truths generalizable across culture, context, and time, processes labelled as basic become candidates for historical and cross-cultural comparison. Here, the emic–etic distinction underlying much cross-cultural work comes to mind. Only through an investigation of phenomena in varying contexts can we discern what is universal and what is culture- or setting-specific, and then only at a particular historical moment.

But if knowledge is so differentiated by culture and context and is so temporally bounded, what is the point? I am taken with the way Cronbach put it in his lovely paper "Social Inquiry by and for Earthlings" (1986):

> Will social knowledge "progress"? Yes. but ... it will be the kind of progress seen in architecture, music, and philosophy. Each of these fields has become richer in each century, the contributions of the past remaining a resource for the present. We are better off for having Descartes and Kant, Beethoven and Bartok, Piranesi and Le Corbusier. We do not store up truth or laws. What social scientists mostly harvest are additional concepts and inquiry skills, along with careful records of events observed. Rather than disparaging such inquiry as unproductive, we should cherish its power to nourish the culture. Mary Hesse put it nicely: "What progresses is the ability to use science to learn the environment. That learning is ever to be done afresh, day by day and generation by generation." (p. 104)

Kingry-Westergaard and Kelly (1990) have shown the relevance of a contextualist epistemology for research and intervention in community psychology more specifically. Tying contextualist epistemology directly to an ecological perspective, they suggest that understanding behavior in context means attending to the varied social constructions of participants in the context, including those of the researcher or interventionist. Achieving such understanding rests on the development of collaborative relationships with setting participants. This, in turn, creates conditions for the authentic exploration of social processes in the setting and the creation of interventions of local relevance.

METHODOLOGY: CONTEXT AND METHODOLOGICAL PLURALISM

To the degree to which behavior is viewed contextually, methods for understanding context become central. To the degree to which any method provides partial and distorted information (Fiske, 1986), diversity of methods becomes important to appreciate and explore. Although the emphasis on quantitative methods still holds sway in psychology more generally and, indeed, in community psychology as well, the call for diversity of methods is now quite widespread. The impetus arises from many sources, including the postmodern critiques of positivism which undergird much feminist literature (e.g., Belenky, Clinchy, Goldberger, & Tarule, 1986; Riger, 1993) and in what Rapapport (1990) referred to as the empowerment social agenda.

They are also found in the swelling literature on the limitations and unintended consequences of quantitative methods more generally. Ten years ago Cronbach (1986) reflected on the unintended consequences of his classic 1955 paper with Meehl "Construct Validity in Psychological Tests." He concluded that while its intent was "to bring together rigorous evaluation to interpretations of psychological tests, particularly personality tests," its long-term effect, while useful in some ways, propelled a movement that has had "a repressive effect.... Taken as a whole," wrote Cronbach, "the paper devalued conjectural interpretations.... Progress requires that we respect poorly formed and even 'untestable ideas' " (pp. 85–86).

Maltz (1994) raised another set of issues in his recent paper "Deviating from the Mean: The Declining Significance of Significance." His focus centered on some of the unintended consequences of significance testing. One involves an overemphasis on hypothesis testing and a relative lack of attention paid to description of phenomena (see also Cohen, 1994, "The Earth is Round: $p < .05$"). Maltz echoed the contextualist hopes of McGuire in recommending that more attention be paid to a descriptive examination of sampling distributions "not only in terms of testing hypotheses, but in terms of generating them as well" (p. 442).

Maltz additionally suggests that the creation of categories central in quantification assumes a unimodality of meaning which decontextualizes phenomena.

> Social scientists tend to employ categories that are almost cartesian in nature, with sharply defined edges that do not overlap. But there are often culturally biased visions of reality implicit deep within these categories. For example, we use terms like dropout, minority, broken homes, lower class, working mothers, and even age, school, and education level as if they are unitary phenomena, notwithstanding the fact that some intact homes are so stressful that a broken home is a welcome alternative (or) that schools affect individuals differently, depending on their temperaments and on family interactions, and that some schools are so bad that the only rational act is to drop out. (p. 449)

And he quotes Stark about the decontextualizing of research in the field of criminology. "Poor neighborhoods disappeared (from the social science literature) to be replaced by individual kids with various levels of family income, but no detectable environment at all.... Yet through it all, social scientists somehow still knew better than to stroll the streets at night in certain parts of town or even to park there." (Stark, 1987, p. 894 as cited in Maltz, 1994, p. 451).

For community psychology, as for many areas of psychology, the primary methods of understanding that have been underrepresented in our research and journals involve qualitative research or studies that include both quantitative and qualitative methods. There are exceptions, of course, such as Watts' (1993) qualitative study of community development programs for young African–American men, Maton's (1994) research on the New Covenant Fellowship, Bond and Keys's (1993) report of empowerment and the functioning of community boards, Hughes and DuMont's (1993) use of focus groups with dual-earner African American families, and my paper with Judy Gruber (Gruber & Trickett, 1986) on the paradoxes of empowerment in the participatory governance of a public school. But in the main, adventuresome research within community psychology has not adventured in this direction.

The relative neglect of qualitative methods, however, has resulted in an enormous loss in our understanding of context. The instinct behind most qualitative work is the interest in social complexity, in nuance, in understanding how different levels of the ecological environment impinge on the way individuals and communities develop a rhythm, order their priorities, and create resources to cope with stressful life events. Such work is more likely to illuminate how lives are led locally and in context. Further, qualitative work encourages, often necessitates, long-term involvement with and commitment to a place, allows a look at how local processes unfold over time, and engenders relationships with citizens which promote the shared social construction of the meaning of data and concepts (Kingry-Westergaard & Kelly, 1990). As an exemplar of the richness of this approach I recommend the work of Burton (1990, 1991; Burton & Dilworth-Anderson, 1991) on the transition to adolescent parenthood among African American adolescents. Her ethnographic description of the norms, networks, and nuances of relationships in which these mothers are embedded shows how this transition cannot be understood without explicit reference to cultural history and current context.

An Ecological Framework: Human Diversity Highlights the Importance of Context

Previous sections have discussed forces that call for an increase in diversity of epistemology and diversity of method in behavioral sciences more generally and psychology in particular. The past 30 years have also witnessed an increased substantive emphasis in psychology on issues of human diversity. This work has progressed through a series of paradigms, each of which brings it closer to an ecological perspective integrating culture and social context.

Rod Watts, Dina Birman, and I have given our perspective on this evolution in our paper "Human Diversity and Community Psychology: Still Hazy After All These Years" (Trickett *et al.*, 1993). First came a transition in consciousness of mainstream psychology about the lives and social circumstances of groups previously rendered invisible or excluded from full participation in the opportunities of the society. Psychology itself, in its representatives and its theories, was seen as mirroring larger issues of social inequality and invisibility. When substantive attention within psychology was directed to understanding the lives of nonrepresented groups, the primary paradigm focused on perceived inadequacies, or "an interpretation of the other (nonrepresented groups) as a deficient or undeveloped version of the self" (Shweder & Sullivan, 1993, p. 501).

More recently, however, as these paradigms have been elaborated, and as the country has itself become increasingly and visibly multicultural, a richer vision of the positive aspects of culture has been added to presumed consequences of disenfranchisement. Culture is increasingly acknowledged as both a community and individual resource, a potential source of strength and resilience, and a buffer against the debilitating effects of discrimination and lack of access to needed resources. As such, it has provided not only a contextualizing influence on our theories and methods but also an intellectual alternative to earlier deficit-driven interpretations of individuals in community.

Jones (1990) has described this shift as one from affirmative action to affirmative diversity. Writing in the context of graduate training, he stated:

> Affirmative diversity is defined as the affirmation of the fundamental value of human diversity in society, with the belief that enhancing diversity increases rather than diminishes quality.... Human diversity is better embodied in the concept of affirmative diversity than in the concept of affirmative action. Although affirmative action addresses questions of social justice, it fails to acknowledge cultural differences (except in a pejorative way) and usually fails to accommodate to implications of these differences in culture for students, faculty, career goals, and the content and development of training. (pp. 18–20)

THE CONTEXTS OF DIVERSITY AND THE DIVERSITY OF CONTEXTS

The emergence of a contextualist philosophy of science, methodological pluralism, and human diversity provides the basis for developing a future community psychology focusing on the contexts of diversity and the diversity of contexts. The distinctive contribution of community psychology is to develop research and intervention based on an appreciation of how sociocultural diversity interacts with diversity in ecological contexts within which individuals live.

"Contexts of diversity" refers to an appreciation of the many varied and differentiated cultural contexts within which individuals develop and are socialized. The concept of culture becomes differentiated and modified by the specific circumstances of varied groups and individuals. Global context-free categories such as Latino, African–American, and gender are situated in the specific ecological circumstances of individual lives. They derive their meaning not from a generalized conception of culture but from an understanding of how the meaning of culture is shaped by localized sets of adaptive requirements. Thus, as Bernal and Echategui-de-Jesus (1994) pointed out, applying the category of "Latino" or "Latina" to immigrants from differing countries minimizes important differences due to differing cultural histories, experiences with colonization, economic status of the country of origin, and the nature of their ethnic communities in the United States.

Further, contexts of diversity highlights the idea that such concepts as ethnic identity are potentially fluid, negotiated in the context of the differing settings of importance, and intimately connected to the complex interdependence of cultural history, current circumstance, and future aspiration. In sum, different contexts shape the different meanings of diversity, and community psychology can refine and enrich our understanding by investigating the many different ways in which diversity reflects people in context.

While contexts of diversity focus on people in context, diversity of contexts refers to the assessment and impact of multiple and differentiated contexts of relevance. These include social institutions, social resources in the community, social norms, and social policies. Here the level of analysis becomes critical, as community psychologists explicitly link differences in individuals to their experience in varied social settings and communities. Of most direct relevance to the current discussion is the value of understanding the implicit and explicit culture of institutions (Sarason, 1972), the ways in which policies differentially influence different cultural groups (Trickett, Birman, & Buchanan, unpublished manuscript), and the degree to which social norms of the broader culture; as reflected in institutions, policies, and norms; converge, diverge, or conflict with the hopes, beliefs, and traditions of varied cultural groups (Tyler, Susswell, & Williams-McCoy, 1985).

Focusing on the interdependence of diverse people and diverse contexts furthers the aspirations of the Swampscott conference in the context of today's increasingly multicultural and interdependent world. Such an ecological prescription requires the use of multiple methods, particularly qualitative research strategies (Agar, 1980; Denzin & Lincoln, 1994; Straus & Corbin, 1990), to capture the complexity and richness of the sociocultural embeddedness of diverse individuals and groups as they cope with varying aspects of their environment.

An Example: Contextualizing Acculturation Theory and Research

In recent years I have attempted to understand how human diversity weaves its way through the adolescent-school transaction (Trickett, 1991b; Trickett & Birman, 1989; Trickett & Buchanan, 1997). Pursuing this goal has led to an interest in research on the concept of acculturation. I use this topic as a brief example of how to develop the "contexts of diversity and diversity of contexts" theme.

Theories Develop in Context

Acculturation refers to change that occurs when individuals or groups from differing cultural contexts come in sustained contact with each other. A contextual perspective suggests that theories describing that process are themselves products of certain contexts. Quoting Birman (1994):

> Acculturation theories are themselves a function of the cultural context within which they were developed. Thus, the range of specific acculturative styles outlined by these models reflects the particular circumstances of cultural contact of the group in question. It is thus argued that acculturation at the individual level cannot be understood without examining the acculturation of the group to which the individual belongs. (p. 267)

From this perspective, it is not happenstance that much of the research involving African–Americans has focused on ethnic identity, an issue made critical by a dominant culture that has historically demeaned, distorted, or attempted to obliterate that identity, whereas interest in the more behaviorally oriented concept of biculturalism has been more prevalent in work involving immigrants or refugees.

An appreciation of the contexts of diversity suggests the acculturation theory must be localized if it is to account for the experiences of individuals of differing cultural backgrounds in varied sociocultural contexts. Such a perspective promotes the investigation of differences within cultural groups living in different ecological contexts. It also suggests that current acculturation theory (Berry, 1994) may not adequately capture the variety of acculturative options or styles because it is based on a limited set of cultural groups in a limited number of ecological contexts (Birman, 1994). Qualitative work, such as the focus groups employed by Cortes, Rogler, and Malgady (1994) in developing an acculturation instrument is useful in localizing such phenomena.

Preferred Acculturative Styles Depend on Context

A second implication of the contextualist position is that the adaptiveness of any individual coping style depends on the context. Within acculturation research, for example, much is made of the value of biculturalism as the adaptive style of choice, at least for those allowed into the dominant culture. Birman (1994), however, suggests in this regard that it is useful to recall the respective roles of Moses and Joseph in Jewish history. "The biblical heroes Moses and Joseph represent different attitudes toward acculturation," she states.

> Joseph's assimilationist attitudes in Egypt allowed him to rise to a high position in Pharaoh's court and to help his family when they came there to survive the famine. Moses, however, was a separatist, leading the Jewish people out of Egypt to escape slavery. Both are heroes in Jewish history, for unless each of them did what they did, the Jewish people would not have survived either the famine in Canaan or slavery in Egypt. These examples serve as reminders that there are times, situations, and contexts when assimilation and separatism, and not biculturalism, are viable, understandable, and preferable acculturation options. (p. 281)

Vinokurov (1995) provided a more current example in his study of acculturation and adaptation among 250 refugees from the former Soviet Union living in New York and Washington, DC. Controlling for education and length of time in the country, both male and female New Yorkers report a greater retention of their Russian culture and less adoption of American culture than do refugees who settle in the Washington, DC area. While selection factors may influence these findings, a contextual interpretation draws attention to differences in the Russian-speaking communities in the two cities. In Brighton Beach, home of the New York sample, the presence of an encompassing social and economic Russian-speaking community, including street signs in both Russian and English, lessens the adaptive necessity of American acculturation compared to the more dispersed community of Russian speakers in the Washington, DC area.

Acculturative Processes Interact with Context

A "diversity of contexts and contexts of diversity" emphasis extends to a contextual examination of the different domains of acculturation as well.

Most current acculturation theorists see acculturation as including different spheres: for example, language acquisition, cultural identity, cultural behavior, and comfort in the host culture (Birman, 1994; Martinez & Mendoza, 1984). Acculturation theorists have posited different paths for these different functions. For example, language acquisition may assume a linear function over time. Comfort in the new culture, however, may follow a curvilinear or U-shaped path, beginning with initial enthusiasm for the new country, followed by disillusionment as hopes inevitably collide with the harsh realities of any society. Eventually a rapproachment occurs between one's initial aspirations and the realization that the new country, as the old, has both appealing and appalling aspects (Portes & Rumbaut, 1990).

A contextualist perspective on such issues tests the premise that these processes play out differently for different groups in different contexts. Thus, language acquisition may be affected by the degree to which the individual is in a community of coculturals versus being a solitary representative of a cultural group forced to participate daily in the new culture (Portes & Rumbaut, 1990); the hypothesized U-shaped curve depicting satisfaction with the new country may take a variety of other forms, depending on such factors as how accepting and supportive members of the host culture are over time, the conditions under which the individual left the country of origin, the solidarity and resources of the local immigrant community, and whether or not the individual can return or plans to return home. The research question thus shifts from an individual-based or group-based frame to one which embeds acculturation in context.

Through attention to the contexts of diversity and the diversity of contexts, community psychology can play a distinctive role in generating knowledge and designing interventions which dignify the complexities of the diversity concept. We can learn about how historical circumstance and current context differentially affect adaptive outcomes, how they are expressed in gender differences in family roles, how they relate to school transitions, and indeed how they are infused across the many substantive areas where community psychologists are currently working. Adopting a contextual perspective on diversity moves us beyond using broad categories such as race and gender without tieing their meaning to specific populations living in specific circumstances at specific historical moments. It cautions us against making generalizations about populations which, at their best, may be inaccurate, and, at their worst, simply perpetuate stereotypes. We need to stop trying to homogenize diversity. It is liberating for us all to do so.

But in so doing we need to pay much more conceptual and empirical attention to the diversity of contexts themselves, for such mediating structures as schools, neighborhoods, churches, governmental programs, and universities provide the arenas where diversity is expressed, supported, or shunned. I return to the concern with "taking the environment into account," a concern that has been the focus of my career as a community psychologist. In my professional years, I have spent considerable time developing frameworks and assessment techniques for understanding the nature of social environments and their multiple and differential effects on people (Trickett, Kelly, & Todd, 1972; Trickett, 1978, 1991b; Trickett & Moos, 1996). I have taught and written about the implications of an ecological perspective for interventions ranging from mental health consultation (O'Neill & Trickett, 1982) to the development of collaborative relationships with schools to promote institutional development (Trickett & Birman, 1989).

Through all these endeavors, I have been privileged to work with a diverse group of individuals who have taught me a great deal about their world views and mine. Working in different settings, in different roles, and with different colleagues has constantly validated the importance of context in shaping behavior, both mine and those with whom I have worked. Integrating this ecological variability in communities, institutions, and local social climate with the rich range of human diversity represents an exciting intellectual and social commitment for the field.

Let me provide just one example of from my own work of how diversity and context intersect. For 14 years I followed the creation and evolution of an inner-city alternative high school in New Haven. It began as a reaction to the bureaucracy and racial tensions prevalent in high schools in the late 1960s, and, as a reaction to these forces, I attempted to create a school based on an empowerment ideology. Because of the school's insistence on the fundamental importance of empowerment, I called the book I wrote on the experience *Living an Idea* (Trickett, 1991b).

In its efforts to empower students, the school allowed students to create their own educational courses in the community and included them in a participatory governance structure which held real power over such domains as the distribution of funds and the hiring of teachers. These structures, in principle, were intended to empower students. However, these structures were based on implicit assumptions about what students wanted, how attractive this kind of empowerment would be, and the notion that the "liberation" of concern involved liberation from an oppressive bureaucracy in the traditional public schools.

Over time, our evaluation of the school suggested that these empowerment structures had differential effects on black and white students, with white students developing more community courses and participating more in governance than blacks. Empirical data and discussions with both teachers and students about this outcome revealed consistent differences between blacks and whites in their perceptions of the educational value and relevance of these structures. Such contrasting perceptions were deeply rooted in differing cultural histories which made such empowerment structures, and the implicit assumptions on which they rested, more meaningful for white students than black students.

Examples such as this suggest that there is no clear link between the best of intentions and the best of outcomes. It further suggests that to translate the relationship between a construct and a social structure which it presumably reflects requires cultural and contextual analysis. A community psychology that focuses on the contexts of diversity and diversity of contexts is uniquely suited to understanding the critical issues that mediate the relationship between good ideas and meaningful social structures reflecting those ideas.

Towards an Integration of Diversity and Context

Let me close by suggesting some potential ways to further integrate the context of diversity with the diversity of context as community psychology begins its next 30 years. These are not new ideas but they may benefit from being renewed. They are also not prescriptions to be offered acontextually. In the words of that early ecologist Ecclesiastes, "To everything there is a season, and a time to every purpose under heaven." Thus, paradoxically, there may be times to ignore what I have said and am about to say about a contextual mind-set. However, let this not be one of those times!

The first set of comments stem from my experience as Editor of the *American Journal of Community Psychology*. In that role I have had the opportunity to read several hundred papers in recent years. I have read much wonderful work, for which the field should be proud. There are also several hidden regularities in many of the papers which, if attended to, could increase our understanding of diversity in context. First, many studies gather data from populations in more than one social setting and do not include setting-level effects in their analyses. The presence of such contextual effects are thus lost as potential information and as avenues for further hypothesis generation. Second, many studies include diverse populations with insufficient numbers of any particular group to enable a group-level analysis. Here we lose the ability to learn whether or not diversity is related to the phenomena of interest. Third, many studies mention the role of context in the research, but only in the discussion section as a post hoc means of explaining what they found but did not expect to find. The first two of these regularities implicitly further a decontextualized understanding of our phenomena of interest; the last explicitly acknowledges that more could have been learned had attention been paid to context in framing the research.

Some of this I attribute to the legacy of positivism in our research socialization, journal practices, and the demand characteristic of academic survival and enhancement. Some of this I attribute to the pervasive individualistic nature of the culture in which we live, an individualism deliciously skewered by Jean Baker Miller in her query "How many women does it take to keep one man independent?". Some of this I attribute to what I have previously called "partial paradigm acquisition" (Trickett, 1984), where we still talk the talk about the importance of context without fully understanding the implications of how to walk the walk. But this decontextualization of research in community psychology is paradoxical at best, given the aspirations of the field.

There are many other ways to contribute to an understanding of the role of culture and context in community psychology. Let me return briefly to some of the implications of my earlier comments on qualitative research, levels of analysis, the contexts of diversity, and the spirit of research in and with communities.

1. I have already mentioned the distinctive advantage of qualitative inquiry for an understanding of culture and context. The inclusion of various qualitative research methods into community psychology, however, confronts not only the more established norms of the profession but the problem that the criteria for assessing qualitative research are not yet consensual. Hope for this effort may be derived from many sources, however, both in the evolution of writings such as the recent *Handbook of Qualitative Research* (Denzin & Lincoln, 1994) and in the growing momentum across different areas of psychology for this work. Further evidence is found in the concern expressed by journal editors about how to deal with the evaluation of qualitative research. Indeed, an NIMH-sponsored consortium of journal editors, in which the *American Journal of Community Psychology* participates, has selected as its topic for discussion next year how to evaluate qualitative work. Because these editors represent such mainstream publications as *Child Development, Journal of Research on Adolescence*, and *Journal of Consulting and Clinical Psychology*, this is a most promising validation of the importance of the topic.

2. The level of analysis issue begins with conceptual work which applies a multilevel framework to the phenomenon or intervention of interest. It may include the systematic sampling of sites as well as people, or the selection of sites for their specific ecological contrasts, as Kelly (1979) did in studying the effects of student turnover rate on the high school coping and adaptation of adolescent boys.

This, in turn, suggests that we must strive for samples of inconvenience rather than working only with the most responsive groups or settings.

Quoting Campbell and Stanley (1972):

> Consider the implications of an experiment on teaching in which the
> researcher has been turned down by nine school systems and accepted by
> a tenth. Thus tenth almost certainly differs from the other nine, and from
> the universe of schools to which we would like to generalize, in many
> specific ways. It is thus, nonrepresentative, and the effects we find, while
> internally valid, may be specific to such schools. (p. 19)

A focus on issues of levels of analysis also means gathering information
about different levels of the ecological environment. And it requires the
development of cross-level strategies of data analysis, both qualitative and
quantitative (see Shinn, 1996).

   3. Developing a better appreciation of human diversity rests on our
ability to look deeply rather than broadly into the ways in which cultural
and subcultural groups interact with their ecological environment. At this
historical moment we should think small and intensive rather than large
and expensive. Without in any way denigrating the currently popular large
scale, multisite projects, to learn more about the contexts of diversity and
diversity of contexts we should localize and deepen our understanding of
varied communities of people. Intensive commitments over time yield the
kind of thick description which clarifies the emic and etic aspects of diverse
groups in diverse contexts. The spirit of such ecological inquiry is to learn
about and appreciate lives of people in context. While research often
involves the measurement of variables, respondents are people, whose variables only make sense in the context of their lives.

   4. Finally, our efforts to develop collaborative and empowering relationships with citizens certainly need conceptual clarification. We would be
helped greatly if we had both settings and publication outlets to write about
our work the way we actually carry it out. To write about our work as we
have been taught to do is to decontextualize our image of how the world
works, how we work, and what we have learned.

   One of my favorite books is called *Reflections on Community Studies*
(Vidich, Bensman, & Stein, 1964), a series of reflections of community
sociologists about their community work. The spirit of the book, found in
its preface, bears repeating:

> This book concerns the methodology of community study, if by methodol-
> ogy we understand something more than the mechanics of research. The
> mood which these essays establish is the personal quality of community
> studies, that is, the intimate connection between the investigator, his [sic]
> methods of investigation, his results, and his own future intellectual devel-
> opment. No one has yet been able to present a formal methodology for the

optimum or proper method for the scientific study of the community. This is necessarily so because there is no way to disentangle the research method from the investigator himself. Anyone who studies a community is as much changed by his work, even while in the midst of it, as the community he studies. (p. vii)

This quote captures the spirit of inquiry as a contextually grounded, ecologically energized process. It suggests a caring, a self-consciousness, an openness to learning, and a commitment to working with those without whose cooperation and collaboration we could not function. It further shows that the process of community research can combine compassion and conceptual insights for future generations of community researchers. Should Jim Kelly's idea of creating a Woods Hole equivalent for community psychology come to fruition (Kelly, 1970), I hope that it serves as a setting where such conversations may occur.

To conclude, I have attempted to make figure out of ground by emphasizing not individuals but the contexts in which we all lead our lives. I have suggested that community psychology can make a distinctive contribution by clarifying the many meanings of the diversity concept through attention to the contexts in which diversity develops and the social milieu in which it is expressed. Such a clarification can support intervention that is both empowering and respectful of the contexts of those with whom we intervene.

The concept of context has long been seen as sensible for community psychology. It grounds us in the real world which we are attempting to understand and improve. It rings true. But it has been slippery to grasp: "The implications of the obvious are not themselves obvious," the power of the prevailing paradigm pervasive. But context is the water in which we fish swim. There are mirrors within mirrors as we attempt to understand its influence and implications. As each new understanding comes, I think of Paul McCartney's description in the song "Penny Lane": "Though she thinks as if she's in a play, she is anyway." I appreciate the opportunity to share with you my journey into diversity and context and my hopes for community psychology. I am particularly grateful to do so under these circumstances.

ACKNOWLEDGMENTS

In receiving this award, I thank four psychologists who have made enduring contributions to my work. To Jim Kelly, Seymour Sarason, Rudolf Moos, and Forrest Tyler my sincere appreciation for the many influences on my life as a community psychologist. Each has created settings and provided support which have challenged and enriched my ideas and my career.

Special thanks are offered to Jim Kelly, whose willingness to introduce my talk represents another supportive act in his 30 years of unconditional mentoring. During the past 10 years my concern about the incorporation of issues of human diversity into community psychology has been greatly influenced by collaboration with Rod Watts and Dina Birman. Their influence is evident in the paper. In addition, I thank Dina Birman for her comments on earlier drafts.

REFERENCES

Agar, M. (1980). *The professional stranger.* New York: Academic Press.

Altman, I. (1987). Community psychology twenty years later: Still another crisis in psychology? *American Journal of Community Psychology, 15*, 613–627.

Barker, R. G. (1968). *Ecological psychology: Concepts and methods for studying the environment of human behavior.* Stanford, CA: Stanford University Press.

Belenky, M. F., Clinchy, B. Mc., Goldberger, N. R., & Tarule, J. M. (1986). *Women's ways of knowing: The development of self voice, and mind.* New York: Basic Books.

Bennett, C. C., Anderson, L. S., Cooper, S., Hassol, L., Klein, D. C., & Rosenblum, G. (Eds.). (1966). *Community psychology: A report of the Boston Conference on the Education of Psychologists for Community Mental Health.* Boston: Boston University Press.

Bernal, G. & Enchautegui-de-Jesus, N. (1994). Latinos and Latinas in community psychology: A review of the literature. *American Journal of Community Psychology, 22*, 531–558.

Berry, J. W. (1994). An ecological perspective on cultural and ethnic psychology. In E. J. Trickett, R. J. Watts, & D. Birman (Eds.), *Human diversity: Perspectives on people in context* (pp. 115–141). San Francisco: Jossey-Bass.

Birman, D. (1994). Acculturation and human diversity in a multicultural society. In E. J. Trickett, R. J. Watts, & D. Birman (Eds.), *Human diversity: Perspectives on people in context* (pp. 261–284). San Francisco: Jossey-Bass.

Bond, M. A. & Keys, C. B. (1993). Empowerment, diversity, and collaboration: Promoting synergy on community boards. *American Journal of Community Psychology, 21*, 37–58.

Burton, L. M. (1990). Teenage childbearing as an alternative life-course strategy in multigeneration black families. *Human Nature, 1*(2), 123–143.

Burton, L. M. (1991). Caring for children. *The American Enterprise*, pp. 34–37.

Burton, L. M. & Dilworth-Anderson, P. (1991). The intergenerational family roles of aged black Americans. *Marriage and Family Review, 16*(3/4), 311–330.

Campbell, D. T. & Stanley, J. C. (1972). *Experimental and quasi-experimental designs for research.* Chicago: Rand McNally.

Caplan, N. & Nelson, S. D. (1973). On being useful: The nature and consequences of psychological research on social problems. *American Psychologist, 28*, 199–211.

Cohen, J. (1994). The earth is round ($p < .05$). *American Psychologist, 49*, 997–1003.

Cortes, D. E., Rogler, L. H., & Malgady, R. G. (1994). Biculturality among Puerto Rican adults in the United States. *American Journal of Community Psychology, 22*, 707–721.

Cowen, E. L. (1980). The wooing of primary prevention. *American Journal of Community Psychology, 8*, 258–284.

Cowen, E. L. (1994). The enhancement of psychological wellness: Challenges and opportunities. *American Journal of Community Psychology, 22*, 149–180.

Cronbach, L. J. (1986). Social inquiry by and for earthlings. In D. W. Fiske & R. A. Shweder (Eds.), *Metatheory in social science* (pp. 83–107). Chicago: University of Chicago Press.

Denzin, N. K. & Lincoln, Y. L. (1994). *Handbook of qualitative research.* Thousand Oaks, CA: Sage.

Fiske, D. W. (1986). Specificity of method and knowledge in social science. In D. W. Fiske & R. A. Shweder (Eds.), *Metatheory in social science* (pp. 61–82). Chicago: University of Chicago Press.

Gibbs, J. T. & Fuery, D. (1994). Mental health and well-being of black women: Toward strategies of empowerment. *American Journal of Community Psychology, 22,* 559–582.

Gruber, J. & Trickett, E. J. (1987). Can we empower others? The paradox of empowerment in the governing of an alternative public school. *American Journal of Community Psychology, 15,* 353–371.

Hughes, D. & DuMont, K. (1993). Using focus groups to facilitate culturally anchored research. *American Journal of Community Psychology, 21,* 775–806.

Jones, J. M. (1990). Who is training our ethnic minority psychologists and are they doing it right? In G. Stricker, E. Davis-Russel, E. Bourg, E. Duran, W. R. Hammond, J. McHolland, K. Polite, & B. E. Vaughn (Eds.), *Toward ethnic diversification in psychology education and training.* Washington, DC: American Psychological Association.

Kelly, J. G. (1970). Antidotes for arrogance: Training for a community psychology. *American Psychologist, 25,* 524–531.

Kelly, J. G. (1979). *Adolescent boys in high school: A psychological study of coping and adaptation.* Hillsdale, NJ: Erlbaum.

Kelly, J. G. (1986). Content and process: An ecological view of the interdependence of practice and research. *American Journal of Community Psychology, 14,* 581–589.

Kelly, J. G. & Hess, R. (1986). *The ecology of prevention: Illustrating mental health consultation.* New York: Haworth.

Kelly, J. G. (Ed.). (1979). *Adolescent boys in high school: A psychological study of coping and adaptation.* Hillsdale, NJ: Erlbaum.

Kingry-Westergaard, C., & Kelly, J. G. (1990). A contextualist epistemology for ecological research. In P. Tolan, C. Keys, F. Chertak, & L. Jason (Eds.), *Researching community psychology: Issues of theory and methods* (pp. 23–31). Washington, DC: American Psychological Association.

Kuhn, T. H. (1970). *The structure of scientific revolutions.* Chicago: University of Chicago Press.

Leidig, M. W. (1977). Women in community psychology: A feminist perspective. In I. Iscoe, B. L. Bloom, & C. D. Spielberger (Eds.), *Community psychology in transition* (pp. 274–277). Washington, DC: Hemisphere.

Loo, C., Fong, K. T., & Iwamasa, G. (1988). Ethnicity and cultural diversity: An analysis of work published in community psychology journals, 1965–1985. *Journal of Community Psychology, 16,* 332–349.

Maltz, M. D. (1994). Deviating from the mean: The declining significance of significance. *Journal of Research in Crime and Delinquency, 31,* 434–463.

Martinez, J. L. Jr. & Mendoza, R. H. (Eds.). (1984). *Chicano psychology.* New York: Academic Press.

Maton, K. I. (1994). A bridge between cultures: Linked ethnographic empirical methodology for culture anchored research. *American Journal of Community Psychology, 21,* 747–774.

McGuire, W. J. (1983). A contextualist theory of knowledge: Its implications for innovation and reform in psychological research. In L. Berkowitz (Ed.), *Advances in experimental social psychology* (Vol. 16, pp. 1–47). New York: Academic Press.

Moos, R. H. (1974). *Evaluating treatment environments: A social ecological approach.* New York: Wiley.

Moos, R. H. (1979). *Evaluating educational environments.* San Francisco: Jossey-Bass.

Myers, E. R. & Pitts, H. (1977). Community psychology and racism. In I. Iscoe, B. L. Bloom, & C. D. Spielberger (Eds.), *Community psychology in transition* (pp. 267–270). Washington, DC: Hemisphere.

Novaco, R. W. & Monahan, J. (1980). Research in community psychology: An analysis of work published in the first six years of the *American Journal of Community Psychology. American Journal of Community Psychology, 8*, 131–145.

O'Neill, P. & Trickett, E. J. (1982). *Community consultation.* San Francisco: Jossey-Bass.

Portes, A. & Rumbaut, R. G. (1990). *Immigrant America: A portrait.* Berkeley: University of California Press.

Rappaport, J. (1977). *Community psychology: Values, research and action.* New York: Holt, Rinehart & Winston.

Rappaport, J. (1990). Research methods and the empowerment social agenda. In P. Tolan, C. Keys, F. Chertok, & L. Jason (Eds.), *Researching community psychology: Issues of theory and methods.* Washington, DC: American Psychological Association.

Riger, S. (1993). What's wrong with empowerment. *American Journal of Community Psychology, 21*, 279–292.

Rosnow, R. & Georgoudi, M. (Eds.). (1986). *Contextualism and understanding in behavioral science: Implications for research and theory.* New York: Praeger.

Ryan, W. (1971). *Blaming the victim.* New York: Vintage Books.

Sarason, S. B. (1981). *Psychology misdirected.* New York: Free Press.

Sarason, S. B. (1972). *The creation of settings and the future societies.* San Francisco: Jossey-Bass.

Shinn, M. (Ed.). (1996). Special issue on ecological assessment. *American Journal of Community Psychology, 24*.

Shweder, R. A. (1990). Cultural psychology: What is it? In J. Stigler, R. Shweder, & G. Herdt (Eds.), *Cultural psychology: Essays on comparative human development* (pp. 1–43). Cambridge, England: Cambridge University Press.

Shweder, R. A. & Sullivan, M. M. (1993). Cultural psychology: Who needs it? *Annual Review of Psychology, 44*, 497–523.

Straus, A. L. & Corbin, J. (1990). *Basics of qualitative research: Grounded theory procedures and technique.* Newbury Park, CA: Sage.

Trickett, E. J. (1978). Towards a social-ecological conception of adolescent socialization: Normative data on contrasting types of public schools. *Child Development, 49*, 408–414.

Trickett, E. J. (1984). Towards a distinctive community psychology: An ecological metaphor for training and the conduct of research. *American Journal of Community Psychology, 12*, 261–279.

Trickett, E. J. (1991a). Paradigms and the research report: Making what actually happens a heuristic for theory. *American Journal of Community Psychology, 19*, 365–370.

Trickett, E. J. (1991b). *Living an idea: Empowerment and the evolution of an inner city alternative high school.* Cambridge, MA: Brookline Books.

Trickett, E. J. (1994). Human diversity and community psychology: Where ecology and empowerment meet. *American Journal of Community Psychology, 22*, 583–592.

Trickett, E. J. (1998). Towards a framework for defining and resolving ethical issues in the protection of communities involved in primary prevention projects. *Ethics and Behavior, 8*, 321–327

Trickett, E. J. & Birman, D. (1989). Taking ecology seriously: A community development approach to individually based interventions. In L. Bond & B. Compas (Eds.), *Primary prevention in the schools.* Hanover, NH: University of New England Press.

Trickett, E. J., Birman, D., & Buchanan, R. M. Immigrant Students in the Schools: Context, culture, and challenge for school psychology. *Journal of School Psychology.* Unpublished manuscript.

Trickett, E. J. & Buchanan, R. M. (1997). The role of personal relationships in transitions: Contributions of an ecological perspective. In S. Duck (Ed.), *Handbook of Personal Relationships*, (pp. 576–593). New York: Wiley.

Trickett, E. J., Dahiyat, C., & Selby, P. (1994). *Primary prevention in mental health 1983–1991: An annotated bibliography.* Washington, DC: U.S. Government Printing Office.

Trickett, E. J., Kelly, J. G., & Todd, D. M. (1972). The social environment of the high school: Guidelines for individual change and organizational development. In S. Golann & C. Eisdorfer (Eds.), *Handbook of community mental health* (pp. 331–406). New York: Appleton-Century-Crofts.

Trickett, E. J., Kelly, J. G., & Vincent, T. A. (1985). The spirit of ecological inquiry in community research. In E. Susskind & D. Klein (Eds.), *Community research: Methods paradigms, and applications.* New York: Praeger.

Trickett, E. J. & Moos, R. H. (1996). *The Classroom Environment Scale Manual (3rd ed.).* Palo Alto, CA: Consulting Psychologists Press.

Trickett, E. J., Watts, R. W., & Birman, D. (1993). Human diversity and community psychology: Still hazy after all these years. *Journal of Community Psychology, 21,* 264–279.

Tyler, F. B. (1978). Individual psychosocial competence: A personality configuration. *Educational and Psychological Measurement, 38,* 309–323.

Tyler, F. B., Susswell, D., & Williams-McCoy, J. (1985). Ethnic validity in psychotherapy. *Psychotherapy, 22,* 311–320.

Vidich, A. J, Bensman, J., & Stein, M. R. (Eds.). (1964). *Reflections on community studies.* New York: Harper and Row.

Vinokurov, A. (1995). *Authoritarianism and the adaptation of Russian-speaking immigrants and refugees.* Unpublished Honors Thesis. University of Maryland, College Park.

Walsh, R. T. (1987a). A social historical note on the formal emergence of community psychology. *American Journal of Community Psychology, 15,* 523–530.

Walsh, R. T. (1987b). The evolution of the research relationship in community psychology. *American Journal of Community Psychology, 15,* 773–788.

Watts, R. J. (1993). Community action through manhood development: A look at concepts and concerns from the frontline. *American Journal of Community Psychology, 21,* 333–360.

24

Family, Peer, and Neighborhood Influences on Academic Achievement among African–American Adolescents: One-Year Prospective Effects

Nancy A. Gonzales, Ana Mari Cauce,
Ruth J. Friedman, and Craig A. Mason

Using a 1-year prospective design, this study examined the influence of family status variables (family income, parental education, family structure), parenting variables (maternal support and restrictive control), peer support, and neighborhood risk on the school performance of 120 African American junior high school students. In addition to main effects of these variables, neighborhood risk was examined as a moderator of the effects of parenting and peer support. Family status variables were not predictive of adolescent school performance as indexed by self-reported grade point average. Maternal support at Time 1 was prospectively related to adolescent grades at Time 2. Neighborhood risk was related to lower grades, while peer support predicted better grades in the prospective analyses. Neighborhood risk also moderated the effects of maternal restrictive control and peer support on adolescent grades in prospective analyses. These findings highlight the importance of an ecological approach to the problem of academic underachievement within the African American community.

Originally published in the *American Journal of Community Psychology*, 24(3) (1996): 365–387.

A Quarter Century of Community Psychology: *Readings from the* American Journal of Community Psychology, edited by Tracey A. Revenson *et al.* Kluwer Academic/Plenum Publishers, New York, 2002.

Academic underachievement among African American youths is a social concern that has reached disturbing proportions. At all levels of schooling and at comparable levels of ability, African American students earn substantially lower grades and attain less education than non-Hispanic white students (Ensminger & Slusarcick, 1992; Mickelson, 1990). In addition to placing severe limits on economic and occupational attainment, academic failure is of concern as it has been tied to a host of problematic consequences including delinquency (Sampson & Laub, 1993), psychopathology (Kurdek, 1987), and substance abuse (Engel, Nordlohne, Hurrelman, & Holler, 1987).

Though the problem of African American underachievement is one of long-standing concern, satisfactory explanations continue to elude educators and social scientists. Theoretical models of academic motivation and achievement have often failed to receive empirical support when applied to African American populations. For example, while family status variables such as parental education, socioeconomic status, and family structure are powerful correlates of achievement in majority populations, they have been less predictive of school success for African American students (Dornbusch, Ritter, & Steinberg, 1991; Gottfredson, 1981; Mickelson, 1990). Parenting practices, and parental values regarding academic achievement, have also been of limited explanatory value (Mickelson, 1990; Steinberg, Dornbusch, & Brown, 1992; Stevenson, Chen, & Uttal, 1990). Patterns of socialization, such as authoritative and authoritarian parenting styles, which have been related consistently and robustly to achievement-related outcomes in non-minority samples (Baumrind, 1971; Maccoby & Martin, 1983), are not as predictive of school success or failure within African American samples (Dornbusch, Ritter, Leiderman, Roberts, & Fraleigh, 1987; Steinberg, Lamborn, Darling, Mounts, & Dornbusch, 1994).

Researchers have therefore begun to examine broader ecological influences, external to the child and his or her immediate family, such as the peer context and aspects of the neighborhoods in which African American children are reared. Although few in number, these efforts suggest that neighborhood and peer influences may exert a more powerful effect on academic achievement within African American communities than that of the immediate family. These influences may also be responsible within some communities for the family's diminished impact (Coleman & Hoffer, 1987; Dornbusch *et al.*, 1991; Steinberg *et al.*, 1992).

Using a 1-year prospective design, the present study examined the combined effects of family, peer, and neighborhood influences on the school performance of African American junior high school students. Consistent with an ecological perspective which suggests that developmental processes may vary depending on the environmental context in which they occur (Bronfenbrenner, 1979), main effects within each of these three domains were examined along with hypothesized interactions among domains.

Neighborhood Context and Academic Achievement

Social disorganization theory (Shaw & McKay, 1969) asserts that three structural neighborhood features—low economic status, ethnic heterogeneity, and residential mobility—lead to the disruption of community social organization, which in turn prevents communities from realizing the common values of residents and maintaining effective social controls for developing youths (Sampson & Groves, 1989). Drawing on social disorganization theory, researchers have recently begun to examine neighborhood variables as risk factors for child and adolescent development (Aber, Mitchell, Garfinkel, Allen, & Seidman, 1992; Dornbusch *et al.*, 1991; Duncan, Brooks-Gunn, & Klebanov, 1994; Sampson & Groves, 1989). This research has focused primarily on census tract indicators of neighborhood poverty—median family income, proportion of single-parent households, absence of middle-class professionals—which have been shown to be related to achievement-related outcomes such as IQ and school grades for young children and adolescents (Aber *et al.*, 1992; Dornbusch *et al.*, 1991; Duncan *et al.*, 1994).

Research on neighborhood context and academic achievement has relied primarily on census tract data to characterize neighborhood structure and composition. However, problems with defining neighborhoods purely geographically and measuring key factors using such data have been noted (Aber, 1993, 1994; Klebanov, Brooks-Gunn, & Duncan, 1993; Sampson & Groves, 1989). First, census data characterize rather large residential areas which may not provide appropriate indicators of functional communities, because adolescents' interactional worlds may not be defined by the "tract." Accordingly, Burton (1993) suggested that neighborhoods should also be conceptualized and measured as associational networks and as phenomenology (subjective perceptions).

Further, as noted by Aber (1993), census tract data only provide distal markers for processes thought to proximally influence adolescent development (Gephart, 1980; Sampson & Groves, 1989). They do not provide information about the more immediate neighborhood characteristics that directly impact adolescent attitudes and behavior. For example, social disorganization theory suggests that low-income, multiethnic communities produce deleterious effects because they are plagued by higher crime rates, lack opportunities for prosocial friendship networks, and are unable to supervise and control teenage peer groups (e.g., gangs). However, few researchers working from this perspective have examined neighborhood characteristics, such as crime and gang activity, as proximal influences on adolescent development (see Sampson & Groves, 1989, for an exception).

Research on neighborhood context has also been limited largely to the examination of main effects, or to a lesser extent to the examination of mediational models (Klebanov *et al.*, 1993), by which neighborhood factors are thought to impact development (Aber, 1993). Yet theory and research in the ecology of adolescent risk suggests that environmental factors within ethnic minority communities may also serve as moderators of development (Aber, 1993, 1994; Baldwin, Baldwin, & Cole, 1990; McLoyd, 1990; Steinberg & Darling, 1993; Trickett, Aber, Carlson, & Cicchetti, 1991). Dornbusch *et al.* (1991), for example, argued that the ethnic mix of a neighborhood operates to modify, or undermine, the influence of authoritative parenting on academic achievement. However, while their argument suggests a moderational model, the interaction between neighborhood and parenting—that is, a direct test of moderation—has not been examined in the literature.

In this study we tested for moderation as well as main effects of neighborhood risk. We proposed that neighborhood risk would have a direct, negative impact on academic achievement in our sample of African American adolescents, and that it would also serve as a moderator of the effects of both parenting and peer support. Further, in recognition of the limitations of census tract data noted above, our assessment of neighborhood risk was based on adolescents' reports (subjective perceptions) of their exposure to specific neighborhood risk activities. These activities included drug trade and drug use, gang-related events (e.g., violerce, shooting), and neighborhood crime (e.g., theft, vandalism), which are viewed as threatening to the safety, organization, and social norms of high risk neighborhoods (Sampson & Groves, 1989; Sampson & Laub, 1993).

Peer Context and African American Achievement

Within the general social support literature, meaningful ties to one's peer group are thought to promote child competence, psychological well-being, and the ability to cope with life stress, and may be specifically related to motivation and academic achievement (Connell & Wellborn, 1991; Cotterell, 1992; Greenberg, Siegel, & Leitch, 1983; Levitt, Guacci-Franio & Levitt, 1993; Ryan, Stiller & Lynch, 1994). However, while developmental theory suggests that strong peer networks promote healthy psychological development, motivation, and competence, African American peer groups are typically viewed as detrimental to academic achievement strivings. Steinberg *et al.* (1992), for example, argued that African American youths are more likely to associate with peers who do not value or encourage achievement, and that the dominant influence of the peer group is powerful enough to offset the positive influence of parental values and effective childrearing strategies. This view is consistent with Obgu's contention that African American youth groups actively discourage academic achievement as a negatively sanctioned form of "acting white" (Fordham, 1991; Fordham & Ogbu, 1986).

Though it is widely assumed that peer associations deter academic achievement for African American students, this assumption has only rarely been tested and the limited evidence is contradictory. Studies have reported a negative relation (Cauce, Felner, & Primavera, 1982), positive relation (Cauce, 1986), and no relation between peer support and academic achievement for African American adolescents (Seidman, Allen, Aber, Mitchell, & Feinman, 1994). Such inconsistencies across studies are difficult to reconcile, particularly since these studies are few in number. The present study therefore provides additional evidence regarding the effects of peer support for African American adolescents.

By also taking into account the larger neighborhood context in which peer support systems are embedded, the study sought in addition to explain previous inconsistencies in the literature. It is possible that the effects of peer support are moderated by characteristics of the neighborhood in which peer associations are maintained. As developmental theory would suggest, support from one's peers may operate to facilitate academic motivation and performance within environments that are conductive to achievement-related outcomes. However, within high-risk neighborhoods, peer support may be inconsequential, or may even undermine academic achievement. Thus, in keeping with an ecological framework, the present study examined the interaction between peer support and neighborhood risk status in addition to the main effects of peer support.

Goals of the Study

The goals of the present study were twofold. First, to test the contention that peer and neighborhood influences are more powerful than family influences (Dornbusch et al., 1991), we examined prospectively the unique and combined contributions to academic performance of family status and parenting variables, peer support, and neighborhood risk. By using a hierarchical regression strategy in which peer support and neighborhood risk were entered into the equation after the effects of the family status and parenting variables, the study also sought to determine whether community level influences could predict academic achievement over and above the effects of the family. Family status variables included (a) family income, (b) parental education level, and (c) number of parental figures in the home. Two socialization variables were chosen to parallel the two primary dimensions of parenting consistently identified as important influences on adolescent development and achievement: (a) parental warmth and

(b) parental control.[1] The parental control measure used in this study was that of restrictive parental control, which is a component of the authoritarian parenting style. Authoritarian parenting has been related to reduced child motivation and achievement; however, this link has not been as robust for African Americans (Dornbusch *et al.*, 1987).

Second, in addition to examining the main effects of these variables, we examined the influence of neighborhood risk as a moderator of the effects of parenting and peer support on academic achievement. According to Baron and Kenny (1986), moderators are variables that "affect the direction or strength of the relation between an independent or predictor variable and a dependent or criterion variable" (p. 1174). Moderated relations are considered significant when the interaction between the moderator and predictor variable is significant. Thus, by comparing a model that includes the hypothesized main effects of parenting and peer support with one that also includes the interactions of these variables with neighborhood context, the study sought to address previous inconsistencies in the literature which, as noted, has been limited primarily to the examination of main effects.

METHOD

Participants and Procedures

This study is part of a larger longitudinal project designed to examine the role of ecological factors in the psychosocial adjustment of African American adolescents. At the beginning of the study, 151 African American adolescents were recruited from diverse neighborhoods in Seattle, Washington. Adolescents were recruited through a variety of formal and informal community systems including, but not limited to, public schools.[2] Adolescents and at least one of their parents were interviewed separately in their homes and completed a set of questionnaires for which each family member received $10.

Data examined in this paper were drawn from the first data collection interview (Time 1), which occurred when the adolescent was in the seventh

---

[1]In our review and discussion of parenting, we will refer to "parental" variables at times because that is how they are described in the literature. Because of the high rates of single-parent families in the sample, however, the present study exclusively included "maternal" childrearing strategies in all analyses.

[2]Because some of the recruitment took place in public places, such as at an African American cultural fair, the exact number of families who were actually "contacted" is unknown. However, figures available for recruitment in school settings indicated that between 75% and 85% of all students eligible for the study expressed an interest in getting further information. Of those, approximately 88% actually participated.

or eighth grade, and follow-up interview which occurred one year later (Time 2). At the start of the study, participating adolescents ranged in age from 12 to 14 with a mean age of 13.7 years. Results are based on interviews with 120 (78 females, 42 males) of the original 151 adolescents who remained in the study and maintained residence within the same neighborhood across the two data collection periods. Five families completed both waves of data collection but were dropped from these analyses because they moved to a different neighborhood in the interim. Additionally, six families were dropped because they were missing data on grades. Twenty families were lost to attrition; approximately one-third of these could not be located after repeated effort by mail, telephone, or through contacts they had provided at Time 1.

Retention/Attrition. The retention rate of 82% was higher than for other longitudinal studies, which have generally reported low retention rates for African American adolescents (Seidman *et al.*, 1994). *T*-tests were conducted to compare the 120 families in this study with those who either left the study or were dropped for reasons described above. These analyses revealed that dropout families reported lower family incomes, $t = -3.27$, $p < .001$, higher levels of restrictive maternal control, $t = 2.76$, $p < .01$, and a higher prevalence of single parenthood, $t = -2.84$, $p < .01$, than those who were retained. There were no differences in retention for any of the remaining independent measures or for gender or grade point average.

Measures

The present analyses are based on maternal reports of family status and parenting variables, and adolescent reports of peer support, neighborhood risk, and grade point average (GPA).[3]

Family Status

Parental Education. Parental education level was coded on a 5-point scale (1 = *Did not complete high school*, 5 = *Graduate degree*). The most commonly endorsed response for this sample was 3, indicating some level of post-high school education or vocational training (56% of the sample).

---

[3] Adolescent reports of maternal control were not obtained at Time 1 of the study. However, adolescent reports of maternal support were obtained and substituted for maternal reports in a parallel set of analyses which were conducted for the sake of cross-informant replication regarding this single variable. When adolescent reports were used in place of maternal reports, the identical pattern of findings was revealed for each analysis that included this variable. These analyses are not presented in the interests of simplicity.

Twelve percent of the sample reported having at least a college degree, while the remaining 32% had a high school degree (or equivalency) or less.

Family Income. Income was assessed on an 8-point scale (1 = *Less than $10,000/year*, 8 = *Greater than $40,000/year*). The median family income level for the sample was between $25,000 and $30,000. While primarily working class, the sample reflected a broad range of income levels that are generally representative of the African American community in the Seattle area: 10% reported earning less than $10,000; 53% reported earning between $10,000 and $30,000; and 37% reported family incomes greater than $30,000.

Family Structure. Family structure was indexed by the number of parental figures in the home environment. This measure was chosen over marital status because a number of families in the study contained father figures who were actively involved with their adolescents, and had been parts of their families for several years, though they were not legally married to the adolescents' mothers. Of the 120 adolescents included in the study, 68 (56%) were living in two-parent homes, and 52 (43%) were living in homes headed by a single mother.

Parenting Variables

Maternal Support and Control. The *Childrearing Practices Report* (CRPR; Block, 1965) is a 91-item questionnaire, completed by the parent, that examines a variety of parenting practices. The CRPR has been used extensively, has been translated into several languages, and has been found to work well in cross-cultural studies. The 40-item two-factor solution—parental nurturance/support and parental restrictive control—recommended by Rickel and Biasatti (1982) was used in the present study. Internal reliabilities based on Cronbach's alpha in the present study were .79 for support and .78 for control.

Peer Support

Peer support was measured with the *Inventory of Parent and Peer Attachment* (IPPA; Armsden & Greenberg, 1987). The IPPA is a self-report questionnaire developed to assess the strength of adolescents' attachments to parents and peers. In the analyses presented, only those 28 items measuring aspects of the adolescents' attachment to their peers were used. Adolescents are asked to indicate on a 5-point scale how true a number of statements are which describe their friends. Factor analysis suggests that three factors are tapped by this measure: trust, communication, and alienation. A composite peer attachment score is computed by summing trust and communication and subtracting from this the alienation raw score. This score has been used as a reliable and valid indicator of peer support in previous research (Armsden & Greenberg, 1987; Greenberg, 1982). High scores reflect higher levels of peer attachment or perceived peer support. Internal consistency reliability for this scale was .92 in the present study.

Neighborhood Risk

The *Neighborhood Environment Scale* (NES) is a 17-item questionnaire developed for this study to assess perceived levels of neighborhood risk. Individual items about problematic behaviors in the neighborhood, such as vandalism, gang activity, and crime, are rated on a scale from 1 to 7 according to "how often each of these things occur in the neighborhood in which you live." The NES was administered at both data collection periods. Internal consistency for the neighborhood risk index was .93 at Time 1 and .92 at Time 2. Time 1 neighborhood risk was correlated .68 with Time 2 neighborhood risk, thus providing evidence for the stability of this measure across a full year test–retest interval.

School Performance

Grade point average was derived from self-reports of the most recently earned grades in adolescents' four core courses on a scale from 0 (E or failing) to 4 (A). Grades have been recommended by educators and researchers as the most appropriate measure of current school performance, more so than scores on standardized achievement tests (Dornbusch *et al.*, 1987). Official records of school grades were available at Time 1 for 52 adolescents, providing a means to examine the validity of self-reported grades. For these adolescents, self-reported GPA was correlated .79 with official grade point average based on grades for all courses taken during a single reporting period.

RESULTS

Means and standard deviations for all measures are presented separately for males and females in Table 1. Females reported significantly higher levels of peer support, $t(118) = -2.29$, $p < .05$, which is consistent with the literature on gender differences in friendship patterns (Berndt, 1982; Buhrmester & Furman, 1987). However, with this one exception, there were no differences between males and females on the predictors or on adolescent grades at either point in time. It was decided, therefore, that gender would not be included as a covariate.

Table 1. Means and Standard Deviations (SD) of Measures by Gender[a]

Variable	Females		Males		t-Value
	Mean	SD	Mean	SD	
Parent education level	2.87	.95	2.91	.95	−.25
Family income	4.65	2.34	4.84	2.59	−.39
Number of parents in home	1.57	.49	1.58	.50	−.17
Maternal support	4.37	.331	4.34	.331	.48
Maternal control	2.78	.525	2.68	.545	.95
Peer support	3.87	.665	3.59	.598	2.29[b]
Neighborhood risk	2.90	1.83	2.77	1.80	.36
Time 1 grade point average	2.91	.887	2.78	.85	1.46
Time 2 grade point average	2.72	.81	2.47	.74	1.56

[a] All measures have been converted to their original scaling units.
[b] Difference between males and females significant at $p < .05$.

Table 2 presents the intercorrelation matrix of all measures used in the study. As expected, family income was related to parental education level, $r = .22$, $p < .05$, and number of parents in the home, $r = .58$, $p < .0001$. Also noteworthy is the negative relation of maternal control with family income, $r = −.26$, $p < .01$, and that of both maternal control, $r = −.29$, $p < .01$, and maternal support, $r = .21$, $p < .05$, with parental education level. This pattern is consistent with other studies that have found low-income families to be less supportive and more restrictive in their parenting style (McLoyd, 1990). Neighborhood risk status was negatively related to family income, $r = −.31$, $p < .001$, and education level, $r = −.25$, $p < .01$, and positively related to maternal control, $r = .19$, $p < .05$. Peer support was unrelated to any of the family status, neighborhood, or parenting measures. When Time 1 predictors were correlated with Time 2 GPA, significant relations were found for maternal support, $r = .24$, $p < .05$, peer support, $r = .25$, $p < .01$, and neighborhood risk, $r = −.26$, $p < .01$. Finally, grade point average was only modestly stable across the two assessment periods, $r = .41$, $p < .001$.

Analysis of Main Effects

Ordinary least-squares regressions were conducted to examine first the main effects and then the hypothesized interactions (moderating effects). These analyses were conducted in two phases to limit the number of lower-order and interaction terms entered in a single equation. Time 1 grades were prospectively controlled in the analyses to provide a more stringent test of the hypothesized causal relations between the predictors and criterion.

Table 2. Intercorrelation Matrix of Variables

	1	2	3	4	5	6	7	8
1. Income								
2. Parental education	+.22^a							
3. Number of parents in home	+.58^d	+.13						
4. Maternal support	+.05	+.21^a	+.14					
5. Maternal control	−.26^b	−.29^b	−.02	−.15				
6. Peer attachment	+.02	−.01	−.12	+.11	+.02			
7. Neighborhood risk	−.31^c	−.25^b	−.05	−.15	+.19^a	−.06		
8. Time 1 grade point average	+.16	+.10	+.11	−.12	−.12	−.00	−.33^b	
9. Time 2 grade point average	+.17	+.16	+.10	+.24^a	−.08	+.25^b	−.26^b	+.41^c

$^a p < .05.$
$^b p < .01.$
$^c p < .001.$
$^d p < .0001.$

The first set of analyses examined the main effects of family status, parenting, peer support, and neighborhood risk. Time 2 grades were regressed on the predictor variables in three blocks following entry of Time 1 grades; the family status variables were entered first, followed by the two parenting variables, and then finally the peer and neighborhood variables, which were entered in the final block. As displayed in Table 3, neither the block of family status variables nor that of parenting were significant when entered into the regression, although maternal support was positively related to Time 2 GPA, beta = .20, $p < .05$, in the model. When entered in the final step, peer support and neighborhood risk uniquely explained a significant proportion of variance in Time 2 GPA, F-change $(7, 112) = 3.02$, $p < .05$, even after controlling for prior grades and all of the family predictors. Peer support was positively related to GPA, beta = .23, $p < .05$, and neighborhood risk was negatively related to GPA, beta = − .19, $p < .05$, in the full model. Together, the combined Time 1 predictors accounted for 27% of the variance, $F(7, 112) = 3.82, p < .001$, in Time 2 GPA.

Test of Interactions: The Moderating Influence of Neighborhood Context

Following the examination of main effects, a second regression was run to test the hypothesized moderating influence of neighborhood risk on the effects of the two parenting and peer support variables. As before,

Table 3. Regression of Time 2 Grade Point Average (GPA) on Time 1 Family Status Variables, Parenting Variables, Peer Relations, and Neighborhood Risk Controlling for Time 1 GPA

Time 1 variables in equation	Hierarchical blocks following entry of Time 1 GPA[a]		
	Block 1 beta	Block 2 beta	Block 3 beta
Time 1 GPA	$.38^d$	$.36^d$	$.35^d$
Family income	.08	.09	.08
Parent education	.12	.07	.09
Number of parents in home	.02	−.03	.02
Maternal support (Support)	—	$.20^b$	.15
Maternal control (Control)	—	.03	.02
Peer support (Peer)	—	—	$.23^b$
Neighborhood risk (Neighborhood)	—	—	$-.19^b$
F-change	.88	1.67	3.02^b
Total R^2	.19	.22	.27
Total *F*	5.01^c	3.95^c	3.82^d

[a] Standardized beta coefficients are reported in table.
[b] $p < .05$.
[c] $p < .01$.
[d] $p < .001$.

Time 2 GPA was regressed on the predictors hierarchically following entry of Time 1 GPA; the lower-order parenting, peer support, and neighborhood risk variables were entered in the first block after entry of Time 1 GPA, followed by the Maternal Support × Neighborhood Risk, Maternal Control × Neighborhood Risk, and Peer Support × Neighborhood Risk interaction terms in the second block. This allowed for a test of the combined and unique effects of the interaction terms.[4] Because no predictions were made about interactions between family status and neighborhood risk, and the family status variables did not account for a significant proportion of variance in the criterion, they were not included in the model. This allowed for a reduction in the total number of predictors in the model and, as a consequence, more stable estimates of the hypothesized interactions.[5]

---

[4] Each interaction term was also examined individually to guard against the potential instability of parameter estimates when the full set of interactions are examined in a single equation. Individual tests yielded the same pattern of findings.
[5] Two-way interactions between neighborhood and family status variables were also conducted but were not significant.

All predictor and moderator variables were first centered to reduce multicollinearity that may occur with product terms. As displayed in Table 4, when all main effects and interactions were included in a full regression model, the block of interaction terms accounted uniquely for an additional 11% of variance, F-change $(7, 112) = 4.70, p < .01$, contributing to a total of 36% of the variance in Time 2 GPA explained in the prospective analysis, $F(7, 112) = 5.95$, $p < .0001$. The interactions of Maternal Control $\times$ Neighborhood Risk, beta $= .24, p < .01$, and Peer Support $\times$ Neighborhood Risk, beta $= -.20, p < .05$, were significant predictors in the model, as was the main effect of peer support, beta $= .25, p < .01$.

To facilitate interpretation of the two significant prospective interaction terms, an analysis of simple slopes was conducted using the procedure recommended by Aiken and West (1992). First, to examine the interaction between maternal restrictive control and neighborhood risk, Time 2 GPA was regressed on maternal restrictive control, controlling for the other predictors in the model shown in Table 4, at 1 standard deviation below the mean of neighborhood risk (high risk) and 1 standard deviation above the mean (low risk). These simple slopes are displayed in Figure 1 in which they

Table 4. Regression of Time 2 Grade Point Average (GPA) on Time 1 Parenting Variables, Peer Support, and Neighborhood Risk Controlling for Time 1 GPA: Main Effects and Interactions

Time 1 variables in equation	Hierarchical steps following entry of Time 1 GPA[a]	
	Block 1 beta	Block 2 beta
Time 1 GPA	.36[d]	.28[c]
Maternal support (Support)	.16	.13
Maternal control (Control)	−.02	−.06
Peer support (Peer)	.22[b]	.25[c]
Neighborhood risk (Neighborhood)	−.14	−.14
Support × Neighborhood	—	−.11
Control × Neighborhood	—	.24[c]
Peers × Neighborhood	—	−.20[b]
F-change	2.67[b]	4.70[c]
Total R^2	.26	.37
Total F	5.93[e]	5.95[e]

[a] Standardized beta coefficients are reported in table.
[b] $p < .05$.
[c] $p < .01$.
[d] $p < .001$.
[e] $p < .0001$.

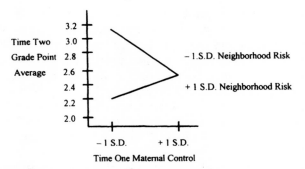

Figure 1. Interaction between Time 1 neighborhood risk and maternal control as predictors of Time 2 grade point average. S.D.=standard deviation.

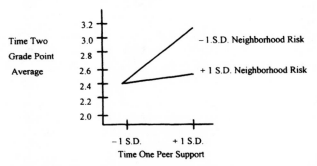

Figure 2. Interaction between Time 1 neighborhood risk and peer support as predictors of Time 2 grade point average. S.D.=standard deviation.

are plotted at 1 standard deviation above and 1 standard deviation below the mean for maternal control. A test of the significance of the simple slopes indicated that, at low levels of neighborhood risk, there was a significant, negative regression of grade point average on maternal control, $t = -2.74$, $p < .01$. At high neighborhood risk, the slope of the regression line was positive but only trending, $t = 1.89, p < .06$. The Neighborhood × Peer Support interaction is displayed in Figure 2. At high neighborhood risk, the regression of Time 2 GPA on peer support was positive, $t = 3.81, p < .001$. In contrast, the slope of the regression line for adolescents at high neighborhood risk was not significantly different from zero, $t = -.121$, n.s.

DISCUSSION

The contribution of family status and parenting variables to academic performance was examined prospectively along with the influence of peer support and perceived neighborhood risk status. When adolescent-reported grade point average was regressed simultaneously onto these predictors, the combined family status and parenting variables did not predict adolescent grade point average. In contrast, the extrafamilial influences of peer support and neighborhood risk did explain a significant proportion of variance in the residualized change in adolescent grades over a 1-year time lag. Peer support at Time 1 was positively related to grade point average while perceived neighborhood risk was negatively related to grades in the prospective analyses.

When looking solely at main effects, these analyses support the view that the peer and neighborhood contexts may be more powerful than that of the family as determinants of school performance for African American adolescents (Dornbusch et al., 1991; Steinberg et al., 1992). However, in the second set of analyses, the moderating effects of neighborhood risk on parenting and peer support were also examined. These analyses revealed significant interactions which modify the study's conclusions regarding the effects of maternal control and peer support.

Whereas maternal restrictive control showed no relation to grades as a main effect, the interactive data revealed a significant, differential impact of maternal control within low- versus high-risk neighborhoods. The positive effect of peer support was also moderated by neighborhood risk; whereas in low-risk neighborhoods peer support was positively related to grades, peer support was not predictive of grades within high-risk neighborhoods. When these moderating influences were included in a combined regression model, the block of interaction terms increased the proportion of explained variance by an additional 11% over that explained by the lower-order terms (main effects) in the prospective model. These findings therefore highlight the importance of ecological models that include multiple contexts and that test for moderation as well as for main effects (Aber, 1993; Bronfenbrenner, 1979). Failure to include these interactive contextual effects would lead, in this study and perhaps others, to an underestimate and mischaracterization of family and peer influences on academic achievement for African American adolescents.

Family Influences on Academic Achievement

The family status variables examined within this study included family income, parent education level, and the number of parental figures in the home. These variables were not significantly predictive of adolescent school performance. This was surprising given the wide range of family incomes and education levels of the families in the study, which should have maximized the power to detect such effects. As others have previously noted, African American children in this study were not achieving at levels consistent with the educational and occupational attainments of their own families (Dornbusch *et al.*, 1991; Gottfredson, 1981; Mickelson, 1990). The lack of association between family structure and school performance is not a novel finding but is worth repeating as it contributes to the growing list of studies that refute the "father absence" explanation of underachievement that once prevailed in the field (see Slaughter-Defoe, Nakagawa, Takanishi, & Johnson, 1990, for a review).

In this study we found a significant prospective effect of maternal support on adolescent grades. These findings are consistent with the larger body of literature that has emphasized a warm, affective parent–child relationship as an important influence on all positive child developmental outcomes, including academic achievement (Maccoby & Martin, 1983; Paulson, 1994). The positive influence of maternal support is best explained as a main effect, as it was not moderated by perceived neighborhood risk. Maternal support apparently contributes to better grades over time for African American adolescents irrespective of the types of neighborhoods in which they reside. In contrast, maternal restrictive control was not significant as a main effect, but the interactive influence of maternal restrictive control with neighborhood risk was significant as a determinant of adolescent grades in the prospective analyses. This finding indicates that maternal control also plays an important role in guiding academic motivation for African American youths during junior high school, but that the effects of control vary substantially depending on the neighborhood context in which they are employed.

Under conditions of low risk, maternal restrictive control demonstrated a strong and negative causal relation with adolescent grades. An elevated level of maternal control was associated with below average grades, while minimum control (i.e., greater autonomy) was associated with grades that were a full letter grade higher. This finding is consistent with theories of motivation which predict maximum motivation in settings that provide ample opportunities for autonomy (Deci & Ryan, 1985; Patrick, Skinner, & Connell, 1993; Ryan & Connell, 1989). It is also consistent with the mainstream socialization literature which has consistently demonstrated a negative relation between authoritarian (restrictive) parental control and adolescent achievement.

However, when we examined the influence of maternal restrictive control on grades within high-risk neighborhoods, the direction of this effect was reverse. Within high-risk neighborhoods, restrictive control was positively associated with grades. Caution is advised in interpreting this effect, however, since the positive slops of the regression line at high levels of neighborhood risk was only marginally significant. Nevertheless, the significant cross-over effect clearly suggests that the impact of restrictive control is substantially modified by neighborhood context, and that it has less negative consequences within high-risk neighborhoods. In another study with African American adolescents, Baldwin et al. (1990) also found higher levels of parental control to be associated with increased academic competence for adolescents within high-risk neighborhoods, while lower levels proved more adaptive within low-risk areas. Similarly, the data of Dornbusch et al. (1987) and Steinberg et al. (1994) showed that authoritarian parenting did not have as detrimental an impact on achievement for African American adolescents as for non-Hispanic Caucasian students. It seems reasonable to suggest that the neighborhood context, which is more likely to be characterized by heightened environmental risks within African American communities, may partially explain the ethnic differences that have been reported in previous studies.

Peer Support and Neighborhood Risk

Peer support was positively related to grades for adolescents living in low-risk neighborhoods. As this finding indicates that supportive peer relationships may facilitate rather than deter achievement for African American adolescents, they provide a more positive view of African American peer groups which are often depicted in a predominantly negative light with respect to academic achievement (Steinberg et al., 1992). This finding is also consistent with the numerous theoretical frameworks which have emphasized the importance of social relatedness and social support as central to motivation, well-being, and academic adjustment (Connell & Well-born, 1991; Levitt et al., 1993; Ryan et al., 1994).

However, we also found that the potential benefits of a strong peer support system were greatly diminished for adolescents in the context of high neighborhood risk. Indeed, at heightened levels of neighborhood risk, peer support demonstrated no relation to achievement. Thus, it seems that neighborhood influences undermine the positive impact of peer support for adolescents, perhaps by preventing the formation of supportive peer groups and prosocial peer activities or by directly shaping the values and activities of the peer group to be less encouraging of academic achievement (Sampson & Groves, 1989). Accordingly, the moderating effects of the neighborhood may also account for the lack of consistent findings in the literature regarding the influence of peer support on academic achievement for African American youths.

However, to better understand the role of peers with respect to academic achievement, future analyses are needed to provide a more comprehensive assessment of adolescents' peer groups than was provided here. In the present study, we examined peer support as one aspect of adolescent peer influence, and we did not include any information about the behaviors or values of the peer groups from which adolescents obtained support. It would be useful to incorporate other dimensions that may be important to academic achievement, such as information about the peers' school orientation, the ethnic mix and ethnic orientation of the peer group, and the type of support or encouragement for achievement that adolescents receive from their peers. It will also be important to examine the effects of peer influence at different developmental periods, and over a longer period of time. The peak in susceptibility to negative peer influence occurs during the middle adolescent years (Berndt, 1979), which is also the period when the largest percentage of African American adolescents begin dropping out of school (Ensminger & Slusarcick, 1992). It is possible that the effects of peer support will reverse in impact as adolescents move into high school (Cauce *et al.*, 1982).

Limitations and Implications

This study adds to the literature on neighborhood context and to our understanding of factors that affect the school performance of African American adolescents. It assesses neighborhood risk as a phenomenological construct and demonstrates a direct and moderating effect of perceived neighborhood risk on the school performance of African American adolescents. These results therefore provide support for social disorganization theory, which maintains that neighborhood crime and gang-related activity produce deleterious effects on adolescent development by disrupting normative socialization processes (i.e., those associated with parents and peers).

The study's findings also highlight the complex interplay between context and individual that are at the heart of ecological models of development, and that are proving to be increasingly important in research with diverse populations (McLoyd, 1990; Steinberg *et al.*, 1992). In doing so, they also underscore the difficulty that parents may face when raising children in high-risk neighborhoods (Garbarino & Sherman, 1980; Spencer & Dornbusch, 1990), particularly during adolescence when children have increased, unsupervised contact with the neighborhood. Our results clearly support those who argue that it is necessary to take environmental considerations into account when theorizing about the potential influence of parents and peers on adolescent development within diverse neighborhoods (Darling & Steinberg, 1993; Dornbusch *et al.*, 1991; Furstenberg, 1992; McLoyd, 1990).

To the extent that the results provide evidence that addresses previous inconsistencies in the literature on African American achievement, the findings are especially noteworthy. Along with these strengths, however, there are limitations which have yet to be addressed. First, our assessment of neighborhood risk was based solely on adolescent reports, rather than an independent source or multiple sources of information. This raises the possibility that adolescent perceptions of the neighborhood may be distorted in a way that could be systematically related to their own achievement. The prospective nature of the study offers some protection against the effects of correlational bias (Kenny & Berman, 1980). Nevertheless, it will be important for future investigations to employ multiple assessment strategies, including more objective, independent measures to assess neighborhood risk.

With regard to sampling, the present study was limited by the fact that our sample included considerably fewer males than females. Analyses assessing gender differences, either as a main effect or in interaction with other predictors, indicate that the study's central findings were consistent across genders. However, future studies should strive to include more males, or at least relatively equal numbers of males and females, to support the generalizability of these findings. The inclusion of African American males is particularly important as they are at greater risk than females for academic difficulties and school dropout (Ensminger & Slusarcick, 1992; Gibbs, 1990).

In conclusion, there are no easy answers to the achievement problem that face the African American community. While parents *do* appear to play an important role with respect to academic success, these results suggest that parental influences may be moderated by the neighborhood context and that parents may be required to make changes in parenting strategies in response to environmental risks. These strategies may or may not be effective, depending on the degree of risk to which their children are exposed within their neighborhoods. Thus, in addition to parent-focused attempts to encourage achievement, our results suggest that it is important to consider the role of peers and the neighborhood context in planning for future research and in the design of interventions to promote academic success for African American youths.

ACKNOWLEDGMENT

This research was supported by a grant (NICHHD: HD24056) awarded to A. M. Cauce. The authors wish to thank Sharlene Wolchik for her comments on this manuscript.

REFERENCES

Aber, J. L. (1993). *The effects of poor neighborhoods on children, youth and families: Theory, research and policy implications*. Background memorandum prepared for the Social

Science Research Council Policy Conference on Persistent Urban Poverty, Nov. 9–10, Washington, DC.

Aber, J. L. (1994). Poverty, violence, and child development: Untangling family and community level effects. In C. A. Nelson (Ed.), *Threats to optimal development: The Minnesota Symposia on Child Psychology* (Vol. 27). Hillsdale, NJ: Erlbaum.

Aber, J. L., Mitchell, G. R., Garfinkel, R., Allen, L., & Seidman, E. (1992, June). *Indices of neighborhood impoverishment: Their associations with adolescent mental health and school achievement.* Paper presented at the Conference on the Urban Underclass: Perspective from the Social Sciences, Ann Arbor.

Aiken, L. S. & West, S. G. (1992). *Multiple regression: Testing and interpreting interactions.* Newbury Park, CA: Sage.

Armsden, G. C. & Greenberg, M. T. (1987). The Inventory of Parent and Peer Attachment: Individual differences and their relationship to psychological well-being in adolescence. *Journal of Youth and Adolescence, 16*, 427–453.

Baldwin, Baldwin, & Cole (1990). Stress-resistant families and stress resistant children. In J. Rolf, A. Masten, D. Cicchetti, K. Nuechterlein, & S. Weintraub (Eds.), *Risk and protective factors in the development of psychopathology.* Cambridge, England: Cambridge University Press.

Baron, R. M. & Kenny, D. A. (1986). The moderator-mediator variable distinction in social psychological research: Conceptual, strategic, and statistical considerations. *Journal of Personality and Social Psychology, 51*, 1173–1182.

Baumrind, D. (1971). Current patterns of parental authority. *Developmental Psychology Monograph, 4*, 1–103.

Berndt, T. (1979). Developmental changes in conformity to peers and parents. *Developmental Psychology, 15*, 608–616.

Berndt, T. (1982). The features and effects of friendships in early adolescence. *Child Development, 53*, 1447–1460.

Block, J. (1965). *The Childrearing Practices Report: A set of parental socialization attitudes and values.* Berkeley: Institute of Human Development, University of California.

Bronfenbrenner, U. (1979). The ecology of the family as a context for human development. *Developmental Psychology, 22*, 723–742.

Buhrmester, D. & Furman, W. (1987). The development of companionship and intimacy. *Child Development, 58*, 1101–1113.

Cauce, A. M. (1986). Social networks and social competence: Exploring the effects of early adolescent friendships. *American Journal of Community Psychology, 14*, 607–628.

Cauce, A. M., Felner, R. D., & Primavera, J. (1982). Social support in high-risk adolescents: Structural components and adaptive impact. *American Journal of Community Psychology, 10*, 417–428.

Coleman, J. & Hoffer, T. (1987). *Public and private high schools: The impact of communities.* New York: Basic Books.

Connell, J. P. & Wellborn, J. G. (1991). Competence, autonomy and relatedness: A motivational analysis of self-system processes. In M. Gunnar & A. Sroufe (Eds.), *Minnesota Symposium on Child Psychology* (Vol. 23, pp. 43–77). Hillsdale, NJ: Erlbaum.

Cotterell, J. L. (1992). The relation of attachments and supports to adolescent well-being and school adjustment. *Journal of Adolescent Research, 7*, 28–42.

Darling, N. & Steinberg, L. (1993). Parenting style as context: An integrative model. *Psychological Bulletin, 113*, 487–496.

Deci, E. L. & Ryan, R. M. (1985). *Intrinsic motivation and self-determination in human behavior.* New York: Plenum Press.

Dornbusch, S. M., Ritter, P. L., Leiderman, P. H., Roberts, D. F., & Fraleigh, M. J. (1987). The relation of parenting style to adolescent school performance. *Child Development, 58*, 1244–1257.

Dornbusch, S. M., Ritter, P. L., & Steinberg, L. (1991). Community influences on the relation of family statuses to adolescent school performance: Differences between African-American and non-Hispanic whites. *American Journal of Education, August*, 543–567.

Duncan, G. J., Brooks-Gunn, J., & Klebanov, P. K. (1994). Economic deprivation and early childhood development. *Child Development, 65*, 296–318.

Engel, U., Nordlohne, E., Hurrelman, K., & Holler, B. (1987). Educational career and substance use in adolescence. *European Journal of Psychological Education, 2*, 365–374.

Ensminger, M. E. & Slusarcick, A. L. (1992). Paths to high school graduation or dropout: A longitudinal study of a first-grade cohort. *Sociology of Education, 65*, 95–113.

Fordham, S. (1991). Peer-proofing academic competition among Black adolescents: "Acting white" Black American style. In C. E. Sleeter (Ed.), *Empowerment through multicultural education.* Albany: State University of New York Press.

Fordham, S. & Ogbu, J. (1986). Black students' school success: Coping with the burden of "acting white." *Urban Review, 18*, 176–206.

Furstenberg, F. (1992, March). *Adapting to difficult environments: Neighborhood characteristics and family strategies.* Symposium paper presented at the Biennial Meeting of the Society for Research on Adolescence, Washington, DC.

Garbarino, J. & Sherman, D. (1980). High-risk neighborhoods and high-risk families: The human ecology of child maltreatment. *Child Development, 51*, 188–198.

Gephart, M. (1980). Neighborhood and communities in concentrated poverty. *Items, 43*, 84–92.

Gibbs, J. T. (1990). Mental health issues of black adolescents: Implications for policy and practice. In A. R. Stiffman & L. E. Davis (Eds.), *Ethnic issues in adolescent mental health.* Newbury Park, CA: Sage.

Gottfredson, D. L. (1981). Black-white differences in the educational attainment process: What have we learned? *American Sociological Review, 46*, 542–557.

Greenberg, M. T. (1982). *Reliability and validity of the Inventory of Adolescent Attachments.* Unpublished manuscript, University of Washington.

Greenberg, M. T., Siegel, J. M., & Leitch, C. J. (1983). The nature and importance of attachment relationships to parents and peers during adolescence. *Journal of Youth and Adolescence, 12*, 373–386.

Kenny, D. A. & Berman, J. S. (1980). Statistical approaches to the correction of correlational bias. *Psychological Bulletin, 88*, 288–295.

Klebanov, P. K., Brooks-Gunn, J. B., & Duncan, G. J. (1993). *Does neighborhood and family poverty affect mother's parenting, mental health, and social support.* Unpublished manuscript.

Kurdek, L. A. (1987). Gender differences in the psychological symptomatology and coping strategies of young adolescents. *Journal of Early Adolescence, 7*, 395–410.

Levitt, M. J., Guacci-Franio, N., & Levitt, J. L. (1993). Convoys of social support in childhood and early adolescence: Structure and function. *Developmental Psychology, 29*, 811–818.

Maccoby, E. E. & Martin, J. A. (1983). Socialization in the context of the family: Parent-child interaction. In P. H. Mussen (Eds.), *Handbook of child psychology* (Vol. 4, pp. 1–101). New York: Wiley.

McLoyd, V. C. (1990). Minority children: Intro to the special issue. *Child Development, 61*, 263–266.

Mickelson, R. (1990). The attitude-achievement paradox among black adolescents. *Sociology of Education, 63*, 44–61.

556   Nancy A. Gonzales *et al.*

Patrick, B. C., Skinner, E. A., & Connell, J. P. (1993). What motivates children's behavior and emotion? Joint effects of perceived control and autonomy in the academic domain. *Journal of Personality and Social Psychology, 65,* 781–791.

Paulson, S. E. (1994). Relations of parenting style and parental involvement with ninth-grade students achievement. *Journal of Early Adolescence, 14,* 250–267.

Rickell, A. U. & Biasatti, L. R. (1982). Modification of the Block Child Rearing Practices Report. *Journal of Clinical Psychology, 39,* 129–134.

Ryan, R. M. & Connell, J. P. (1989). Perceived locus of causality and internalization: Examining reasons for acting in two domains. *Journal of Personality and Social Psychology, 57,* 749–761.

Ryan, R. M., Stiller, J. D., & Lynch, J. H. (1994). Representations of relationships to teachers, parents, and friends as predictors of academic motivation and self-esteem. *Journal of Early Adolescence, 14,* 226–249.

Sampson, R. J. & Groves, W. B. (1989). Community structure and crime: Testing social disorganization theory. *American Journal of Sociology, 94,* 774–802.

Sampson, R. J. & Laub, J. H. (1993). *Crime in the making: Pathways and turning points through life.* Cambridge, MA: Harvard University Press.

Seidman, E., Allen, L., Aber, J. L., Mitchell, C., & Feinman, J. (1994). The impact of school transitions in early adolescence on the self-system and perceived social context of poor urban youth. *Child Development, 65,* 507–522.

Shaw, C., & McKay, H. (1969). *Juvenile delinquency and urban area.* Chicago: University of Chicago Press.

Slaughter-Defoe, D. T., Nakagawa, K., Takanishi, R., & Johnson, D. J. (1990). Toward cultural/ecological perspectives on schooling and achievement in African-American and Asian-American children. *Child Development, 61,* 363–383.

Spencer, M. B. & Dornbusch, S. M. (1990). Challenges in studying minority youth. In S. S. Feldman & G. R. Elliott (Eds.), *At the Threshold: The developing adolescent.* Cambridge, MA: Harvard University Press.

Steinberg, L. & Darling, N. (1993). The broader context of social influence in adolescence. In R. Silbereisen & E. Todt (Eds.), *Adolescence in context.* New York: Springer.

Steinberg, L., Dornbusch, S. M., & Brown, B. B. (1992). Ethnic differences in adolescent achievement: An ecological perspective. *American Psychologist, 47,* 723–729.

Steinberg, L., Mounts, N. S., Lamborn, S. D., & Dornbusch, S. M. (1991). Authoritative parenting and adolescent adjustment across varied ecological niches. *Journal of Research on Adolescence, 1,* 19–36.

Steinberg, L., Lamborn, S. D., Darling, N., Mounts, N. S., & Dornbusch, S. (1994). Over-time changes in adjustment and competence among adolescent from authoritative, authoritarian, indulgent, and neglectful families. *Child Development, 64,* 754–770.

Stevenson, H. W., Chen, C., & Uttal, D. H. (1990). Beliefs and achievement: A study of black, white, and Hispanic children. *Child Development, 61,* 508–523.

Trickett, P., Aber, M. L., Carlson, V., & Cicchetti, D. (1991). The relationship of socioeconomic status to the etiology and developmental sequelae of physical child abuse. *Developmental Psychology, 27,* 148–158.

Appendices

A. Reprinted Articles Categorized by Community Psychology Topics, Settings, and Constructs

	Children and adolescents	Diversity	Community settings	Social systems and groups	Poverty and structural inequality	Stress, coping, and social support
Cherniss (1976)			X	X		
Dohrenwend (1978)						X
Rappaport (1981)						
Felner, Ginter, & Primavera (1982)	X		X	X		
Blakely et al. (1987)				X		
Seidman (1988)			X			X
Maton (1989)				X		X
Martin, Dean, García, & Hall (1989)		X		X		
Chavis & Wandersman (1990)			X			
DeFour & Hirsch (1990)		X	X	X		X
Weinstein et al. (1991)	X		X			
Shinn (1992)					X	
Phillips, Howes, & Whitebook (1992)	X			X		
Riger (1993)		X				
Wolchik et al. (1993)	X					X
Cowen (1994)						X
Vinokur, Price, & Schul (1995)					X	X
Trickett (1996)		X				
Gonzales, Cauce, Friedman, & Mason (1996)	X	X	X			

A. Continued

	Prevention	Empowerment	Social change and social policy	Innovation and evaluation	Values and epistemology
Cherniss (1976)				X	
Dohrenwend (1978)					
Rappaport (1981)		X	X		X
Felner, Ginter, & Primavera (1982)	X			X	
Blakely et al. (1987)				X	
Seidman (1988)			X		X
Maton (1989)					
Martin, Dean, García, & Hall (1989)					
Chavis & Wandersman (1990)		X			
DeFour & Hirsch (1990)					
Weinstein et al. (1991)	X			X	
Shinn (1992)			X		
Phillips, Howes, & Whitebook (1992)	X		X		
Riger (1993)		X	X		X
Wolchik et al. (1993)	X			X	
Cowen (1994)	X				
Vinokur, Price, & Schul (1995)	X				X
Trickett (1996)				X	
Gonzales, Cauce, Friedman, & Mason (1996)					X

B. The Society for Community Research and Action Award for Distinguished Contribution to Theory and Research in Community Psychology, Published in the *American Journal of Community Psychology*[a]

Year	Award recipient(s)	Title	Year	Volume	Pages
1974	Robert Reiff	Of Cabbages and Kings	1975	3(3)	187–196
1975	John C. Glidewell	A Theory of Induced Social Change	1976	4(3)	227–242
1975	Seymour B. Sarason	Community Psychology and the Anarchist Insight	1976	4(3)	246–261
1976	Ira Iscoe	Realities and Trade-Offs in a Viable Community Psychology	1977	5(2)	137–154
1977	Bernard Bloom	Community Psychology: Midstream and Middream	1978	6(3)	205–217
1978	James G. Kelly	'Tain't What You Do, It's the Way That You Do It	1979	7(3)	244–261
1979	Emory L. Cowen	The Wooing of Primary Prevention	1980	8(3)	258–284
1980	Barbara Snell Dohrenwend & Bruce P. Dohrenwend	Socioenvironmental Factors, Stress, and Psychopathology	1981	9(2)	129–164
1981	George W. Albee	The Politics of Nature and Nurture	1982	10(1)	4–36
1983	Rudolf H. Moos	Context and Coping: Toward a Unifying Conceptual Framework	1984	12(1)	5–36
1984	George Spivack & Myrna B. Shure	ICPS and Beyond: Centripetal and Centrifugal Forces	1985	13(3)	226–244
1986	George W. Fairweather	The Need for Uniqueness	1996	14(2)	128–137
1986	Julian Rappaport	Terms of Empowerment/Exemplars of Prevention: Toward a Theory for Community Psychology	1987	15(2)	121–145
1987	Murray Levine	An Analysis of Mutual Assistance	1988	16(2)	167–188
1988	Richard H. Price	Bearing Witness	1989	17(2)	151–167
1989	Edward Zigler	Shaping Child Care Policies and Programs in America	1990	18(2)	183–216
1990	Edward Seidman	Growing Up the Hard Way: Pathways of Urban Adolescents	1991	19(2)	173–205
1991	Kenneth Heller	Ingredients for Effective Community Change: Some Field Observations	1992	20(2)	143–163

B. *Continued*

Year	Award recipient(s)	Title	Publication reference		
			Year	Volume	Pages
1992	Irwin Altman	Challenges and Opportunities of a Transactional World View: Case Study of Contemporary Mormon Polygynous Families	1993	21(2)	135–163
1993	William Ryan	Many Cooks, Brave Men, Apples, and Oranges: How People Think About Equality	1994	22(1)	25–35
1994	J. R. Newbrough	Toward Community—A Third Position	1995	23(1)	9–37
1995	Edison J. Trickett	A Future for Community Psychology: The Contexts of Diversity and the Diversity of Contexts	1996	24(2)	209–229
1996	Marybeth Shinn	Family Homelessness: State or Trait?	1997	25(6)	755–769
1997	Leonard A. Jason	Tobacco, Drug, and HIV Prevention Media Interventions	1998	26(2)	151–188
1998	N. Dickon Reppucci	Adolescent Development and Juvenile Justice	1999	27(3)	307–326
1999	Irwin Sandler	Quality and Ecology of Adversity as Common Mechanisms of Risk and Resilience	2001	29(1)	19–61
2000	Stephanie Riger	Transforming Community Psychology	2001	29(1)	69–81
2001	Rhona Weinstein	Overcoming Inequality in Schooling: A Call to Action for Community Psychology	2002	30(1)	21–42

*a*The 1982 awardee, Charles D. Spielberger, did not publish his talk in *AJCP*.

C. The Society for Community Research and Action Award for Distinguished Practice in Community Psychology, Published in the *American Journal of Community Psychology*[a]

Year	Award recipient(s)	Title	Publication reference		
			Year	Volume	Pages
1985	Thomas Wolff	Community Psychology and Empowerment: An Activist's Insights	1987	15(2)	151–166
1987	Donald C. Klein	The Power of Appreciation	1988	16(3)	302–324
1988	Betty Tableman	Installing Prevention Programming in the Public Mental Health System	1989	17(2)	171–183
1989	Frank Riessman	Restructuring Help: A Human Services Paradigm for the 1990s	1990	18(2)	221–230
1991	Beverly B. Long	Developing a Constituency for Prevention	1992	20(2)	169–178
1992	David M. Chavis	A Future for Community Psychology Practice	1993	21(2)	171–183
1993	Maurice J. Elias	Capturing Excellence in Applied Settings: A Participant Conceptualizer and Praxis Explicator Role for Community Psychologists	1994	22(3)	293–318
1995	Bill Berkowitz	Personal and Community Sustainability	1996	24(4)	441–445
1996	Joseph Galano	Academic on a Mission: Run and Run and Run	1996	24(6)	681–695
2000	J. Wilbert Edgerton	The Community Is It!	2001	29(1)	87–96

[a]Other award recipients include Saul Cooper (1983), Carolyn Swift (1984), Anthony Broskowski (1986), John Morgan (1990), Gloria Levin (1994), Steven Fawcett (1997), Vivian Barnett-Brown (1998), and Thomas Gulotta (1999).

D. Special Issues/Special Sections Published in the *American Journal of Community Psychology*

Special issue/Section	Publication reference		
	Year	Volume	Issue editor(s)
Developing Trends in Community Mental Health Centers	1978	6(2)	Morton A. Lieberman and John C. Glidewell
The Helping Process	1978	6(5)	
Stressful Life Events	1979	7(4)	
Research in Primary Prevention in Mental Health	1982	10(3)	Emory L. Cowen
Training in Community Psychology	1984	12(2)	Raymond P. Lorion and David E. Stenmark
Children's Environments and Mental Health	1985	13(4)	Irwin Sandler
Rural Mental Health	1986	14(5)	Steven R. Heyman
Organizational Perspectives in Community Psychology	1987	15(3)	Christopher B. Keys and Susan Frank
Swampscott Anniversary Symposium	1987	15(5)	James G. Kelly
Community Psychology and the Law	1988	16(4)	Ronald Roesch
Community Psychology in Asia	1989	17(1)	Murray Levine
Citizen Participation, Voluntary Organizations and Community Development: Insights for Empowerment Through Research	1990	18(1)	Abraham Wandersman and Paul Florin
Preventive Intervention Research Centers	1991	19(4)	Doreen Spillon Koretz
Self-Help Groups	1991	19(5)	Thomasina J. Borkman
Methodological Issues in Prevention Research	1993	21(5)	Edward Seidman
Cultural Phenomena and the Research Enterprise: Toward a Culturally Anchored Methodology	1993	21(6)	Edward Seidman, Diane Hughes, and Nathaniel Williams
Empowering the Silent Ranks	1994	22(4)	Irma Serrano-García and Meg A. Bond
Empowerment Theory, Research, and Application	1995	23(5)	Marc A. Zimmerman and Douglas D. Perkins
Ecological Assessment	1996	24(1)	Marybeth Shinn
Meta-Analysis of Primary Prevention Programs for Children and Adolescents	1997	25(2)	Irwin Sandler

D. *Continued*

Special issue/Section	Publication reference		Issue editor(s)
	Year	Volume	
Prevention Research in Rural Settings	1997	25(4)	Peter Muehrer
Women of Color: Social Challenges of Dual Minority Status and Competing Community Contexts	1997	25(5)	Melvin N. Wilson
HIV/AIDS Prevention through Community Psychology	1998	26(1)	John L. Peterson
Qualitative Research in Community Psychology	1998	26(4)	Kenneth E. Miller and Victoria L. Banyard
Adolescent Risk Behavior	1999	27(2)	LaVome Robinson, Ana Mari Cauce, Craig A. Mason, and Gary W. Harper
Prevention Science: Part I	1999	27(4)	Sheppard G. Kellam, Doreen Koretz, and Eve K. Mościcki
Prevention Science: Part II	1999	27(5)	Sheppard G. Kellam, Doreen Koretz, and Eve K. Mościcki
Minority Issues in Prevention	2000	28(2)	Mark W. Roosa and Nancy A. Gonzales
Feminism and Community Psychology: Part I	2000	28(5)	Meg A. Bond, Jean Hill, Anne Mulvey, and Marion Terenzio
Feminism and Community Psychology: Part II	2000	28(6)	Meg A. Bond, Jean Hill, Anne Mulvey, and Marion Terenzio
Community Coalition Building—Contemporary Practice and Research	2001	29(2)	Thomas J. Wolff

About the Editors

Tracey A. Revenson (Senior Editor) is Associate Professor of Psychology at the Graduate Center of the City University of New York, where she is the former director of the Health Psychology Concentration. In addition to this volume and its companion (*Ecological Research to Promote Social Change: Methodological Advances from Community Psychology*, Kluwer Academic/Plenum Publications, 2002), Revenson is the co-author or co-editor of three other books: *The Handbook of Health Psychology* (Erlbaum, 2001), *Understanding Rheumatoid Arthritis* (Routledge, 1996), and *A Piaget Primer: How a Child Thinks* (revised edition, Penguin, 1996). From 1995–1999, Dr. Revenson was the founding Editor-in-Chief of the journal, *Women's Health: Research on Gender, Behavior and Policy*, and has served on the Editorial Board of *AJCP*. Her primary research interests include stress and coping processes among individuals, couples, and families facing chronic physical illnesses and psychosocial aspects of women's health. Her current work examines long-term adaptation among breast cancer survivors and the interactive effects of gender, discrimination, and ethnic identity on smoking among African Americans.

Anthony R. D'Augelli is Professor of Human Development at Pennsylvania State University. In 1999 he received the Distinguished Scientific Contribution Award from the Society for the Psychological Study of Lesbian, Gay, and Bisexual Issues (Division 44 of APA) and an award from the Society for Community Research and Action for Outstanding Contribution to Education and Training in Community Research and Action. He is currently on the Editorial Board of *AJCP*. He is co-editor of three books reviewing psychological research on sexual orientation: *Lesbian, Gay, and Bisexual Identities over the Lifespan* (1995), *Lesbian, Gay, and Bisexual Identities in Families* (1998), and *Lesbian, Gay, and Bisexual Identities and Adolescence* (2001), all published by Oxford University Press. His primary research interests concern sexual orientation and human development in community settings.

Sabine E. French is Assistant Professor of Psychology at the University of California, Riverside. She has conducted research on the development of racial and ethnic identity in ethnically diverse urban adolescents and its impact on self-esteem and academic achievement. Her current research includes longitudinal studies examining the development of racial and ethnic identity, racial socialization, experiences of discrimination, and adjustment to school after the transitions to senior high school and college.

Diane L. Hughes is Associate Professor of Psychology at New York University. She is an Associate of the MacArthur Network on Successful Mid-life Development, and Chair-elect of the Black Caucus of the Society for Research in Child Development and of the Council of Program Directors in Community Psychology. In 1997, she was a Visiting Scholar at the Russell Sage Foundation. She co-edited a special issue of *AJCP* on *Culturally Anchored Methods* (1993). Her continuing research has been in the areas of ecological influences on family processes and children's development, cultural diversity, and exposure to racial bias and race-related socialization among African American and Latino families. She received a grant from the Carnegie Corporation to improve intergroup relations among youth, and serves nationally as a peer reviewer of articles and grants related to minority youth and families. Her recent research focuses on how parents' and children's experiences with race-related prejudice and discrimination in workplaces and schools influence family process and psychosocial adjustment.

David Livert is a doctoral candidate in Social-Personality Psychology at the Graduate Center of the City University of New York and a Research Associate for the national impact evaluation of the Fighting Back program, sponsored by the Robert Wood Johnson Foundation. His research has examined attributional influences on support for public assistance, and social support processes among clinical psychologists. Current projects include a longitudinal study of friendship formation and intergroup attitudes, neighborhood influences on political attitudes and crime concerns, and physicians' age and gender stereotyping of patients.

Edward Seidman is Professor of Psychology at New York University. He has received international recognition as a Scholar in Residence at the Rockefeller Foundation's Bellagio Center (2001) and Senior Fulbright-Hays Research Scholar (1977), and is the recipient of several awards from the Society for Community Research and Action (SCRA), including Outstanding Contribution to Education and Training in Community Research and Action (1999), Distinguished Contribution to Theory and Research in Community Psychology (1990), and Ethnic Minority Mentoring (2001). He served as President of SCRA in 1998, as Associate Editor for Methodology of *AJCP* from 1988–1992, and co-editor for the special issue,

Culturally Anchored Methods (1993). He is co-editor of the *Handbook of Community Psychology* (2000), *Redefining Social Problems* (1986), the *Handbook of Social Intervention* (1983), and the author of the forthcoming *Risky School Transitions, Engagement, and Educational Reform* (Harvard University Press). His current research focuses on understanding developmental trajectories of economically at-risk urban adolescents and how these trajectories are altered by the social contexts of family, peer, school, neighborhood, and their interactions.

Marybeth Shinn is Professor of Psychology at New York University. She is a former president of the Society for Community Research and Action and received its awards for Distinguished Contributions to Theory and Research (1996) and for Ethnic Minority Mentoring (1997). She has co-authored several books on childcare, and edited or co-edited special issues of the *Journal of Social Issues (JSI)* and *AJCP* on *Institutions and Alternatives (JSI,* 1981), *Urban Homelessness (JSI,* 1990), and *Ecological Assessment (AJCP,* 1996). She has served two terms as Associate Editor of *AJCP,* and on various scientific and policy panels including the NIMH Child/Adolescent Risk and Prevention Review Committee, The NIMH Behavioral Science Task Force, and the Task Force on Integrating Behavioral/Social Science into Public Health for the New York City Department of Health. Her current research interests are in homelessness, welfare reform, and methods for assessing the social and policy contexts of people's lives.

Hirokazu Yoshikawa is Assistant Professor of Psychology at New York University. He received the award for best dissertation in community psychology from the Society for Community Research and Action in 1999 and the Louise Kidder Early Career Award from the Society for the Psychological Study of Social Issues and the APA Minority Fellowship Program Early Career Award in 2001. He co-authored, with Jane Knitzer, a monograph on mental health in Head Start, *Lessons from the Field: Head Start Mental Health Strategies to Meet Changing Needs* (1997). He is a member of the Committee on Family Work Policies of the Board on Children, Youth, and Families of the National Academy of Sciences. He has conducted research on long-term effects of early childhood programs, mental health, and family support in Head Start, and competence among urban adolescents in poverty. His current projects examine the effects of welfare and anti-poverty policies on children and families and community-based HIV prevention among Asian/Pacific Islander immigrants to the U.S.

Index

Catholic churches, 55
Caucasians: *see* Whites
Center for Epidemiological Studies-Depression
  Scale (CES-D), 299, 304
CES: *see* Classroom Environment Scale
CES-D: *see* Center for Epidemiological
  Studies-Depression Scale
Change: *see* Social change
Child Assessment Schedule (CAS), 415
Child Assessment Schedule-Revised (CAS),
  418–419, 429–430
Child Behavior Checklist, 419
Child care centers, 36, 67, 367–390
  auspices (profit-nonprofit) and, 368, 370,
    372, 373, 376, 383–385, 388–389, 390
  classrooms of, 373–374
  compliance with regulations, 368–370, 375–
    376, 380–383, 385, 386–387
  description of, 372–373
  ecological paradigm of study, 368–369, 386
  legal context of, 370
  quality assessments of, 371–372, 374–375
  regulatory context of, 369–370
  regulatory effects on, 378–380, 386–388
  teachers in, 373–374, 382
Child Depression Inventory, 418, 430
Childhood resilience, 465
Childrearing Practice Report (CRPR), 548
Children in Need, 312
Children of Divorce Intervention Project, 412
Children's Inventory of Social Support, 417
Children's Manifest Anxiety Scale-Revised,
  418
Children's Perception Questionnaire, 417
Child Report of Parenting Behavior Inventory,
  416, 417
Child's Contact with Father Scale, 418
Child's Depression Inventory, 415
Christian Fellowship, 209, 210, 211, 229
Churches: *see* Religious congregations
Church of Christ, 209–210, 211
Civil rights movement, 8, 15, 37, 131
Classroom Environment Scale (CES), 153
Clinical psychologists, 114–115
Coalition building, 36, 38, 41, 43, 52
Cocaine, 250–251
Cognitive behavior modification, 134
Collaborative preventive intervention, 311–339
  data sources and analysis, 324–325

Collaborative preventive intervention (*cont.*)
  design of, 318–320
  entry, 317–318
  intervention procedures, 321–324
  overview of school failure, 312–313
  participants in, 320–321
  researchers and, 325–326
  school policy and, 329–331
  students and, 331–334
  teachers and, 326–329
  transition as opportunity for, 316–317
Collective efficacy, 58, 269
Communion, 401
Community Arbitration Project (CAP), 168t,
  173, 175f
Community development: *see* Block
  associations
Community mental health, 5, 6, 9, 84–85, 86,
  130, 131
Community Mental Health Act, 8
Community Mental Health Movement, 4
Community organizations, 398–399
*Community Psychology: Values, Research, and
  Action* (Rappaport), 8–9
Compassionate Friends, 215–222, 229–230
Competence building, 10, 40
  empowerment and, 132, 134
  psychological wellness and, 451–452, 454,
    456, 457–460, 466
Competent community, 7
Compositional qualities of settings, 54
Condom use, 247–248
Consciousness raising, 198
Conservative politics, 131, 132, 133, 134, 400
Consultation, 7, 85, 86, 89–100
  appropriate situations for, 90–95
  constituency issue in, 95–96
  defined, 90
  economic considerations in, 91
  primary focus of, 96–99
Contexts, 513–530
  of acculturation theory, 523–527
  cultural, 16, 41–43
  of diversity, 514, 521–530
  diversity highlighting of, 520–521
  diversity integration with, 527–530
  diversity of, 66–68, 514, 521–530
  methodological pluralism and, 518–521
  originating vision and, 514–516

575

CPSIA information can be obtained at www.ICGtesting.com
Printed in the USA
LVOW10s1551070715

445279LV00001B/5/P

9 780306 467301